TO OUR STUDENTS

MATHEMATICS
FOR
HEALTH
OCCUPATIONS

MATHEMATICS
FOR
HEALTH
OCCUPATIONS

Dennis Bila

Washtenaw Community College

Ralph Bottorff

Washtenaw Community College

Paul Merritt

Highland Community College

Donald Ross

Washtenaw Community College

Instructional Technologies Inc
P.O. Box 6146
Plymouth, MI 48170-0146
248-423-3459

Copyright © 1986 by Instructional Technologies, Inc.

Library of Congress Catalog Card No. 82-21674

ISBN 0-935115-04-8

27 26 25 24

Printed in the United States of America.

CONTENTS

PREFACE

Mathematics for Health Occupations is designed for a wide range of students with diverse mathematical backgrounds and abilities. It presumes knowledge of basic arithmetic (whole numbers, fractions, and decimals) and is presented in a semiprogrammed worktext format that allows students to proceed at their own pace. Students who have retained some knowledge from previous study in mathematics can go rapidly through the material that is familiar to them, thereby gaining the benefit of a useful review of their skills. Students without this advantage will want to proceed at a slower pace. *Mathematics for Health Occupations* can be used in a course for the general health student who will not continue on to more advanced mathematics. For students who do not have the necessary background to enter introductory algebra or more advanced courses in health, this text provides all the skills and knowledge necessary to prepare them for such courses.

Mathematics for Health Occupations is also intended for use as the introductory mathematics course in one- and two-year vocational programs in allied health areas. Such programs might include:

Dental Assistant   Firemen Paramedic Emergency
Radiologic Technology   Dietetics and Food Service
Respiratory Therapist   Medical Laboratory Technician
Medical Office Specialist   Orthotics Prosthetics
Practical Nurse   Urological Technology
Veterinary Science

This list is not complete, but simply represents the broad range of programs for which the text is intended.

Although *Mathematics for Health Occupations* is meant primarily for use in a laboratory with an instructor, its format is also well suited for use in a more traditional classroom.

For many years we have struggled with the problem of providing well-written programmed materials with appropriate applications for those students who wish to learn mathematics relating to their field of interest. Many of these students have had poor experiences in their earlier mathematics courses and are reluctant to take further courses. Our attempts to help them have been hindered by the lack of adequate text material. As a result, we began writing semiprogrammed booklets on single-concept ideas to supplement the material we were using. The positive reactions of students to our materials were encouraging. As a result, we decided to develop a series of semiprogrammed texts written specifically for those who need this level of instruction. *Mathematics for Health Occupations* is one in this series. Others include *Core Mathematics* (for the general student who has not identified a specific occupational interest), *Mathematics for Business Occupations* (for the student interested in general business areas), *Mathematics for Technical Occupations* (for those interested in technically related fields not requiring intermediate algebra or higher), and *Introductory Algebra* and *Intermediate Algebra* (for those pursuing a more traditional course of study leading to precalculus and calculus). We sincerely hope that your experiences with these texts will be as rewarding as ours have been.

Core Mathematics, Introductory Algebra, and *Intermediate Algebra* are all available from Worth Publishers, Inc., N.Y. We would like to thank Worth Publishers for their permission to use excerpts from *Core Mathematics* and *Introductory Algebra* in this text.

We feel that the use of hand-held calculators should be permitted, if not encouraged. The use of the calculator during the study of the text will permit the student to focus attention on the mastery of the content and minimize much of the drudgery associated with the study of the topics included in the text.

The symbols and notation used in the chapters on the metric system are those of the International System of Units (SI). The National Bureau of Standards has adopted the SI in all its research work and publications, except where use of these units would impair communications or reduce the usefulness of the material. Chapter 4 has been reviewed by the National Bureau of Standards. We have used the "metre" and "litre" spelling, though this is still a controversial issue. If conventions are adopted in the United States which conflict with those used in this text, appropriate changes will be made in subsequent editions.

FEATURES OF *Mathematics for Health Occupations*

FORMAT

Each unit of material (a single concept or a few closely related concepts) is presented in a section. Within a section, short, boxed, numbered frames contain all instructional material, including sample problems and sample solutions. Frames are followed by practice problems, with workspace provided. Answers immediately follow, with numerous solutions and supplementary comments.

EXERCISES

Exercises at the end of each section are quite traditional in nature. However, they are generally shorter than those found in most texts because the student has already done numerous problems and answered many questions during the study of the section. Hence, the exercises serve as a review of the content of the section and as a guide that will help students to recognize whether they have mastered the material. Answers to the problems are provided immediately, permitting the student to advance through the text without having to turn to the back of the text to check answers. Word problems are used throughout.

SAMPLE CHAPTER TESTS

At the end of each chapter we have provided a Sample Chapter Test. It is keyed to each section with the answers provided immediately for student convenience. It may also serve as a pretest for each chapter. However, if an instructor wishes to pretest without the availability of the answers (to the student), one form of the post-test for the chapter (provided in the *Test Manual*) could be used for this purpose.

Upon finishing the chapter, the student should complete the Chapter Sample Test, and the results should be shown to the instructor and discussed with the student. If the instructor and student are confident about mastery of the content of the chapter, a post-test can then be administered. Used in this manner, outstanding results can be anticipated on the first attempt for each post-test.

OBJECTIVES

The Sample Chapter Tests serve as objectives for both student and instructor. The instructor can readily ascertain the objectives of any chapter by examining the sample test at its end, and the student is in a good position to see what is expected of him by examining problems and questions that are going to be asked at the completion of the chapter. We believe that objectives stated verbally are of less benefit to the student than the statement of a problem that must be solved.

GLOSSARY

The glossary at the back of the text provides the student with the pronunciation and the definition of all mathematical words and phrases used in the text. This is particularly important wherever the text is used in a laboratory situation where the student will not hear the words used in class discussions.

SUPPLEMENTS

A *Test Manual* and an *Instructional Kit* are available separately for instructors using *Mathematics for Health Occupations*. The *Test Manual* contains a reproducible master copy of each of three forms of a post-test for each chapter of the text. Each post-test contains ample workspace and answer blanks. Answers to the tests are given at the end of the *Test Manual*. The *Instructional Kit* discusses the text format in detail and describes at length both the lecture-recitation and laboratory methods of instruction. Sample schedule guidelines and progress records are given, along with a Mathematics Inventory Test which the instructor may give at the start of the course. The kit also includes the authors' chapter-by-chapter rationale for the procedures used in the text.

ACKNOWLEDGMENTS

We would like to thank those whose reviews were particularly helpful in the writing of this text: Yvonne Abdoo, University of Michigan Medical Center; John L. Lawson, Shelby State Community College; Marilyn Slotfeldt, M.S., Assistant Professor of Clinical Pharmacy, University of Michigan Hospital; and John Snyder, Sinclair Community College. Since Mathematics for Health Occupations contains material from Core Mathematics, we would like to extend another expression of gratitude to the reviewers of that text who originally were so helpful in its preparation.

We would like to express our thanks to our colleagues at Washtenaw Community College and Highland Park Community College for their contributions, with special thanks to Jerry Baker, Carl Hammond, and Robert Nelson for their detailed analysis of course requirements relating to vocational programs in the health fields. Also to student reviewers Joyce Awosika and Terri Ross who worked each and every problem in the text. Their suggestions (and corrections) were invaluable. Certainly we owe a debt of gratitude to all the students who participated in the class testing. Our thanks also to our typists, Nancy Hayes, Marcia Joiner (now Mrs. Paul Merritt), Marilyn Myers, Terri Ross, Diane Torrance, Carolyn Williams, and Carol Wilson. How they were able to read our handwriting is still a mystery.

John Covell, the production editor at Winthrop Publishers, must receive special accolades. His patience, attention to detail, unflappable nature, and support contributed more than words can describe to the successful outcome of this text.

Special thanks are also due to Ken Tennity, Dorothy Werner, Walt Kirby, and Greg Wood of the Prentice-Hall fieldstaff for their invaluable marketing research assistance.

To all those unnamed who participated, we are eternally thankful.

Dennis Bila
Ralph Bottorff
Paul Merritt
Donald Ross

TO THE STUDENT

You are about to brush up on some skills you may already have learned in a previous course; but they may be a bit rusty. You will learn some new techniques, too. This book is designed to help pinpoint those areas where you need to sharpen your skills and to permit you to move quickly through those topics you know well.

If you follow the suggestions below, you will make best use of your time, proceeding through the course as quickly as possible, and you will have mastered all the material in this book.

CHAPTER SAMPLE TESTS

The Chapter Sample Test at the end of each chapter will help you to determine whether you can skip certain sections of the chapter. It is a cumulative review of the entire chapter, and questions are keyed to the individual sections of the chapter. To use this test to best advantage we suggest this procedure:

1. Work the solutions to all problems neatly on your own paper to the best of your ability. You want to determine what you know about the material without help from someone else. If you receive help in completing this self-test, the result will show another person's knowledge rather than your own.
2. Once you have done as much as you can, check the test with the answers provided. On the basis of errors made, determine the most appropriate course of study. You may need to study all sections in the chapter or you may be able to skip one or two sections.
3. When you have completed the chapter, rework all problems originally missed on the Chapter Sample Test and review the entire test in preparation for the post-test that will cover the entire chapter.

INSTRUCTIONAL SECTIONS

To use each section most effectively:

1. Study the boxed frames carefully.
2. Following each frame are questions based on the information presented in the frame. When completing these questions, do the work in the spaces provided.
3. Use a blank piece of paper as a mask to cover the answers below the divider rule. For example:

Q1   How many eggs can 21 chickens lay in 1 hour, if 1 chicken can lay 7 eggs in $\frac{1}{2}$ hour?

(Work space)

＃＃＃ • ＃＃＃ • ＃＃＃ • ＃＃＃ • ＃＃＃ • ＃＃＃ • ＃＃＃ • ＃＃＃ • ＃＃＃ • ＃＃＃

Paper Mask

4. After you have written your calculations and response in the workspace, slide the paper mask down, uncovering the correct solution, and check your response with the correct answer given. In this way you can check your progress as you go without accidentally seeing the response before you have completed the necessary thinking or work.

Q1   How many eggs can 21 chickens lay in 1 hour, if 1 chicken can lay 7 eggs in $\frac{1}{2}$ hour?

$$7 \times 2 = 14 \qquad \begin{array}{r} 14 \\ \times 21 \\ \hline 14 \\ 28 \\ \hline 294 \end{array}$$

＃＃＃ • ＃＃＃ • ＃＃＃ • ＃＃＃ • ＃＃＃ • ＃＃＃ • ＃＃＃ • ＃＃＃ • ＃＃＃ • ＃＃＃

A1   294: 1 chicken can lay 14 in 1 hour; hence, 21 chickens can lay 21(14) in 1 hour.

Paper Mask

Notice that the answer is often followed by a colon (:). The information following the colon is one of the following:
a. The complete solution,
b. A partial solution, possibly a key step frequently missed by many students,
c. A remark to remind you of an important point, or
d. A comment about the solution.
If your answer is correct, advance immediately to the next step of instruction.
5. Space is provided for you to work in the text. However, you may prefer to use the paper mask to work out your solutions. If you do, be sure to show complete solutions to all problems, clearly numbered, on the paper mask. When both sides of the paper are full, file it in a notebook for future reference.
6. Make all necessary corrections before continuing to next frame or problem.
7. If something is not clear, talk to your instructor immediately. Do not accept any answers just because the text says so. Make sure you are convinced of the logic behind the work.

8. If difficulty arises when you are studying outside of class, be sure to note the difficulty so that you can ask about it at your earliest convenience.
9. When preparing for a chapter post-test, the frames of each section serve as an excellent review of the chapter.

SECTION EXERCISES

The exercises at the end of each section are provided for additional practice on the content of the section. For your convenience, answers are given immediately following the exercises. However, detailed solutions to these problems are not shown.

You should:

1. Work all problems neatly on your own paper.
2. Check your responses against the answers given.
3. Rework any problem with which you disagree. If you cannot verify the response given, discuss the result with your instructor.
4. In the process of completing the exercise, use the instructional material in the section for review when necessary.

Problems marked with an asterisk (*) are considered more difficult than examples in the instructional section. They are intended to challenge the interested student. Problems of this difficulty will not appear on the Chapter Sample Test or the post-test.

You should realize that the zero is placed to the left of a decimal number in the text to eliminate confusion over the placement of the decimal point. However, it is not incorrect to omit the zero when performing a calculation or expressing an answer, that is, $0.16 = .16$.

This three-part learning program has proven successful in situations where there have been students with many different backgrounds. With conscientious effort, you will have success with it too.

CHAPTER 1

HEALTH APPLICATIONS FOR BASIC MATHEMATICS

1.1 APPLICATIONS FOR WHOLE NUMBERS

1 The need for a thorough knowledge of the mathematics of health occupations will be apparent to students when they obtain their first employment, and secondly, for adequate job performance.

Much of the mathematics that health students will encounter deals with business mathematics. The success of a medical practice depends to a large degree on the efficient operation of the business end of the practice. Nothing will upset patients more than an incorrect billing.

Applications are the most difficult types of mathematics problems for most students. Practice and an organized plan will aid in solving application problems. The following organization of a problem may be helpful.

Step 1: Decide what the problem asks you to find.

Step 2: Decide the correct mathematical operation to be used.

Step 3: Estimate the answer.

Step 4: Solve and check the problem.

Step 3 is an important part in the solution of a problem. You are really answering the question, "What is a reasonable answer?"

Example: Estimate the following sum by rounding off each number to the hundreds place.

$$\begin{array}{r} 236 \\ 754 \\ 891 \\ \underline{148} \end{array}$$

Solution:
$$\begin{array}{r} 200 \\ 800 \\ 900 \\ \underline{100} \\ 2000 \end{array}$$

The estimated sum of 2,000 illustrates that the actual sum of 2,029 is a reasonable answer.

Q1 Estimate the sum by rounding off to the tens place:
a. $23+65+12$ **b.** $219+47+8$

• # # # • # # # • # # # • # # # • # # # • # # # • # # # • # #

A1   **a.** 100: $20+70+10$ **b.** 280: $220+50+10$

Q2   Estimate the difference by rounding off to the hundreds place:
    a. $1450 - 248$ **b.** $7988 - 4003$

\# \# \# • \# \# \# • \# \# \# • \# \# \# • \# \# \# • \# \# \# • \# \# \# • \# \# \# • \# \# \#

A2   **a.** 1,300: $1500 - 200$ **b.** 4,000: $8000 - 4000$

Q3   Estimate the product by rounding off to the tens place:
    a. 84×36 **b.** 19×8

\# \# \# • \# \# \# • \# \# \# • \# \# \# • \# \# \# • \# \# \# • \# \# \# • \# \# \# • \# \# \#

A3   **a.** 3,200: 80×40 **b.** 200: 20×10

Q4   Estimate the quotient by rounding off to the hundreds place:
    a. $623 \div 219$ **b.** $681 \div 82$

\# \# \# • \# \# \# • \# \# \# • \# \# \# • \# \# \# • \# \# \# • \# \# \# • \# \# \# • \# \# \#

A4   **a.** 3: $600 \div 200$ **b.** 7: $700 \div 100$

---

2   When estimating problems involving multiplication and division, the different numbers are often rounded off to different places. Recall that estimation is a technique to determine whether or not the answer is reasonable. The key to estimation is ease of use, speed, and a reasonably accurate result.

Example 1: 523×6 is estimated as $500 \times 6 = 3,000$. 523 was rounded off to the hundreds place and the 6 was left alone.

Example 2: 685×9 is estimated as $700 \times 9 = 6,300$

Example 3: 685×13 is estimated as $700 \times 10 = 7,000$. 685 was rounded off to the hundreds place and 13 was rounded off to the tens place.

Example 4: 685×13 is estimated as $690 \times 10 = 6,900$. Here 685 was rounded off to the tens place. The actual product 685×13 is 8,905, so either estimate of examples 3 and 4 would be appropriate.

Q5   Estimate the product:
    a. 623×8 **b.** 46×843

\# \# \# • \# \# \# • \# \# \# • \# \# \# • \# \# \# • \# \# \# • \# \# \# • \# \# \# • \# \# \#

A5   Possible answers:
    a. $600 \times 8 = 4,800$ **b.** $50 \times 800 = 40,000$
           $600 \times 10 = 6,000$ $50 \times 840 = 42,000$
           $620 \times 10 = 6,200$

Q6   Estimate the quotient:
    a. $1372 \div 7$ **b.** $419 \div 21$

\# \# \# • \# \# \# • \# \# \# • \# \# \# • \# \# \# • \# \# \# • \# \# \# • \# \# \# • \# \# \#

A6   **a.** 200: $1400 \div 7$ **b.** 20: $400 \div 20$

---

3   Step 2 in solving a problem is determining the correct mathematical operation to be used. Key words often indicate the operation involved. Some key words are shown on the next page under the operation they usually indicate.

Addition	Subtraction	Multiplication	Division
plus	difference	product	quotient
added to	take away	times	divided by
more than	reduced by	double	
sum of	less	twice	
increased by	diminished	triple	
	decreased	of	
	minus		
	depreciate		

Q7   Indicate the correct mathematical operation (addition, subtraction, multiplication, division):

a. The sum of _____   **d.** Two less than _____

b. Three times as much _____   **e.** Depreciated by 5% _____

c. The difference between _____   **f.** Divided equally amongst _____

\# # # • # # # • # # # • # # # • # # # • # # # • # # # • # # # • # # #

A7   **a.** addition   **b.** multiplication   **c.** subtraction
      d. subtraction   **e.** subtraction   **f.** division

Q8   In the following problems, *only* indicate the correct mathematical operation to be used:
      a. At a recent sale of excess dental equipment, total sales amounted to $112. If the money is to be divided equally between Sharon, Dave, Dick, and Nancy, how much should each receive?
      b. Collections this week for Dr. Kesches were $4,217. Last week's collections were $482 less. What were last week's collections?

\# # # • # # # • # # # • # # # • # # # • # # # • # # # • # # # • # # #

A8   **a.** division   **b.** subtraction

4	The combined steps in solving a problem will now be illustrated using Q8a.

Step 1: Decide what the problem asks you to find.

Solution: The amount each of the four people is to receive.

Step 2: Decide the correct mathematical operation to be used.

Solution: "divided equally" indicates division.

Step 3: Estimate the answer.

Solution: $112 ÷ 4$ is estimated as $100 ÷ 4 = 25$, so $25 is the estimated answer.

Step 4: Solve and check the problem.

Solution: $112 ÷ 4 = 28$

The estimate indicates that the answer is a reasonable one. Each person receives $28.

Q9   Collections this week for Dr. Kesches were $4,217. Last week's collection were $482 less. What were last week's collections?

a. Step 1: What are you to find? _____

b. Step 2: What operation? _____

c. Step 3: Estimate the answer. _____

d. Step 4: Solve and check.

\# # # • # # # • # # # • # # # • # # # • # # # • # # # • # # # • # # #

A9   **a.** last week's collections   **b.** subtraction
      c. $4,000 − $500 = $3,500   **d.** $4,217 − $482 = $3,735

Q10   Kallie is on a liquid diet. Her lunch consisted of 280 ml of soup, 120 ml of jello, and 95 ml of hot tea. What was the total amount of fluids for this meal? (The symbol "ml" is a metric unit of measurement for millilitre and will be explained in Chapter 4. One millilitre is approximately $\frac{1}{30}$ of an ounce).

• # # # • # # # • # # # • # # # • # # # • # # # • # # # • # #

A10   495 ml: Step 2: "total number" indicates addition.

Q11   Ken's annual salary is $19,836. He is offered a new job at an annual salary of $22,500. What would be his increase in salary?

• # # # • # # # • # # # • # # # • # # # • # # # • # # # • # #

A11 $2,664:   Step 2: "increase" usually indicates addition; however, you are actually finding the difference between the salaries and "difference" indicates subtraction.

Q12   Dick receives $820 per month in his position as junior accountant for a local industry. What is his annual salary?

• # # # • # # # • # # # • # # # • # # # • # # # • # # # • # #

A12 $9,840

Q13   Betty Kisabeth wrote checks for the following items: Tuition $183, books $43, and supplies $18. If this money was deducted from a checkbook balance of $372, what is her new balance?

• # # # • # # # • # # # • # # # • # # # • # # # • # # # • # #

A13 $128:   Step 1: You are looking for the new balance after the total for the checks has been deducted.
            Step 2: Use addition to find the total and subtraction to find the difference between the check total and the balance of $372.
            Step 3: total ($200 + $40 + $20 = $260)
                    new balance ($370 − $260 = $110)
            Step 4: total ($183 + $43 + $18 = $244)
                    new balance ($372 − $244 = $128)

Q14   An optical supplies company decided to distribute excess profits of $21,315 equally to each of 245 employees. How much would each employee receive?

• # # # • # # # • # # # • # # # • # # # • # # # • # # # • # #

A14 $87:   Step 2: "distribute equally" indicates division.

---

5   When working with various office forms it is often necessary or convenient, to add, subtract, and multiply horizontally instead of vertically. When adding or subtracting horizontally it is especially

important to add or subtract like place values. That is, units added to units, tens to tens, hundreds to hundreds, and so on.

Example: Add $217 + 823 + 8$.

Solution: First add the units digits.

$$217 + 823 + 8 = 8$$

Now add the ten's digits, remembering to carry the 1 from the units place.

$$217 + 823 + 8 = 48$$

Finally, add the hundred's digits.

$$217 + 823 + 8 = 1,048$$

Q15   Add horizontally:

   a. $19 + 23 + 56 + 7 + 14 =$ _____

   b. $\$2,619 + \$586 + \$4,012 + \$89 =$ _____

•   # # #   •   # # #   •   # # #   •   # # #   •   # # #   •   # # #   •   # # #   •   # #

A15   **a.** 119   **b.** $7,306

Q16   Add:

   a. $461 + 38 + 692 =$ _____

   b. $\$83,394 + \$705 + \$192,647 + \$315 =$ _____

•   # # #   •   # # #   •   # # #   •   # # #   •   # # #   •   # # #   •   # # #   •   # #

A16   **a.** 1,191   **b.** $277,061

6   Errors are often made when subtracting horizontally by forgetting to borrow.

Example: Subtract: $6423 - 456$

Solution: It may be helpful not to borrow mentally.

$$6\,4\,\overset{1}{2}\,{}^{1}3 = 456 = 7$$

$$13 - 6$$

$$6\,\overset{3}{4}\,\overset{11}{2}\,{}^{1}3 - 456 = 67$$

$$11 - 5$$

$$\overset{5}{6}\,\overset{13}{4}\,\overset{11}{2}\,{}^{1}3 - 456 = 967$$

$$13 - 4$$

$$\overset{5}{6}\,\overset{13}{4}\,\overset{11}{2}\,{}^{1}3 - 456 = 5,967$$

$$5 - 0$$

Q17   Subtract horizontally:

    a. $875 - 354 =$ _____   **b.** $215 - 164 =$ _____

\# \# \# • \# \# \# • \# \# \# • \# \# \# • \# \# \# • \# \# \# • \# \# \# • \# \# \# • \# \# \#

A17   **a.** 521   **b.** 51

Q18   Subtract:

    a. $8,095 - 3,381 =$ _____   **b.** $2,476 - 873 =$ _____

\# \# \# • \# \# \# • \# \# \# • \# \# \# • \# \# \# • \# \# \# • \# \# \# • \# \# \# • \# \# \#

A18   **a.** 4,714   **b.** 1,603

Q19   Find:

    a. $\$6,408 - \$2,463 =$ _____   **b.** $\$2,463 + \$3,945 =$ _____

\# \# \# • \# \# \# • \# \# \# • \# \# \# • \# \# \# • \# \# \# • \# \# \# • \# \# \# • \# \# \#

A19   **a.** $3,945   **b.** $6,408

Q20   Record the total caloric intake for each patient:

Caloric Intake

Patient	Breakfast	Lunch	Dinner	Total
Jane	225	480	925	**a.** _____
Mary	320	618	1,018	**b.** _____
Sue	175	215	823	**c.** _____
Gayle	525	766	1,289	**d.** _____

\# \# \# • \# \# \# • \# \# \# • \# \# \# • \# \# \# • \# \# \# • \# \# \# • \# \# \# • \# \# \#

A20   **a.** 1,630   **b.** 1,956   **c.** 1,213   **d.** 2,580

Q21   Determine the new balance for each patient:

Patient	Old Balance	Payment	New Balance
A	$72	$9	**a.** _____
B	213	28	**b.** _____
C	103	74	**c.** _____
D	1,004	825	**d.** _____

\# \# \# • \# \# \# • \# \# \# • \# \# \# • \# \# \# • \# \# \# • \# \# \# • \# \# \# • \# \# \#

A21   **a.** $63   **b.** $185   **c.** $29   **d.** $179

Q22   Multiply horizontally:

    a. $413 \times 5 =$ _____   **b.** $1,084 \times 3 =$ _____

\# \# \# • \# \# \# • \# \# \# • \# \# \# • \# \# \# • \# \# \# • \# \# \# • \# \# \# • \# \# \#

A22   **a.** 2,065   **b.** 3,252

Q23 The Chesaning Health Clinic received a bill for the following items. Find the total cost:

Item Stock No.	Cost per Item	No. Purchased	Cost Total
218	$23	8	a. _____
036	17	6	b. _____
087	127	5	c. _____
113	98	3	d. _____
		Total	e. _____

• # # # • # # # • # # # • # # # • # # # • # # # • # # # • # #

A23   **a.** $184   **b.** $102   **c.** $635   **d.** $294   **e.** $1,215

---

7 *Calories* are units of energy found in all foods. If you eat more calories than your body can use in its normal daily activities, the excess is stored as fat. To reduce this storehouse of fat it is necessary to eat fewer calories than your body uses.

Most people leading moderately active lives need 15 calories per pound to maintain their desired weight. So, if you weigh 140 pounds, you should consume foods containing no more than 2,100 calories each day.

Q24 How many calories should be consumed daily to maintain the desired weight?
   a. 115 pounds   **b.** 150 pounds

• # # # • # # # • # # # • # # # • # # # • # # # • # # # • # #

A24   **a.** 1,725   **b.** 2,250

---

8 If you are above your desired weight, you will have to cut down on your caloric intake. There are approximately 3,500 calories in each stored pound of fat. So to lose one pound a week, consume 500 fewer calories each day (7×500 calories = 3,500 calories).

Example 1: William's desired weight is 150 pounds. He wishes to lose one pound per week until he reaches his desired weight. How many calories should he consume daily?

Solution: 150 pounds (desired weight)
             $\times 15$
             2,250 (calories needed to maintain desired weight)
             -500 (calories daily to lose one pound per week)
             1,750 (maximum daily calories)

Example 2: Sally's desired weight is 120 pounds. She wishes to lose *two* pounds per week. How many calories should she consume daily?

Solution: 120 pounds (desired weight)
             $\times 15$
             1,800 (calories needed to maintain desired weight)
             $-1,000$ (calories needed to lose two pounds per week)
             800 (maximum daily calories)

The above formulas will vary from individual to individual, especially as exercise varies. The American Medical Association recommends that one not try to lose more than two pounds per week.

Q25   To arrive at the following desired weight, losing one pound per week, what should be the daily caloric intake?

a. 110 pounds   **b.** 165 pounds

\# \# \#   •   \# \# \#   •   \# \# \#   •   \# \# \#   •   \# \# \#   •   \# \# \#   •   \# \# \#   •   \# \# \#   •   \# \# \#

A25   **a.** 1,150: $110 \times 15 = 1,650$ (calories needed to maintain desired weight)
$1,650 - 500 = 1,150$ (maximum daily calories)
b. 1,975: $165 \times 15 = 2,475$ $2,475 - 500 = 1,975$

Q26   To arrive at the following desired weight, losing two pounds per week, what should be the daily caloric intake?

a. 140 pounds   **b.** 118 pounds

\# \# \#   •   \# \# \#   •   \# \# \#   •   \# \# \#   •   \# \# \#   •   \# \# \#   •   \# \# \#   •   \# \# \#   •   \# \# \#

A26   **a.** 1,100: $2,100 - 1,000$ **b.** 770: $1,770 - 1,000$

Q27   A patient is urged to drink 4000 ml of fluid daily. Yesterday she drank three glasses of juice which were 220 ml each, two glasses of milk at 230 ml each, and four glasses of water at 250 ml each. How many more ml are needed to reach 4000 ml?

\# \# \#   •   \# \# \#   •   \# \# \#   •   \# \# \#   •   \# \# \#   •   \# \# \#   •   \# \# \#   •   \# \# \#   •   \# \# \#

A27   1880 ml:
$3 \times 220 \text{ ml} = 660 \text{ ml}$
$2 \times 230 \text{ ml} = 460 \text{ ml}$
$4 \times 250 \text{ ml} = 1000 \text{ ml}$
total $= 2120$ ml
$4000 \text{ ml} - 2120 \text{ ml} = 1880 \text{ ml}$

9   The numerals 0, 1, 2, 3, 4, 5, 6, 7, 8, 9 are called the *Hindu–Arabic numerals*. Most of your mathematical training and experience will be with these numerals. However, it is necessary for many people in the medical area to understand *Roman numerals*. The seven basic Roman numerals are assigned the following values (lower case Roman numerals are usually used in the medical area):

i = 1   v = 5   x = 10   l = 50
c = 100   d = 500   m = 1,000

Q28   Indicate the Roman numerals that would be used to represent the following numerals:

     a. 5 = _____   **b.** 1 = _____   **c.** 10 = _____

     d. 50 = _____   **e.** 500 = _____   **f.** 100 = _____

\# \# \# • \# \# \# • \# \# \# • \# \# \# • \# \# \# • \# \# \# • \# \# \# • \# \# \# • \# \# \#

A28   **a.** v   **b.** i   **c.** x   **d.** l   **e.** d   **f.** c

---

10   The Roman numeral system employs three basic principles for writing numerals other than the seven mentioned above. The first is the addition principle. If smaller-valued numerals are placed to the right of larger-valued numerals, or if numerals are repeated, the values represented by the numerals are to be added.

Examples:

     1. vi = 5 + 1 = 6   **2.** vii = 5 + 1 + 1 = 7   **3.** xi = 10 + 1 = 11

     4. xx = 10 + 10 = 20   **5.** xxvii = 10 + 10 + 5 + 1 + 1 = 27

Q29   Give the Hindu–Arabic numeral represented by the following Roman numerals:

     a. viii____   **b.** xv____   **c.** li____   **d.** xviii____

     e. lxv____   **f.** lxxvii____   **g.** clv____   **h.** mc____

\# \# \# • \# \# \# • \# \# \# • \# \# \# • \# \# \# • \# \# \# • \# \# \# • \# \# \# • \# \# \#

A29   **a.** 8   **b.** 15   **c.** 51   **d.** 18   **e.** 65   **f.** 77   **g.** 155   **h.** 1,100

Q30   Give the Roman numeral represented by the following Hindu–Arabic numeral:

     a. 3____   **b.** 12____   **c.** 28____   **d.** 101____

     e. 30____   **f.** 35____   **g.** 52____   **h.** 505____

\# \# \# • \# \# \# • \# \# \# • \# \# \# • \# \# \# • \# \# \# • \# \# \# • \# \# \# • \# \# \#

A30   **a.** iii   **b.** xii   **c.** xxviii   **d.** ci

        e. xxx   **f.** xxxv   **g.** lii   **h.** dv

---

11   The second basic principle for writing Roman numerals is the *subtraction principle.* If a smaller-valued numeral is placed to the *left* of a larger-valued numeral, the value represented by the smaller numeral is to be subtracted.

Example:

     1. iv = 5 − 1 = 4   **2.** ix = 10 − 1 = 9

     3. xl = 50 − 10 = 40   **4.** cm = 1,000 − 100 = 900

Only one smaller-valued numeral is allowed to precede a larger-valued one.

Q31   Give the Hindu–Arabic numeral represented by the following Roman numerals:

     a. xc____   **b.** cd____   **c.** xl____   **d.** ix____

\# \# \# • \# \# \# • \# \# \# • \# \# \# • \# \# \# • \# \# \# • \# \# \# • \# \# \# • \# \# \#

A31   **a.** 90   **b.** 400   **c.** 40   **d.** 9

Q32   **a.** Why would iix be inadmissible for 8? _____

     b. Write 8 using Roman numerals._____

\# \# \# • \# \# \# • \# \# \# • \# \# \# • \# \# \# • \# \# \# • \# \# \# • \# \# \# • \# \# \#

A32   **a.** Only one smaller numeral is allowed to precede a larger one.
      b. viii

---

12   When a larger numeral has smaller numerals to the left and right the subtraction is performed first. When a smaller numeral is between two larger numerals, the subtraction principle also takes precedence. That is, xix would be evaluated

$$xix = x + \underset{\text{evaluated first}}{\underline{ix}} = 10 + 9 = 19$$

Examples:

1. xxix = 10 + 10 + 9 = 29   **2.** xlii = 40 + 2 = 42
3. lix = 50 + 9 = 59   **4.** lxxix = 70 + 9 = 79

Q33   Give the Hindu–Arabic numeral represented by the following Roman numerals:

a. xiv_____   **b.** xix_____   **c.** lix_____

d. cxli_____   **e.** ccx_____   **f.** xxiv_____

• # # # • # # # • # # # • # # # • # # # • # # # • # # # • # #

A33   **a.** 14   **b.** 19   **c.** 59   **d.** 141   **e.** 210   **f.** 24

Q34   Give the Roman numeral represented by the Hindu–Arabic numeral:

a. 9_____   **b.** 75_____

• # # # • # # # • # # # • # # # • # # # • # # # • # # # • # #

A34   **a.** ix: 10 − 1   **b.** lxxv: 50 + 10 + 10 + 5

---

13   Placing a numeral to the left of another to indicate subtraction is limited to the following instances:

1. i may be deducted only from v or x.
2. x may be deducted only from l or c.
3. c may be deducted only from d or m.
4. The Roman numerals v, l, d, and m are not used to indicate subtraction.

Example 1: 49 would be written xlix, not il.

Example 2: 45 would be written xlv, not vl.

Q35   Give the Roman numeral represented by the Hindu–Arabic numeral:

a. 99_____   **b.** 990_____   **c.** 490_____

• # # # • # # # • # # # • # # # • # # # • # # # • # # # • # #

A35   **a.** xcix not ic   **b.** cmxc   **c.** cdxc

Q36   Give the Roman numeral represented by the Hindu–Arabic numeral:

a. 154_____   **b.** 28_____   **c.** 549_____

• # # # • # # # • # # # • # # # • # # # • # # # • # # # • # #

A36   **a.** cliv   **b.** xxviii   **c.** dxlix

14	If there seem to be two acceptable ways of writing with Roman numerals, the shorter form should be used. That is, lvv should be written lx.

Q37   Convert each of the following:

    a. xliv_____   **b.** 942_____   **c.** cdix_____

    d. 88_____   **e.** 1977_____   **f.** xlix_____

\# # # • # # # • # # # • # # # • # # # • # # # • # # # • # # # • # # #

A37   **a.** 44   **b.** cmxlii   **c.** 409   **d.** lxxxviii   **e.** mcmlxxvii   **f.** 49

15	A horizontal line over a Roman numeral indicates that its value is to be multiplied by 1,000 (uppercase numerals will be used in the following problems).

    Examples: $\bar{V} = 5{,}000\ (5 \times 1{,}000)$

                     $\bar{X} = 10{,}000\ (10 \times 1{,}000)$

                     $\overline{XI} = 11{,}000\ (11 \times 1{,}000)$

                     $\overline{XX} = 20{,}000\ (20 \times 1{,}000)$

Q38   Write using Hindu–Arabic numerals:

    a. $\bar{L}$_____   **b.** $\bar{C}$_____   **c.** $\bar{M}$_____

    d. $\overline{XIV}$_____   **e.** $\overline{XIX}$_____   **f.** $\overline{CC}$_____

\# # # • # # # • # # # • # # # • # # # • # # # • # # # • # # # • # # #

A38   **a.** 50,000   **b.** 100,000   **c.** 1,000,000

       d. 14,000   **e.** 19,000   **f.** 200,000

This completes the instruction for this section.

1.1   EXERCISE

1. Mr. Fred Smith works 42 hours each week. If he receives $6 per hour, how much does he earn per week?
2. Which is the better wage?
   a. $6,400 per year or $540 per month?
   b. $90 per week or $4,500 per year (50 weeks)?
   c. $250 per month or $3,200 per year?
3. Before Glee left on a trip the odometer of her automobile read 36,708 miles. At the end of the trip the odometer reading was 44,519. How far did Glee travel?
4. William received Demerol IM the following times: 150 mg (milligrams) at 6 AM, 100 mg at noon, and 75 mg at 6 PM. What was the total amount given?
5. Ms. Shea is to receive para-aminosalicylic acid 6 tablets t.i.d. (three times a day). How many tablets should be ordered for a weeks supply?
6. Determine Mary's caloric intake for breakfast. Jelly roll: 200 calories; coffee, cream, and sugar: 65 calories; $\frac{3}{4}$ cup of milk: 125 calories; 6 oz orange juice: 75 calories.
7. To qualify for a home loan your monthly income should be 5 times your monthly payment. For a monthly payment of $283, what must your minimum monthly income be?

8. Find the total cost:

No. of Items Purchased	Cost per Item	Total Cost
1,118	$8	a._____
982	5	b._____
2,036	7	c._____
	Grand total	d._____

9. One dose of aspirin is grain v. How many doses of aspirin are there in grain xxxv?

10. A patient is receiving injections of 20,000 units of penicillin every four hours. How many units will he receive in 24 hours?

11. How many calories should be consumed daily to maintain a desired weight of 185 pounds (using the formula of Frame 7)?

12. How many calories should be consumed daily to arrive at a desired weight of 112 pounds, losing one pound a week?

13. A patient is urged to drink 3000 ml of fluids daily. The daily intake was 2 glasses of juice at 220 ml each; 1 glass of milk at 230 ml; and 6 glasses of water at 250 ml each. How many more ml are needed to reach 3000 ml?

14. Convert to Hindu–Arabic numerals:

    a. vi   **b.** iv   **c.** xliv   **d.** cmxlvii

15. Write the Roman numerals 1–20.

16. Dave reduced his cholesterol level to 253 milligrams from a high of 310 milligrams. What was his change in cholesterol readings?

17. In the past few years the number of women in medical schools has increased from 3,894 to 7,824. Find the actual increase.

1.1   EXERCISE ANSWERS

1. $252   **2. a.** $540 per month   **b.** no difference   **c.** $3,200 per year   **3.** 7,811
4. 325 mg   **5.** 126   **6.** 465   **7.** $1,415
8. a. $8,944   **b.** $4,910   **c.** $14,252   **d.** $28,106
9. 7   **10.** 120,000   **11.** 2,775   **12.** 1,180
13. 830
14. a. 6   **b.** 4   **c.** 44   **d.** 947
15. i, ii, iii, iv, v, vi, vii, viii, ix, x, xi, xii, xiii, xiv, xv, xvi, xvii, xviii, xix, xx.
16. 57   **17.** 3,930

1.2   APPLICATIONS FOR FRACTIONS

> **1**   Numbers that are expressed in terms of a standard unit of measure are called *denominate numbers*. The number 3 by itself is an abstract number. But 3 weeks, 3 days, 3 dollars, 3 feet, and 3 centimetres are denominate numbers; they identify the measures of quantity.

Q1   Which of the following are denominate numbers?_____

    a. 5 ounces   **b.** $6\frac{1}{2}$ **c.** 2 seconds   **d.** 7 houses   **e.** 18,000   **f.** 1 pint

\# \# \# • \# \# \# • \# \# \# • \# \# \# • \# \# \# • \# \# \# • \# \# \# • \# \# \# • \# \# \#

A1   **a, c,** and **f:**   Houses is not a standard unit of measure.

2 Denominate numbers are generally expressed in the largest unit of measure possible. That is, 68 minutes would be expressed as 1 hour 8 minutes (60 minutes = 1 hour).

Example 1: 90 seconds = 1 minute 30 seconds

Example 2: 26 days = 3 weeks 5 days

Standard units of measure to be used in this section, and their abbreviations are given below.

1 yr (year) = 52 wk (weeks)
1 yr = 12 mo (months)
1 yr = 365 da (days)
1 yr = 360 da (commonly used for business computations)
1 wk = 7 da
1 da = 24 hr (hours)
1 hr = 60 min (minutes)
1 min = 60 sec (seconds)

Q2 Express in larger units of measure:
a. 83 min   **b.** 65 sec

• # # # • # # # • # # # • # # # • # # # • # # # • # # # • # #

A2   **a.** 1 hr 23 min   **b.** 1 min 5 sec

3 When adding or subtracting abstract numbers, it is necessary to add like place values; that is, units to units, tens to tens, hundreds to hundreds, and so on. Likewise, in the addition or subtraction of denominate numbers, the numbers of like denomination (unit of measure) are arranged in vertical columns with the smallest denomination on the right. The like denominations are then added or subtracted a column at a time from right to left.

Example:

$$
\begin{array}{rrr}
7\,\text{hr} & 30\,\text{min} & 17\,\text{sec} \\
+3\,\text{hr} & 42\,\text{min} & 50\,\text{sec} \\
\hline
10\,\text{hr} & 72\,\text{min} & 67\,\text{sec}
\end{array}
$$

Working from right to left, each denomination should be expressed as a larger denomination, where possible. That is, 67 sec = 1 min 7 sec. The 1 min is added to 72 min leaving a sum of 10 hr 73 min 7 sec. However, the 73 min = 1 hr 13 min. The 1 hr is added to 10 hr leaving the final sum 11 hr 13 min 7 sec.

Q3 Add and simplify by writing denominations as larger denominations, where possible:

a.

7 hr	23 min
4 hr	58 min

b.

2 wk	3 da	6 hr
1 wk	6 da	23 hr

• # # # • # # # • # # # • # # # • # # # • # # # • # # # • # #

A3   **a.** 12 hr 21 min:

7 hr	23 min
4 hr	58 min
11 hr	81 min
or 12 hr	21 min

b. 4 wk 3 da 5 hr:

2 wk	3 da	6 hr
1 wk	6 da	23 hr
3 wk	9 da	29 hr
or 3 wk	10 da	5 hr
or 4 wk	3 da	5 hr

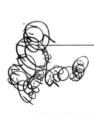

Q4   Add:

a. 8 hr   17 min   46 sec
    10 hr   39 min   42 sec
    26 hr   51 min   35 sec

b. 6 wk   12 da   7 hr
    7 wk   35 da   3 hr
    8 wk   12 da   16 hr

• ### • ### • ### • ### • ### • ### • ### • ### •

A4   **a.** 1 da 21 hr 49 min 3 sec   **b.** 29 wk 4 da 2 hr

---

4   Subtraction of denominate numbers is similar to addition; however, it may be necessary to express a larger denomination as a smaller denomination when borrowing.

Example: 7 hr   23 min
             −2 hr   56 min

To subtract 56 min from 23 min it is first necessary to borrow 1 hr (60 min) from 7 hr. The 60 min borrowed is then added to 23 min giving 83 min. The subtraction is now completed:

    6 hr   83 min
   −2 hr   56 min
    4 hr   27 min

Q5   Subtract:

a. 18 min   15 sec
    −6 min   45 sec

b. 3 da   14 hr   6 min
    −1 da   21 hr   36 min

• ### • ### • ### • ### • ### • ### • ### • ### •

A5   **a.** 11 min 30 sec: 17 min   75 sec
                          −6 min   45 sec

b. 1 da 16 hr 30 min: 3 da   13 hr   66 min
                        1 da   21 hr   36 min

                                or

                            2 da   37 hr   66 min
                            1 da   21 hr   36 min

Q6   Subtract:

a. 8 hr   15 min
    −5 hr   25 min

b. 88 hr   36 min   24 sec
    −69 hr   49 min   48 sec

• ### • ### • ### • ### • ### • ### • ### • ### •

A6   **a.** 2 hr 50 min   **b.** 18 hr 46 min 36 sec

---

5   When multiplying a denominate number by an abstract number, first multiply each denomination separately and then change the product to larger denominations, where possible.

Example: 3 hr   17 min
            ×   6
            18 hr   102 min
       or   19 hr   42 min

To divide a denominate number by an abstract number, divide each denomination separately; rewriting partial remainders as smaller denominations. The rewritten smaller denominations are added to like denominations and the division is continued.

Example:

$$\begin{array}{r} 2\text{ hr }\ \ 12\text{ min} \\ 6\overline{)13\text{ hr }\ \ 12\text{ min}} \end{array}$$

add

$$\begin{array}{r} 12\text{ hr} \\ \overline{1\text{ hr}=60\text{ min}} \\ \overline{72\text{ min}} \\ 72\text{ min} \\ \overline{0} \end{array}$$

Q7   Complete:
   a. 12 min   13 sec
             ×   7

   b. 5)23 hr   10 min

＃＃＃ • ＃＃＃ • ＃＃＃ • ＃＃＃ • ＃＃＃ • ＃＃＃ • ＃＃＃ • ＃＃＃ • ＃＃＃

A7   **a.** 1 hr 25 min 31 sec   **b.** 4 hr 38 min

6   Hours are sometimes expressed as fractional parts of an hour. For example, $7\frac{3}{4}$ hours. It may be convenient to express these fractional numbers as denominate numbers, in terms of hours and minutes. This is accomplished by recalling that an hour is 60 minutes and $\frac{3}{4}$ of an hour is $\frac{3}{4}$ of 60 minutes.

Example: Change $7\frac{3}{4}$ to hours and minutes.

Solution: $\frac{3}{4}$ of 60 minutes $=\frac{3}{4}\times\frac{60}{1}$ min $=45$ min

Hence, $7\frac{3}{4}$ hours = 7 hours 45 minutes.

Q8   Express as hours and minutes:
   a. $\frac{1}{4}$ hr   **b.** $3\frac{1}{2}$ hr

＃＃＃ • ＃＃＃ • ＃＃＃ • ＃＃＃ • ＃＃＃ • ＃＃＃ • ＃＃＃ • ＃＃＃ • ＃＃＃

A8   **a.** 15 min   **b.** 3 hr 30 min

Q9   Express as hours and minutes:
   a. $7\frac{2}{5}$ hr   **b.** $8\frac{3}{10}$ hr

＃＃＃ • ＃＃＃ • ＃＃＃ • ＃＃＃ • ＃＃＃ • ＃＃＃ • ＃＃＃ • ＃＃＃ • ＃＃＃

A9   **a.** 7 hr 24 min   **b.** 8 hr 18 min

7   Generally, hours worked are expressed as fractional or decimal numbers. Therefore, it will be necessary to express denominate numbers as fractional numbers.

Example 1: Express 7 hours 25 minutes as a fractional part of an hour.

Solution: It is necessary to express 25 minutes as a fractional part of an hour. Since 1 hour = 60 minutes, 25 minutes is $\frac{25}{60}$ of an hour. Hence, 7 hours 25 minutes $=7\frac{25}{60}$ hr. The fraction is reduced when possible. That is, $7\frac{25}{60}$ hr $=7\frac{5}{12}$ hr.

Example 2: Express 8 hr 40 min as a fractional part of an hour.

Solution: 8 hr 40 min $= 8\dfrac{40}{60}$ hr $= 8\dfrac{2}{3}$ hr.

Q10   Express as a fractional part of an hour:
a. 6 hr 15 min

b. 10 hr 12 min

\# \# \#   •   \# \# \#   •   \# \# \#   •   \# \# \#   •   \# \# \#   •   \# \# \#   •   \# \# \#   •   \# \# \#   •   \# \# \#

A10   **a.** $6\dfrac{1}{4}$ hr: 6 hr 15 min $= 6\dfrac{15}{60}$ hr

b. $10\dfrac{1}{5}$ hr

Q11   Express as a fractional part of an hour:
a. 7 hr 42 min

b. 5 hr 33 min

\# \# \#   •   \# \# \#   •   \# \# \#   •   \# \# \#   •   \# \# \#   •   \# \# \#   •   \# \# \#   •   \# \# \#   •   \# \# \#

A11   **a.** $7\dfrac{7}{10}$ hr

b. $5\dfrac{11}{20}$ hr

Q12   Sally worked the following hours this past week. Mon 7 hr 20 min, Tue 6 hr 35 min, and Wed 8 hr 50 min. Change each denominate number to a fractional part of an hour and find the total hours worked.

\# \# \#   •   \# \# \#   •   \# \# \#   •   \# \# \#   •   \# \# \#   •   \# \# \#   •   \# \# \#   •   \# \# \#   •   \# \# \#

A12 $22\dfrac{3}{4}$ hr: 7 hr   20 min $= 7\dfrac{1}{3}$ hr $= 7\dfrac{4}{12}$ hr

$\qquad\qquad$ 6 hr   35 min $= 6\dfrac{7}{12}$ hr $= 6\dfrac{7}{12}$ hr

$\qquad\qquad$ 8 hr   50 min $= 8\dfrac{5}{6}$ hr $= 8\dfrac{10}{12}$ hr

$\qquad\qquad\qquad\qquad\qquad$ _____   _____

Q13   In Q12, find the total hours worked by adding the denominate numbers.

\# \# \#   •   \# \# \#   •   \# \# \#   •   \# \# \#   •   \# \# \#   •   \# \# \#   •   \# \# \#   •   \# \# \#   •   \# \# \#

A13   22 hr 45 min: 7 hr   20 min

$\qquad\qquad\qquad\quad$ 6 hr   35 min

$\qquad\qquad\qquad\quad$ 8 hr   50 min

$\qquad\qquad\qquad\quad$ ─────────────

$\qquad\qquad\qquad\quad$ 21 hr 105 min

Q14 Nancy worked $6\frac{3}{8}$ hours on Monday, $7\frac{1}{2}$ hours on Tuesday, $8\frac{3}{4}$ hours on Wednesday, $7\frac{3}{8}$ hours on Thursday, and $9\frac{1}{4}$ hours on Friday. How many hours did she work during the week?

\#\#\# • \#\#\# • \#\#\# • \#\#\# • \#\#\# • \#\#\# • \#\#\# • \#\#\# • \#\#\#

A14 $39\frac{1}{4}$ hr

Q15 The following is a dental patient's record for 10 visits.
a. Determine the total time (in fractional parts of an hour) and
b. the total fee.

Visits		Time Required	Fee
1.	Root canal therapy (started)	20 minutes	$30
2.	Root canal therapy (continued)	30 minutes	30
3.	Root canal therapy (completed)	30 minutes	30
4.	Lingual adaptic for RCT tooth	15 minutes	11
5.	#2 MO Amalgam	25 minutes	14
6.	#12 MOD Amalgam	35 minutes	21
7.	#13 MOD Amalgam	35 minutes	21
8.	#14 MO Amalgam	25 minutes	20
9.	#18 O Amalgam	15 minutes	8
10.	#20 MOD Amalgam	35 minutes	21

\#\#\# • \#\#\# • \#\#\# • \#\#\# • \#\#\# • \#\#\# • \#\#\# • \#\#\# • \#\#\#

A15 **a.** $4\frac{5}{12}$ hr: 265 min $= 4\frac{5}{12}$ hr   **b.** $206

---

8 Earnings per hour is determined by dividing the total fee by the total number of hours worked.

Example: A dentist worked a total of 12 hours and charged his patient $696. Determine the dentist's gross earnings per hour.

Solution: earnings per hour = total fee ÷ hours worked
earnings per hour = $696 ÷ 12 hours
earnings per hour = $58 per hour

Q16 The total fee, for 10 visits, in Q15 was $206. The dentist worked $4\frac{5}{12}$ hours. Find the earnings per hour (round off to the nearest dollar).

\#\#\# • \#\#\# • \#\#\# • \#\#\# • \#\#\# • \#\#\# • \#\#\# • \#\#\# • \#\#\#

A16 $47 per hour: $206 ÷ $4\frac{5}{12}$ hours

[handwritten: Of = multiply (×) = "total meds. questions"]

---

9   Exposure to x-rays is measured in units called *roentgens*. For every minute a patient is being examined by means of a fluorescent screen ("fluoroscopy" or "screening"), 6 roentgens of x-rays are received. For a single x-ray picture ("radiograph") $\frac{1}{2}$ a roentgen is received. Hence, the total amount of roentgens received by a patient is given by:

Screening = 6 roentgens per minute

Radiograph = $\frac{1}{2}$ roentgens per picture

Example: Find the total number of roentgens received by a patient who is "screened" for 4 minutes, and of whom 5 radiographs are taken.

Solution: screening = 6 roentgens $\times 4 = 24$ roentgens

radiograph = $\frac{1}{2}$ roentgens $\times 5 = 2\frac{1}{2}$ roentgens

total = $24 + 2\frac{1}{2} = 26\frac{1}{2}$ roentgens

Q17   Find the total number of roentgens received by a patient who is screened for 5 minutes, and of whom 7 radiographs are taken.

● ### ● ### ● ### ● ### ● ### ● ### ● ### ●

A17 $33\frac{1}{2}$ roentgens: screening = 6 roentgens $\times 5$

radiograph = $\frac{1}{2}$ roentgens $\times 7$

Q18   **a.** Screening = _____ roentgens per minute of screening.

b. Radiograph = _____ roentgens per picture.

● ### ● ### ● ### ● ### ● ### ● ### ● ### ●

A18   **a.** 6   **b.** $\frac{1}{2}$

Q19   The label reads Morphine gr $\frac{1}{8}$. How many tablets would be needed to give Morphine gr $\frac{3}{4}$? (Hint: How many $\frac{1}{8}$ gr are contained in $\frac{3}{4}$ gr?) Note that gr is the symbol for grain, a unit of weight in the apothecaries' system (see Chapter 5).

● ### ● ### ● ### ● ### ● ### ● ### ● ### ●

A19   6 tablets: $\frac{3}{4} \div \frac{1}{8}$

Q20   About two-thirds of a person's body weight is represented by water. What is the weight of the water in a 150-pound person?

\# \# \#   •   \# \# \#   •   \# \# \#   •   \# \# \#   •   \# \# \#   •   \# \# \#   •   \# \# \#   •   \# \# \#   •   \# \# \#

A20   100 pounds: $\frac{2}{3} \times 150$ pounds

Q21   In the early 1900s *encephalitis lethargica* (sleeping sickness) swept Europe. Of nearly 5 million people infected, a third died. How many survived?

\# \# \#   •   \# \# \#   •   \# \# \#   •   \# \# \#   •   \# \# \#   •   \# \# \#   •   \# \# \#   •   \# \# \#   •   \# \# \#

A21 $3\frac{1}{3}$ million: $\frac{2}{3} \times 5$ million

Q22   Determine the calories consumed:

Food	Calories Aver. Serving	Size of Serving	Calories Consumed
Danish pastry	200	$\frac{1}{4}$	a._____
Doughnut	150	$\frac{2}{3}$	b._____
1 Egg (fried)	125	1	c._____
Milk	130	$\frac{3}{4}$	d._____
		Total	e._____

\# \# \#   •   \# \# \#   •   \# \# \#   •   \# \# \#   •   \# \# \#   •   \# \# \#   •   \# \# \#   •   \# \# \#   •   \# \# \#

A22   **a.** 50   **b.** 100   **c.** 125   **d.** $97\frac{1}{2}$ **e.** $372\frac{1}{2}$

---

10   One of the more important applications of fractions to health-related areas is *medication problems*. There is little room for error when determining the amount of medication or number of tablets given a patient. The following formula can be used to determine the total medication given a patient.

total medication = number of tablets × medication per tablet

Example: If a nurse gave $\frac{1}{2}$ of a $\frac{3}{4}$-grain morphine sulfate tablet to a patient, how much drug did the patient receive?

Solution: total medication $= \frac{1}{2}$ tablet $\times \frac{3}{4}$ grain

total medication $= \frac{3}{8}$ grain

Q23   A patient was given $\frac{1}{4}$ of a $\frac{1}{4}$-grain atropine sulfate tablet. How much medication did the patient receive?

\# \# \#   •   \# \# \#   •   \# \# \#   •   \# \# \#   •   \# \# \#   •   \# \# \#   •   \# \# \#   •   \# \# \#   •   \# \# \#

A23 $\frac{1}{16}$ grain: $\frac{1}{4}$ tablet $\times \frac{1}{4}$ grain

Q24   Helen was given $\frac{3}{4}$ of a $\frac{1}{2}$ grain codeine sulfate tablet. How much medication did she receive?

\# \# \#   •   \# \# \#   •   \# \# \#   •   \# \# \#   •   \# \# \#   •   \# \# \#   •   \# \# \#   •   \# \# \#   •   \# \# \#

A24 $\frac{3}{8}$ grain: $\frac{3}{4}$ tablet $\times \frac{1}{2}$ grain

Q25   Jack received $\frac{1}{4}$ of a $\frac{3}{8}$-grain ephedrine sulfate ampul. How much medication did he receive?

\# \# \#   •   \# \# \#   •   \# \# \#   •   \# \# \#   •   \# \# \#   •   \# \# \#   •   \# \# \#   •   \# \# \#   •   \# \# \#

A25 $\frac{3}{32}$ grain: $\frac{1}{4}$ tablet $\times \frac{3}{8}$ grain

Q26   Total medication given = _____ × _____.

\# \# \#   •   \# \# \#   •   \# \# \#   •   \# \# \#   •   \# \# \#   •   \# \# \#   •   \# \# \#   •   \# \# \#   •   \# \# \#

A26   number of tablets × medication per tablet

---

11   The number of tablets given a patient can be determined by dividing the amount of drug desired by the amount of drug available. That is,

$$\text{number of tablets} = \frac{\text{desired amount}}{\text{available amount}}$$

Example: A nurse wishes to give 8 mg of morphine sulfate from 15-mg morphine sulfate tablets. How many tablets should be used*?

Solution: $\text{number of tablets} = \frac{8 \text{ mg}}{15 \text{ mg}}$

$\text{number of tablets} = \frac{1}{2} \text{ tablet}$

*Tablets can only be easily divided into units of $\frac{1}{2}$ or $\frac{1}{4}$. For this reason the tablet dosage is usually rounded off to the nearest $\frac{1}{4}$ tablet.

Q27 To give 25 mg of ascorbic acid from 100-mg tablets, how many tablets would you use?

• # # # • # # # • # # # • # # # • # # # • # # # • # # # • # # # • # #

A27 $\frac{1}{4}$ tablet: number of tablets = $\dfrac{\text{desired amount}}{\text{amount available}} = \dfrac{25 \text{ mg}}{100 \text{ mg}}$

Q28 A patient requires $\frac{1}{2}$ mg of Digoxin. How many tablets of $\frac{1}{4}$-mg Digoxin should be given?

$$\frac{\frac{1}{2}}{\frac{1}{4}} = \frac{1}{2} \div \frac{1}{4} = \frac{1}{2} \times \frac{4}{1} = \frac{4}{2} = 2$$

• # # # • # # # • # # # • # # # • # # # • # # # • # # # • # # # • # #

A28 2 tablets: number of tablets = $\dfrac{\frac{1}{2} \text{ mg}}{\frac{1}{4} \text{ mg}}$

Q29 A nurse wishes to give tetracycline, 125 mg from 250-mg tetracycline tablets. How many tablets should be given?

• # # # • # # # • # # # • # # # • # # # • # # # • # # # • # # # • # #

A29 $\frac{1}{2}$ tablet

Q30 How many tablets of digitalis, $1\frac{1}{2}$ grain, would you use to give $\frac{1}{2}$ grain of digitalis?

• # # # • # # # • # # # • # # # • # # # • # # # • # # # • # # # • # #

A30 $\frac{1}{4}$ tablet: number of tablets = $\dfrac{\frac{1}{2} \text{ grain}}{1\frac{1}{2} \text{ grain}} = \frac{1}{2} \div \frac{3}{2} = \frac{1}{3}$ (round off to nearest $\frac{1}{4}$ tablet)

Q31 A patient is to receive $\frac{3}{4}$ grain of vitamin B_1. If the tablets are $1\frac{1}{2}$ grains, how many tablets should be taken?

• # # # • # # # • # # # • # # # • # # # • # # # • # # # • # # # • # #

A31 $\frac{1}{2}$ tablet

Q32 The number of tablets given a patient is equal to

_____ medication divided by _____ .

\# \# \# • \# \# \# • \# \# \# • \# \# \# • \# \# \# • \# \# \# • \# \# \# • \# \# \# • \# \# \#

A32 desired amount, amount available

---

12 One method of determining a child's dosage of medication from an adult dosage, is through the use of the child's weight. The following formula is called *Clark's Rule*, which states:

$$\text{child's dosage} = \frac{\text{weight of child (pounds)}}{150} \times \text{adult dosage}$$

The 150 in the denominator represents the weight of an average adult.

Example: If an adult dosage of aspirin is 5 grains, what is the dosage for a 30-pound child?

Solution: child's dosage $= \dfrac{30}{150} \times 5$ grains $= \dfrac{1}{5} \times 5$ grains $= 1$ grain

---

Q33 If the adult dosage of medication is 2 tablets (5 grains each), what is the dosage of a child weighing 50 pounds?

\# \# \# • \# \# \# • \# \# \# • \# \# \# • \# \# \# • \# \# \# • \# \# \# • \# \# \# • \# \# \#

A33 $\dfrac{3}{4}$ tablet: child's dosage $= \dfrac{\text{weight of child}}{150} \times \text{adult dosage}$

$= \dfrac{50}{150} \times 2$ tablets

$= \dfrac{1}{3} \times 2$ (round off to the nearest $\dfrac{1}{4}$ tablet)

Q34 If the adult dosage of a drug is 50 mg, how much should a 100-pound child receive?

\# \# \# • \# \# \# • \# \# \# • \# \# \# • \# \# \# • \# \# \# • \# \# \# • \# \# \# • \# \# \#

A34 $33\dfrac{1}{3}$ mg: child's dosage $= \dfrac{100}{150} \times 50$ mg

---

Q35 If the adult dosage of a drug is $5\dfrac{1}{2}$ grains, how much should a 60-pound child receive?

\# \# \# • \# \# \# • \# \# \# • \# \# \# • \# \# \# • \# \# \# • \# \# \# • \# \# \# • \# \# \#

A35 $2\dfrac{1}{5}$ grains: child's dosage $= \dfrac{60}{150} \times 5\dfrac{1}{2}$ grains

---

Q36   The adult dosage of Histaspan-D is one capsule twice a day. What is the dosage of a 80-pound child?

• # # # • # # # • # # # • # # # • # # # • # # # • # # # • # #

A36 $\frac{1}{2}$ capsule twice a day: child's dosage $= \frac{80}{150} \times 1$ capsule

$\left(\text{Note: } \frac{8}{15} \text{ capsule is approximately } \frac{1}{2} \text{ capsule.} \right)$

---

13   More practical dosage problems will be presented in Chapter 8. The problems in this first chapter are primarily intended to give the student review with basic mathematics while working with health-related concepts.

This completes the instruction for this section.

1.2   EXERCISE

1. Change to a fractional part of an hour:
   - **a.** 8 hr 10 min
   - **b.** 7 hr 25 min
   - **c.** 6 hr 12 min
   - **d.** 15 hr 6 min
   - **e.** 10 hr 33 min
   - **f.** 2 hr 50 min

2. Change to a denominate number in hours and minutes:
   - **a.** $8\frac{2}{3}$ hr
   - **b.** $7\frac{1}{10}$ hr
   - **c.** $8\frac{1}{5}$ hr
   - **d.** $9\frac{3}{4}$
   - **e.** $8\frac{5}{6}$
   - **f.** $7\frac{3}{10}$ hr

3. Perform the indicated operation and simplify:
   - **a.** 8 hr   10 min
        − 3 hr   45 min
   - **b.** 3 hr 20 min × 8
   - **c.** 8 hr 14 min ÷ 2
   - **d.** 6 hr   10 min
        − 2 hr   17 min

4. Seven employees of the Plymouth Health Clinic worked the following hours. Find the total hours worked for each employee.

M	T	W	Th	F	S	Total
7	$8\frac{1}{4}$	$7\frac{1}{4}$	$7\frac{1}{2}$	9	—	**a.**_____
8	8	7	—	7	7	**b.**_____
$7\frac{1}{4}$	$7\frac{1}{2}$	$7\frac{1}{4}$	$7\frac{3}{4}$	$6\frac{1}{2}$	—	**c.**_____
$7\frac{1}{4}$	$7\frac{1}{2}$	$7\frac{1}{2}$	$3\frac{1}{4}$	$8\frac{1}{2}$	$4\frac{1}{2}$	**d.**_____
8	8	$7\frac{1}{2}$	—	8	$7\frac{1}{2}$	**e.**_____
$8\frac{1}{2}$	$7\frac{1}{2}$	$7\frac{3}{4}$	—	7	$7\frac{1}{4}$	**f.**_____
$7\frac{1}{2}$	$8\frac{1}{2}$	8	7	5	4	**g.**_____

5. A dentist, his wife, and 2 children want to fly to Cleveland. The price of a regular ticket is $72. Before tax, what is the total cost of the tickets for the family?

One Way Airlines

Special Family Rates for Tickets

Husband—pays regular price

Wife—pays $\frac{2}{3}$ of regular price

Child—pays $\frac{1}{2}$ of regular price

6. A chemist ordered $255\frac{3}{4}$ litres of distilled water which he divided into $\frac{1}{2}$ litre containers. How many $\frac{1}{2}$-litres of distilled water did he have?

7. The following is a dental patient's record for 11 visits.
    a. Determine the total time (in fractional parts of an hour) and **b.** the total fee.

Visits	Time Required	Fee
#30 DO Amalgam	25 minutes	14
#19 VC prep, band imp & Temp crown	40 minutes	44
#19 Imp with coping & bite registration	30 minutes	43
#19 Insert VC & bite adjustment	25 minutes	43
#5 POG prep, band imp & temp crown	40 minutes	150
#3 POG prep, band imp & temp crown	40 minutes	150
Imp with copings, bite registration	30 minutes	150
Castings try in	30 minutes	—
Biscuit bake try in	30 minutes	—
Insertion 3 unit POG bridge	30 minutes	—
#16 extraction	15 minutes	15

8. Determine the earnings per hour in Problem 7 (round off to the nearest dollar).

9. Find the total number of roentgens received by a patient who is screened for 3 minutes, and of whom 9 radiographs are taken.

10. Find the total number of roentgens received by a patient if 11 radiographs are taken.

11. Approximately one-half of the total calcium and one-third of the total phosphorus in a baby's body at birth are deposited during the last 6 weeks of pregnancy. If a baby's body contains 25 grams of calcium and 13 grams of phosphorus at birth, how much was deposited in the last 6 weeks?

12. Determine the calories consumed:

Food	Calories in Average Serving	Size of Serving	Calories Consumed
1 slice pizza	225	$2\frac{1}{2}$ slices	**a.**_____
beer	150	$3\frac{1}{3}$ bottles	**b.**_____
ice cream	150	$\frac{1}{2}$ scoop	**c.**_____
		Total	**d.**_____

13. A patient was given $\frac{1}{2}$ of a $\frac{1}{4}$-grain atropine sulfate tablet. How much medication did the patient receive?

14. A patient was given $\frac{3}{4}$ of a $\frac{1}{2}$-grain codeine sulfate tablet. How much medication did the patient receive?

15. A patient receives $\frac{3}{4}$ grain of ephedrine from $\frac{3}{8}$-grain tablets. How many tablets did he receive?

16. To give $\frac{1}{4}$ grain of digitalis from $\frac{1}{2}$-grain tablets, how many tablets should you use?

17. If you gave $\frac{1}{2}$ of a $\frac{1}{4}$-grain morphine sulfate tablet, how much medication did you give?

18. If an aspirin tablet contains $7\frac{1}{2}$ grains of acetylsalicylic acid, how much would $\frac{3}{4}$ of a tablet contain?

19. A nurse is requested to give a patient 8 mg of morphine sulfate. How many tablets should be given if each tablet is 10 mg (round off to the nearest $\frac{1}{4}$ tablet)?

20. If the adult dosage of a drug is 2 tablets (100 mg each), how much should be given a 45-pound child (round off to the nearest $\frac{1}{4}$ tablet)?

21. If the adult dosage of a medication is $\frac{1}{8}$ grain, how much should a 60-pound child receive?

22. If the adult dosage of a drug is 50 mg, how much should a 100-pound child receive?

23. If the adult dosage is 2 tablets of 5-grain aspirin, what is the dosage for a 80-pound child in tablets and grains (round off to the nearest $\frac{1}{4}$ tablet)?

1.2 EXERCISE ANSWERS

1. a. $8\frac{1}{6}$ hr   **b.** $7\frac{5}{12}$ hr   **c.** $6\frac{1}{5}$ hr   **d.** $15\frac{1}{10}$ hr   **e.** $10\frac{11}{20}$ hr   **f.** $2\frac{5}{6}$ hr

2. a. 8 hr 40 min   **b.** 7 hr 6 min   **c.** 8 hr 12 min
   d. 9 hr 45 min   **e.** 8 hr 50 min   **f.** 7 hr 18 min

3. a. 4 hr 25 min   **b.** 26 hr 40 min   **c.** 4 hr 7 min   **d.** 3 hr 53 min

4. a. 39 hr   **b.** 37 hr   **c.** $36\frac{1}{4}$ hr   **d.** $38\frac{1}{2}$ hr

   e. 39 hr   **f.** 38 hr   **g.** 40 hr

5. $192   **6.** $511\frac{1}{2}$ **7. a.** $5\frac{7}{12}$ hr   **b.** $609

8. $109   **9.** $22\frac{1}{2}$ roentgens   **10.** $5\frac{1}{2}$ roentgens

11. $12\frac{1}{2}$ grams calcium, $4\frac{1}{3}$ grams phosphorus

12. a. $562\frac{1}{2}$ **b.** 500   **c.** 75   **d.** $1,137\frac{1}{2}$

13. $\frac{1}{8}$ grain   **14.** $\frac{3}{8}$ grain   **15.** 2 tablets   **16.** $\frac{1}{2}$ tablet

17. $\frac{1}{8}$ grain   **18.** $5\frac{5}{8}$ grains   **19.** $\frac{3}{4}$ tablet   **20.** $\frac{1}{2}$ tablet

21. $\frac{1}{20}$ grain   **22.** $33\frac{1}{3}$ mg   **23.** 1 tablet, $5\frac{1}{3}$ grains

1.3   APPLICATIONS FOR DECIMALS

<table>
<tr><td>1</td><td>

The ability to make proper change is an important concern for anyone dealing with sums of money. For that matter all consumers should be familiar with change making procedures.

    The *addition method* is a popular and accurate method of making change. To make change using the addition method, one starts with the amount of the fee (or sale) and adds as few pieces of money as possible until the amount presented in payment is reached. For example, assume that a receptionist is presented a ten-dollar bill in payment for a $2.73 fee to a patient. The receptionist should start with the amount of the fee, $2.73, and count out two pennies to make $2.75; one quarter to make $3.00; two one-dollar bills to make $5.00; and one five-dollar bill to make $10.00, the amount presented.*

Examples:

Amount Presented	Amount of Sale	Amount of Change							
		1¢	5¢	10¢	25¢	50¢	$1	$5	$10
1. $10	$2.63	2		1	1		2	1	
2. 1	0.82	3	1	1					
3. 5	2.54	1		2	1		2		

* The government is encouraging the use of the two-dollar bill. Hence, for every two one-dollar bills needed, one two-dollar bill could be used. However, the use of the two-dollar bill has been omitted from the examples and problems of this section.

</td></tr>
</table>

Q1   Show the pieces of change that should be given. Use as few pieces of money as possible:

Amount Presented	Amount of Sale	Amount of Change							
		1¢	5¢	10¢	25¢	50¢	$1	$5	$10
a. $1	$0.43								
b. 3	2.18								
c. 5	3.79								
d. 6	5.32								
e. 10	2.45								
f. 10	5.58								
g. 10	7.01								
h. 20	11.15								
i. 20	15.93								
j. 20	1.75								
k. 50	25.08								

• # # # • # # # • # # # • # # # • # # # • # # # • # # # • # # # • # #

A1

		1¢	5¢	10¢	25¢	50¢	$1	$5	$10
a.		2	1			1			
b.		2	1		1	1			
c.		1		2			1		
d.		3	1	1		1			
e.			1			1	2	1	
f.		2	1	1	1		4		
g.		4		2	1	1	2		
h.				1	1	1	3	1	
i.		2	1				4		
j.						1	3	1	1
k.		2	1	1	1	1	4		2

2 Many people and businesses find it both convenient and safe to deposit money in a bank and then write checks directing the bank to pay out certain sums of money. The amounts to be paid out cannot exceed the amounts deposited minus any previous checks written, so it is important that an accurate record of all deposits and checks be kept. This record is usually kept in a *check register*. Note from the illustration that check number 101 for $27.56 was subtracted from the balance $249.87, leaving $222.31 as the new balance. The deposit of $500 was added to $222.31, leaving a new balance of $722.31.

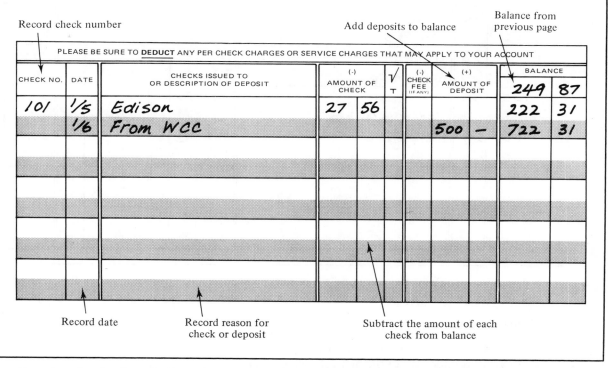

Record check number   Add deposits to balance   Balance from previous page

Record date   Record reason for check or deposit   Subtract the amount of each check from balance

Q2 Complete the check register on the next page (each item should be added or subtracted separately):

Check No.	Date	Description	Amount	Deposit
101	1/5	Edison	$27.56	
102	1/6	Wiltse	14.04	
103	1/6	F. Jack	10.00	
104	1/7	J. Lawson	6.52	
105	1/8	Kresge	12.36	
	1/8	Sales receipts		$492.18
106	1/9	Colony Co.	100.92	

Complete the check register on the next page (each item should be added or subtracted separately):

PLEASE BE SURE TO **DEDUCT** ANY PER CHECK CHARGES OR SERVICE CHARGES THAT MAY APPLY TO YOUR ACCOUNT

CHECK NO.	DATE	CHECKS ISSUED TO OR DESCRIPTION OF DEPOSIT	(-) AMOUNT OF CHECK		√ T	(-) CHECK FEE (IF ANY)	(+) AMOUNT OF DEPOSIT	BALANCE 249	87

\#\#\# • \#\#\# • \#\#\# • \#\#\# • \#\#\# • \#\#\# • \#\#\# • \#\#\# • \#\#\#

A2

PLEASE BE SURE TO **DEDUCT** ANY PER CHECK CHARGES OR SERVICE CHARGES THAT MAY APPLY TO YOUR ACCOUNT

CHECK NO.	DATE	CHECKS ISSUED TO OR DESCRIPTION OF DEPOSIT	(-) AMOUNT OF CHECK		√ T	(-) CHECK FEE (IF ANY)	(+) AMOUNT OF DEPOSIT	BALANCE 249	87
101	1/5	Edison	27	56				222	31
102	1/6	Wiltse	14	04				208	27
103	1/6	F. Jack	10	—				198	27
104	1/7	J. Lawson	6	52				191	75
105	1/8	Kresge	12	36				179	39
	1/8	Sales Receipts					492 18	671	57
106	1/9	Colony Co	100	92				570	65

---

3 Application problems for rounding off decimals often involve rounding off to the nearest cent or dollar; however, for purposes of estimation it may be necessary to round off to other place values.

Examples

1. $7.025 rounded off to the nearest cent is $7.03.
2. $187.49 rounded off to the nearest dollar is $187.
3. $187.49 rounded off to the nearest hundred dollars is $200.

Q3   Round off to the nearest cent:

a. $17.253＿＿＿＿＿   b. $187.066＿＿＿＿＿＿＿

c. $0.333＿＿＿＿＿   d. $23.1692＿＿＿＿＿＿＿

\#\#\# • \#\#\# • \#\#\# • \#\#\# • \#\#\# • \#\#\# • \#\#\# • \#\#\# • \#\#\#

A3   a. $17.25   b. $187.07   c. $0.33   d. $23.17

Q4   Round off $1,905.495 as indicated:

    a. nearest cent_____

    b. nearest dollar_____

    c. nearest hundred dollars_____

    d. nearest $1,000_____

\# \# \# • \# \# \# • \# \# \# • \# \# \# • \# \# \# • \# \# \# • \# \# \# • \# \# \# • \# \# \#

A4   **a.** $1,905.50   **b.** $1,905   **c.** $1,900   **d.** $2,000

---

4   Errors with decimals often involve the placement of the decimal point in the final result. For this reason it is especially important, when working decimal problems, to estimate the answer.

Examples:

1. 8.7×0.34 is estimated as $9 \times 0.3 = 2.7$
2. 16.582×2.18 is estimated as $17 \times 2 = 34$
3. $17.6 \div 0.2$ is estimated as $18 \div 0.2 = 180 \div 2 = 90$ (Note that the decimal point in the divisor and the dividend was moved one place to the right.)
4. $47 \div 0.63$ is estimated as $48 \div 0.6 = 480 \div 6 = 80$

Q5   Estimate:
    a. 19.5×0.41 **b.** $2.6 \div 0.16$ **c.** $\$39.05 \times 8.35$ **d.** $0.061 \div 0.2$

\# \# \# • \# \# \# • \# \# \# • \# \# \# • \# \# \# • \# \# \# • \# \# \# • \# \# \# • \# \# \#

A5   **a.** 8: 20×0.4 **b.** 13: $2.6 \div 0.2 = 26 \div 2$
        c. $320: 40×8 **d.** 0.3: $0.06 \div 0.2 = 0.6 \div 2$

Q6   Choose the best estimate:

    a. 4.2×7.1 is approximately; 0.28, 28, 280, 2.8_____

    b. 0.03×9.8 is approximately; 0.3, 30, 3, 0.03_____

    c. 782×2.438 is approximately; 160, 0.16, 1,600, 16,000_____

    d. 2.9×0.11 is approximately; 30, 290, 0.3, 3_____

    e. $19.5 \div 2.5$ is approximately; 38, 8, 40, 17_____

    f. $0.7 \div 0.04$ is approximately; 0.028, 18, 2, 1.7_____

    g. 0.26×728 is approximately; 500, 200, 14, 1.6_____

\# \# \# • \# \# \# • \# \# \# • \# \# \# • \# \# \# • \# \# \# • \# \# \# • \# \# \# • \# \# \#

A6   **a.** 28   **b.** 0.3   **c.** 1600   **d.** 0.3   **e.** 8   **f.** 18   **g.** 200

Q7   Estimate in hundreds, the sum of $265.32, $413.78, $837.60, and $572.91.

\# \# \# • \# \# \# • \# \# \# • \# \# \# • \# \# \# • \# \# \# • \# \# \# • \# \# \# • \# \# \#

A7 $2,100

Q8   Horton had $4,183.72 in his checking account. He wrote a check for $1,982.79. Determine approximately how much he has left in his account by estimating in thousands.

\# \# \# • \# \# \# • \# \# \# • \# \# \# • \# \# \# • \# \# \# • \# \# \# • \# \# \# • \# \# \#

A8 $2,000

Q9   Find the new bank balance if the previous monthly balance was $582.07, deposits during the month were $406.53, $92.87, $396.34, $155.91, and $268.43. Checks drawn were $309.23, $127.87, $435.80, and $75.63.

•   # # #   •   # # #   •   # # #   •   # # #   •   # # #   •   # # #   •   # # #   •   # #

A9 $953.62:   Add the deposits to the previous monthly balance and subtract the total of the checks written.

Q10   The office manager orders a gross (gross = 144) of pencils. If the pencils are $3.50 a gross, what is the price of one pencil (round off to the nearest cent)?

•   # # #   •   # # #   •   # # #   •   # # #   •   # # #   •   # # #   •   # # #   •   # #

A10 $0.02: $3.50 ÷ 144

Q11   A young girl is to receive 0.025 g(gram) of Furoxone 4 times daily. How many grams will she receive in 1 week?

•   # # #   •   # # #   •   # # #   •   # # #   •   # # #   •   # # #   •   # # #   •   # #

A11   0.7 g: $0.025 \times 4 \times 7$

Q12   The oxidation of carbohydrates is a process in which oxygen unites with carbohydrates to form carbon dioxide, water, and heat. One ounce of carbohydrate oxidized by the body requires 1.19 ounces of oxygen for its combustion. The end products are 1.63 ounces of carbon dioxide, 0.55 ounces of water, and 119 calories of heat. How much oxygen is needed, and what quantities of carbon dioxide, water, and heat would be created in the oxidation of 12 ounces of carbohydrates?

•   # # #   •   # # #   •   # # #   •   # # #   •   # # #   •   # # #   •   # # #   •   # #

A12   14.28 ounces of oxygen: 1.19×12
19.56 ounces of carbon dioxide: 1.63×12
6.6 ounces of water: 0.55×12
1,428 calories of heat: 119×12

5   The height of a child as an adult depends on many factors. Heredity, nutrition, and general health are factors that are hard to estimate; however, a chart for predicting the adult height of a person is given below. It should be remembered that these figures are correct for averages, but who's average? The chart gives general figures for different ages.

Age	Boys	Girls	
6 months	37.67	39.84	
12 months	42.23	44.67	
24 months	48.57	52.15	The numbers do not represent height, but are used
5 years	61.60	66.64	to help find height.
10 years	78.74	84.76	
15 years	94.60	99.31	

To estimate the adult height take the child's height in inches at any of the given ages, multiply it by 100, and then divide by the corresponding figure in the chart. The answer is in inches.

Example: R. Hayes is 43 inches tall and is 5 years old. Estimate his height as an adult.

Solution: Multiply his height by 100:

$43 \times 100 = 4,300$

Divide this result by the figure in the chart.
$4,300 \div 61.60 = 69.8$ inches (nearest tenth).

Height is usually given in terms of feet and inches; hence, his adult height will be 5 feet 10 inches (69.8 is 70 rounded off to the nearest inch).

Q13   Determine the adult height of a boy 15 years of age and 5 feet 6 inches tall (round off to the nearest inch).

•   # # #   •   # # #   •   # # #   •   # # #   •   # # #   •   # # #   •   # # #   •   # #

A13   5 feet 10 inches: 5 feet 6 inches = 66 inches
$66 \times 100 = 6,600$
$6,600 \div 94.60 = 70$ inches (nearest inch)

Q14   Determine the adult height of a girl 15 years of age and 5 feet 6 inches tall (round off to the nearest inch).

•   # # #   •   # # #   •   # # #   •   # # #   •   # # #   •   # # #   •   # # #   •   # #

A14   5 feet 6 inches: $6,600 \div 99.31 = 66$ (nearest inch)

Q15   The thiamine requirement is related to caloric intake. The approximate minimum daily need is given by thiamine need $= \dfrac{\text{caloric intake}}{1,000} \times 0.22$ mg. What are the thiamine requirements for an intake of 1,750 calories?

\# \# \#   •   \# \# \#   •   \# \# \#   •   \# \# \#   •   \# \# \#   •   \# \# \#   •   \# \# \#   •   \# \# \#   •   \# \# \#

A15   0.385 mg: $\dfrac{1,750}{1,000} \times 0.22$ mg

---

6   Three important medication formulas introduced in Section 2 were:

1. Total medication = number of tablets × medication per tablet

2. Number of tablets $= \dfrac{\text{desired amount}}{\text{available amount}}$

3. Child's dosage $= \dfrac{\text{child's weight}}{150} \times$ adult dosage

---

Q16   A patient received 0.25 of a 0.5-grain codeine sulfate tablet. How much medication did he receive?

\# \# \#   •   \# \# \#   •   \# \# \#   •   \# \# \#   •   \# \# \#   •   \# \# \#   •   \# \# \#   •   \# \# \#   •   \# \# \#

A16   0.125 grain: Total medication = number of tablets × medication per tablet
Total medication = 0.25 × 0.5 grain

Q17   If you gave 0.75 of a 0.02-grain atropine sulfate tablet, how much medication did you give?

\# \# \#   •   \# \# \#   •   \# \# \#   •   \# \# \#   •   \# \# \#   •   \# \# \#   •   \# \# \#   •   \# \# \#   •   \# \# \#

A17   0.015 grain: 0.75 × 0.02 grain

Q18   A patient received 0.25 of a 0.375-grain ephedrine sulfate ampul. How much medication did he receive?

\# \# \#   •   \# \# \#   •   \# \# \#   •   \# \# \#   •   \# \# \#   •   \# \# \#   •   \# \# \#   •   \# \# \#   •   \# \# \#

A18   0.09375 grain: 0.25 × 0.375 grain

Q19 A nurse wishes to give 8 mg of morphine sulfate from 15-mg morphine sulfate tablets. How many tablets should be used?

\# \# \# • \# \# \# • \# \# \# • \# \# \# • \# \# \# • \# \# \# • \# \# \# • \# \# \# • \# \# \#

A19 0.5 tablets: Number of tablets $= \dfrac{\text{desired amount}}{\text{available amount}} = \dfrac{8\text{ mg}}{15\text{ mg}}$

Q20 To give 0.5 mg of Digoxin from 0.25-mg Digoxin tablets, how many tablets would you use?

\# \# \# • \# \# \# • \# \# \# • \# \# \# • \# \# \# • \# \# \# • \# \# \# • \# \# \# • \# \# \#

A20 2 tablets: $0.5\text{ mg} \div 0.25\text{ mg}$

Q21 How many tablets of 1.5 grain digitalis would you use to give 0.5 grain of digitalis?

\# \# \# • \# \# \# • \# \# \# • \# \# \# • \# \# \# • \# \# \# • \# \# \# • \# \# \# • \# \# \#

A21 $\dfrac{1}{4}$ tablet: $0.5 \div 1.5$

Q22 If the adult dosage of medication is 2 tablets, what is the dosage of a child weighing 50 pounds?

\# \# \# • \# \# \# • \# \# \# • \# \# \# • \# \# \# • \# \# \# • \# \# \# • \# \# \# • \# \# \#

A22 $\dfrac{3}{4}$ tablet: Child's dosage $= \dfrac{\text{weight of child}}{150} \times$ adult dosage

Child's dosage $= \dfrac{50}{150} \times 2$ tablets

Q23 If the adult dosage of a drug is 5.5 grains, how much should a 60-pound child receive?

\# \# \# • \# \# \# • \# \# \# • \# \# \# • \# \# \# • \# \# \# • \# \# \# • \# \# \# • \# \# \#

A23 2.2 grains: $\dfrac{60}{150} \times 5.5$ grains

Q24 A survey conducted by economists for a large bank revealed the worth of tasks performed by an average housewife. Listed on page 34 are the twelve tasks a housewife might be called upon to perform daily, the numbers of hours she spends on each, and the usual rate of pay for these jobs. Find out how much she could earn in a week and write the results in the column on the right. Round off answers to the nearest cent.

Job	Hours per Week	Rate per Hour	Value per Week
Nursemaid	44.5	$2.50	a. $_____
Dietitian	1.2	3.85	b. _____
Food Buyer	3.3	2.15	c. _____
Cook	13.1	4.25	d. _____
Dishwasher	6.2	2.00	e. _____
Housekeeper	17.5	2.50	f. _____
Laundress	5.9	2.60	g. _____
Seamstress	1.3	3.25	h. _____
Practical Nurse	0.6	3.75	i. _____
Maintenance Person	1.7	3.20	j. _____
Gardener	2.3	2.10	k. _____
Chauffeur	2.0	3.65	l. _____
Total	99.6		m. $_____

\# \# \# • \# \# \# • \# \# \# • \# \# \# • \# \# \# • \# \# \# • \# \# \# • \# \# \# • \# \# \#

A24　　a. 111.25　　　　b. 4.62　　　　c. 7.10　　　　d. 55.68
　　　　e. 12.40　　　　f. 43.75　　　　g. 15.34　　　　h. 4.23
　　　　i. 2.25　　　　j. 5.44　　　　k. 4.83　　　　l. 7.30
　　　　m. 274.19

Q25　　What would the yearly salary be of the housewife in the above problem (52 weeks in one year)?

\# \# \# • \# \# \# • \# \# \# • \# \# \# • \# \# \# • \# \# \# • \# \# \# • \# \# \# • \# \# \#

A25　　$14,257.88

This completes the instruction for this section.

1.3　EXERCISE

1. Show the pieces of change that should be given. Use as few pieces of money as possible:

Amount Presented	Amount of Sale	1¢	5¢	10¢	25¢	$1	$5	$10	$20
a. $1.00	$0.14								
b. 2.00	1.10								
c. 5.00	0.68								
d. 5.00	1.26								
e. 8.00	6.15								
f. 10.00	2.32								
g. 10.00	5.57								
h. 20.00	12.74								
i. 20.00	6.95								
j. 100.00	46.93								

2. Complete the check register if the balance brought forward is $1,503.17:

Check No.	Date	Description	Amount	Deposits
131	8/2	Edison	$193.17	
132	8/2	Consumers	215.36	
133	8/3	H. Hopkins	28.15	
	8/3	Sales Receipts		432.08
134	8/4	First National	483.92	
135	8/5	Office Supplies	56.17	
	8/5	Sales Receipts		199.16
136	8/6	S. Bebe	800.00	

PLEASE BE SURE TO **DEDUCT** ANY PER CHECK CHARGES OR SERVICE CHARGES THAT MAY APPLY TO YOUR ACCOUNT

CHECK NO.	DATE	CHECKS ISSUED TO OR DESCRIPTION OF DEPOSIT	(-) AMOUNT OF CHECK	√ T	(-) CHECK FEE (IF ANY)	(+) AMOUNT OF DEPOSIT	BALANCE	

3. Round off to the nearest cent:

    a. $18 \div 7$ **b.** 12.23×0.76 **c.** $\frac{1}{3} \times \$5$ **d.** $17.25 \div 2$

4. Choose the best estimate:

    a. 23×2.75:   0.60, 600, 60, 6   **b.** 8.16×9.77:   0.0008, 80, 800, 0.08

    c. $3.17 \div 0.2$:   15, 0.15, 150, 1.50   **d.** $0.96 \div 5.17$: $2, $20, $0.20, $0.02

5. The telephone bills for the Westland Dental Clinic, for 6 months, were: $43.17, $59.25, $60.77, $29.86, $51.01, $72.55.

    a. Find the expenses for the 6-month period.

    b. Find the yearly bill if the expenses remain the same.

6. For each litre of oxygen absorbed in the oxidation of fat, 0.707 litres of carbon dioxide and 4.686 calories of heat are produced. How many litres of carbon dioxide and how many calories of heat are produced when 8.2 litres of oxygen are absorbed in the oxidation of fat?

7. A patient was given 0.5 of a 0.25-grain ephedrine sulfate tablet. How much medication did the patient receive?

8. A patient receives 0.75 grain of ephedrine from 0.375-grain tablets. How many tablets did he receive?

9. A dentist charges $1,095.75 for a total of 18.5 hours of dental work. What are the gross earnings per hour?

10. To give 0.25 grain of digitalis from a 1.0-grain tablet, how many tablets should you use?

11. The people in the District of Columbia, on the average, drink more alcoholic beverages than the people in any other state. The average yearly consumption per person is 9.9 gallons of distilled spirits, 6.3 gallons of wine, and 30.5 gallons of beer. Determine the average consumption of alcoholic beverages per person.

12. A patient was given 0.75 grains of a 0.5-grain codeine sulfate tablet. How many tablets did the patient receive?

13. If you gave 0.3 of a 0.75-grain morphine sulfate tablet, how much medication did you give?

14. A nurse wishes to give 0.006 grain of atropine sulfate from 0.01-grain tablets. How many tablets should be given?

15. A patient receives 0.016 gram of codeine sulfate from 0.032-gram codeine sulfate tablets. How many tablets does the patient receive?

16. A nurse gives 0.64 gram of acetylsalicylic acid from 0.32-gram acetylsalicylic acid tablets. How many tablets were given?

17. A patient receives 0.5 gram of Terramycin from 0.25-gram Terramycin capsules. How many capsules did he receive?

18. If the adult dosage of a medication is 0.125 grains, how much should a 60-pound child receive?

19. If the adult dosage of a drug is one tablet (5 grains) t.i.d. (3 times a day), what is the dosage for a 75-pound child?

20. If the adult dosage of a drug is 0.35 mg, what is the dosage for a 110-pound child (round off to the nearest hundredth)?

1.3   EXERCISE ANSWERS

1.

	1¢	5¢	10¢	25¢	$1	$5	$10	$20
a.	1		1	3				
b.		1	1	3				
c.	2	1		1	4			
d.	4		2	2	3			
e.			1	3	1			
f.	3	1	1	2	2	1		
g.	3	1	1	1	4			
h.	1			1	2	1		
i.		1		3		1		
j.	2	1		3		1	2	

2.

PLEASE BE SURE TO **DEDUCT** ANY PER CHECK CHARGES OR SERVICE CHARGES THAT MAY APPLY TO YOUR ACCOUNT

CHECK NO.	DATE	CHECKS ISSUED TO OR DESCRIPTION OF DEPOSIT	(-) AMOUNT OF CHECK		√ T	(-) CHECK FEE (IF ANY)	(+) AMOUNT OF DEPOSIT		BALANCE	
									1,503	17
131	8/2	Edison	193	17					1,310	00
132	8/2	Consumers	215	36					1,094	64
133	8/3	H. Hopkins	28	15					1,066	49
	8/3	Sales Receipts					432	08	1,498	57
134	8/4	First National	483	92					1,014	65
135	8/5	Office Supplies	56	17					958	48
	8/5	Sales Receipts					199	16	1,157	64
136	8/6	S. Bebe	800	00					357	64

3. a. $2.57   **b.** $9.29   **c.** $1.67   **d.** $8.63
4. a. 60   **b.** 80   **c.** 15   **d.** $0.20
5. a. $316.61   **b.** $633.22

6. 5.7974 litres carbon dioxide, 38.4252 calories of heat
7. 0.125 grains
8. 2 tablets
9. $59.23
10. 0.25 tablets
11. 46.7 gallons
12. 1.5 tablets
13. 0.225 grains
14. 0.5 tablets
15. 0.5 tablets
16. 2 tablets
17. 2 capsules
18. 0.05 grains
19. 0.5 tablets t.i.d.
20. 0.26 mg

CHAPTER 1 SAMPLE TEST

At the completion of Chapter 1 you should be able to work the following problems.

1.1 APPLICATIONS FOR WHOLE NUMBERS

1. Determine the caloric total for the following meal.

T-bone steak	200 calories
Baked potato	125 calories
Roll	100 calories
Peas	110 calories
Cherry pie	350 calories

2. If a patient drinks 2430 ml of fluids daily, how many ml will be consumed in two weeks?
3. One dose of aspirin is grain v. How many doses are there in grain xxv?
4. Convert to Hindu–Arabic numerals: **a.** xiv **b.** cdxcii
5. Convert to Roman numerals: **a.** 46 **b.** 688

1.2 APPLICATIONS FOR FRACTIONS

6. A patient was given $\frac{3}{4}$ of $\frac{5}{8}$-grain ephedrine sulfate. How much medication did the patient receive?
7. A patient receives $\frac{1}{2}$ grain of ephedrine from a $\frac{3}{8}$-grain tablet. How many tablets did he receive (round off to the nearest $\frac{1}{4}$ tablet)?
8. If the adult dosage of medication is 30 mg, how much should a 50-pound child receive?
9. A doctor receives $723 for $8\frac{1}{2}$ hours of work. What are the gross earnings (before deductions) per hour (round off to the nearest dollar)?

1.3 APPLICATIONS FOR DECIMALS

10. A patient received 0.75 of a 0.125-grain codeine sulfate tablet. How much medication did he receive?

11. A patient receives 0.75 grains of ephedrine sulfate from a 0.5-grain tablet. How many tablets did she receive?

12. If the adult dosage of a drug is 75 mg, what is the dosage for a 25-pound child?

CHAPTER 1 SAMPLE TEST ANSWERS

1. 885 calories   **2.** 34 020 ml   **3.** 5 doses

4. a. 14   **b.** 492   **5. a.** xlvi   **b.** dclxxxviii

6. $\frac{15}{32}$ grains   **7.** $1\frac{1}{4}$ tablets   **8.** 10 mg   **9.** $85

10. 0.09375 grains   **11.** 1.5 tablets   **12.** 12.5 mg

CHAPTER 2

OPERATIONS WITH PERCENTS

2.1 PERCENTS

---

1 Fractions with a denominator of 100 are called decimal fractions. Fractions with a denominator of 100 are also called *percents*. The word percent means "hundredths." Thus, $\dfrac{7}{100}$ is equivalent to 7 percent. The symbol % is an abbreviation for the word "percent" and is derived from the denominator of 100. Therefore,

$$\frac{7}{100} \longrightarrow 7\%$$

The symbol 7% is read "7 percent" and means 7 hundredths.

Q1   Write the fractions using the % symbol:

     a. $\dfrac{23}{100} = $ _____   **b.** $\dfrac{3}{100} = $ _____   **c.** $\dfrac{25}{100} = $ _____   **d.** $\dfrac{50}{100} = $ _____

\# \# \#   •   \# \# \#   •   \# \# \#   •   \# \# \#   •   \# \# \#   •   \# \# \#   •   \# \# \#   •   \# \# \#   •   \# \# \#

A1   **a.** 23%   **b.** 3%   **c.** 25%   **d.** 50%

Q2   Write the percents as fractions:

     a. 29% = _____   **b.** 9% = _____   **c.** 53% = _____   **d.** 97% = _____

\# \# \#   •   \# \# \#   •   \# \# \#   •   \# \# \#   •   \# \# \#   •   \# \# \#   •   \# \# \#   •   \# \# \#   •   \# \# \#

A2   **a.** $\dfrac{29}{100}$ **b.** $\dfrac{9}{100}$ **c.** $\dfrac{53}{100}$ **d.** $\dfrac{97}{100}$

Q3   Write the percents as fractions and reduce to lowest terms:

     a. 25% = _____   **b.** 20% = _____   **c.** 75% = _____   **d.** 44% = _____

\# \# \#   •   \# \# \#   •   \# \# \#   •   \# \# \#   •   \# \# \#   •   \# \# \#   •   \# \# \#   •   \# \# \#   •   \# \# \#

A3   **a.** $\dfrac{1}{4}$ **b.** $\dfrac{1}{5}$ **c.** $\dfrac{3}{4}$ **d.** $\dfrac{11}{25}$

---

2 Some percents can also be expressed as mixed numbers. For example,

$$225\% = \frac{225}{100} = 2\frac{25}{100} = 2\frac{1}{4}$$

Fractional percents can be expressed as a fraction as follows:

$$\frac{1}{2}\% = \frac{\frac{1}{2}}{100} = \frac{1}{2} \div \frac{100}{1} = \frac{1}{2} \times \frac{1}{100} = \frac{1}{200}$$

Q4   Change 250% to a mixed number.

\# \# \#   •   \# \# \#   •   \# \# \#   •   \# \# \#   •   \# \# \#   •   \# \# \#   •   \# \# \#   •   \# \# \#   •   \# \# \#

A4 $2\frac{1}{2}$: $250\% = \frac{250}{100} = 2\frac{50}{100} = 2\frac{1}{2}$

Q5   Change to a mixed number:
a. 480%   **b.** 333%

\# \# \#   •   \# \# \#   •   \# \# \#   •   \# \# \#   •   \# \# \#   •   \# \# \#   •   \# \# \#   •   \# \# \#   •   \# \# \#

A5   **a.** $4\frac{4}{5}$ **b.** $3\frac{33}{100}$

Q6   Change $\frac{1}{4}\%$ to a fraction.

\# \# \#   •   \# \# \#   •   \# \# \#   •   \# \# \#   •   \# \# \#   •   \# \# \#   •   \# \# \#   •   \# \# \#   •   \# \# \#

A6 $\frac{1}{400}$: $\frac{1}{4}\% = \frac{\frac{1}{4}}{100} = \frac{1}{400}$

Q7   Change $\frac{2}{3}\%$ to a fraction.

\# \# \#   •   \# \# \#   •   \# \# \#   •   \# \# \#   •   \# \# \#   •   \# \# \#   •   \# \# \#   •   \# \# \#   •   \# \# \#

A7 $\frac{1}{150}$: $\frac{2}{3}\% = \frac{\frac{2}{3}}{100} = \frac{2}{300}$

3   To change a mixed-number percent to a fraction it is necessary to write the mixed number as an improper fraction over 100. Consider this example:

$$66\frac{2}{3}\% = \frac{66\frac{2}{3}}{100} = \frac{\frac{200}{3}}{100} = \frac{200}{3} \div \frac{100}{1} = \frac{200}{3} \times \frac{1}{100} = \frac{200}{300} = \frac{2}{3}$$

Q8   Change $33\frac{1}{3}\%$ to a fraction.

\# \# \# • \# \# \# • \# \# \# • \# \# \# • \# \# \# • \# \# \# • \# \# \# • \# \# \# • \# \# \#

A8 $\frac{1}{3}$: $33\frac{1}{3}\% = \frac{33\frac{1}{3}}{100} = \frac{\frac{100}{3}}{100} = \frac{100}{300} = \frac{1}{3}$

Q9   Change $12\frac{1}{2}\%$ to a fraction.

\# \# \# • \# \# \# • \# \# \# • \# \# \# • \# \# \# • \# \# \# • \# \# \# • \# \# \# • \# \# \#

A9 $\frac{1}{8}$: $12\frac{1}{2}\% = \frac{12\frac{1}{2}}{100} = \frac{\frac{25}{2}}{100} = \frac{25}{200} = \frac{1}{8}$

Q10   Change to fractions:
   a. $16\frac{2}{3}\%$ **b.** $37\frac{1}{2}\%$

\# \# \# • \# \# \# • \# \# \# • \# \# \# • \# \# \# • \# \# \# • \# \# \# • \# \# \# • \# \# \#

A10   **a.** $\frac{1}{6}$ **b.** $\frac{3}{8}$

Q11   Change $3\frac{1}{8}\%$ to a fraction.

\# \# \# • \# \# \# • \# \# \# • \# \# \# • \# \# \# • \# \# \# • \# \# \# • \# \# \# • \# \# \#

A11 $\frac{1}{32}$: $3\frac{1}{8}\% = \frac{3\frac{1}{8}}{100} = \frac{\frac{25}{8}}{100} = \frac{25}{800} = \frac{1}{32}$

4   Fractions with a denominator of 100 can be written as decimals. Since percents are written as a fraction with denominator of 100, they can also be expressed as a decimal. For example,

$$18\% = \frac{18}{100} = 0.18$$

Q12   Express 23% as a fraction and a decimal._____

• # # # • # # # • # # # • # # # • # # # • # # # • # # # • # #

A12 $23\% = \dfrac{23}{100} = 0.23$

---

5   A number can be divided by 100 by simply moving the decimal point two places to the left. Hence, to change a percent to a decimal, remove the percent sign and move the decimal point two places to the left.

Examples:

$23\% = 0.23$ because $23\% = 23. \div 100$
$7\% = 0.07$ because $7\% = 7. \div 100$
$17.5\% = 0.175$ because $17.5\% = 17.5 \div 100$

Notice that the decimal point, for a number written without a decimal point, is placed after the last digit. Hence, $8 = 8$.

Q13   Express 23.7% as a decimal. _____

• # # # • # # # • # # # • # # # • # # # • # # # • # # # • # #

A13   0.237:   23.7% = 0.237 (drop the percent sign and move the decimal point two places to the left).

Q14   Express as a decimal:

a. 13% = _____   **b.** 75% = _____

• # # # • # # # • # # # • # # # • # # # • # # # • # # # • # #

A14   **a.** 0.13   **b.** 0.75

Q15   Express as a decimal:

a. 19.8% = _____   **b.** 2.75% = _____   **c.** 250% = _____

• # # # • # # # • # # # • # # # • # # # • # # # • # # # • # #

A15   **a.** 0.198   **b.** 0.0275   **c.** 2.50 or 2.5

Q16   Express as a decimal:

a. 700% = _____   **b.** 0.03% = _____
c. 1% = _____   **d.** 5% = _____

• # # # • # # # • # # # • # # # • # # # • # # # • # # # • # #

A16   **a.** 7   **b.** 0.0003   **c.** 0.01   **d.** 0.05

---

6   To change a decimal to a percent, move the decimal two places to the right and append the percent sign. For example,

$0.28 = 28\%$ because $0.28 = \dfrac{28}{100} = 28\%$

Examples:

$0.04 = 4\%$
$0.15 = 15\%$
$1.86 = 186\%$
$0.002 = 0.2\%$

Q17   Change 0.617 to a percent. _____

\# \# \# • \# \# \# • \# \# \# • \# \# \# • \# \# \# • \# \# \# • \# \# \# • \# \# \# • \# \# \#

A17   61.7%:   0.617 = 61.7% (move the decimal point two places to the right and append the % sign).

Q18   Change to a percent:

    a. 0.93 = _____   **b.** 0.0015 = _____

    c. 1.72 = _____   **d.** 0.473 = _____

\# \# \# • \# \# \# • \# \# \# • \# \# \# • \# \# \# • \# \# \# • \# \# \# • \# \# \# • \# \# \#

A18   **a.** 93%   **b.** 0.15%   **c.** 172%   **d.** 47.3%

---

7   It may be necessary to use zeros as placeholders when changing a decimal to a percent. For example, change 0.8 to a percent:

0.8 = 0.80 = 80%

Q19   Change 0.7 to a percent. _____

\# \# \# • \# \# \# • \# \# \# • \# \# \# • \# \# \# • \# \# \# • \# \# \# • \# \# \# • \# \# \#

A19   70%:   0.7 = 0.70 = 70%

Q20   Change 17 to a percent. _____

\# \# \# • \# \# \# • \# \# \# • \# \# \# • \# \# \# • \# \# \# • \# \# \# • \# \# \# • \# \# \#

A20   1,700%:   17 = 17.00 = 1,700%

Q21   Change to a percent:

    a. 0.2 = _____   **b.** 5 = _____   **c.** 0.1 = _____   **d.** 213 = _____

\# \# \# • \# \# \# • \# \# \# • \# \# \# • \# \# \# • \# \# \# • \# \# \# • \# \# \# • \# \# \#

A21   **a.** 20%   **b.** 500%   **c.** 10%   **d.** 21,300%

---

8   To change a fraction to a percent, first change the common fraction to a decimal and then change the decimal to a percent. Consider these examples:

$$\frac{3}{4} = 0.75 = 75\%$$

$$\frac{1}{8} = 0.125 = 12.5\%$$

    Recall that to change a fraction to a decimal the numerator is divided by the denominator.

Q22   Change $\frac{3}{8}$ to a percent.

\# \# \# • \# \# \# • \# \# \# • \# \# \# • \# \# \# • \# \# \# • \# \# \# • \# \# \# • \# \# \#

A22   37.5%: $8\overline{)3.000}$; 0.375

Q23   Change to a percent:

a. $\dfrac{1}{4} = \underline{\qquad}_{\text{(decimal)}} = \underline{\qquad}_{\text{(percent)}}$ **b.** $\dfrac{5}{8} = \underline{\qquad}_{\text{(decimal)}} = \underline{\qquad}_{\text{(percent)}}$

• # # # • # # # • # # # • # # # • # # # • # # # • # # # • # #

A23   **a.** 0.25, 25%   **b.** 0.625. 62.5%

---

9   A fraction represented by a repeating decimal is usually changed to a percent by completing the division to two decimal places and writing the remainder in fraction form. That is, $\dfrac{1}{3} = 0.33\dfrac{1}{3} = 33\dfrac{1}{3}\%$. The problem could be stated $\dfrac{1}{3} = 0.33\bar{3} = 33.\bar{3}\%$; however, the first method is preferred*.

It should be noted that when moving the decimal point two places to the right, only digits count as places. Fractions do not hold a place. Hence, $0.3\dfrac{1}{3}$ *does not* equal $3\dfrac{1}{3}\%$. The division must be carried out to at least two decimal places before the remainder is written as a fraction.

* Bar indicates that digit(s) under bar repeat endlessly.

Q24   Express $\dfrac{1}{6}$ as a percent.

• # # # • # # # • # # # • # # # • # # # • # # # • # # # • # #

A24 $16\dfrac{2}{3}\%:$ $6\overline{)1.00}$ with quotient $0.16\dfrac{2}{3}$

Q25   Change to a percent:

a. $\dfrac{2}{3}$ **b.** $\dfrac{2}{7}$

• # # # • # # # • # # # • # # # • # # # • # # # • # # # • # #

A25   **a.** $66\dfrac{2}{3}\%$ **b.** $28\dfrac{4}{7}\%$

This completes the instruction for this section.

2.1   **EXERCISE**

Fill the blanks with the proper equivalents, as shown in problem 1.

	Fraction	Decimal	Percent		Fraction	Decimal	Percent
1.	$\dfrac{1}{2}$	0.5	50%	2.	_____	0.25	_____%
3.	$\dfrac{1}{3}$	_____	_____%	4.	_____	_____	10%

Fraction	Decimal	Percent
5. _____	0.125	_____%
7. _____	_____	$66\frac{2}{3}$%
9. $\frac{3}{10}$	_____	_____%
11. _____	0.0625	_____%
13. _____	_____	80%
15. _____	0.90	_____%
17. $\frac{1}{6}$	_____	_____%
19. $\frac{11}{20}$	_____	_____%
21. $\frac{3}{5}$	_____	_____%
23. _____	_____	95%
25. _____	0.875	_____%
27. $1\frac{7}{8}$	_____	_____%
29. _____	_____	200%
31. _____	0.08	_____%
33. $4\frac{4}{5}$	_____	_____%
35. _____	_____	180%
37. _____	6.166	_____%
39. $3\frac{3}{4}$	_____	_____%
41. $2\frac{1}{2}$	_____	_____%
43. _____	_____	$166\frac{2}{3}$%
45. $1\frac{5}{8}$	_____	_____%

Fraction	Decimal	Percent
6. $\frac{2}{5}$	_____	_____%
8. _____	0.75	_____%
10. _____	_____	5%
12. $\frac{3}{8}$	_____	_____%
14. _____	0.625	_____%
16. _____	_____	100%
18. _____	_____	20%
20. _____	0.375	_____%
22. _____	0.166	_____%
24. $\frac{7}{10}$	_____	_____%
26. _____	_____	225%
28. _____	$0.16\frac{2}{3}$	_____%
30. $\frac{1}{100}$	_____	_____%
32. _____	_____	$16\frac{2}{3}$%
34. _____	5.00	_____%
36. $\frac{1}{50}$	_____	_____%
38. _____	_____	110%
40. _____	0.2	_____%
42. _____	4.08	_____%
44. _____	2.125	_____%
46. _____	3.875	_____%

2.1 EXERCISE ANSWERS

1. given

2. $\frac{1}{4}$, 25%

3. $0.33\frac{1}{3}$, $33\frac{1}{3}$%

4. $\frac{1}{10}$, 0.1 or 0.10

5. $\frac{1}{8}$, 12.5%

6. 0.4 or 0.40, 40%

7. $\frac{2}{3}$, $0.66\frac{2}{3}$

8. $\frac{3}{4}$, 75%

9. 0.3 or 0.30, 30%

10. $\frac{1}{20}$, 0.05

11. $\frac{1}{16}$, 6.25%

12. 0.375, 37.5%

13. $\frac{4}{5}$, 0.8 or 0.8

14. $\frac{5}{8}$, 62.5%

15. $\frac{9}{10}$, 90%

16. 1, 1 or 1.00

17. $0.16\frac{2}{3}$, $16\frac{2}{3}$%

18. $\frac{1}{5}$, 0.2 or 0.20

19. 0.55, 55%

20. $\frac{3}{8}$, 37.5%

21. 0.6 or 0.60, 60%

22. $\frac{83}{500}$, 16.6%

23. $\frac{19}{20}$, 0.95

24. 0.7 or 0.70, 70%

25. $\frac{7}{8}$, 87.5%

26. $2\frac{1}{4}$, 2.25

27. 1.875, 187.5%

28. $\frac{1}{6}$, $16\frac{2}{3}$%

29. 2, 2 or 2.00

30. 0.01, 1%

31. $\frac{2}{25}$, 8%

32. $\frac{1}{6}$, $0.16\frac{2}{3}$

33. 4.8 or 4.80, 480%

34. 5, 500%

35. $1\frac{4}{5}$, 1.8 or 1.80

36. 0.02, 2%

37. $6\frac{83}{500}$, 616.6%

38. $1\frac{1}{10}$, 1.1 or 1.10

39. 3.75, 375%

40. $\frac{1}{5}$, 20%

41. 2.5 or 2.50, 250%

42. $4\frac{2}{25}$, 408%

43. $1\frac{2}{3}$, $1.66\frac{2}{3}$

44. $2\frac{1}{8}$, 212.5%

45. 1.625, 162.5%

46. $3\frac{7}{8}$, 387.5%

2.2   WRITING AND SOLVING MATHEMATICAL SENTENCES

1   When such a statement as "2% of 100 is 2" is written in the form $0.02 \times 100 = 2$, it is said to be written mathematically. Written mathematically, 6% of 20 is 1.2 would become: $0.06 \times 20 = 1.2$. Notice that "of" means "multiply" and is replaced by the multiplication symbol, ×. "Is" means "is equal to" and is replaced by the equal sign, =.

Q1   Write "10% of 20 is 2" mathematically. _____

•   # # #   •   # # #   •   # # #   •   # # #   •   # # #   •   # # #   •   # # #   •   # #

A1 $0.10 \times 20 = 2$, or $\frac{1}{10} \times 20 = 2$

Q2   Write mathematically:

    a. 2% of 14 is 0.28   _____

    b. 20% of 50 is 10   _____

    c. 14% of 40 is 5.6   _____

d. 200% of 4 is 8   _____

e. $66\frac{2}{3}$% of 24 is 16   _____

\# \# \# • \# \# \# • \# \# \# • \# \# \# • \# \# \# • \# \# \# • \# \# \# • \# \# \# • \# \# \#

A2   **a.** $0.02 \times 14 = 0.28$, or $\frac{1}{50} \times 14 = 0.28$ **b.** $0.20 \times 50 = 10$, or $\frac{1}{5} \times 50 = 10$

c. $0.14 \times 40 = 5.6$, or $\frac{7}{50} \times 40 = 5.6$ **d.** $2 \times 4 = 8$

e. $0.66\frac{2}{3} \times 24 = 16$, or $\frac{2}{3} \times 24 = 16$

---

2   Consider the question: 5% of 12 is what number? Written mathematically: $0.05 \times 12 =$ what number?

When we use letter N to "hold the place" of the missing number, the statement becomes: $0.05 \times 12 = N$? Any letter can be used for the missing (unknown) number. N is a popular choice, because "number" begins with the letter n.

Q3   Write mathematically: 75% of 116 is what number?   _____

\# \# \# • \# \# \# • \# \# \# • \# \# \# • \# \# \# • \# \# \# • \# \# \# • \# \# \# • \# \# \#

A3 $0.75 \times 116 = N$? or $\frac{3}{4} \times 116 = N$?

Q4   Write mathematically:

a. 420% of 7 is what number?   _____

b. What number is 420% of 7?   _____

c. 62% of 19 is what number?   _____

d. What number is 62% of 19?   _____

\# \# \# • \# \# \# • \# \# \# • \# \# \# • \# \# \# • \# \# \# • \# \# \# • \# \# \# • \# \# \#

A4   **a.** $4.2 \times 7 = N$?   **b.** $N = 4.2 \times 7$?   **c.** $0.62 \times 19 = N$?   **d.** $N = 0.62 \times 19$?

---

3   In the following question a different part of the problem is missing:

4.1% of what number is 7.3?

$0.041 \times N = 7.3$ (written mathematically)

Notice that "of" is replaced by "×," "what number" by "N," and "is" by "=." (4.1% = 0.041.)

Q5   Write mathematically: 7% of what number is 0.09?   _____

\# \# \# • \# \# \# • \# \# \# • \# \# \# • \# \# \# • \# \# \# • \# \# \# • \# \# \# • \# \# \#

A5 $0.07 \times N = 0.09$?

Q6   Write mathematically:

a. 22% of what number is 12?   _____

b. 15 is 35% of what number?   _____

    c. 320% of what number is 400? _____

    d. $37\frac{1}{2}$% of what number is 54? _____

    e. 23.5 is 10% of what number? _____

#　•　# # #　•　# # #　•　# # #　•　# # #　•　# # #　•　# # #　•　# # #　•　# #

A6   **a.** $0.22 \times N = 12$?   **b.** $15 = 0.35 \times N$?   **c.** $3.2 \times N = 400$?

        d. $0.37\frac{1}{2} \times N = 54$? or $\frac{3}{8} \times N \times 54$?   **e.** $23.5 = 0.10 \times N$?

---

4   Consider still another type of percent question:

    What percent of 90 is 7?
$$P \quad \times 90 = 7?$$

    Notice that the percent is missing; hence, the letter P was used as a reminder that the missing number is a percent.

Q7   Write mathematically: What percent of 70 is 203? _____

#　•　# # #　•　# # #　•　# # #　•　# # #　•　# # #　•　# # #　•　# # #　•　# #

A7 $P \times 70 = 203$?

Q8   Write mathematically:

    a. What percent of 12 is 0.6? _____

    b. What percent of 9 is 24? _____

    c. 23 is what percent of 19? _____

    d. 14 is what percent of 30? _____

    e. What percent of 30 is 14? _____

#　•　# # #　•　# # #　•　# # #　•　# # #　•　# # #　•　# # #　•　# # #　•　# #

A8   **a.** $P \times 12 = 0.6$?   **b.** $P \times 9 = 24$?   **c.** $23 = P \times 19$?   **d.** $14 = P \times 30$?
    e. $P \times 30 = 14$?

---

5   In a multiplication problem the numbers that are multiplied together to form the *product* are called the *factors*. In the example $4 \times 3 = 12$, 4 and 3 are the factors and 12 is the product.
        Two division problems can be formed from any multiplication problem. For example, $4 \times 3 = 12$ implies that $4 = 12 \div 3$ and $3 = 12 \div 4$.

Q9   Write two division problems that can be formed from $3 \times 5 = 15$.

    _____ and _____

#　•　# # #　•　# # #　•　# # #　•　# # #　•　# # #　•　# # #　•　# # #　•　# #

A9 $3 = 15 \div 5$, $5 = 15 \div 3$ (either order)

Q10   Write two division problems that can be formed from $5 \times 9 = 45$.

    _____ and _____

#　•　# # #　•　# # #　•　# # #　•　# # #　•　# # #　•　# # #　•　# # #　•　# #

A10 $5 = 45 \div 9, 9 = 45 \div 5$ (either order)

---

6   Generally, a multiplication problem can be represented as: *factor* × *factor* = *product*. From the previous example this statement can be written *one factor* = *product* ÷ *other factor*. For example, if $4 \times 8 = 32$, *what number* = $32 \div 8$ or $N = 32 \div 8$? The answer is that $4 = 32 \div 8$; hence $N = 4$.

Q11   Determine the missing factor represented by the letter N:

    a. If $4 \times 8 = 32$, then $N = 32 \div 4$; $N =$ _____

    b. If $2 \times 3 = 6$, then $N = 6 \div 3$; $N =$ _____

    c. If $45 = 5 \times 9$, then $N = 45 \div 5$; $N =$ _____

    d. If $25 \times N = 1,200$, then $N = 1,200 \div 25$; $N =$ _____

\# # # • # # # • # # # • # # # • # # # • # # # • # # # • # # # • # # #

A11   **a.** 8   **b.** 2   **c.** 9   **d.** 48

---

7   Often one of the factors of a product will be unknown. That is, *unknown factor* × *known factor* = *product*. This statement could be written *unknown factor* = *product* ÷ *known factor*. For example, if $N \times 15 = 60$, then $N = 60 \div 15$. N represents the unknown factor, 15 the known factor, and 60 the product.

Q12   Write the unknown factor as the quotient of the product and the known factor:

    a. $N \times 7 = 42$ _____   **b.** $7 \times N = 42$ _____

\# # # • # # # • # # # • # # # • # # # • # # # • # # # • # # # • # # #

A12   **a.** $N = 42 \div 7$ **b.** $N = 42 \div 7$

Q13   Solve for N by writing the unknown factor as a quotient of the product and the known factor:
    a. $0.03 \times N = 15$ **b.** $2.5 = 0.06 \times N$

\# # # • # # # • # # # • # # # • # # # • # # # • # # # • # # # • # # #

A13   **a.** 500: $N = 15 \div 0.03 = 500$ **b.** $41\frac{2}{3}$: $N = 2.5 \div 0.06 = 41\frac{2}{3}$

Q14   Solve for N:
    a. $0.1 \times N = 2.4$ **b.** $\$1.62 = 0.06 \times N$

\# # # • # # # • # # # • # # # • # # # • # # # • # # # • # # # • # # #

A14   **a.** 24: $N = 2.4 \div 0.1$ **b.** $\$27$: $N = \$1.62 \div 0.06$

Q15 Solve for N:
    a. $N \times \$21 = \$0.42$ **b.** $\$0.12 \times N = \$2.40$

\#\#\# • \#\#\# • \#\#\# • \#\#\# • \#\#\# • \#\#\# • \#\#\# • \#\#\# • \#\#\#

A15   **a.** 0.02: $N = \$0.42 \div \$21$ **b.** 20: $N = \$2.40 \div \$0.12$

This completes the instruction for this section.

2.2   **EXERCISE**

1. Write mathematically:
   a. 6% of 10 is what number?   **b.** What number is 17.3% of 92?
   c. 520% of what number is 62?   **d.** What percent of 17 is 9?
   e. 17 is 43% of what number?

2. If factor $\times$ factor = product, one factor = _____ $\div$ _____ .

3. If known factor $\times$ unknown factor = product, _____ = product $\div$ _____ .

4. If $75 = N \times 3$, $N =$ _____ $\div$ _____ .

5. Solve for N or P:
   a. $5.2 \times N = 62$ **b.** $17 = 0.43 \times N$ **c.** $0.06 \times 10 = N$
   d. $\$13 = P \times \$52$ **e.** $\$0.21 = 0.03 \times N$

2.2   **EXERCISE ANSWERS**

1. **a.** $0.06 \times 10 = N$ **b.** $N = 0.173 \times 92$ **c.** $5.2 \times N = 62$
   d. $P \times 17 = 9$ **e.** $17 = 0.43 \times N$
2. product, other factor
3. unknown factor, known factor
4. 75, 3
5. **a.** $11\frac{12}{13}$ **b.** $39\frac{23}{43}$ **c.** 0.6   **d.** 0.25 or 25%
   e. \$7

2.3   SOLVING PERCENT PROBLEMS

1   Problems involving percents usually occur in three forms:

    1. Finding a percent of a number or quantity. *Example:* What number is 6% of 12?
    2. Finding what percent one number is of another. *Example:* 18 is what percent of 36?
    3. Finding a number when a certain percent of it is known. *Example:* 12 is 15% of what number?

    These questions can be solved by first writing them mathematically.

    Example: What number is 6% of 12?

Solution:

$N = 0.06 \times 12$*
$N = 0.72$

$$\begin{array}{r} 12 \\ \times\, 0.06 \\ \hline 0.72 \end{array}$$

(show work
where necessary)

Therefore, 0.72 is 6% of 12.

* It is common to omit the "?" mark.

Q1   What number is 3% of 7?

\# \# \#   •   \# \# \#   •   \# \# \#   •   \# \# \#   •   \# \# \#   •   \# \# \#   •   \# \# \#   •   \# \# \#   •   \# \# \#

A1   0.21: $N = 0.03 \times 7$

Q2   0.3% of 63 is what number?

\# \# \#   •   \# \# \#   •   \# \# \#   •   \# \# \#   •   \# \# \#   •   \# \# \#   •   \# \# \#   •   \# \# \#   •   \# \# \#

A2   0.189: $0.003 \times 63 = N$

Q3   0.4% of 210 is what number?

\# \# \#   •   \# \# \#   •   \# \# \#   •   \# \# \#   •   \# \# \#   •   \# \# \#   •   \# \# \#   •   \# \# \#   •   \# \# \#

A3   0.84: $0.004 \times 210 = N$

Q4   What number is 520% of 92?

\# \# \#   •   \# \# \#   •   \# \# \#   •   \# \# \#   •   \# \# \#   •   \# \# \#   •   \# \# \#   •   \# \# \#   •   \# \# \#

A4   478.4: $N = 5.2 \times 92$

---

2   Recall that a mixed-number percent is simplified in the following manner:

$$23\frac{1}{3}\% = \frac{70}{3} \times \frac{1}{100} = \frac{7}{30}$$

Example: $23\frac{1}{3}\%$ of 900 is what number?

Solution:

$$\frac{7}{30} \times 900 = N$$

$$210 = N$$

Therefore, $23\frac{1}{3}\%$ of 900 is 210.

Q5   **a.** What number is 200% of 4?   **b.** 24% of 30 is what number?

c. 0.5% of 18 is what number?   **d.** What is $15\frac{1}{3}\%$ of 600?

•   # # #   •   # # #   •   # # #   •   # # #   •   # # #   •   # # #   •   # # #   •   # #

A5   **a.** 8   **b.** 7.2   **c.** 0.09   **d.** 92

---

3   The second type of percent problem is finding what percent one number is of another.

Example: 18 is what percent of 36?

Solution:
$18 = P \times 36$ (written mathematically)

Recall that *factor $\times$ factor = product* and *unknown factor = product $\div$ known factor*. Hence,

$18 \div 36 = P$ [18 (product) $\div$ 36 (known factor)]
$0.5 = P$
$50\% = P$

Therefore, 18 is 50% of 36.

Q6   17 is what percent of 68?

•   # # #   •   # # #   •   # # #   •   # # #   •   # # #   •   # # #   •   # # #   •   # #

A6   25%: $17 = P \times 68$
$17 \div 68 = P$
$0.25 = P$

Q7   24 is what percent of 30?

•   # # #   •   # # #   •   # # #   •   # # #   •   # # #   •   # # #   •   # # #   •   # #

A7   80%: $24 = P \times 30$
$$24 \div 30 = P$$
$$0.8 = P$$

Q8   21 is what percent of 300?

\# \# \#   •   \# \# \#   •   \# \# \#   •   \# \# \#   •   \# \# \#   •   \# \# \#   •   \# \# \#   •   \# \# \#   •   \# \# \#

A8   7%: $21 = P \times 300$
$$21 \div 300 = P$$
$$0.07 = P$$

Q9   80 is what percent of 64?

\# \# \#   •   \# \# \#   •   \# \# \#   •   \# \# \#   •   \# \# \#   •   \# \# \#   •   \# \# \#   •   \# \# \#   •   \# \# \#

A9   125%: $80 = P \times 64$
$$80 \div 64 = P$$
$$1.25 = P$$

Q10   What percent of 6 is 4?

\# \# \#   •   \# \# \#   •   \# \# \#   •   \# \# \#   •   \# \# \#   •   \# \# \#   •   \# \# \#   •   \# \# \#   •   \# \# \#

A10 $66\frac{2}{3}$%: $P \times 6 = 4$
$$P = 4 \div 6$$
$$P = 0.66\frac{2}{3}$$

Q11   What percent of 25 is 30?

\# \# \#   •   \# \# \#   •   \# \# \#   •   \# \# \#   •   \# \# \#   •   \# \# \#   •   \# \# \#   •   \# \# \#   •   \# \# \#

A11   120%: $P \times 25 = 30$
$$P = 30 \div 25$$
$$P = 1.2$$

Q12   **a.** What percent of 300 is 45?   **b.** 38 is what percent of 304?

         c. What percent of 12 is 4.6?   **d.** 66.6 is what percent of 74?

\# \# \# • \# \# \# • \# \# \# • \# \# \# • \# \# \# • \# \# \# • \# \# \# • \# \# \# • \# \# \#

A12   **a.** 15%   **b.** 12.5%   **c.** $38\frac{1}{3}\%$ **d.** 90%

---

4   The third type of percent problem is finding a number when a certain percent of it is known.

Example: 12 is 15% of what number?

Solution:
$$12 = 0.15 \times N$$
$$12 \div 0.15 = N$$
$$80 = N$$

Therefore, 12 is 15% of 80.

Q13   27 is 5% of what number?

\# \# \# • \# \# \# • \# \# \# • \# \# \# • \# \# \# • \# \# \# • \# \# \# • \# \# \# • \# \# \#

A13   540: $27 = 0.05 \times N$
              $27 \div 0.05 = N$

Q14   17 is 4% of what number?

\# \# \# • \# \# \# • \# \# \# • \# \# \# • \# \# \# • \# \# \# • \# \# \# • \# \# \# • \# \# \#

A14   425: $17 = 0.04 \times N$
              $17 \div 0.04 = N$

Q15   34 is 125% of what number?

\# \# \# • \# \# \# • \# \# \# • \# \# \# • \# \# \# • \# \# \# • \# \# \# • \# \# \# • \# \# \#

A15   27.2: $34 = 1.25 \times N$
              $34 \div 1.25 = N$

Q16   91 is 70% of what number?

•   # # #   •   # # #   •   # # #   •   # # #   •   # # #   •   # # #   •   # # #   •   # #

A16   130: $91 = 0.7 \times N$
                   $91 \div 0.7 = N$

Q17   5% of what number is 8?

•   # # #   •   # # #   •   # # #   •   # # #   •   # # #   •   # # #   •   # # #   •   # #

A17   160: $0.05 \times N = 8$
              $N = 8 \div 0.05$

Q18   16% of what number is 10?

•   # # #   •   # # #   •   # # #   •   # # #   •   # # #   •   # # #   •   # # #   •   # #

A18   62.5: $0.16 \times N = 10$
               $N = 10 \div 0.16$

Q19   **a.** 78 is 15.6% of what number?   **b.** 8% of what number is 24?

       c. 5 is 0.2% of what number?   **d.** $33\frac{1}{3}$% of what number is 12.5?

•   # # #   •   # # #   •   # # #   •   # # #   •   # # #   •   # # #   •   # # #   •   # #

A19   **a.** 500   **b.** 300   **c.** 2,500   **d.** 37.5

This completes the instruction for this section.

2.3   EXERCISE

1. 15 is what percent of 70?
2. 69% of $21 is what number?
3. 6 is 30% of what number?
4. What number is 19% of 20?
5. 152% of 5 is what number?
6. What percent of 320 is 500?
7. 8 is what percent of 15?
8. 32 is 64% of what number?

9. 75% of what number is 4.65?

10. 3.6 is 18% of what number?

11. What number is $33\frac{1}{3}$% of 60?

12. 12.5% of 28 is what number?

13. $63\frac{1}{3}$% of 3 is what number?

14. 122.5 is what percent of 98?

15. 2 is what percent of 400?

2.3 EXERCISE ANSWERS

1. $21\frac{3}{7}$%

2. $14.49

3. 20

4. 3.8

5. 7.6

6. 156.25%

7. $53\frac{1}{3}$%

8. 50

9. 6.2

10. 20

11. 20

12. 3.5

13. 1.9

14. 125%

15. 0.5%

2.4 APPLICATIONS

1   Some of the more difficult types of percent problems are those dealing with a rate of change. When working rate of change problems it is necessary to remember that:

rate of change = the change ÷ original amount

Example: A doctor's basic office fee was increased from $6 to $7.50. Find the percent increase.

Solution: Rate of change = the change ÷ original amount. In this case the change represents an increase ($1.50); hence,

rate of increase = increase ÷ original fee
rate of increase = $1.50 ÷ $6
rate of increase = 0.25

Since the rate of change is usually expressed as a percent, the rate of increase is 25%.

Q1   Rate of change = _____ ÷ _____.

\# \# \# • \# \# \# • \# \# \# • \# \# \# • \# \# \# • \# \# \# • \# \# \# • \# \# \# • \# \# \#

A1   the change (increase or decrease) ÷ original amount

Q2   Eyeglass frames priced at $18.20 are to be remarked $14.56 because of a style change.

    a. Original price = _____

    b. The change = _____

    c. Is the change an increase or decrease? _____

\# \# \# • \# \# \# • \# \# \# • \# \# \# • \# \# \# • \# \# \# • \# \# \# • \# \# \# • \# \# \#

A2   **a.** $18.20   **b.** $3.64   **c.** decrease

Q3   Determine the rate of decrease in Q2.

\# \# \# • \# \# \# • \# \# \# • \# \# \# • \# \# \# • \# \# \# • \# \# \# • \# \# \# • \# \# \#

A3   20%:   rate of decrease = decrease ÷ original price = \$3.64 ÷ \$18.20 = 0.2

Q4   Find the rate of decrease if Thomson's income is \$13,400 one year and \$11,800 the next year (round off the percent to one decimal place).

\# \# \#   •   \# \# \#   •   \# \# \#   •   \# \# \#   •   \# \# \#   •   \# \# \#   •   \# \# \#   •   \# \# \#   •   \# \# \#

A4   11.9%:   rate of decrease = \$1,600 ÷ \$13,400

Q5   Rate of decrease = _____ ÷ _____.

\# \# \#   •   \# \# \#   •   \# \# \#   •   \# \# \#   •   \# \# \#   •   \# \# \#   •   \# \# \#   •   \# \# \#   •   \# \# \#

A5   decrease ÷ original amount

Q6   Find the rate of increase if a person's pulse rate increases from 80 beats per minute to 100 beats per minute.

\# \# \#   •   \# \# \#   •   \# \# \#   •   \# \# \#   •   \# \# \#   •   \# \# \#   •   \# \# \#   •   \# \# \#   •   \# \# \#

A6   25%:   rate of increase = 20 ÷ 80

Q7   Find the rate of increase in the systolic blood pressure of a patient if the blood pressure increased from 176 to 192 (round off the percent to one decimal place).

\# \# \#   •   \# \# \#   •   \# \# \#   •   \# \# \#   •   \# \# \#   •   \# \# \#   •   \# \# \#   •   \# \# \#   •   \# \# \#

A7   9.1%:   rate of increase = 16 ÷ 176

Q8   A patient's temperature increased from 98.6 to 103. Find the rate of increase (round off the percent to one decimal place).

\# \# \#   •   \# \# \#   •   \# \# \#   •   \# \# \#   •   \# \# \#   •   \# \# \#   •   \# \# \#   •   \# \# \#   •   \# \# \#

A8   4.5%:   rate of increase = 4.4 ÷ 98.6

Q9   In two months Gayla's weight went from 182 pounds to 156 pounds. Find the rate of decrease (round off the percent to one decimal place).

\# \# \#   •   \# \# \#   •   \# \# \#   •   \# \# \#   •   \# \# \#   •   \# \# \#   •   \# \# \#   •   \# \# \#   •   \# \# \#

A9   14.3%:   rate of decrease ≐ 26 ÷ 182

2   As was the case with other types of problems, it will be helpful to estimate the answer when working percent problems. Since percents are easily converted to decimals, the technique for estimation will be similar to that developed in the previous chapter.

Example 1: 92% of 582 is estimated nearest to 52.38, 500, 0.535, or 58.2?

Solution: Since 100% of a quantity represents the entire amount, 92% of 582 must be close to 582, but a little less. The best estimate would then be 500.

Example 2: Estimate 4% of 392.

Solution: 4% is the same as $4 \times 1\%$, so
4% of 392 is the same as
$4 \times 1\%$ of 392. $1\% = .01$, giving
$4 \times .01 \times 392$
4×3.92

Now, 4×3.92 can be estimated as $4 \times 4 = 16$. In summary, 4% of 392 is estimated by first taking 1% of 392 (move the decimal point two places to the left) and then multiplying by 4.

Q10   Estimate 6% of 721.

•   # # #   •   # # #   •   # # #   •   # # #   •   # # #   •   # # #   •   # # #   •   # #

A10   42: $6 \times 1\% \times 721 = 6 \times 7.21 = 6 \times 7$

Q11   Choose the best estimate:

    a. 5% of 3,956 is approximately: 18,000, 200, 1,900, 15 _____

    b. 20% of 324 is approximately: 628, 65, 6, 0.06 _____

    c. 90% of 438 is approximately: 500, 400, 43, 5 _____

    d. 12% of 329 is approximately: 360, 40, 20, 1,000 _____

    e. 3% of $14.95 is approximately: $45, $4.48, $0.45, $14.85 _____

    f. 60% of 2.38 is approximately: 1.2, 0.12, 23.8, 0.1428 _____

•   # # #   •   # # #   •   # # #   •   # # #   •   # # #   •   # # #   •   # # #   •   # #

A11   **a.** 200   **b.** 65   **c.** 400   **d.** 40   **e.** $0.45   **f.** 1.2

---

3   Percent estimation can be conveniently used when one is trying to determine the proper tip to leave after dinner in a restaurant. When the bill arrives it would be rather embarrassing to compute the tip using paper and pencil. However, the tip can be determined mentally using the following technique. The usual rate for dinner tipping is 15%. Assume that the dinner bill is $12.40.

Step 1: Multiply by 10% (move the decimal point one place to the left).
$10\% \times \$12.40 = \$1.24$

Step 2: Find $\frac{1}{2}$ of the result of Step 1.
$\frac{1}{2} \times \$1.24 = \$0.62$

Step 3: Add the result of Steps 1 and 2 for the proper tip.
$\$1.24 + \$0.62 = \$1.86$

The procedure works because multiplying by 10% and adding $\frac{1}{2}$ of 10% is the same as multiplying by 15%

Step 4: In actual practice, one rarely leaves the exact change as a tip. The amount is usually rounded off to the nearest nickel or dime. Hence, the tip left would be $1.85.

Q12   Determine the proper tip (at 15%) for a meal costing $8.16.

$10\% \times \$8.16 =$ _____

$\dfrac{1}{2} \times$ _____ $=$ _____

tip $=$ _____

$=$ _____ (rounded off)

\# \# \# • \# \# \# • \# \# \# • \# \# \# • \# \# \# • \# \# \# • \# \# \# • \# \# \# • \# \# \#

A12 $10\% \times \$8.16 = \$0.82$ (nearest cent)

$\dfrac{1}{2} \times \$0.82 = \$0.41$

tip $= \$1.23$
tip $= \$1.25$

Q13   Determine the proper tip (at 15%) for the following priced meals:
a. $4.21   **b.** $16.81

\# \# \# • \# \# \# • \# \# \# • \# \# \# • \# \# \# • \# \# \# • \# \# \# • \# \# \# • \# \# \#

A13   **a.** $0.65: $10\% \times \$4.21 = \$0.42$ **b.** $2.50: $10\% \times \$16.81 = \$1.68$

$\dfrac{1}{2} \times \$0.42 = \$0.21$ $\dfrac{1}{2} \times \$1.68 = \$0.84$

Note that the intermediate answers were rounded off to the nearest cent.

---

4   Percent applications can be presented in a number of different situations. The variety of situations is what generally causes the most difficulty when working with percents. The following plan should prove helpful when solving percent problems:

Step 1: Decide what the problem asks you to find.

Step 2: State the problem mathematically.

Step 3: Estimate the answer.

Step 4: Solve and check the problem.

Example: Steve saved $576 from his annual income of $6,400. What percent of his income did he save?

Step 1: The savings ($576) is what percent of his annual income ($6,400)?

Step 2: $576 is what percent of $6,400?

$\$576 = P \times \$6,400$

Step 3: Observe that 10% of the annual income would be $640 saved; hence, the answer should be slightly less than 10%.

Step 4: The problem is solved by recalling that the unknown factor = product ÷ known factor.

$P = \$576 \div \$6,400$
$P = 0.09$
$P = 9\%$

Check: $9\% \times \$6,400 = \$576$.

Hence, Steve saved 9% of his income.

Q14   A solution weighs 18 g (grams). If the solution contains 3.96 g of alcohol, what percent of the solution is the alcohol (complete each step)?

Step 1: Decide what the problem asks you to find. _____

_____

Step 2: State the problem mathematically. _____

_____

Step 3: Estimate the answer. _____

Step 4: Solve and check.

•   # # #   •   # # #   •   # # #   •   # # #   •   # # #   •   # # #   •   # # #   •   # #

A14   Step 1: The alcohol is what percent of the total weight.

Step 2: 3.96 g is what percent of 18 g.

$3.96 = P \times 18$

Step 3: 10% of 18 is 1.8, so the answer is a little more than double 10% or approximately 20%.

Step 4: $P = 3.96 \div 18$
$P = 22\%$

Check: $22\% \times 18 = 3.96$

Q15   Of 36 babies born recently in a large hospital, 3 were premature births. What percent of the births were premature?

Step 1: _____

Step 2: _____

Step 3: _____

Step 4:

•   # # #   •   # # #   •   # # #   •   # # #   •   # # #   •   # # #   •   # # #   •   # #

A15   Step 1: The premature births are what percent of the total?

Step 2: 3 is what percent of 36?

$3 = P \times 36$

Step 3: 10% of 36 is 3.6, so the answer should be slightly less than 10%.

Step 4: $P = 3 \div 36$
$P = 8\frac{1}{3}\%$

Q16   A mixture contains 12 pounds of water, 23 pounds of alcohol, and 8 pounds of glycerine. What percent is the alcohol of the total mixture (round off the percent to one decimal place)?

Step 1: _____

Step 2: _____

Step 3: _____

Step 4:

\# \# \# • \# \# \# • \# \# \# • \# \# \# • \# \# \# • \# \# \# • \# \# \# • \# \# \# • \# \# \#

A16   Step 1: The alcohol is what percent of the total mixture (43 pounds)?

Step 2: 23 pounds is what percent of 43 pounds?

$23 = P \times 43$

Step 3: 23 is approximately $\frac{1}{2}$ of 43, so the percent should be approximately 50%.

Step 4: $P = 23 \div 43$
$P = 53.5\%$

---

5   In the remaining problems only certain steps will be presented in the solution; however, you should complete all steps as outlined in Frame 4. An organized plan is a necessity when solving application problems.

Q17   Nancy paid $1.65 for the 10% tax on gasoline. What was the total cost of the gasoline?

\# \# \# • \# \# \# • \# \# \# • \# \# \# • \# \# \# • \# \# \# • \# \# \# • \# \# \# • \# \# \#

A17 $16.50:   Step 2: $1.65 is 10% of total cost
$1.65 = 0.1 \times C$

Q18   A mixture contains 6 kilograms salt, 23 kilograms water, and 17 kilograms glycerine. What percent of the total is the salt (round off the percent to one decimal place)?

\# \# \# • \# \# \# • \# \# \# • \# \# \# • \# \# \# • \# \# \# • \# \# \# • \# \# \# • \# \# \#

A18   13%:   Step 2:   6 is what percent of 46?
$6 = P \times 46$

Q19 $2,400 is 8% of the price of a house. What is the price of the house?

\# \# \# • \# \# \# • \# \# \# • \# \# \# • \# \# \# • \# \# \# • \# \# \# • \# \# \# • \# \# \#

A19 $30,000:   Step 2: $2,400 = 0.08 \times$ price

Q20   Ice shrinks $8\frac{1}{3}\%$ of its volume in melting to form water. If a block of ice is 27 cubic inches, what is the volume after the ice melts?

\# \# \# • \# \# \# • \# \# \# • \# \# \# • \# \# \# • \# \# \# • \# \# \# • \# \# \# • \# \# \#

A20   24.75 cubic inches: Step 2:   shrinkage $= 8\frac{1}{3}\% \times 27$

$$\text{shrinkage} = \frac{25}{300} \times 27$$

Step 4: 27 cubic inches $-$ 2.25 cubic inches

Q21   Calcium, the most abundant mineral in the body, comprises about 1.75% of the weight of an adult's body. Approximately how many pounds of calcium are in the body of a 150 pound adult?

•   # # #   •   # # #   •   # # #   •   # # #   •   # # #   •   # # #   •   # # #   •   # #

A21   2.625 pounds: Calcium $= 1.75\% \times 150$ pounds

Q22   If you gave 20% of a 50-grain tablet, how much medication did you give?

•   # # #   •   # # #   •   # # #   •   # # #   •   # # #   •   # # #   •   # # #   •   # #

A22   10 grains: total medication $= 20\% \times 50$ grains

Q23   A nurse gave 75% of a 40-ml ampul (a small sealed glass vessel used to hold a solution for hypodermic injection). How much medication by volume did she give?

•   # # #   •   # # #   •   # # #   •   # # #   •   # # #   •   # # #   •   # # #   •   # #

A23   30 ml

Q24   In a recent study, 61 questionnaires were sent to chief technologists and chief radiologists in the Minneapolis–St. Paul area. Twenty-nine of the questionnaires were returned. What percent were returned (round off to the nearest percent)?

•   # # #   •   # # #   •   # # #   •   # # #   •   # # #   •   # # #   •   # # #   •   # #

A24   48%:   Step 2:   29 is what percent of 61?
$29 = P \times 61$

Q25   Eighteen out of a possible 32 replies were from chief technologists and 11 out of a possible 29 replies were from chief radiologists. What percent of each group replied (round off to the nearest percent)?

•   # # #   •   # # #   •   # # #   •   # # #   •   # # #   •   # # #   •   # # #   •   # #

A25   Chief technologists 56%; chief radiologists 38%

Q26 To the question, "Do you feel that radiologic technologists in your department are adequately compensated for their work?", 80 percent of the technologists responded "no." What actual number responded no (see Q25)?

\# \# \# • \# \# \# • \# \# \# • \# \# \# • \# \# \# • \# \# \# • \# \# \# • \# \# \# • \# \# \#

A26 14: 18 technologists responded. Step 2: $N = 80\%$ of 18

Q27 The following is a partial table taken from *Respiratory Care*, July 1974, Vol. 19, No. 7. Determine the percentage of orders filled for each year and month (nearest percent):

Month	IPPB Treatments Ordered		IPPB Treatments Given		Percentage of Orders Filled	
	1972	1973	1972	1973	1972	1973
Feb	390	329	321	310		
Mar	224	419	166	409		
Apr	328	487	302	477		
May	489	508	476	482		

\# \# \# • \# \# \# • \# \# \# • \# \# \# • \# \# \# • \# \# \# • \# \# \# • \# \# \# • \# \# \#

A27 Feb. 82%, 94%, Mar. 74%, 98%, Apr. 92%, 98%, May 97%, 95%.

This completes the instruction for this section.

2.4 EXERCISE

1. Choose the best estimate:
   a. 15% of 88 mg: 0.13, 13, 1.32, 8.8
   b. 7% of 195:   140, 0.14, 14, 1.365
   c. 10% of 6.03:   0.6, 6, 60, 0.06
   d. 2% of 19.6:   39.2, 0.4, 4, 40
2. A patient's pulse rate increased from 72 beats per minute to 108 beats per minute. Find the rate of increase.
3. A patient's weight decreased from 186 pounds to 115 pounds. Find the rate of decrease (round off to one decimal place).
4. A radiologist's salary was increased from $1,000 to $1,200 per month. Find the percent of increase (round off to one decimal place).
5. Jim's salary was raised from $850 to $900 per month. Find his percent increase and new yearly salary (round off to one decimal place).
6. The following is a table taken from *Respiratory Care*, July 1974, Vol. 19, No. 7. Determine the percentage of orders filled for each year and month (round off to nearest percent).

Month	IPPB Treatments Ordered		IPPB Treatments Given		Percentage of Orders Filled	
	1972	1973	1972	1973	1972	1973
Feb	6,813	8,919	2,235	2,634		
Mar	7,025	9,007	2,128	2,772		
Apr	8,047	8,905	1,331	2,364		
May	8,374	10,200	1,272	2,641		
Jun	8,300	10,300	1,174	2,452		
Jul	8,481	10,390	1,181	2,902		
Aug	8,800	10,680	1,712	2,919		

7. In a local election, 411,700 people cast their votes. If this number of voters represented a gain of 15% over the last election, what was the number of voters in the last election?

8. An article costs $17.60. If the price is increased 15%, find the new price.

9. Find the percent increase in a price increase from $7.20 to $8.

10. Find the percent decrease if Frank's pay falls from $96 to $91.50 (round off to one decimal place).

11. Ann's income this year is $7,800. If this is an increase of 20% over last year's income, find last year's income.

12. A mixture contains 13 pounds of water, 25 pounds of borax, and 10 pounds of alcohol. What percent of the total is water (round off to one decimal place)?

13. A popular cereal has a total weight of 567 grams. The cereal contains 2.5% of nonnutritive crude fiber by weight. How many grams of crude fiber are in the box of cereal?

14. If there are 20 average servings (about $\frac{1}{2}$ cup) in the box (problem 13), how many grams are in each serving (round off to the nearest gram)?

15. Each average serving (problem 14) contains protein 2 grams, carbohydrate 22 grams, fat 1 gram. Find the percentage of each in the average serving (round off to the nearest percent).

16. A mixture contains 6 kilograms of water, 13 kilograms of alcohol, and 12 kilograms of glycerine. What percent of the total is the alcohol (round off to one decimal place)?

17. Exercise serves to promote better circulation throughout the body. A recent study indicated the average pulse rate of marathon runners was 59, long distance runners 63, and sprinters 66. If 75 is the normal heart beat rate, what percent of the normal heart beat rate is each of the above (round off to the nearest percent)?

18. A 4% tax is added to the selling price of an article. Find the amount of the tax on an article that sells for $18.60.

19. Sue saved $1.25 by buying a blanket at a reduction of 10%. What was the regular price?

20. A crowd of 62,094 fans filled 85% of the Ponmet Stadium Saturday to view the Lion's first game in their new home. What is the capacity of the Ponmet Stadium?

21. Mr. Graves contributed 9% of a $180 Red Cross Fund. How much did he contribute?

22. Gordon worked 9 of 14 weeks of his vacation. What percent of his vacation did he work (round off to one decimal place)?

23. During the first 6 months, Mary gained 25% of her weight at birth. If she gained $2\frac{1}{2}$ pounds during this period, how much did she weigh at birth?

24. If you gave 75% of a 30-ml ampul, how much did you give?

25. If you gave 5% of a 60-mg tablet, how much did you give?

2.4   EXERCISE ANSWERS

1. a. 13   **b.** 14   **c.** 0.6   **d.** 0.4
2. 50%   **3.** 38.2%   **4.** 20%   **5.** 5.9%, $10,800
6. Feb. 33%, 30%, Mar. 30%, 31%, Apr. 17%, 27%, May 15%, 26%, Jun. 14%, 24%, Jul. 14%, 28%, Aug. 19%, 27%.

7. 358,000   **8.** $20.24   **9.** $11\frac{1}{9}$%   **10.** 4.7%

11. $6,500   **12.** 27.1%   **13.** 14.175 grams   **14.** 28 grams
15. protein 7%, carbohydrate 79%, fat 4%   **16.** 41.9%
17. marathon runners 79%, long distance runners 84%, sprinters 88%
18. $0.74   **19.** $12.50   **20.** 73,052   **21.** $16.20
22. 64.3%   **23.** 10 pounds   **24.** 22.5 ml   **25.** 3 mg

CHAPTER 2 SAMPLE TEST

At the completion of Chapter 2 you should be able to work the following problems.

2.1   PERCENTS

1. Change to a decimal:
a. 24%   **b.** 7.3%

2. Change to a percent:
a. 0.8   **b.** 1.25

3. Change to a fraction:
a. $16\frac{2}{3}$%   **b.** $12\frac{1}{2}$%

4. Change to a percent:
a. $\frac{9}{40}$ **b.** $\frac{5}{6}$

2.2   WRITING AND SOLVING MATHEMATICAL SENTENCES

5. Write the following mathematically:
a. 17% of 61 is 10.37   **b.** 5% of 30 is what number?

6. a. If $4 \times 5 = 20$, $5 = $ _____ $\div$ _____.

  b. If $0.5 \times A = \$2.70$, $A = $ _____ $\div$ _____.

2.3   SOLVING PERCENT PROBLEMS

7. a. 15 is 30% of what number?   **b.** 336 is what percent of 16?

2.4   APPLICATIONS

8. Solve the following problems:
  a. Mr. Knox's rent during the past year amounted to $780 per year. His rent was 20% of his income. Find his income for last year.

    b. If you gave 25% of a 40-mg tablet, how much medication did you give?

    c. A patient's heart beat increased from 75 beats per minute to 88 beats per minute, find the percent of increase (round off to one decimal place).

    d. An average serving of cereal contains 3 grams of protein, 20 grams of carbohydrate, and 2 grams of fat. Find the percent of carbohydrates of the total.

CHAPTER 2 SAMPLE TEST ANSWERS

1. a. 0.24   **b.** 0.073   **2. a.** 80%   **b.** 125%

3. a. $\dfrac{1}{6}$ **b.** $\dfrac{1}{8}$ **4. a.** 22.5%   **b.** $83\dfrac{1}{3}\%$

5. a. $0.17 \times 61 = 10.37$ **b.** $0.05 \times 30 = N$

6. a. 20, 4   **b.** \$2.70, 0.5   **7. a.** 50   **b.** 2,100%

8. a. \$3,900   **b.** 10 mg   **c.** 17.3%   **d.** 80%

CHAPTER 3

GEOMETRY

We live in a geometric world. A technician in the health fields can use geometric properties to better understand the world in which they work. This chapter will introduce fundamental geometric objects and some of their properties.

3.1 POINTS, LINES, AND ANGLES

1	The most fundamental notion in geometry is a *point*. A point is a location in space and has no thickness. Although a point is represented with a dot on paper, the dot is much too large to actually be a point. The dot helps in thinking about the point.

Q1   Which dot is the best representation of a point?_____
      a. ●   **b.** •   **c.** ·

• # # # • # # # • # # # • # # # • # # # • # # # • # # # • # #

A1   **c:**   It looks most like a location with no dimensions.

Q2   Is the presentation in part **c** of Q1 actually a point?_____

• # # # • # # # • # # # • # # # • # # # • # # # • # # # • # #

A2   no: It is still too large and is actually many, many points all very close together.

2	Another geometric object which is so fundamental that other objects depend on its properties is a *line*. A line is a set of points and is represented with a picture such as: ←——————————————→ Notice the arrowheads on the end of the representation. They are placed there to remind you that a line extends forever in each direction, even though the representation of the line stops. A line has no thickness and is always straight. Therefore, it is not necessary to say "straight line."

Q3   If the following words describe a line write true, if it does not write false:
      a. extends forever_____   **b.** curved_____   **c.** has end points_____
      d. definite length_____   **e.** straight _____   **f.** no thickness_____

• # # # • # # # • # # # • # # # • # # # • # # # • # # # • # #

A3   **a.** true   **b.** false   **c.** false   **d.** false   **e.** true   **f.** true

---

3   A point is named with a capital letter. Two points on the line below are P and Q.

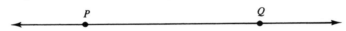

A line is named by writing the names of two points on the line side by side and placing a double headed arrow over them. The line above would be named $\overleftrightarrow{PQ}$.

In the figure below $\overleftrightarrow{AB}$ intersects $\overleftrightarrow{PQ}$ at the point R.

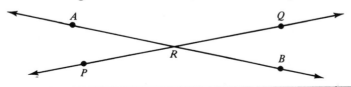

Q4   **a.** Name two lines that intersect $\overleftrightarrow{PQ}$._____

       b. Name the intersection of $\overleftrightarrow{AB}$ and $\overleftrightarrow{PQ}$._____

       c. Name the line that intersects $\overleftrightarrow{CD}$ at S._____

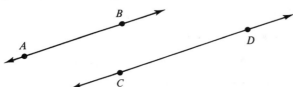

•   # # #   •   # # #   •   # # #   •   # # #   •   # # #   •   # # #   •   # # #   •   # #

A4   **a.** $\overleftrightarrow{AB}, \overleftrightarrow{CD}$ **b.** R **c.** $\overleftrightarrow{PQ}$

---

4   A plane is a flat surface that extends forever in every direction. If two lines in a plane do not intersect, they are *parallel*. $\overleftrightarrow{AB}$ and $\overleftrightarrow{CD}$ are parallel. We write $\overleftrightarrow{AB} \| \overleftrightarrow{CD}$, and read it "line AB is parallel to line CD."

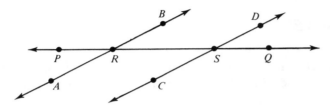

     If two lines intersect and all four angles formed by the lines are equal, each angle is a *right* angle and the lines are said to be *perpendicular lines*. $\overleftrightarrow{PQ}$ is perpendicular to $\overleftrightarrow{RS}$ in the figure below. We write $\overleftrightarrow{PQ} \perp \overleftrightarrow{RS}$, and read it "line PQ is perpendicular to line RS". The small square in the corner tells you that the angle formed is a right angle.

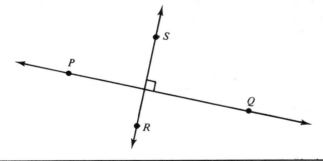

Q5   Fill in the appropriate symbol ∥ or ⊥ on the blank:

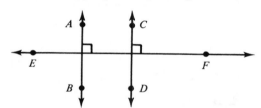

a. $\overleftrightarrow{AB}$_____$\overleftrightarrow{CD}$ b. $\overleftrightarrow{AB}$_____$\overleftrightarrow{EF}$ c. $\overleftrightarrow{CD}$_____$\overleftrightarrow{EF}$

\#\#\# • \#\#\# • \#\#\# • \#\#\# • \#\#\# • \#\#\# • \#\#\# • \#\#\# • \#\#\#

A5   a. ∥   b. ⊥   c. ⊥

Q6   a. From the figure below, write which lines appear to be parallel. Use the appropriate symbolism._____

b. Write two pairs of perpendicular lines. Use the appropriate symbolism._____

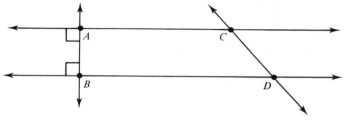

\#\#\# • \#\#\# • \#\#\# • \#\#\# • \#\#\# • \#\#\# • \#\#\# • \#\#\# • \#\#\#

A6   a. $\overleftrightarrow{AC}\|\overleftrightarrow{BD}$ b. $\overleftrightarrow{AC}\perp\overleftrightarrow{AB}$ and $\overleftrightarrow{AB}\perp\overleftrightarrow{BD}$

---

5   A *line segment* (sometimes referred to as a segment) is the portion of a line between two points including the endpoints. A line segment is referred to with the symbol $\overline{AB}$, where A and B are its endpoints. Segment $\overline{CD}$ is shown as

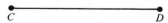

In the next figure $\overleftrightarrow{AB}$ is drawn, but $\overline{AB}$ refers only to the points A and B and those between A and B. The segment is a part of the line.

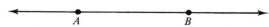

Refer to the figure below for the following examples:

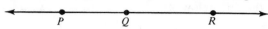

1. P is on $\overleftrightarrow{QR}$.
2. P is not on $\overline{QR}$ (because P is not between Q and R).
3. Q is on $\overline{PR}$.
4. Q is on $\overleftrightarrow{PR}$.
5. R is on $\overleftrightarrow{PQ}$.
6. R is not on $\overline{PQ}$.
7. P is on $\overleftrightarrow{PR}$.

Q7   Indicate whether the symbolism represents a segment, a line, or neither:

a. $\overline{AB}$_____   b. $\overleftrightarrow{PQ}$_____   c. RS_____

\#\#\# • \#\#\# • \#\#\# • \#\#\# • \#\#\# • \#\#\# • \#\#\# • \#\#\# • \#\#\#

A7   **a.** segment   **b.** line   **c.** neither

Q8   Label the statements true or false:

a. A is on $\overleftrightarrow{CD}$. _____   **b.** A is on $\overline{CD}$. _____

c. B is on $\overline{AC}$. _____   **d.** B is on $\overrightarrow{AC}$. _____

e. C is on $\overrightarrow{AB}$. _____   **f.** C is on $\overline{AB}$. _____

g. B is on $\overline{BC}$. _____

• # # # • # # # • # # # • # # # • # # # • # # # • # # # • # #

A8   **a.** true   **b.** false   **c.** true   **d.** true   **e.** true   **f.** false   **g.** true

Q9   Refer to the figure to answer the following:

a. Name a line parallel to $\overleftrightarrow{AB}$. _____

b. Name a segment which intersects $\overleftrightarrow{AB}$. _____

c. Name a segment on $\overleftrightarrow{CD}$. _____

d. Name a line not parallel to $\overleftrightarrow{AB}$. _____

• # # # • # # # • # # # • # # # • # # # • # # # • # # # • # #

A9   **a.** $\overleftrightarrow{CD}$ **b.** $\overline{DB}$ **c.** $\overline{CD}$ **d.** $\overrightarrow{DB}$

---

6   If two line segments are equal, they have the same endpoints. Therefore, there are three line segments, none of which equals another on the line below. The line segments are $\overline{AB}$, $\overline{AC}$ and $\overline{BC}$.

Q10   Name all possible different line segments on the line below. _____

• # # # • # # # • # # # • # # # • # # # • # # # • # # # • # #

A10 $\overline{AB}$, $\overline{AC}$, $\overline{AD}$, $\overline{BC}$, $\overline{BD}$, $\overline{CD}$: $\overline{BA}$ is the same segment as $\overline{AB}$, so it is not listed separately.

---

7   Line segments may be measured to determine their length. To measure a line segment, an instrument, such as a ruler, marked in graduations of a standard unit is used. In the English system, inches, feet, yards, and miles are common units of length. The relationships among the English units are:

1 mile = 5,280 feet
1 yard = 3 feet
1 yard = 36 inches
1 foot = 12 inches

A ruler with its scale marked in $\frac{1}{2}, \frac{1}{4}, \frac{1}{8}, \frac{1}{16}$ inch marks is shown with some examples of how to read it. Study the examples.

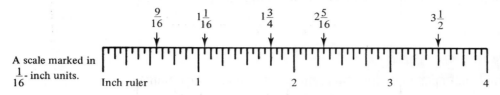

A scale marked in $\frac{1}{16}$- inch units.

Q11   Read the scale at the places marked:

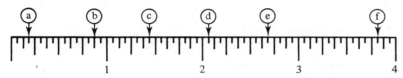

a. _____   b. _____   c. _____   d. _____

e. _____   f. _____

• # # # • # # # • # # # • # # # • # # # • # # # • # # # • # #

A11   a. $\frac{3}{16}$ inches   b. $\frac{7}{8}$ inches   c. $1\frac{7}{16}$ inches   d. $2\frac{1}{16}$ inches

e. $2\frac{11}{16}$ inches   f. $3\frac{13}{16}$ inches

---

8   The common units of measurement in the metric system are millimetre, centimetre, metre, and kilometre. Their relationships follow:

1 kilometre (km) = 1000 metres (m)*
1 metre = 100 centimetres (cm)
1 centimetre = 10 millimetres (mm)

Notice that each unit is a multiple of 10 times another unit. This makes conversion of units easier in the metric system. Illustrated is a 10-centimetre ruler further subdivided into millimetres. When a centimetre ruler is also marked in millimetres, a measurement can be read to the nearest millimetre. A millimetre is one tenth of a centimetre. The following measurements are reported two ways. The two results are equal.

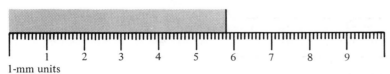

1-mm units

58 millimetres or 5.8 centimetres

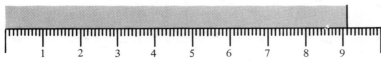

1-mm units

91 millimetres or 9.1 centimetres

*In some countries a comma is used to represent a decimal point. To avoid confusion in all countries of the world, a number with a metric unit with more than four digits in it will be written with no commas but with a space every 3 digits from the decimal. The number that we have been writing in the United States as 3,462,241. will be written 3 462 241.

Q12   Read the scales to the nearest millimetre:

a.

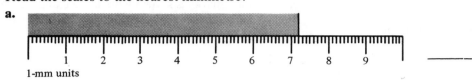

1-mm units

b.

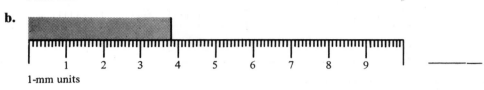

1-mm units

\# \# \#   •   \# \# \#   •   \# \# \#   •   \# \# \#   •   \# \# \#   •   \# \# \#   •   \# \# \#   •   \# \# \#   •   \# \# \#

A12   **a.** 72 millimetres   **b.** 38 millimetres

Q13   Read the scales below to the nearest $\frac{1}{10}$ of a centimetre:

a.

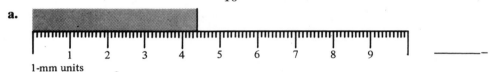

1-mm units

b.

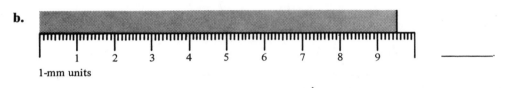

1-mm units

\# \# \#   •   \# \# \#   •   \# \# \#   •   \# \# \#   •   \# \# \#   •   \# \# \#   •   \# \# \#   •   \# \# \#   •   \# \# \#

A13   **a.** 4.4 centimetres   **b.** 9.5 centimetres

---

9   The part of the line on one side of a point that includes the endpoint is called a *ray*. A ray is represented by noting its endpoint first along with another point on the ray with a single-headed arrow extending to the right above them. The name of the following rays would be $\overrightarrow{DC}$:

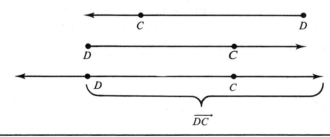

$$\overrightarrow{DC}$$

Q14   Name five rays on the figures below. _____

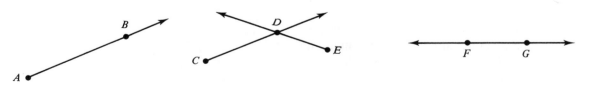

\# \# \#   •   \# \# \#   •   \# \# \#   •   \# \# \#   •   \# \# \#   •   \# \# \#   •   \# \# \#   •   \# \# \#   •   \# \# \#

A14 $\overrightarrow{AB}$, $\overrightarrow{CD}$, $\overrightarrow{ED}$, $\overrightarrow{FG}$, and $\overrightarrow{GF}$

10 The same ray can be named in several ways. For example, in the figure below $\overrightarrow{BC}$ and $\overrightarrow{BD}$ represent the same ray. We therefore say $\overrightarrow{BC} = \overrightarrow{BD}$ since they contain the same points.

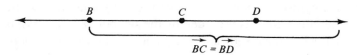

$$\overrightarrow{BC} = \overrightarrow{BD}$$

Notice, however, that $\overrightarrow{BC} \neq \overrightarrow{CB}$.* They do not contain the same points. For example, D is on $\overrightarrow{BC}$ but D is not on $\overrightarrow{CB}$.

*The symbol $\neq$ says "is not equal to."

Q15 Name a ray on the figure in two different ways. _____

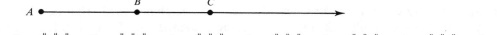

• # # # • # # # • # # # • # # # • # # # • # # # • # # # • # #

A15 $\overrightarrow{AB}$, $\overrightarrow{AC}$

Q16 Name four rays on the figure using the letters A, B, C. _____

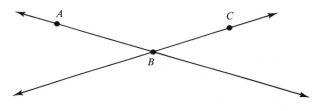

• # # # • # # # • # # # • # # # • # # # • # # # • # # # • # #

A16 $\overrightarrow{AB}$, $\overrightarrow{BA}$, $\overrightarrow{BC}$, and $\overrightarrow{CB}$

Q17 Are any of the rays listed in A16 equal?_____

• # # # • # # # • # # # • # # # • # # # • # # # • # # # • # #

A17 no

11 An *angle* consists of two rays with a common endpoint. The common endpoint is called the *vertex* of the angle. The rays are the *sides* of the angle. A representation of an angle is shown. The two rays are $\overrightarrow{BA}$ and $\overrightarrow{BC}$, with the vertex being the point B. Sometimes a curved line connects the two sides of an angle.

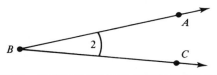

Q18 **a.** Name the vertex of the angle._____

b. Name the two sides of the angle._____

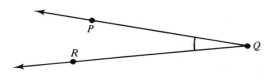

• # # # • # # # • # # # • # # # • # # # • # # # • # # # • # #

A18   **a.** Q

b. $\overrightarrow{QP}$, $\overrightarrow{QR}$: $\overrightarrow{PQ}$ and $\overrightarrow{RQ}$ are incorrect because the rays (sides) of the angle start at the vertex.

---

12   An angle can most easily be named by using the letter at its vertex or by a number written at the vertex between the sides. The name of the angle is preceded by the symbol "∡". The symbol ∡A is read "angle A". Thus, two names for the angle shown are ∡Q and ∡2. However, if there is more

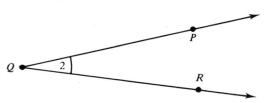

than one angle at a vertex, a more complicated scheme is sometimes used. That is, three letters follow the ∡ symbol. For example, ∡2 in the figure below is named ∡ACD or ∡DCA. ∡3 is named ∡ACB or ∡BCA. Notice that the vertex is *always* the middle letter.

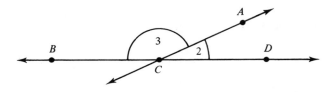

Q19   Write another name for each angle, using 1 letter or number.

a. ∡ABC = _____

b. ∡BCA = _____

c. ∡CAB = _____

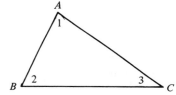

• # # # • # # # • # # # • # # # • # # # • # # # • # # # • # #

A19   **a.** ∡B or ∡2   **b.** ∡C or ∡3   **c.** ∡A or ∡1

Q20   Name the angles in the following figure by using the easiest method (fewest letters) and the points shown. (The letter C names the *point* of intersection of the lines.)

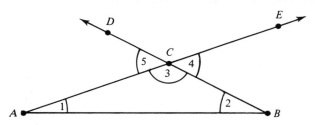

a. ∡1 = _____   **b.** ∡4 = _____   **c.** ∡2 = _____

d. ∡5 = _____   **e.** ∡3 = _____

• # # # • # # # • # # # • # # # • # # # • # # # • # # # • # #

A20   **a.** ∡1 = ∡A **b.** ∡4 = ∡ECB or ∡BCE **c.** ∡2 = ∡B
       d. ∡5 = ∡DCA or ∡ACD **e.** ∡3 = ∡ACB or ∡BCA

13   The *measurement of an angle* is a number assigned to the amount of rotation required to swing one ray of the angle to the other ray. The unit of measure will be the *degree* (°), which is based upon the division of 1 complete revolution into 360 parts. Each of these parts is a degree. You should become familiar with the measure of angles so you can tell the approximate size of an angle by inspection. Some frequently used angles are shown. A curved line with an arrow on the end will sometimes be placed inside an angle to show the direction of rotation.

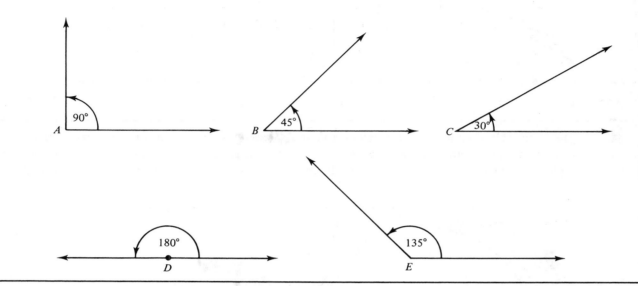

Q21   Compare the angles shown to the examples in Frame 13 to estimate the approximate measure of the angle:

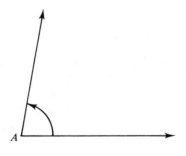

a. 40°, 80°, or 100° _____

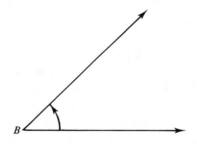

b. 20°, 45°, or 60° _____

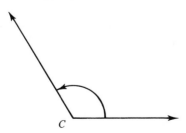

c. 80°, 160°, or 120° _____

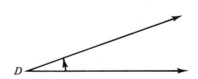

d. 20°, 45°, or 60° _____

• # # # • # # # • # # # • # # # • # # # • # # # • # # # • # #

A21   **a.** 80°   **b.** 45°   **c.** 120°   **d.** 20°

Q22   A patient placed in a full Trendelenburg position is placed with their feet elevated to 45° so that the abdominal organs are pushed upward toward the chest. Which of the positions below is the full Trendelenburg position? _____

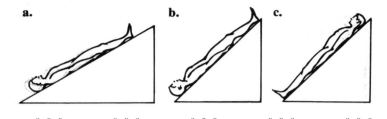

a.   b.   c.

• # # # • # # # • # # # • # # # • # # # • # # # • # # # • # #

A22   **b**

14   The instrument used to measure angles is called a *protractor*. A protractor is needed to complete this section. The protractor is shown as it would be used to measure an angle. The base of the protractor is placed along one ray of the angle with the center mark on the protractor at the vertex. The other

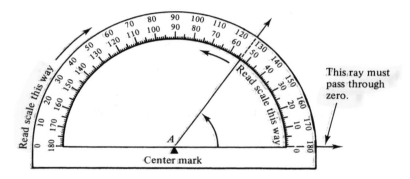

ray of the angle will pass under the scale of the protractor and the degree measure is read from the scale. The measure of the angle shown is approximately 54° to the nearest degree. Notice that each scale mark has two numbers beside it. The numbers larger than 90 are used if an angle over 90° is being measured. Write $m\angle A = 54°$ (read "the measure of angle A is equal to 54 degrees"). If a side of an angle does not pass under the outer edge of the protractor, extend the side with your pencil. This will not affect the measure of the angle.

   The construction of protractors vary in the placement of the centermark. Check your own protractor to make sure that when the centermark is on the vertex, one ray runs through 0° on the edge of the protractor.

Q23   Use a protractor to measure the angles (extend sides of angle if necessary):

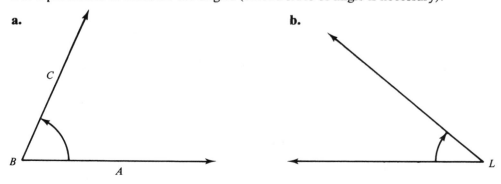

a.   b.

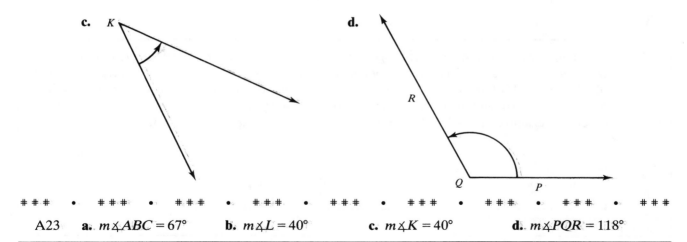

c. *K*   **d.**   *R*   *Q*   *P*

\# \# \# • \# \# \# • \# \# \# • \# \# \# • \# \# \# • \# \# \# • \# \# \# • \# \# \# • \# \# \#

A23   **a.** $m \angle ABC = 67°$ **b.** $m \angle L = 40°$ **c.** $m \angle K = 40°$ **d.** $m \angle PQR = 118°$

Q24   When the central ray (C.R.) of an x-ray beam is positioned to pass through two checkpoints on the skull, the angle the C.R. makes with a vertical line varies between the two angles shown below. Measure these angles.

a.   C.R.   **b.**   C.R.

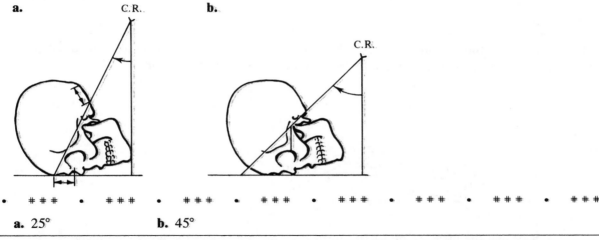

\# \# \# • \# \# \# • \# \# \# • \# \# \# • \# \# \# • \# \# \# • \# \# \# • \# \# \# • \# \# \#

A24   **a.** 25°   **b.** 45°

Q25   Measure the angle formed by the axis of the femur and the axis of the shaft neck where it connects in the joint of the hip.

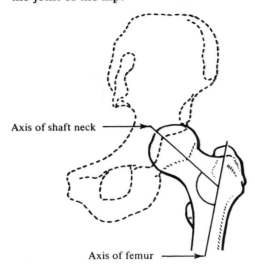

Axis of shaft neck →

Axis of femur →

\# \# \# • \# \# \# • \# \# \# • \# \# \# • \# \# \# • \# \# \# • \# \# \# • \# \# \# • \# \# \#

A25   122°

---

15   Two angles whose measures added together result in a sum of 90° or a right angle are said to be *complementary* angles. Each is the complement of the other. For example, if $m\angle 1 = 35°$ and $m\angle 2 = 55°$, angles 1 and 2 are complementary. Two angles whose measures added together result in a sum of 180° (straight angle) are said to be *supplementary* angles. Each is the supplement of the other. For example, if $m\angle 3 = 36°$ and $m\angle 4 = 144°$, angles 3 and 4 are supplementary.

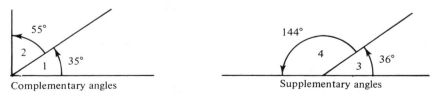

Q26   **a.** The supplement of an angle of 50° would have what measure? _____

b. The complement of an angle of 50° would have what measure? _____

\# \# \#   •   \# \# \#   •   \# \# \#   •   \# \# \#   •   \# \# \#   •   \# \# \#   •   \# \# \#   •   \# \# \#   •   \# \# \#

A26   **a.** 130°   **b.** 40°

Q27   **a.** When the measure of $\angle ABC$ shown below is 60°, what is the measure of its supplement $\angle CBD$, which is the angle formed by the femur and tibia (do not measure)?

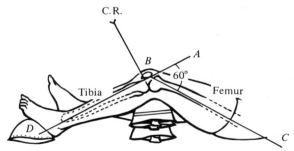

b. When the measure of $\angle ABC$ formed by the femur and the horizontal plane is 70° what is the measure of its complement $\angle CBD$ which is the angle between the femur and the central ray focused in a vertical direction into the knee (do not measure)?

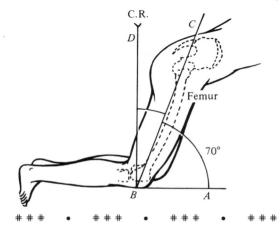

\# \# \#   •   \# \# \#   •   \# \# \#   •   \# \# \#   •   \# \# \#   •   \# \# \#   •   \# \# \#   •   \# \# \#   •   \# \# \#

A27   **a.** 120°   **b.** 20°

This completes the instruction for this section.

3.1   EXERCISE

1. Name the four segments that are the four sides of Figure 1.

Figure 1

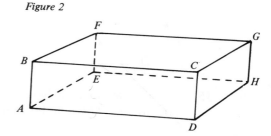

2. In Figure 1, name two line segments that intersect at *B*.

3. In Figure 1, name two line segments that appear to be part of parallel lines (there are two possibilities).

4. Figure 2 has the shape of a brick. The dashed lines would not be visible.

Figure 2

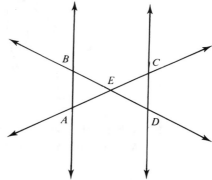

  a. Name a pair of edges that have the common point *C* in the plane closest to you.

  b. Name a pair of edges that appear to be part of parallel lines in the plane farthest from you (there are two possibilities).

  c. Name an edge that is not in the plane of the top or the plane of the bottom of the figure.

5. Use the figure at the right to answer the following:

  a. Name two lines that appear to be parallel.

  b. $\overleftrightarrow{AC}$ and $\overleftrightarrow{BD}$ intersect at what point?

  c. Name eight line segments on the figure.

  d. Are there any perpendicular lines in the figure?

6. Which is the best model of a point: the sun, a bowling ball, a grain of sand, or a marble?

7. Name two rays with endpoints at *B*.

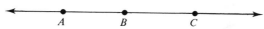

8. Give two other ways of naming the ray *AC*.

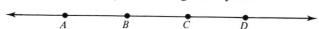

9. What is the name of the intersection of the two rays that make up an angle?

10. What is the geometric name for the sides of an angle?

11. Name the angle in three ways.

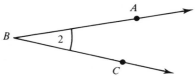

12. Name four angles in the figure.

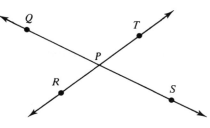

13. How many degrees are in one complete revolution?

14. Without measuring the angles, choose the most likely number of degrees in the angle:

a.

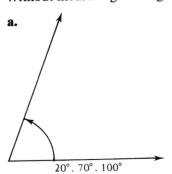

20°, 70°, 100°

b.

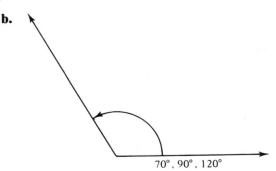

70°, 90°, 120°

15. Arm slings are made to hold the forearm at various angles with the upper arm. Match the angles 120°, 90°, and 60° with the appropriate figure.

a.

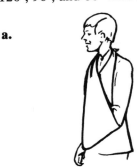

b.

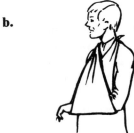

c.

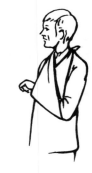

16. What is the name of the instrument used to measure angles?

17. Measure the angles below to the nearest degree:

a.

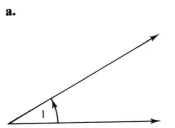

b.

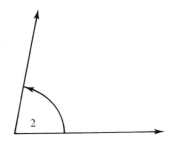

c.

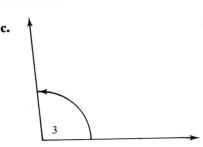

d.

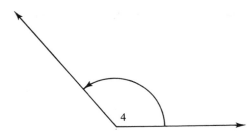

18. Measure the angles formed by the apophysial joints ∡*ABC* and ∡*CBD* in the figure below.

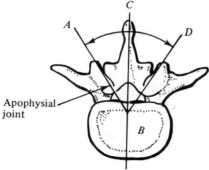

Direction of lumbar apophysial joints

19. The diagram below shows the position of the table and the central ray for a particular x-ray.
a. Measure ∡1, the angle of elevation of the table. **b.** Measure ∡2, the angle the central ray makes with the vertical.

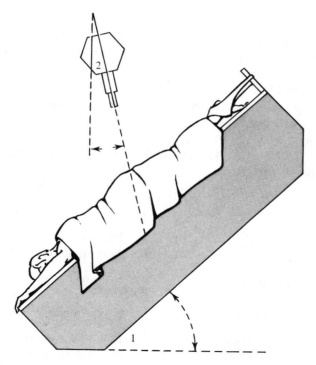

20. The angle, ∡*ABC* formed by the thumb nail and the top of the thumb in a healthy person is between 140° and 170°. If the angle falls outside this range there is a possibility of disease. Which of the following are healthy?

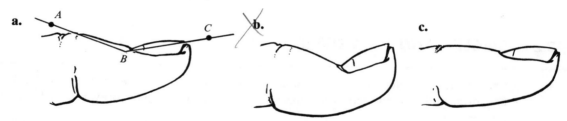

21. What does it mean to say two angles are complementary?
22. What does it mean to say two angles are supplementary?

23. Read the inch ruler at each of the arrows:

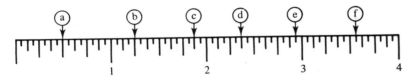

24. Read the centimetre ruler at each of the arrows in tenths of a centimetre.

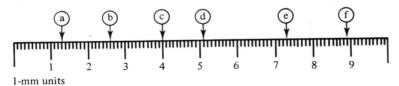

1-mm units

25. Read the centimetre ruler for each arrow in problem 24 in millimetres.

3.1 EXERCISE ANSWERS

1. $\overline{AB}, \overline{BC}, \overline{CD}$, and $\overline{DA}$ **2.** $\overline{AB}$ and $\overline{BC}$ **3.** $\overline{AB} \| \overline{CD}$ and $\overline{BC} \| \overline{AD}$

4. a. $\overline{BC}$ and $\overline{CD}$ **b.** $\overline{FG} \| \overline{EH}$ and $\overline{EF} \| \overline{GH}$ **c.** $\overline{AB}, \overline{CD}, \overline{GH}$, or $\overline{FE}$

5. a. $\overleftrightarrow{AB} \| \overleftrightarrow{CD}$ **b.** E

c. $\overline{AB}, \overline{AE}, \overline{BE}, \overline{EC}, \overline{ED}, \overline{CD}, \overline{AC}$, and $\overline{BD}$ **d.** no

6. A grain of sand. However, something as large as the sun, such as a star, appears to be a point if you are far enough away.

7. $\overrightarrow{BC}$ and $\overrightarrow{BA}$ **8.** $\overrightarrow{AB}$ and $\overrightarrow{AD}$ **9.** vertex **10.** rays

11. $\angle ABC, \angle B, \angle 2$, or $\angle CBA$ **12.** $\angle QPR, \angle RPS, \angle SPT$, and $\angle TPQ$

13. $360°$ **14. a.** $70°$ **b.** $120°$

15. a. $120°$ **b.** $90°$ **c.** $60°$ **16.** protractor

17. a. $31°$ **b.** $78°$ **c.** $95°$ **d.** $130°$

18. $m\angle ABC = 33°$, $m\angle CBD = 33°$

19. a. $43°$ **b.** $14°$ **20. a, c**

21. The sum of their measures is $90°$. **22.** The sum of their measures is $180°$.

23. a. $\frac{1}{2}$ inch **b.** $1\frac{1}{4}$ inches **c.** $1\frac{7}{8}$ inches

d. $2\frac{3}{8}$ inches **e.** $2\frac{15}{16}$ inches **f.** $3\frac{9}{16}$ inches

24. a. 1.3 centimetres **b.** 2.6 centimetres **c.** 4.0 centimetres

d. 5.1 centimetres **e.** 7.3 centimetres **f.** 8.9 centimetres

25. a. 13 millimetres **b.** 26 millimetres **c.** 40 millimetres

d. 51 millimetres **e.** 73 millimetres **f.** 89 millimetres

3.2 CIRCLES AND POLYGONS

1   One of the fundamental ideas of geometry is the notion of a *plane*. A plane can be thought of as a flat surface, like a table top, which has no edges. A plane extends forever in each direction and has no thickness.

The geometric objects that will be discussed in this section are contained in a plane. We say circles and polygons are plane figures because all of their points are in one plane. In a physical sense you might say that a circle or polygon could be completely constructed or drawn on the flat surface of a piece of paper.

Q1 Answer true or false:

a. A plane extends forever in each direction. _____

b. A plane has the thickness of a piece of paper. _____

c. A table top is a helpful but imperfect representation of a plane. _____

d. In geometry a plane figure means that it is a very ordinary figure. _____

• # # # • # # # • # # # • # # # • # # # • # # # • # # # • # #

A1 **a.** true **b.** false **c.** true **d.** false

---

2 A *circle* is a set of all points in a plane whose distance from a given point, *P*, is equal to a positive number, *r*. The point *P* is the *center* of the circle. The positive number *r* is the *radius* of the circle. Twice the radius is the *diameter* of the circle.

The instrument used to draw circles is the *compass*. It can also be used to compare distances.

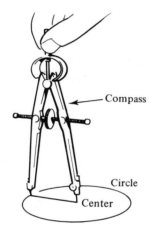

Compass

Circle

Center

Example 1: The radius of a circle is 12 inches. What is the diameter?

Solution: 24 inches: The diameter is twice the radius.

Example 2: The diameter of a circle is 37 centimetres. What is the radius?

Solution: $18\frac{1}{2}$ centimetres: If the diameter is twice the radius, the radius must be $\frac{1}{2}$ the diameter.

Q2 **a.** If a circle has a radius of 3 inches, its diameter must be _____.

b. If a circle has a diameter of 5 inches, its radius must be _____.

• # # # • # # # • # # # • # # # • # # # • # # # • # # # • # #

A2 **a.** 6 inches **b.** $2\frac{1}{2}$ inches

---

3 The word "radius" (plural form is radii) is also used to refer to a line segment with one endpoint at the center and the other on the circle. Likewise, the word "diameter" has two meanings. It is a line segment with endpoints on the circle containing the center, as well as being used to represent the length of such a line segment. It is common in geometry to let a word represent both a line segment and its length. You will be able to tell which meaning is intended from the context of the statement.

Q3   **a.** Identify the line segments that are radii. _____

b. Identify the line segments that are diameters. _____

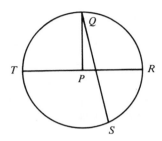

\# \# \#   •   \# \# \#   •   \# \# \#   •   \# \# \#   •   \# \# \#   •   \# \# \#   •   \# \# \#   •   \# \# \#   •   \# \# \#

A3   **a.** $\overline{TP}$, $\overline{PR}$, and $\overline{PQ}$ **b.** $\overline{TR}$

4   A *polygon* is a plane figure made up of line segments connected at their endpoints. Each endpoint is a *vertex* of the polygon. Some examples of polygons follow. Polygons are named for the number of

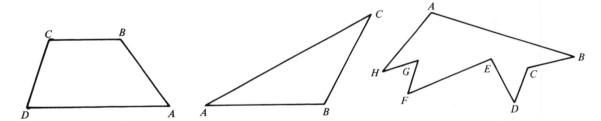

sides they have. In this text, three-sided polygons, called *triangles*, and four-sided polygons, called *quadrilaterals*, will be studied. You will probably not need to know the names of polygons with more sides, but each has a name. For example, a six-sided polygon is a hexagon, and an eight-sided polygon is a octagon.

Q4   Indicate whether each of the figures shown is a polygon:

a. _____   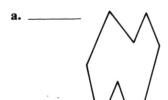   **b.** _____   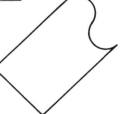   **c.** _____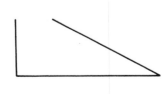

\# \# \#   •   \# \# \#   •   \# \# \#   •   \# \# \#   •   \# \# \#   •   \# \# \#   •   \# \# \#   •   \# \# \#   •   \# \# \#

A4   **a.** yes   **b.** no   **c.** no

Q5   Indicate whether each polygon is a triangle or a quadrilateral:

a. _____   **b.** _____   **c.** _____   **d.** _____

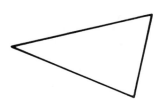 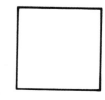 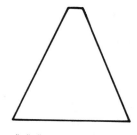 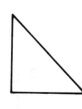

•   # # #   •   # # #   •   # # #   •   # # #   •   # # #   •   # # #   •   # # #   •   # #

A5   **a.** triangle   **b.** quadrilateral   **c.** quadrilateral   **d.** triangle

---

5   If one of the angles of a triangle is a right angle, the triangle is called a *right triangle*. Some examples of right triangles follow. The small square is placed in the angle which is the right angle.

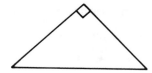

Q6   Measure the angles of the triangles to see if they are right triangles (indicate yes or no).

a. 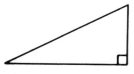   **b.**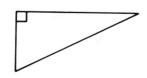

•   # # #   •   # # #   •   # # #   •   # # #   •   # # #   •   # # #   •   # # #   •   # #

A6   **a.** yes: $m \angle B = 90°$ **b.** no: $m \angle C = 100°$

---

6   If all three sides of a triangle have the same length, the triangle is *equilateral*.

If *two or more* sides of a triangle have the same length, it is *isosceles*. Notice by this definition that an equilateral triangle is also an isosceles triangle. Frequently we indicate the equal sides of a polygon by marking them with a short line through the sides.

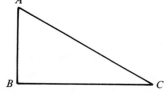

Equilateral triangle
and isosceles triangle

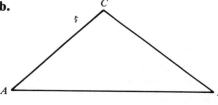

Isosceles triangle

Q7   **a.** By measuring the sides, determine which of the following triangles are equilateral. _____

b. Which triangles are isosceles? _____

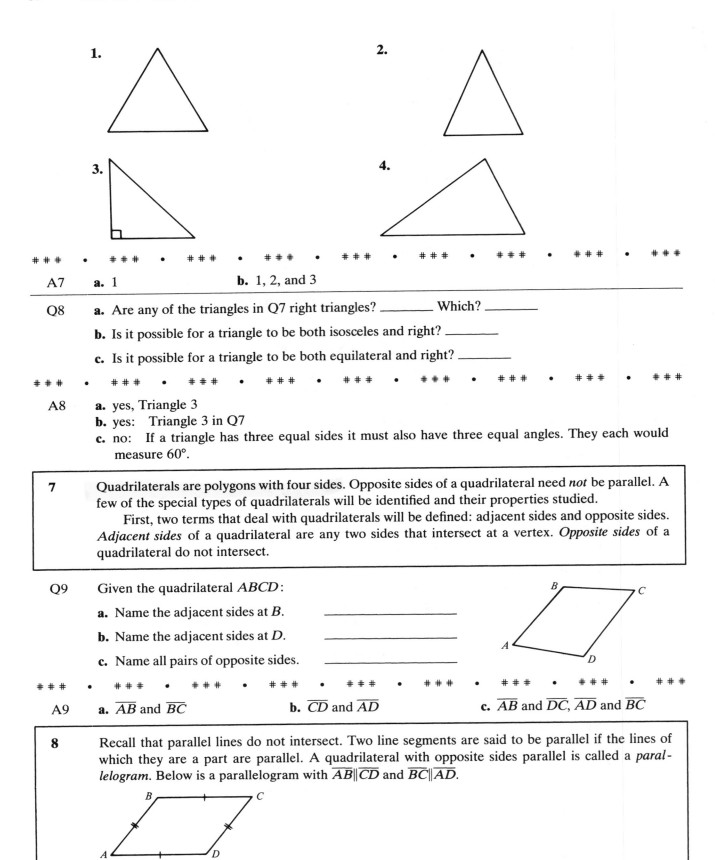

1.

2.

3.

4.

•   # # #   •   # # #   •   # # #   •   # # #   •   # # #   •   # # #   •   # # #   •   # #

A7   **a.** 1   **b.** 1, 2, and 3

Q8   **a.** Are any of the triangles in Q7 right triangles? _____ Which? _____

b. Is it possible for a triangle to be both isosceles and right? _____

c. Is it possible for a triangle to be both equilateral and right? _____

•   # # #   •   # # #   •   # # #   •   # # #   •   # # #   •   # # #   •   # # #   •   # #

A8   **a.** yes, Triangle 3
b. yes: Triangle 3 in Q7
c. no: If a triangle has three equal sides it must also have three equal angles. They each would
measure 60°.

---

7   Quadrilaterals are polygons with four sides. Opposite sides of a quadrilateral need *not* be parallel. A
few of the special types of quadrilaterals will be identified and their properties studied.

First, two terms that deal with quadrilaterals will be defined: adjacent sides and opposite sides.
Adjacent sides of a quadrilateral are any two sides that intersect at a vertex. *Opposite sides* of a
quadrilateral do not intersect.

Q9   Given the quadrilateral *ABCD*:

a. Name the adjacent sides at *B*.   _____

b. Name the adjacent sides at *D*.   _____

c. Name all pairs of opposite sides.   _____

•   # # #   •   # # #   •   # # #   •   # # #   •   # # #   •   # # #   •   # # #   •   # #

A9   **a.** $\overline{AB}$ and $\overline{BC}$ **b.** $\overline{CD}$ and $\overline{AD}$ **c.** $\overline{AB}$ and $\overline{DC}$, $\overline{AD}$ and $\overline{BC}$

---

8   Recall that parallel lines do not intersect. Two line segments are said to be parallel if the lines of
which they are a part are parallel. A quadrilateral with opposite sides parallel is called a *paral-
lelogram*. Below is a parallelogram with $\overline{AB}\|\overline{CD}$ and $\overline{BC}\|\overline{AD}$.

Parallelogram

Q10   The line segments $\overline{AB}$ and $\overline{CD}$ do not intersect. Why are they not considered parallel?

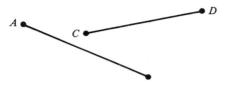

•   # # #   •   # # #   •   # # #   •   # # #   •   # # #   •   # # #   •   # # #   •   # #

A10   They are not parallel, because the lines of which they are a part are not parallel.

Q11   Which of the following figures appear to be parallelograms? _____

   a. 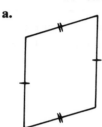   **b.** 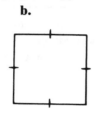   **c.** 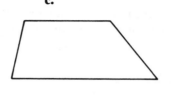   **d.**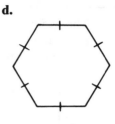

•   # # #   •   # # #   •   # # #   •   # # #   •   # # #   •   # # #   •   # # #   •   # #

A11   **a** and **b**: Notice that the opposite sides of figure **d** appear to be parallel. However, a parallelogram must first be a quadrilateral.

---

9   If the sides of a parallelogram meet at right angles, it is a *rectangle*. If the parallelogram's sides meet at right angles and are of equal length, it is a *square*. Notice that a square is a rectangle.
        The following quadrilateral is a rectangle as well as being a parallelogram:

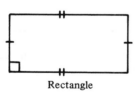

Rectangle

        The following quadrilateral is a square as well as being a rectangle and a parallelogram:

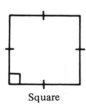

Square

Q12   List (in blanks on page 88) the letters of the appropriate geometric figures:

  a.   **b.**   **c.**   **d.**   **e.**

 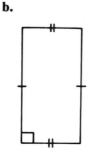 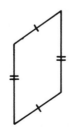 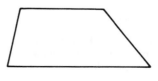 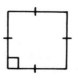

polygons   _____   rectangles   _____

quadrilaterals _____   squares   _____

parallelograms _____

•   # # #   •   # # #   •   # # #   •   # # #   •   # # #   •   # # #   •   # # #   •   # #

A12   polygons   **a, b, c, d, e**
       quadrilaterals   **b, c, d, e**
       parallelograms   **b, c, e**
       rectangles   **b, e**
       squares   **e**

---

10   The *perimeter* of a polygon is the total length of all its sides. For any geometric figure in a plane, the perimeter is the length of the boundary of the geometric figure. Notice that perimeter is a measure of length (distance). The perimeter, *p*, of a rectangle can be found by adding the lengths of the sides:

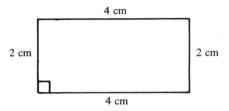

The perimeter of the rectangle would be

$p = 2 + 4 + 2 + 4$

$p = 12$

Therefore, the perimeter of the rectangle is 12 cm.

Q13   Which would have a larger perimeter, a triangle with each side 2 inches or a square with each side 2 inches? _____

•   # # #   •   # # #   •   # # #   •   # # #   •   # # #   •   # # #   •   # # #   •   # #

A13   square

Q14   Find the perimeter of the figures:

a.

b.

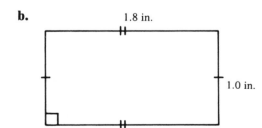

Note: It is the publisher's convention to abbreviate inch or inches as in. (with the period) to avoid confusion with the word *in*. Other English abbreviations (ft, yd, mi) will be used without the period. The units m, cm, and mm are metric symbols, not abbreviations; they are written without the period.

•   # # #   •   # # #   •   # # #   •   # # #   •   # # #   •   # # #   •   # # #   •   # #

A14   **a.** 12 cm: $p = 3 + 4 + 5$ **b.** 5.6 in.: $p = 1.8 + 1.0 + 1.8 + 1.0$
              $p = 12$ $p = 5.6$

---

11   For some geometric figures, formulas can be used to find the perimeter. A formula is an equation involving variables (letters) which tells what arithmetic operations must be performed to obtain the perimeter. For example, to find the perimeter of a rectangle, two lengths and two widths must be added together. This can be written as follows:

$p = 2l + 2w$

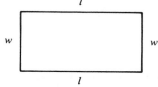

When a number and a variable are written side by side it means to multiply. Therefore $2w$ means 2 times w. The formula can be used as the example below shows.

Example: Find the perimeter of a rectangle with a length of 8 inches and a width of 3 inches.

Solution: First write the formula that you will use, then substitute the numbers for the corresponding variables and simplify.

$p = 2l + 2w$
$p = 2 \times 8 + 2 \times 3$*
$p = 16 + 6$
$p = 22$ inches

*2×8 can also be written 2(8) or (2)(8).

Q15   Find the perimeters of the following rectangles by substituting in the appropriate formula:

a.   8.0 mi   **b.**   1.6 ft

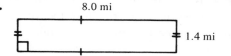   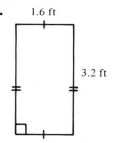

1.4 mi   3.2 ft

•   # # #   •   # # #   •   # # #   •   # # #   •   # # #   •   # # #   •   # # #   •   # #

A15   **a.** 18.8 mi: $p = 2l + 2w$ **b.** 9.6 ft: $p = 2l + 2w$
                  $p = 2(8.0) + 2(1.4)$ $p = 2(3.2) + 2(1.6)$
                  $p = 16.0 + 2.8$ $p = 6.4 + 3.2$
                  $p = 18.8$ $p = 9.6$

---

12   Since a square is a rectangle, the formula $p = 2l + 2w$ may be used. However, a shorter formula may be used also. Since all four sides of a square are the same length, the perimeter is four times the length of a side.

$p = 4s$

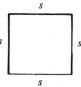

Q16   Find the perimeters of the square by using the formula $p = 4s$.

a.   22.0 cm

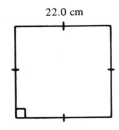

b. $1\frac{3}{4}$ in.

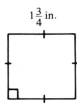

•   # # #   •   # # #   •   # # #   •   # # #   •   # # #   •   # # #   •   # # #   •   # #

A16   **a.** 88.0 cm: $p = 4s$

$p = 4(22.0)$

$p = 88.0$

b. 7 in.: $p = 4s$

$p = 4\left(1\frac{3}{4}\right)$

$p = 4\left(\frac{7}{4}\right)$

$p = 7$

---

13   The perimeter of a circle is called its *circumference*. The circumference of a circle is found with another formula. To obtain the circumference it is necessary to know the diameter of the circle and the value of the number π (pi). The number π is the ratio of the circumference to the diameter of a circle. The value of π is a constant; that is, it never changes. However, it is impossible to write a decimal or fraction that is exactly equal to π. Since all rational numbers* can be written as fractions, we conclude that π is not a rational number. One is therefore forced to use approximations of π rounded off to various numbers of decimal places. Since it is not possible to say that π *equals* another number, the symbol "$\doteq$" is used to mean approximately equal. The symbol "$\doteq$" says "is approximately equal to." Various approximations follow:

1. $\pi \doteq 3.14159265$, precise to 8 decimal places.

2. $\pi \doteq 3.14$, precise to 2 decimal places. This approximation is acceptable for calculations in this book.

3. $\pi \doteq 3\frac{1}{7}$, also precise to 2 decimal places. This value is commonly used when calculating with fractions.

4. $\pi \doteq \frac{355}{113}$, precise to 6 decimal places. This is an easy approximation to remember (think 1, 1, 3, 3, 5, 5) for use with an electronic calculator.

*See Section 6.6.

Q17   Is π a variable or a constant? _____

•   # # #   •   # # #   •   # # #   •   # # #   •   # # #   •   # # #   •   # # #   •   # #

A17   constant

Q18   **a.** Give two approximations of π that are precise to two decimal places. _____ and _____

b. Give two approximations of π that are precise to six decimal places. _____ and _____

•   # # #   •   # # #   •   # # #   •   # # #   •   # # #   •   # # #   •   # # #   •   # #

A18   **a.** 3.14 and $3\frac{1}{7}$ **b.** 3.141593 and $\frac{355}{113}$

Q19   Can an exact value for π be written as a decimal? _____

•   # # #   •   # # #   •   # # #   •   # # #   •   # # #   •   # # #   •   # # #   •   # #

A19   no

---

14   The circumference of a circle is found by using the formula $c = \pi d$, where d is the diameter. Since the diameter is twice the radius ($d = 2r$), a second formula for the circumference is $c = 2\pi r$, where r is the radius:

$c = 2\pi r = \pi d$

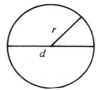

Example: If the diameter of a circle is 2.5 inches, what is its circumference? Round off to tenths.

Solution : $c = \pi d$
        $c = (3.14)(2.5)$
        $c = 7.850$

$d = 2.5$ in.

Therefore, the circumference is 7.9 in.

Use $\pi \doteq \frac{22}{7}$ when measurements are given as common fractions. Use $\pi \doteq 3.14$ when measurements are given as decimal fractions.

Q20   Find the circumference of a circle with diameter 8.5 cm (use $\pi \doteq 3.14$). Round off to ones.

•   # # #   •   # # #   •   # # #   •   # # #   •   # # #   •   # # #   •   # # #   •   # #

A20   27 cm: $c = \pi d$
          $c = (3.14)(8.5)$
          $c = 26.690$

Q21   What is the circumference of a circle whose *radius* is $4\frac{3}{4}$ ft? Use $c = 2\pi r$ and $\pi \doteq 3\frac{1}{7}$. Round off to ones.

•   # # #   •   # # #   •   # # #   •   # # #   •   # # #   •   # # #   •   # # #   •   # #

A21   30 ft: $c = 2\pi r$

$$c = 2\left(3\frac{1}{7}\right)\left(4\frac{3}{4}\right)$$

$$c = \frac{2}{1}\left(\frac{22}{7}\right)\left(\frac{19}{4}\right)$$

$$c = 29\frac{6}{7}$$

---

15   The *area* of a polygon or circle is a measure of the region inside it. The units used to measure area are square units.

A square with all four sides 1 inch long is said to have an area of 1 square inch. This area is considered to be a unit, and areas of other closed figures are given as some number of square inches. "Square inch" will be symbolized as in.^{2} Other square units will be symbolized in a similar manner, that is, square feet as ft^2, square centimeters as cm^2, and so on. The figures below show a square inch, and also a rectangle with an area of 6 square inches. This area may be obtained by counting.

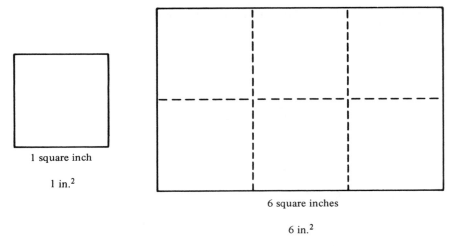

1 square inch

1 in.^{2}

6 square inches

6 in.^{2}

The area of the rectangle can also be obtained by a formula. To find the area of a rectangle, multiply the length times the width. The formula is $A = lw$.

$A = lw$
$A = 2 \cdot 3$*
$A = 6$

Therefore, the area of the rectangle is 6 in.^{2}

*The raised dot also indicates multiplication.

Q22   Find the area of a rectangular floor with one dimension 10.5 ft and the other dimension 12.0 ft. Round off to a whole number.

\# \# \#   •   \# \# \#   •   \# \# \#   •   \# \# \#   •   \# \# \#   •   \# \# \#   •   \# \# \#   •   \# \# \#   •   \# \# \#

A22   126 ft^2: $A = lw$
$A = 12.0 \cdot 10.5$
$A = 126.00$

Q23 Find the area in square yards of a rectangular lot with dimensions 30 yd 2 ft by 53 yd 1 ft.

\# \# \# • \# \# \# • \# \# \# • \# \# \# • \# \# \# • \# \# \# • \# \# \# • \# \# \# • \# \# \#

A23 $1,635\frac{5}{9}$ yd^2: 30 yd 2 ft $= 30\frac{2}{3}$ yd $A = lw$

$\qquad\qquad\qquad$ 53 yd 1 ft $= 53\frac{1}{3}$ yd $A = 53\frac{1}{3} \cdot 30\frac{2}{3}$

$\qquad\qquad\qquad\qquad\qquad\qquad\qquad\qquad$ $A = 1,635\frac{5}{9}$

---

16 The formula for the area of a square is a special case of the formula for the area of a rectangle. If $l = w$ in the formula $A = lw$, then it becomes $A = ww = w^2$. Rather than using w for the width of a square, the variable s is usually used. Therefore, the area of a square is computed with the formula

$A = s^2$ (Note: s^2 means $s \times s$ and is read "s squared.")

Example: Find the area of a square card table that is 30 inches on a side.

Solution: $A = s^2$
$\qquad\quad$ $A = 30^2$
$\qquad\quad$ $A = 900$

Therefore, the area is 900 in^2.

Q24 Find the area of a field that is 45 yards square. Round off to hundreds.

\# \# \# • \# \# \# • \# \# \# • \# \# \# • \# \# \# • \# \# \# • \# \# \# • \# \# \# • \# \# \#

A24 2,000 yd^2: $A = s^2$
$\qquad\qquad\qquad$ $A = 45^2$
$\qquad\qquad\qquad$ $A = 2,025$

---

17 The following figure is a parallelogram. The opposite sides are parallel. The bases of a parallelogram are any two opposite sides (usually the longest side is considered a base). The altitude, h, of a parallelogram is the perpendicular distance between the bases.

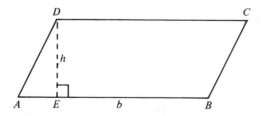

Example 1: Name the bases of the parallelogram.

Solution: $\overline{AB}$ and $\overline{DC}$ ($\overline{AD}$ and $\overline{BC}$ could be considered bases, but it would not be as convenient to find the altitude.)

Example 2: The altitude of parallelogram *ABCD* is the length of what line segment?

Solution: $\overline{DE}$

The area of a parallelogram is found by multiplying the length of a base, *b*, times the altitude (height), *h*. The formula is

$A = bh$

Example 3: Find the area of a parallelogram with base 22 cm and altitude 14 cm.

Solution: $A = bh$
 $A = 22(14)$
 $A = 308$ Therefore, the area is 308 cm^2.

Q25   **a.** Find the area of a parallelogram with base 202 m and altitude 26 m. (Round off to hundreds.)

 **b.** Find the area of the parallelogram. (Round off to tens.)

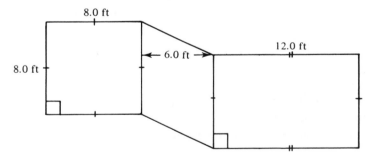

•   # # #   •   # # #   •   # # #   •   # # #   •   # # #   •   # # #   •   # # #   •   # #

A25   **a.** 5300 m^2: $A = bh$ **b.** 210 ft^2: $A = bh$
 $A = 202(26)$ $A = 26(8)$
 $A = 5252$ $A = 208$

Q26   Find the total area of the space enclosed in the following floor plan:

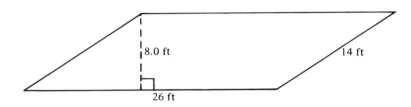

•   # # #   •   # # #   •   # # #   •   # # #   •   # # #   •   # # #   •   # # #   •   # #

A26   208 ft^2: $A = s^2$ $A = bh$ $A = lw$
 $A = 8.0^2$ $A = (8.0)(6.0)$ $A = (12.0)(8.0)$
 $A = 64$ $A = 48$ $A = 96$

18   The formula for the area of the triangle *ABC* with base *b* and altitude *h* may be found by drawing another triangle with the same size and shape upside down above it.

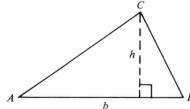
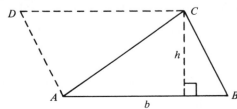

Since triangles ABC and ACD have the same area, the area of triangle ABC is equal to one half the area within parallelogram $ABCD$.

area of triangle $ABC = \dfrac{1}{2}$ area of parallelogram $ABCD = \dfrac{1}{2}bh$

The formula for the area of a triangle with base b and altitude h is $A = \dfrac{1}{2}bh$.

Example: Find the area of a triangle with base 10.5 m and altitude 5.6 m. Round off to a whole number.

Solution: $A = \dfrac{1}{2}bh$

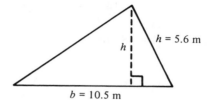

$A = \dfrac{1}{2}(10.5)(5.6)$

$A = 29.40$

Therefore, the area of the triangle is 29 m².

Q27 Find the area of a triangle with base 4.6 cm and altitude 3.7 cm. Round off to tenths.

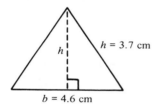

• # # # • # # # • # # # • # # # • # # # • # # # • # # # • # #

A27 8.5 cm²: $A = \dfrac{1}{2}bh$

$A = \dfrac{1}{2}(4.6)(3.7)$

$A = 8.51$

Q28 Find the area of a triangle with base 4.2 ft and altitude 4.0 yd. Round off to a whole number.

• # # # • # # # • # # # • # # # • # # # • # # # • # # # • # #

A28 25 ft²: $A = \dfrac{1}{2}bh$

$A = \dfrac{1}{2}(4.2)(12.0)$

$A = 25.2$

19 The area of a circle is found with a formula that contains the constant π. The values of 3.14 or $3\dfrac{1}{7}$ may be used for the problems of this section.

The area of a circle with radius r is given by

$A = \pi r^2$

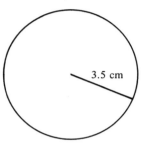

Example: If the radius of a circle is 3.5 cm, find the area of the circle. Round off to a whole number.

Solution: $A = \pi r^2$
$A = (3.14)(3.5)^2$
$A = (3.14)(12.25)$
$A = 38.4650$

3.5 cm

Therefore, the area is 38 cm².

Q29   Find the area of a circle with radius 2.5 feet (use $\pi \doteq 3.14$ when you are given a measurement in decimal form). Round off to a whole number.

•   # # #   •   # # #   •   # # #   •   # # #   •   # # #   •   # # #   •   # # #   •   # #

A29   20 ft²: $A = \pi r^2$
$A = (3.14)(2.5)(2.5)$
$A = 19.6250$

Q30   Find the area of the following region. (*Hint*: To find the area of a semicircular region, take $\frac{1}{2}$ the area of a circular region of the same radius.) Round off to a whole number of square feet.

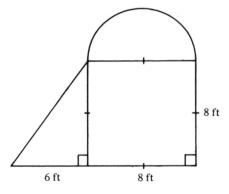

8 ft

6 ft   8 ft

•   # # #   •   # # #   •   # # #   •   # # #   •   # # #   •   # # #   •   # # #   •   # #

A30   113 ft²: $A = \frac{1}{2}bh$ $A = s^2$ $A = \frac{1}{2}\pi r^2$

$A = \frac{1}{2}(6)(8)$ $A = 8^2$ $A = \frac{1}{2}(3.14)(4)^2$

$A = 24$ $A = 64$ $A = 25.12$
                        $A = 25$

total area $= 24 + 64 + 25 = 113$ ft²

20   This section will be concluded with a summary of the formulas that are used to compute area and perimeters.

Geometric figures	Formula for area	Formula for perimeter
Triangle	$A = \frac{1}{2}bh$	$p = a + b + c$
Square	$A = s^2$	$p = 4s$
Rectangle	$A = lw$	$p = 2l + 2w$
Parallelogram	$A = bh$	$p = 2a + 2b$
Circle	$A = \pi r^2$	$c = 2\pi r$ or $c = \pi d$

This completes the instruction for this section.

3.2   EXERCISE

1. A patient's waist is measured and found to be a circle with diameter 7 inches. A tumor is located at the center of the circle. How far below the surface of the skin is the tumor?

2. Use the figure at the right to identify the following by name:

   a. The point P is called the _____.

   b. $\overline{PB}$ is a _____.

   c. $\overline{AC}$ is a _____.

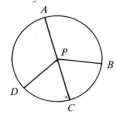

3. Name the following goemetric figures.

   a.   **b.**   **c.**   **d.**

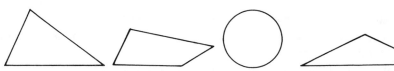

4. In medicine, many regions of the body are named as a triangle. For example, Alsberg's triangle is formed by a line drawn through the long axis of the neck of the femur, a second through the center of the diaphysis and continued upward, and a third transversely at the level of the base of the femoral head. This triangle is sometimes an equilateral triangle. Measure to see if the pictured Alsberg's triangle is equilateral.

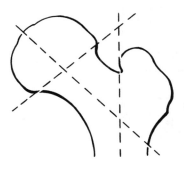

Alsberg's triangle

5. List the letters of the appropriate triangles:

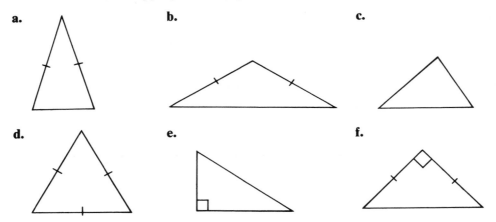

a.   **b.**   **c.**

d.   **e.**   **f.**

     a. equilateral triangles   **b.** isosceles triangles   **c.** right triangles

6. How many pairs of parallel sides are contained in a parallelogram?

7. Is a square a rectangle?

8. Is a rectangle a parallelogram?

9. Is a square a parallelogram?

10. Is a square a polygon?

11. Is a rectangle a square?

12. Is a parallelogram a rectangle?

13. A square is rectangle with what further restriction?

14. A rectangle is a parallelogram with what further restriction?

15. A person must walk $\frac{1}{2}$ mile on a rectangular path as a part of their physical therapy.

     a. If the path is 20 ft × 40 ft, how far does the person walk in traversing the perimeter one time?

     b. If a person makes 25 rounds will they have surpassed their $\frac{1}{2}$ mile (2,640 ft)?

16. Find the perimeter of a square that has a side of 0.5 centimetres.

17. Assuming the head of a newborn child is circular (which it is not), find the circumference based on a diameter of 9.2 centimetres.

18. Find the area of a rectangular shaped burn with dimensions 4.5 cm × 9.0 cm.

19. A hemocytometer is a glass instrument used to hold diluted blood in order to count blood cells under a microscope. It consists of a "large" square 3 millimetres (mm) on a side which is subdivided into 9 squares (cells) each with side 1 mm (Figure 1). In Figure 2 it can be seen that cells 1, 2, 3, and 4 are further subdivided into smaller squares with sides of 0.25 mm. Cell 5 is subdivided into smaller squares of 0.2 mm on a side. A scale drawing is shown below:

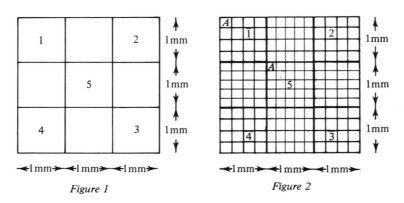

Figure 1   *Figure 2*

a. Find the area of the 3 mm × 3 mm square in Figure 1.
b. Find the area of square number 1 in Figure 1.
c. Find the area of square number 5 in Figure 1.
d. Find the area of square 1A in Figure 2.
e. Find the area of square 5A in Figure 2.

20. Because of the small air chambers in the lungs the surface area between the body and the environment is much greater in the lungs than other portions of the body. It requires approximately one square metre of lung surface for each kilogram (kg) of body weight in order to sustain life processes. This, in common language, is said to be the area of a tennis court. Check this conjecture for a man that weighs 90 kilograms (198 lb). A singles court is 8.2 m × 23.8 m.

21. Find the area of a circular x-ray with diameter 9 inches. (Use $\pi = 3.14$.)

3.2 EXERCISE ANSWERS

1. 3.5 inches   **2. a.** center   **b.** radius   **c.** diameter
3. a. triangle   **b.** quadrilateral   **c.** circle   **d.** triangle
4. It is not.   **5. a.** d   **b.** a, b, d, and f   **c.** e and f
6. two pairs   **7.** yes   **8.** yes   **9.** yes
10. yes   **11.** no, not necessarily   **12.** no, not necessarily
13. All sides are of equal measure.   **14.** The angles at the vertices have measure 90°.
15. a. 120 feet   **b.** yes   **16.** 2.0 centimetres
17. 28.888 centimetres   **18.** 40.5 square centimetres
19. a. 9 mm^2 **b.** 1 mm^2 **c.** 1 mm^2 **d.** 0.0625 mm^2 **e.** 0.04 mm^2

20. not true: The area of the lung of a 90 kg man is closer to $\frac{1}{2}$ a tennis court. The area of the court is 195.16 m^2 while the area of the lung of a 90 kg man is 90 m^2.

21. 63.585 in^2.

3.3 SOLID GEOMETRIC FIGURES

1   There is a geometric term for solid shapes with flat surfaces. They are called polyhedra. A *polyhedron* is defined as a geometric solid whose surfaces are polygons. Some examples of polyhedra are shown.

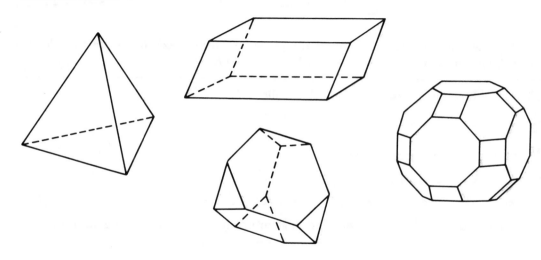

The polygons which form the surface of the polyhedron are called *faces*. The sides of the faces are now called *edges* of the polyhedron. The vertices of the faces are the *vertices* of the polyhedron.

Q1   One common polyhedron is the cube. Examine the cube shown next. You see seven of its eight vertices. Suppose the one you do not see is labeled *E*. Use your imagination to complete the following:

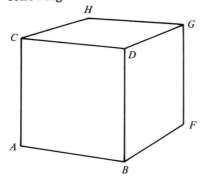

vertices = _____

edges   = _____

\# \# \# • \# \# \# • \# \# \# • \# \# \# • \# \# \# • \# \# \# • \# \# \# • \# \# \# • \# \# \#

A1   vertices = *A, B, C, D, E, F, G, H*
      edges   = $\overline{AB}, \overline{BD}, \overline{DC}, \overline{CA}, \overline{BF}, \overline{DG}, \overline{CH}, \overline{AE}, \overline{EF}, \overline{FG}, \overline{GH}, \overline{HE}$

2   The polyhedra discussed in this text will be limited to prisms and pyramids. A prism is a polyhedron with two faces which are polygons of the same size and shape and which lie in parallel planes; the remaining faces are parallelograms. The two faces that are parallel to each other are called *bases*. The remaining faces are called *lateral* faces. Some examples:

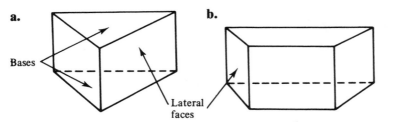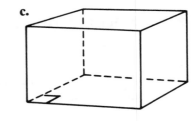

The base determines the name of the prism. A prism whose bases are triangles is called a *triangular prism*; a prism whose bases are hexagons is a *hexangular prism*; and so on.

Q2   What would the three prisms in Frame 2 be called?

a. _____

b. _____

c. _____

\# \# \# • \# \# \# • \# \# \# • \# \# \# • \# \# \# • \# \# \# • \# \# \# • \# \# \# • \# \# \#

A2   **a.** triangular prism   **b.** quadrangular prism   **c.** rectangular prism

Q3   Give the descriptive name of each prism; otherwise, indicate "not a prism":

a.   **b.**   **c.**   **d.**   **e.**

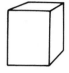 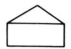 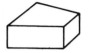 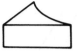

a. _____   b. _____

c. _____   d. _____

e. _____

• # # # • # # # • # # # • # # # • # # # • # # # • # # # • # #

A3   **a.** rectangular prism (any of the rectangular faces could be considered the base)
      b. triangular prism
      c. quadrangular prism
      d. not a prism: The base is not a polygon.
      e. not a prism: The base is not a polygon.

---

3   The following polyhedra are pyramids. A *pyramid* is formed by a polygon called the *base* and a point outside the plane containing the base called the *apex*. A pyramid is the solid formed by all the points in the polygon of the base and all triangles formed by segments between the vertices of the base and the apex.

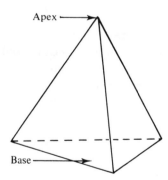 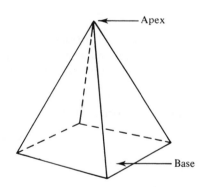

The *altitude* of a pyramid is a segment from the apex perpendicular to the base. The altitude also is the length of this segment. The apex along with the vertices of the base are the vertices of the pyramid. Pyramids are classified and named according to the shape of their base. One with a triangular base is a triangular pyramid; one with a rectangular base is a rectangular pyramid; and so on.

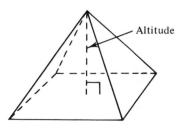

Q4   Name the polyhedra below:

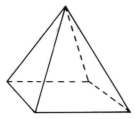   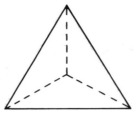

a. _____   **b.** _____

＃＃＃ • ＃＃＃ • ＃＃＃ • ＃＃＃ • ＃＃＃ • ＃＃＃ • ＃＃＃ • ＃＃＃ • ＃＃＃

A4   **a.** rectangular pyramid   **b.** triangular pyramid

---

4   Although cylinders, cones, and spheres are geometric solids they are not polyhedra because of their curved surfaces. Circular cylinders are not difficult to recognize. Some examples are shown here.

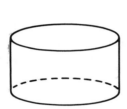 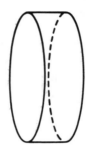 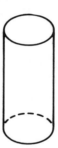

A right-circular cylinder is a solid formed by two circles with the same radius, called bases, connected by line segments perpendicular to the planes of the two circles. Because only right-circular cylinders are discussed in this text, we shall refer to them simply as "cylinders."

Q5   Which of the following have a cylindrical shape?   _____

a. round pencil

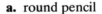

b. wastebasket

c. section of a water pipe

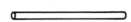

d. beer can

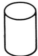

e. cigarette

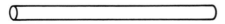

f. cigar

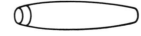

＃＃＃ • ＃＃＃ • ＃＃＃ • ＃＃＃ • ＃＃＃ • ＃＃＃ • ＃＃＃ • ＃＃＃ • ＃＃＃

A5   **a, c, d**, and **e: b** is not because the circles do not have the same radius; **f** is not because the bases are not connected with line segments.

---

5   The curved surface connecting the bases is called the *lateral surface*. The *axis* of a cylinder is the line segment that connects the centers of the bases of the cylinder. The length of the axis is the *altitude* of a cylinder. The radius of the circular base is the radius of the cylinder.

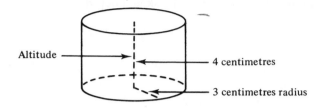

Altitude ⟶ 4 centimetres

3 centimetres radius

Q6   **a.** The radius of the cylinder is _____.

b. The altitude of the cylinder is _____.

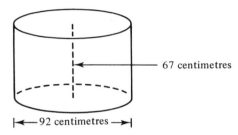

67 centimetres

|←—92 centimetres —→|

• # # # • # # # • # # # • # # # • # # # • # # # • # # # • # #

A6   **a.** 46 cm   **b.** 67 cm

---

6   A right-circular *cone* is a solid formed by a circle and the line segments connecting the circle with a point located on a line through the center of the circle and perpendicular to the plane of the circle.

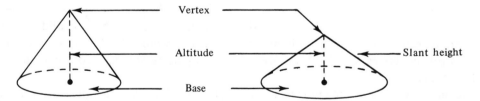

Vertex

Altitude   Slant height

Base

The circle is called the *base*. The point to which the base is connected is the *vertex*. The line segment connecting the vertex to the center of the base is the *altitude*. The *slant height* of a right-circular cone is a line segment from the vertex to a point on the circle of the base. The attitude and slant height also sometimes represent the length of these respective segments.

Q7   Use the sketch to complete the sentences below:

a. $\overline{OP}$ is the _____ of the right-circular cone.

b. The length of $\overline{PQ}$ is the _____ of the cone.

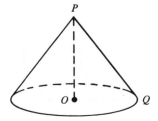

• # # # • # # # • # # # • # # # • # # # • # # # • # # # • # #

A7   **a.** altitude   **b.** slant height

---

7   A *sphere* is the solid formed by all points in space at some fixed distance from a fixed point called the *center*. A *radius* of the sphere is a line segment connecting a point on the sphere with the center. A *diameter* of the sphere is a line segment containing the center with endpoints on the sphere. "Radius" and "diameter" also are used to represent the lengths of these segments. A sketch of a sphere is shown. Notice how the dashed lines are used to give the sketch depth.

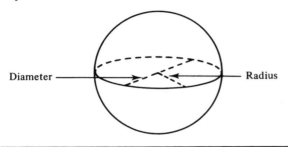

Diameter ——————— Radius

Q8   **a.** Name a diameter of the sphere. ————

   b. Name a radius of the sphere. ————

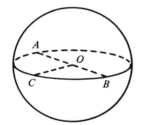   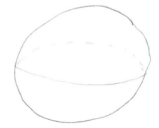

   c. If $\overline{AB}$ is 12 metres long, how long is $\overline{OC}$? ————

• # # # • # # # • # # # • # # # • # # # • # # # • # # # • # #

A8   **a.** $\overline{AB}$ **b.** $\overline{OA}$, $\overline{OB}$, or $\overline{OC}$ **c.** 6 metres

---

8   *Volume* is a measure of the space within a closed solid figure. Irregular-shaped solid figures have volume, but the measurement of these volumes is difficult to obtain. The volumes of certain solid figures, such as prisms, cones, and spheres, are obtained by using standard formulas that will be studied in this chapter.

   One basic unit of volume is the cubic inch. This is a cube with each edge measuring 1 inch. To find the volume of a rectangular prism in cubic inches, think of the number of cubes, 1 inch on each edge, that could be stacked inside the prism.

l = length, 5 in.
h = height, 4 in.
w = width, 3 in.
V = volume, 60 in.^{3}

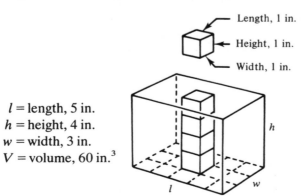

Length, 1 in.

Height, 1 in.

Width, 1 in.

The prism shown above would have 15 cubes on the bottom level. This is the same number as the area of the rectangular base. Above *each* of these bottom cubes would be three more, making a stack 4 cubes high. Therefore, the total volume would be 60 cubic inches. "Cubic inch" will be symbolized by "in.^{3}" Other cubic units will be symbolized in a similar manner, that is, cubic centimetres as cm^3, cubic yards as yd^3, and so on.

Q9   Use the method of Frame 8 to determine the volume of the prism at the right. _____

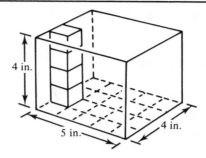

\# \# \# • \# \# \# • \# \# \# • \# \# \# • \# \# \# • \# \# \# • \# \# \# • \# \# \# • \# \# \#

A9   80 in.^{3}

9   The volume of a prism can be obtained from the dimensions: the length (l), width (w), and height (h). Just as the volume of the rectangular prism in Frame 8 could be found by multiplying the length times the width to get the area of the base and then multiplying that times the height, the volume of any rectangular prism may be found the same way. The formula would be $V = lwh$.

Example: Find the volume of the prism. Round off to tens.

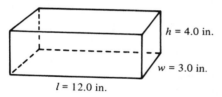

$h = 4.0$ in.

$w = 3.0$ in.

$l = 12.0$ in.

Solution: $V = lwh$
    $V = (12.0)(3.0)(4.0)$
    $V = 144.000$

Therefore, the volume is 140 cubic inches.

Q10   Find the volumes of the following prisms:
    a. Round off to tens.

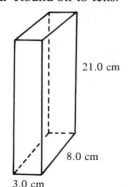

21.0 cm

8.0 cm

3.0 cm

    b. Round off to tenths.

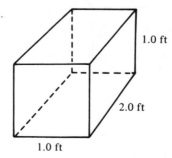

1.0 ft

2.0 ft

1.0 ft

\# \# \# • \# \# \# • \# \# \# • \# \# \# • \# \# \# • \# \# \# • \# \# \# • \# \# \# • \# \# \#

A10   **a.** 500 cm^3: $V = lwh$
                        $V = (3.0)(8.0)(21.0)$
                        $V = 504.000$

b. 2.0 ft^3: $V = lwh$
                $V = (1.0)(2.0)(1.0)$
                $V = 2.000$

---

10   The formula for the volume of a rectangular prism fits a general form that can also be used for all prisms and cylinders. The volume of each is found by multiplying the area of the base B by the altitude (height perpendicular to the base) h:

$$V = Bh$$

More specific formulas follow:

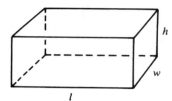

Rectangular prism
$V = Bh$
$V = lwh$

Area of the base
$B = lw$

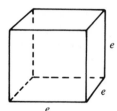

Cube
$V = Be$
$V = e^2 e$
$V = e^3$

Area of the base
$B = e^2$

(Note: e^3 means $e \times e \times e$ and is read "e cubed.")

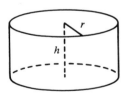

Cylinder
$V = Bh$
$V = \pi r^2 h$

Area of the base
$B = \pi r^2$

Q11   Find the volume of each of the prisms (round answer off to the nearest tens):

   a.

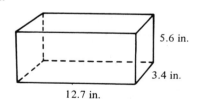

5.6 in.

3.4 in.

12.7 in.

   b.

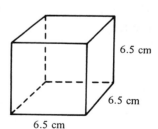

6.5 cm

6.5 cm

6.5 cm

•   # # #   •   # # #   •   # # #   •   # # #   •   # # #   •   # # #   •   # # #   •   # #

A11   **a.** 240 in.^3: $V = lwh$
                      $V = (12.7)(3.4)(5.6)$
                      $V = 241.808$

b. 270 cm^3: $V = e^3$
               $V = 6.5^3$
               $V = 274.625$

Q12   Find the volume of the following cylinders:

    a. Round off to tens.   **b.** Round off to hundreds.

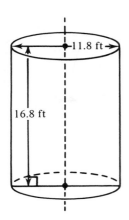

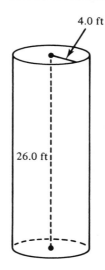

\# \# \# • \# \# \# • \# \# \# • \# \# \# • \# \# \# • \# \# \# • \# \# \# • \# \# \# • \# \# \# • \# \# \#

A12   **a.** $1,840 \text{ ft}^3$: $V = \pi r^2 h = (3.14)(5.9)(5.9)(16.8)$
$$V = 1,836.29712$$

        b. $1,300 \text{ ft}^3$: $V = \pi r^2 h = (3.14)(4.0)(4.0)(26.0)$
$$V = 1,306.24$$

---

11   The volume of pyramids and cones are related to the volume of the prism or cylinder with the same base and altitude. Consider the following figures:

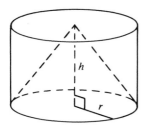   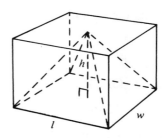

Volume of cylinder: $V = \pi r^2 h$ Volume of prism: $V = lwh$

Volume of cone: $V = \dfrac{1}{3}\pi r^2 h$ Volume of pyramid: $V = \dfrac{1}{3}lwh$

The volume of a pyramid or cone is always one-third of the area of the base times the altitude. This applies to all pyramids, no matter what the shape of the base.

$$V = \frac{1}{3}Bh$$

Q13   Find the volume of the following figures:
      a. Round off to tens.   **b.** Round off to thousands.

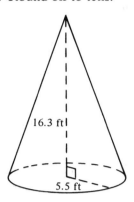

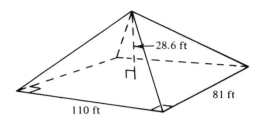

\# \# \# • \# \# \# • \# \# \# • \# \# \# • \# \# \# • \# \# \# • \# \# \# • \# \# \# • \# \# \#

A13   **a.** 520 ft^3: $V = \dfrac{1}{3}\pi r^2 h$ **b.** $85{,}000\text{ ft}^3$: $V = \dfrac{1}{3}lwh$

$$V = \frac{1}{3}(3.14)(5.5)(5.5)(16.3) \qquad\qquad V = \frac{1}{3}(110)(81)(28.6)$$

$$V = 516.08517 \qquad\qquad\qquad\qquad\qquad V = 84{,}942$$

---

12   The volume of a sphere is found with the formula

$$V = \frac{4}{3}\pi r^3$$

r = 2.4 ft

Example: Find the volume of the sphere above with $r = 2.4$ ft. Round off to a whole number.

Solution: $V = \dfrac{4}{3}\pi r^3$

$$V = \frac{4}{3}(3.14)(2.4)(2.4)(2.4)$$

$$V = 57.87648$$

Therefore, the volume is 58 ft^3.

Q14   Find the volume of a sphere with radius 8.4 in. Round off to hundreds.

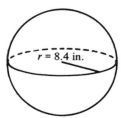

\# \# \# • \# \# \# • \# \# \# • \# \# \# • \# \# \# • \# \# \# • \# \# \# • \# \# \# • \# \# \#

A14   2,500 in.^{3}: $V = \frac{4}{3}\pi r^3$

$V = \frac{4}{3}(3.14)(8.4)(8.4)(8.4)$

$V = 2,481.4540$

---

13   This section will close with a summary of the formulas for volume.

Geometric figure	Formula for volume
Prism or cylinder	$V = Bh$, where B is the area of the base
Cube	$V = e^3$
Rectangular prism	$V = lwh$
Cylinder	$V = \pi r^2 h$
Cone	$V = \frac{1}{3}\pi r^2 h$
Pyramid	$V = \frac{1}{3}Bh$, where B is the area of the base
Sphere	$V = \frac{4}{3}\pi r^3$

This completes the instruction for this section.

3.3   EXERCISE

1. Specifically name each polyhedron:

a. 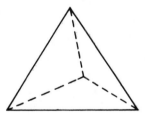   b. 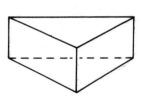   c.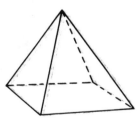

d. 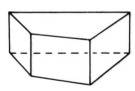   e. 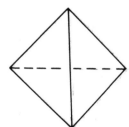   f.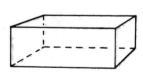

2. Below is a rectangular prism:
   a. How many faces does it have?
   b. How many edges does it have?
   c. How many vertices does it have?

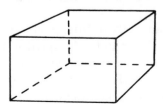

3. Find the volume of a rectangular prism that is 5 cm by 3 cm by 10 cm.

4. The hemocytometer mentioned in Exercise 3.2, problem 19, is actually a prism. The length and width are 3 mm each and the depth is 0.1 mm. The diagram below indicates a view from the top as you would see through a microscope, but each rectangular area is actually the top of a prism 0.1 mm deep, thus holding a volume of diluted blood. The squares 1, 2, 3, and 4 are subdivided into squares 0.25 mm on a side and square 5 is subdivided into squares 0.2 mm on a side. Refer to the following scale drawings.

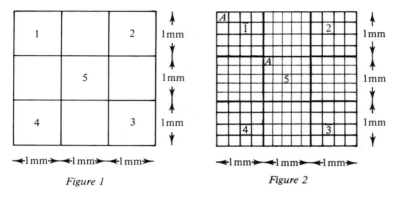

Figure 1   Figure 2

  a. What is the volume of prism 1?
  b. What is the volume of prisms 1, 2, 3, 4, and 5 combined?
  c. What is the volume of prism 1A?
  d. What is the volume of prism 5A?

5. If 21% of air is oxygen at sea level, how many cubic feet of pure oxygen is there in a room with dimensions 10 ft by 15 ft by 8 ft?

6. Name each of the geometric solids:

  a.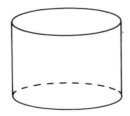

  b.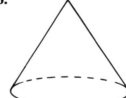

  c.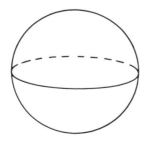

7. In a test tube of diameter 1.0 cm, what is the volume of a column of blood 6.0 cm long? Round off to tenths.

8. Find the volume of a cone with radius 5.0 cm and altitude 8.0 cm. Round off to tens.

9. In a typical positive-pressure, time-cycled ventilator the gas to be delivered to the patient is drawn into a cylindrical bellows of radius 8 cm (section D, next page) and then forced out of the bellows with pressure below it which raises the bellows. How much gas is delivered to the patient when the bottom of the bellows is raised 12 cm? Round off to hundreds.

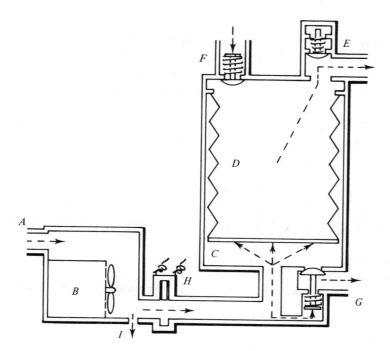

10. In a double-circuit, time-cycled piston ventilating machine, a spherical breathing bag fills with patient gas when a negative pressure is created in section 2 of the diagram. When a positive pressure is created in section 2 the balloon is diminished. What volume of air is contained in a breathing bag with a radius of 6.2 cm? Round off to tens.

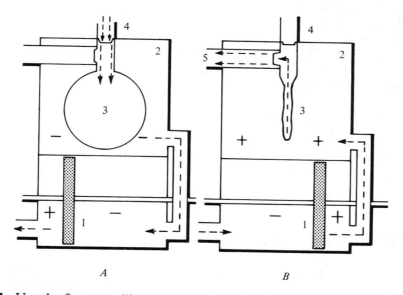

11. Use the figures to identify the line segments or points (see top of page 112):

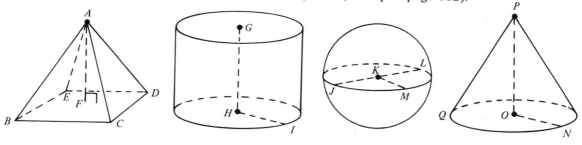

a. vertex of a cone
c. diameter of a sphere
e. radius of a cylinder
g. center of a sphere
i. slant height of a cone
k. altitude of a cylinder

b. radius of a sphere
d. radius of a cone
f. altitude of a cone
h. apex of a pyramid
j. altitude of a pyramid

12. The beam of x-radiation is delimited so as to irradiate only the area under examination. The diameter of the beam of radiation is reduced to the required area through the use of x-ray proof cones. The circular end of a cone of an x-ray machine has a diameter of 4.8 inches. What is its radius?

13. When the distance from the focus to the film (focus-film distance) increases, the area of the exposed surface increases also. If the focus–film distance changes from 10 inches to 20 inches (on the figure this is $\overline{IK}$ and $\overline{IJ}$), the side of the square exposed changes from 6 inches to 12 inches.
   a. Find the original area of exposure $ABCD$.
   b. Find the new area of exposure $EFGH$.
   c. When the focus–film distance was made twice as great, how many times greater was the new area?

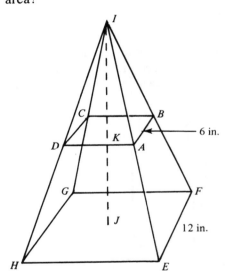

3.3   EXERCISE ANSWERS

1. a. triangular pyramid
   d. quadrangular prism

   b. triangular prism
   e. triangular pyramid

   c. rectangular pyramid
   f. rectangular prism

2. a. 6   b. 12   c. 8   3. 150 cm³

4. a. 0.1 mm³   b. 0.5 mm³   c. 0.00625 mm³   d. 0.004 mm³

5. 252 ft³   6. a. cylinder   b. cone   c. sphere

7. 4.7 cm³   8. 210 cm³   9. 2400 cm³   10. 1000 cm³

11. a. P b. $\overline{KM}$, $\overline{KJ}$, or $\overline{KL}$ c. $\overline{JL}$
    d. $\overline{ON}$ e. $\overline{HI}$ f. $\overline{PO}$
    g. K h. A i. $\overline{PQ}$ or $\overline{PN}$
    j. $\overline{AF}$ k. $\overline{GH}$

12. 2.4 inches   13. a. 36 in.²   b. 144 in.²   c. 4 times

CHAPTER 3 SAMPLE TEST

At the completion of Chapter 3 you should be able to work the following problems.

3.1 POINTS, LINES, AND ANGLES

1. **a.** Name the line that intersects $\overleftrightarrow{AE}$ at B.
   b. Name the line that appears to be parallel to $\overleftrightarrow{AC}$.
   c. Name the intersection of $\overleftrightarrow{AC}$ and $\overleftrightarrow{BC}$.
   d. Name the intersection of $\overleftrightarrow{AE}$ and $\overleftrightarrow{DB}$.
   e. Name a line segment that includes E.
   f. Name a point on $\overrightarrow{BE}$ that is not on $\overline{BE}$.
   g. Name three segments on $\overrightarrow{CB}$.

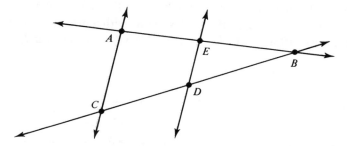

2. Fill in the blank with the appropriate symbol to indicate parallel or perpendicular:

   a. $\overleftrightarrow{AB}$_____$\overleftrightarrow{CD}$

   b. $\overleftrightarrow{EF}$_____$\overleftrightarrow{AB}$

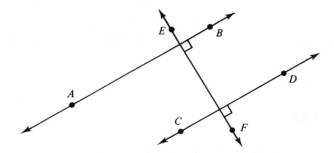

3. Read the measurements at the letters indicated in either inches or centimetres:

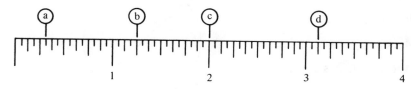

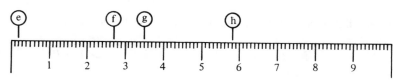

1-mm units

4. Name four rays on the line below.

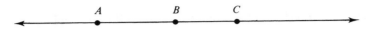

5. a. Name ∡*DBE* in another way.

    b. ∡*DBF* is a _____ angle.
    c. Name ∡1 using three letters.
    d. Name two supplementary angles.
    e. Name two complementary angles.

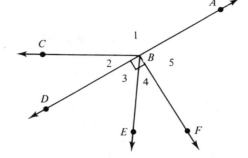

6. To prepare a dry smear of blood, one slide is held at a 30° angle to the other and moved in the direction of the arrow. If the angle is too great the blood collects in front and if the angle is too small the blood collects behind. Measure the angles below with a protractor to find the example which is being held correctly. (Source: *Color Atlas and Textbook of Hematology.*)

a.

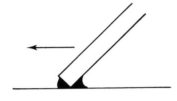

b.

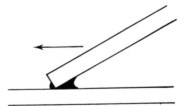

c.

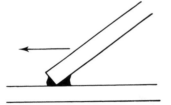

d.

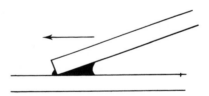

3.2 CIRCLES AND POLYGONS

Formulas may be found immediately preceding the sample test answers.

7. a. Line segment $\overline{AB}$ is called a _____.

    b. $\overline{CD}$ is called a _____.

    c. If $\overline{AB}$ is 4 inches, $\overline{CB}$ is _____.

    d. If $\overline{AB}$ is 4 inches, $\overline{CD}$ is _____.

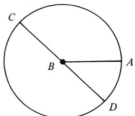

8. Indicate whether each figure is a triangle, quadrilateral, or not a polygon:

a. 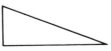   **b.** 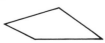   **c.**   **d.**

9. a. Indicate the triangles which are equilateral.
   b. Indicate the triangles which are isosceles.
   c. Indicate the triangles which are right triangles.

1. 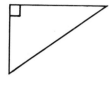   **2.** 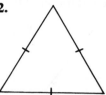   **3.**    **4.**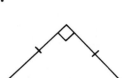

10. List the letters of the appropriate geometric figures:

a.    **b.** 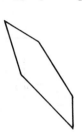   **c.** 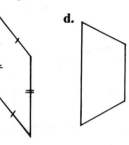   **d.** 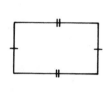   **e.**

    1. squares
    2. rectangles
    3. parallelograms
    4. quadrilaterals
    5. polygons

11. Find the perimeters of the figures.

a.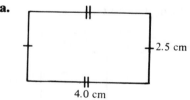
4.0 cm, 2.5 cm

b.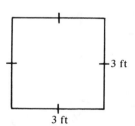
3 ft, 3 ft

12. Find the areas of the figures in problem 11. Round off to ones.

13. Suppose a circle has a radius of 5.0 centimetres:
    a. Find its circumference. Round off to ones.
    b. Find its area. Round off to ones.

14. Find the area of the parallelogram. Round off to tens.

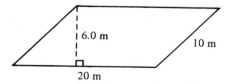
6.0 m, 10 m, 20 m

15. The accompanying triangle is an equilateral triangle:
    a. Find the perimeter.
    b. Find the area.
       Round off to ones.

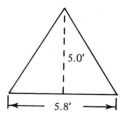
5.0′, 5.8′

3.3 SOLID GEOMETRIC FIGURES

Formulas are included immediately preceding the sample test answers.

16. Give the descriptive name of each geometric solid below:

a.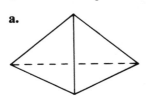

b.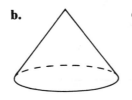

c.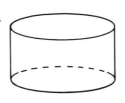

d.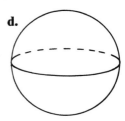

e.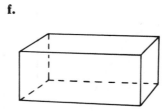

f.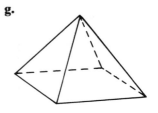

g.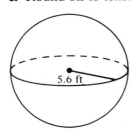

17. Find the volumes of the geometric solids below:

a. Round off to tenths

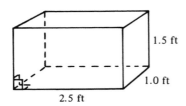

1.5 ft
1.0 ft
2.5 ft

b. Round off to tens.

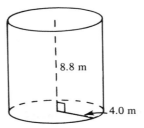

8.8 m
4.0 m

c. Round off to tens.

5.6 ft

d. Round off to tens.

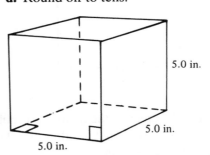

5.0 in.
5.0 in.
5.0 in.

e. Round off to hundreds.

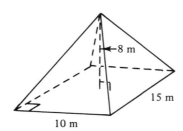

8 m
15 m
10 m

f. Round off to tens.

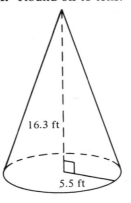

16.3 ft
5.5 ft

18. Use the figures to match the line segment or point to the appropriate name:

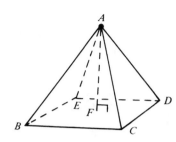
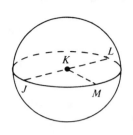
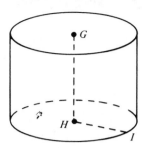
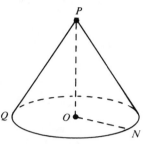

<table>
<tr><td>

a. vertex of a cone
b. radius of a sphere
c. diameter of a sphere
d. radius of a cone
e. radius of a cylinder
f. altitude of a cone
g. center of a sphere
h. apex of a pyramid
i. slant height of a cone
j. altitude of a pyramid
k. altitude of a cylinder

</td><td>

1. $\overline{HI}$
2. $\overline{PO}$
3. A
4. $\overline{JL}$
5. $\overline{AB}$
6. P
7. K
8. $\overline{KM}$
9. $\overline{PQ}$
10. $\overline{ON}$
11. $\overline{AF}$
12. $\overline{GH}$

</td></tr>
</table>

Summary of Formulas

Geometric Figure	Perimeter	Area
Triangle	$p = a + b + c$	$A = \frac{1}{2}bh$
Quadrilateral	$p = a + b + c + d$	—
Rectangle	$p = 2l + 2w$	$A = lw$
Square	$p = 4s$	$A = s^2$
Circle	$c = 2\pi r = \pi d$	$A = \pi r^2$
Parallelogram	$p = 2a + 2b$	$A = bh$

Formula for volume

Prism or cylinder	$V = Bh$, where B is the area of the base
Cube	$V = e^3$
Rectangular prism	$V = lwh$
Cylinder	$V = \pi r^2 h$
Cone	$V = \frac{1}{3}\pi r^2 h$
Pyramid	$V = \frac{1}{3}Bh$, where B is the area of the base
Sphere	$V = \frac{4}{3}\pi r^3$

CHAPTER 3 SAMPLE TEST ANSWERS

1. **a.** $\overleftrightarrow{CB}$ **b.** $\overleftrightarrow{ED}$ **c.** C **d.** B
   e. $\overline{AB}$ or $\overline{AE}$ or $\overline{DE}$ or $\overline{EB}$ **f.** A **g.** $\overline{CD}$, $\overline{DB}$, and $\overline{CB}$

2. **a.** ∥ **b.** ⊥

3. **a.** $\frac{5}{16}$ in. **b.** $1\frac{1}{4}$ in. **c.** 2 in. **d.** $3\frac{1}{8}$ in.
   e. 0.2 cm **f.** 2.7 cm **g.** 3.5 cm **h.** 5.8 cm

4. $\overrightarrow{AB}$ (same as $\overrightarrow{AC}$), $\overrightarrow{CB}$ (same as $\overrightarrow{CA}$), $\overrightarrow{BA}$, and $\overrightarrow{BC}$

5. **a.** ∡3 **b.** right **c.** ∡ABC or ∡CBA **d.** ∡1 and ∡2
   e. ∡3 and ∡4 **6.** b

7. **a.** radius **b.** diameter **c.** 4 inches **d.** 8 inches

8. **a.** triangle **b.** quadrilateral **c.** not a polygon
   d. quadrilateral

9. **a.** 2 **b.** 2, 3, 4 **c.** 1, 4

10. **1.** a
    2. a, e
    3. a, c, e
    4. a, c, d, e
    5. a, b, c, d, e

11. **a.** 13 cm **b.** 12 ft **12. a.** $10 \, cm^2$ **b.** $9 \, ft^2$

13. **a.** 31 cm **b.** $79 \, cm^2$ **14.** $120 \, m^2$

15. **a.** 17.4 ft **b.** $15 \, ft^2$

16. **a.** triangular pyramid **b.** cone **c.** cylinder
    d. sphere **e.** triangular prism **f.** rectangular prism
    g. rectangular pyramid

17. **a.** $3.8 \, ft^3$ **b.** $440 \, m^3$ **c.** $740 \, ft^3$
    d. $130 \, in.^3$ **e.** $400 \, m^3$ **f.** $520 \, ft^3$

18. **a.** 6 **b.** 8 **c.** 4 **d.** 10
    e. 1 **f.** 2 **g.** 7 **h.** 3
    i. 9 **j.** 11 **k.** 12

CHAPTER 4

THE METRIC SYSTEM

Before entering a profession in the health sciences it is important to gain a basic understanding of the systems used for weighing and measuring drugs. One system that is currently used throughout the world for this purpose is the metric system of measurement.

4.1 UNITS OF LENGTH AND AREA

1   The base unit of length in the metric system is the *metre*.* The word, metre, comes from the Greek word metron, meaning "a measure." One metre is slightly longer than a yard and is approximately equal to 39.37 inches. The following diagrams are drawn to scale.

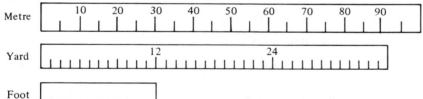

* Another spelling for metre is meter. The -re spelling is the International System of Units (SI) spelling. Both spellings are accepted by the United States National Bureau of Standards.

Q1   Answer true or false:

a. The metre is the base unit of length in the metric system. _____

b. A yard is longer than a metre. _____

c A metre is slightly longer than a yard. _____

\# \# \# • \# \# \# • \# \# \# • \# \# \# • \# \# \# • \# \# \# • \# \# \# • \# \# \# • \# \# \#

A1   **a.** true   **b.** false   **c.** true

2   Metric measurement is based on a decimal system which means that its units are related by multiples of ten (such as 10, 100, 1000) or divisions of ten $\left(\text{such as } \frac{1}{10}, \frac{1}{100}, \frac{1}{1000}\right)$. The multiples of ten are denoted by Greek derived prefixes. The most common prefixes are:

kilo — 1000
hecto — 100
deka — 10

The divisions (fractions) of ten are denoted by Latin derived prefixes. The most common are:

deci — 0.1   or $\dfrac{1}{10}$

centi — 0.01   or $\dfrac{1}{100}$

milli — 0.001   or $\dfrac{1}{1000}$

Metric measurements of length are written using any of the designated prefixes in front of the base unit metre.

Examples:

1. 1 dekametre = 10 metres
2. 1 millimetre = 0.001 metre

Q2   A sphygmomanometer is an instrument used to measure blood pressure. Its scale is calibrated in millimetres. Thus, each division of length on the scale represents _____ of a metre.

\# \# \#   •   \# \# \#   •   \# \# \#   •   \# \# \#   •   \# \# \#   •   \# \# \#   •   \# \# \#   •   \# \# \#   •   \# \# \#

A2   0.001 or $\dfrac{1}{1000}$

Q3   Use the prefixes of Frame 2 to write each of the following in terms of the base unit metre.

a. 1 hectometre = _____   **b.** 1 decimetre = _____

c. 1 centimetre = _____   **d.** 1 kilometre = _____

e. 1 millimetre = _____   **f.** 1 dekametre = _____

\# \# \#   •   \# \# \#   •   \# \# \#   •   \# \# \#   •   \# \# \#   •   \# \# \#   •   \# \# \#   •   \# \# \#   •   \# \# \#

A3   **a.** 100 metres   **b.** 0.1 or $\dfrac{1}{10}$ metre   **c.** 0.01 or $\dfrac{1}{100}$ metre

d. 1000 metres   **e.** 0.001 or $\dfrac{1}{1000}$ metre   **f.** 10 metres

3   For simplicity, symbols are used to stand for each of the units of length in Frame 2. These are as follows:

kilometre   — km
hectometre — hm
dekametre — dam
metre   — m
decimetre — dm
centimetre — cm
millimetre — mm

The symbols are not considered abbreviations and thus are written without periods.

Q4   Write the symbol for each of the following:

a. centimetre _____   **b.** kilometre _____   **c.** millimetre _____   **d.** decimetre _____

\# \# \#   •   \# \# \#   •   \# \# \#   •   \# \# \#   •   \# \# \#   •   \# \# \#   •   \# \# \#   •   \# \# \#   •   \# \# \#

A4   **a.** cm   **b.** km   **c.** mm   **d.** dm

Q5   Complete each of the following equations by filling in the correct multiple or division of ten:

    a. 1 cm = _____ m   **b.** 1 km = _____ m

    c. 1 dm = _____ m   **d.** 1 mm = _____ m

• # # # • # # # • # # # • # # # • # # # • # # # • # # # • # #

A5   **a.** 0.01   **b.** 1000   **c.** 0.1   **d.** 0.001

---

4   The most frequently used multiples and divisions of the metre from Frames 2 and 3 are summarized as follows:

    1 kilometre (km) = 1000 metres (m)
    1 hectometre (hm) = 100 metres
    1 dekametre (dam) =   10 metres
    1 decimetre (dm) = 0.1 metre
    1 centimetre (cm) = 0.01 metre
    1 millimetre (mm) = 0.001 metre

Q6   Complete each of the following equations:

    a. 1 m = _____ mm   **b.** 1 cm = _____ m

    c. 1 km = _____ m   **d.** 1 dm = _____ m

• # # # • # # # • # # # • # # # • # # # • # # # • # # # • # #

A6   **a.** 1000   **b.** 0.01   **c.** 1000   **d.** 0.1

---

5   The metric units most used in hospital terminology are the metre, decimetre, centimetre, and millimetre. The sizes of the latter three units are shown.

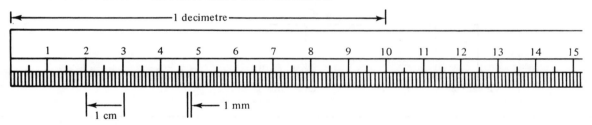

The relationships demonstrated by the metric ruler are:

1 dm = 10 cm   or   1 cm = 0.1 dm
1 cm = 10 mm   or   1 mm = 0.1 cm

Ten decimetres placed end to end equal 1 metre. Thus, the decimetre and metre are related as follows:

1 m = 10 dm   or   1 dm = 0.1 m

Notice that a centimetre is about the width of your little finger, while a decimetre is approximated by measuring across the knuckles of your clenched fist.

Q7   Approximate the following lengths in the unit given:

    a. (cm)   _____

    b. (dm)   _____

c. (mm) _____

d. (cm) _____

\# \# \#　•　\# \# \#　•　\# \# \#　•　\# \# \#　•　\# \# \#　•　\# \# \#　•　\# \# \#　•　\# \# \#　•　\# \# \#

A7　　**a.** 4 cm　　　　　**b.** 1 dm　　　　　**c.** 15 mm　　　　　**d.** 7 cm

---

Q8　　Complete each of the following equations:

a. 1 mm = _____ cm　　　**b.** 1 cm = _____ mm　　　**c.** 1 dm = _____ cm

d. 1 m = _____ dm　　　**e.** 1 cm = _____ m　　　**f.** 1 m = _____ cm

\# \# \#　•　\# \# \#　•　\# \# \#　•　\# \# \#　•　\# \# \#　•　\# \# \#　•　\# \# \#　•　\# \# \#　•　\# \# \#

A8　　**a.** 0.1　**b.** 10　**c.** 10　**d.** 10　**e.** 0.01　**f.** 100

6　　Conversion within the metric system is simplified if the similarity between metric units and our decimal number system is pointed out. Examine the following place value diagram.

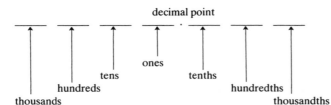

Using its prefix, each metric unit of length can be appropriately placed in the above diagram. For example, since kilometre has prefix "kilo" (1000), kilometre (km) is placed in the thousands place. Since centimetre has prefix "centi" $\left(\frac{1}{100}\right)$, centimetre (cm) is placed in the hundredths place.

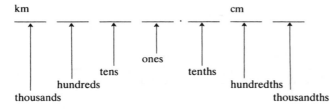

Q9　　Complete the diagram below by filling in the appropriate metric units of length.

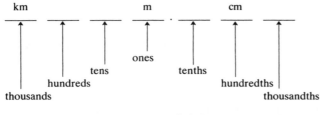

\# \# \#　•　\# \# \#　•　\# \# \#　•　\# \# \#　•　\# \# \#　•　\# \# \#　•　\# \# \#　•　\# \# \#　•　\# \# \#

A9　　__km__　__hm__　__dam__　__m__　.　__dm__　__cm__　__mm__

7　　Notice that the place values and metric units of length in the diagram of Q9 are related by 10's in the following ways:

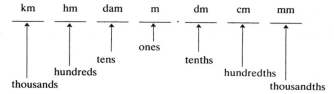

(1) Each unit is equal to 10 times the unit to its right.

Examples:

1 km = 10 hm
1 hm = 10 dam
1 dam = 10 m

(2) Each unit is equal to 0.1 times $\left(\frac{1}{10}\text{ of}\right)$ the unit to its left.

Examples:

1 mm = 0.1 cm
1 cm = 0.1 dm
1 dm = 0.1 m

Q10   Fill in 10 or 0.1 to complete each of the following:

    a. 1 km = _____ hm   **b.** 1 cm = _____ dm

    c. 1 dm = _____ cm   **d.** 1 dm = _____ m

\# \# \# • \# \# \# • \# \# \# • \# \# \# • \# \# \# • \# \# \# • \# \# \# • \# \# \# • \# \# \#

A10   **a.** 10   **b.** 0.1   **c.** 10   **d.** 0.1

---

8   The diagram of Frame 7 can be simplified in the following chart:

$$\text{km}\overset{10}{—}\text{hm}\overset{10}{—}\text{dam}\overset{10}{—}\text{m}\overset{10}{—}\text{dm}\overset{10}{—}\text{cm}\overset{10}{—}\text{mm}$$

The 10's indicate that any unit is equal to the unit on its right multiplied by 10 and the unit on its left divided by 10.

Multiplying or dividing by 10 in a decimal number system is done by moving the decimal point one place to the right or one place to the left. Thus, conversions between units in the metric system can be made by moving the decimal point in the following ways:

1. To convert any unit to a unit on its *right, multiply* by the number of 10's separating the two units. (Move the decimal point to the right the same number of places as there are 10's.)
2. To convert any unit to a unit on its *left, divide* by the number of 10's separating the two units. (Move the decimal point to the left the same number of places as there are 10's.)

Q11   Fill in the blank:

    a. Any two consecutive metric units on the chart in Frame 8 are related by the number _____.

    b. To convert any unit to a unit on its right, _____ by the number of 10's separating the two units.

    c. To convert any unit to a unit on its left, _____ by the number of 10's separating the two units.

\# \# \# • \# \# \# • \# \# \# • \# \# \# • \# \# \# • \# \# \# • \# \# \# • \# \# \# • \# \# \#

A11   **a.** 10   **b.** multiply   **c.** divide

---

9   Consider the following examples:

Example 1:   45.8 dm = _____ m

$$\text{km} \overset{10}{-} \text{hm} \overset{10}{-} \text{dam} \overset{10}{-} \text{m} \overset{10}{\underset{\smile}{-}} \text{dm} \overset{10}{-} \text{cm} \overset{10}{-} \text{mm}$$

Solution: "m" is *one* 10 to the *left* of "dm" on the chart. Move the decimal point *one* place to the *left* (45.8). Thus, 45.8 dm = 4.58 m.

Example 2:   0.5 m = _____ mm

$$\text{km} \overset{10}{-} \text{hm} \overset{10}{-} \text{dam} \overset{10}{-} \text{m} \overset{10}{\underset{\smile}{-}} \text{dm} \overset{10}{\underset{\smile}{-}} \text{cm} \overset{10}{\underset{\smile}{-}} \text{mm}$$

Solution: "mm" is *three* 10's to the *right* of "m" on the chart. Move the decimal point *three* places to the *right* (0.500). Thus, 0.5 m = 500 mm.

Q12   15.5 cm = _____ mm

\# \# \#   •   \# \# \#   •   \# \# \#   •   \# \# \#   •   \# \# \#   •   \# \# \#   •   \# \# \#   •   \# \# \#   •   \# \# \#

A12   155: $\text{km} \overset{10}{-} \text{hm} \overset{10}{-} \text{dam} \overset{10}{-} \text{m} \overset{10}{-} \text{dm} \overset{10}{-} \text{cm} \overset{10}{\underset{\smile}{-}} \text{mm}$. "mm" is *one* 10 to the *right* of "cm" on the

chart. Move the decimal point *one* place to the *right* (15.5).

Q13   80 km = _____ m

\# \# \#   •   \# \# \#   •   \# \# \#   •   \# \# \#   •   \# \# \#   •   \# \# \#   •   \# \# \#   •   \# \# \#   •   \# \# \#

A13   80 000:* $\text{km} \overset{10}{\underset{\smile}{-}} \text{hm} \overset{10}{\underset{\smile}{-}} \text{dam} \overset{10}{\underset{\smile}{-}} \text{m} \overset{10}{-} \text{dm} \overset{10}{-} \text{cm} \overset{10}{-} \text{mm}$. "m" is *three* 10's to the *right* of "km" in the

chart. Move the decimal point *three* places to the *right* (80.000).

*In the metric system when there are more than four digits to the right or left of the decimal point, the numerals are separated by a space into groups of three digits, starting at the decimal point. No commas are inserted.

Q14   A patient's height is recorded as 175 cm. What is the height in metres?

\# \# \#   •   \# \# \#   •   \# \# \#   •   \# \# \#   •   \# \# \#   •   \# \# \#   •   \# \# \#   •   \# \# \#   •   \# \# \#

A14   1.75 m: $\text{km} \overset{10}{-} \text{hm} \overset{10}{-} \text{dam} \overset{10}{-} \text{m} \overset{10}{\underset{\smile}{-}} \text{dm} \overset{10}{\underset{\smile}{-}} \text{cm} \overset{10}{-} \text{mm}$. "m" is two 10's to the *left* of "cm" on the

chart. Move the decimal point two places to the *left* (175.).

Q15   The length of a hospital hall is 125 metres. What is the length in kilometres?

\# \# \#   •   \# \# \#   •   \# \# \#   •   \# \# \#   •   \# \# \#   •   \# \# \#   •   \# \# \#   •   \# \# \#   •   \# \# \#

A15   0.125 km: $\text{km} \overset{10}{\underset{\smile}{-}} \text{hm} \overset{10}{\underset{\smile}{-}} \text{dam} \overset{10}{\underset{\smile}{-}} \text{m} \overset{10}{-} \text{dm} \overset{10}{-} \text{cm} \overset{10}{-} \text{mm}$. "km" is *three* 10's to the *left* of "m" on

the chart. Move the decimal point three places to the *left* (125.).

Q16   Complete each of the following:

a. 35 cm = _____ mm   **b.** 2.25 m = _____ cm

c. 130 cm = _____ m   **d.** 0.5 km = _____ m

• # # # • # # # • # # # • # # # • # # # • # # # • # # # • # #

A16   **a.** 350 (35.0.)   **b.** 225   **c.** 1.3   **d.** 500

---

10   In the metric system, as in the U.S. customary system* of measurement, area is measured using square units. A common metric unit of area is the *square metre* (m²) or the area covered by a square with sides equal to 1 metre. The illustration which follows gives an idea of the approximate size of one square metre. A common use of the square metre in the health sciences is to express the surface area of the human body.

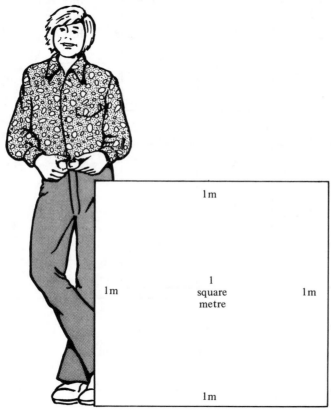

After J. R. Smart, *Metric Math: The Modernized Metric System* (1974).

*The system of measurement historically used for most everyday measurements in the United States is called the U.S. customary or the English system of measurement.

Q17   Answer true or false:

a. Area is measured in square units. _____

b. A common unit of area in the metric system is the square metre. _____

• # # # • # # # • # # # • # # # • # # # • # # # • # # # • # #

A17   **a.** true   **b.** true

---

11   Metric units of area for measuring areas smaller than one square metre are the square decimetre (dm²), square centimetre (cm²), and the square millimetre (mm²). The relationships between dm²,

cm^2, and mm^2 can be seen in the accompanying actual-size drawing. The relationships demonstrated by the drawing are:

$1\ dm^2 = 100\ cm^2$ or $1\ cm^2 = 0.01\ dm^2$
$1\ cm^2 = 100\ mm^2$ or $1\ mm^2 = 0.01\ cm^2$

Notice that consecutive units of area from m^2 to mm^2 are related by multiples or divisions of 100.

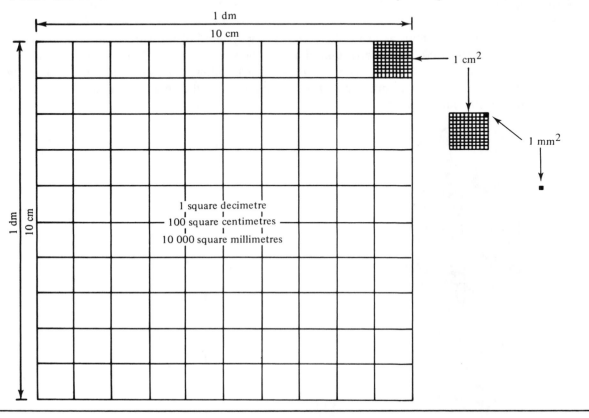

Q18   Complete each of the following using the information of Frame 11.

    a. $1\ cm^2 = $ _____ mm^2 **b.** $1\ mm^2 = $ _____ cm^2

\# \# \#   •   \# \# \#   •   \# \# \#   •   \# \# \#   •   \# \# \#   •   \# \# \#   •   \# \# \#   •   \# \# \#   •   \# \# \#

    A18   **a.** 100   **b.** 0.01 or $\dfrac{1}{100}$

12   The chart which follows can be used to simplify conversion between metric units of area. The 100's separating units indicate that consecutive units of area differ by a multiple or division of 100. Since consecutive units of area differ by 100 and not 10 as is the case with units of length (Frame 8), each space now involves a movement of the decimal point *two* places right or left instead of one.

$$m^2 \xrightarrow{100} dm^2 \xrightarrow{100} cm^2 \xrightarrow{100} mm^2$$

Example 1: $25\ m^2 = $ _____ dm^2

Solution "dm^2" is *one* space to the *right* of "m^2." Move the decimal point *two* places to the *right* (25.00). Thus, $25\ m^2 = 2500\ dm^2$.

Example 2: $350\,\text{mm}^2 = \underline{\hspace{1.5cm}} \text{cm}^2$

Solution "cm^2" *is one* space to the *left* of "mm^2." Move the decimal point *two* places to the *left* ($3.50.$). Thus, $350\,\text{mm}^2 = 3.5\,\text{cm}^2$.

Q19 Complete each of the following:

    a. $15.2\,\text{cm}^2 = \underline{\hspace{1.5cm}} \text{mm}^2$ **b.** $3.7\,\text{dm}^2 = \underline{\hspace{1.5cm}} \text{m}^2$

\# \# \# • \# \# \# • \# \# \# • \# \# \# • \# \# \# • \# \# \# • \# \# \# • \# \# \# • \# \# \#

A19   **a.** 1520   **b.** 0.037

Q20 The area of burns on a patient's body was estimated as $4.5\,\text{dm}^2$. What is the area of burns in square centimetres?

\# \# \# • \# \# \# • \# \# \# • \# \# \# • \# \# \# • \# \# \# • \# \# \# • \# \# \# • \# \# \#

A20 $450\,\text{cm}^2$: $4.5\,\text{dm}^2 = \underline{\hspace{1.5cm}} \text{cm}^2$

This completes the instruction for this section.

4.1 EXERCISE

1. The base unit of length in the metric system is the _____.

2. The base metric unit of length is slightly _____ than a yard.
                                 (shorter/longer)

3. Write symbols for each of the following:

    a. kilometre _____   **b.** metre _____

    c. centimetre _____   **d.** millimetre _____

4. Complete each of the following equations by filling in the correct multiple or division of ten:

    a. $1\,\text{m} = \underline{\hspace{1cm}} \text{cm}$ **b.** $1\,\text{mm} = \underline{\hspace{1cm}} \text{m}$

    c. $1\,\text{mm} = \underline{\hspace{1cm}} \text{cm}$ **d.** $1\,\text{km} = \underline{\hspace{1cm}} \text{m}$

5. Approximate the following lengths in the units given:

    a. cm _____

    b. mm _____

    c. dm _____

6. Complete each of the following equations:

    a. $152\,\text{cm} = \underline{\hspace{1cm}} \text{m}$ **b.** $50\,\text{dm} = \underline{\hspace{1cm}} \text{m}$

    c. $1000\,\text{m} = \underline{\hspace{1cm}} \text{km}$ **d.** $25\,\text{cm} = \underline{\hspace{1cm}} \text{mm}$

7. A baby's length is 450 mm. What is the length in centimetres?

8. A patient's height is recorded as 1.95 metres. What is the height in centimetres?

9. Perform each of the following conversions:

    a. $15\,\text{cm}^2 = \underline{\hspace{1cm}} \text{mm}^2$ **b.** $500\,\text{mm}^2 = \underline{\hspace{1cm}} \text{cm}^2$

10. The burn area on a patient's body was estimated as $7\,\text{dm}^2$. What is the burn area in square centimetres?

4.1 EXERCISE ANSWERS

1. metre   **2.** longer

3. a. km   **b.** m   **c.** cm   **d.** mm

4. a. 100   **b.** 0.001   **c.** 0.1   **d.** 1000

5. a. 5 cm   **b.** 30 mm   **c.** 0.5 dm

6. a. 1.52   **b.** 5   **c.** 1   **d.** 250

7. 45 cm   **8.** 195 cm   **9. a.** 1500   **b.** 5

10. 700 cm^2

4.2 UNITS OF VOLUME

1   The volume or capacity of an object can be thought of as the amount that the object holds. Volume can be expressed in units of liquid measure or in cubic units. A cube that has edges of length 1 cm is

1 cm   1 cm   1 cm

1 cubic centimetre (cm^3)

The volume of
this figure is:

1 litre
or
1000 cubic centimetres
or
1 cubic decimetre

1 decimetre
10 centimetres

1 decimetre
10 centimetres

1 decimetre
10 centimetres

said to have a volume of 1 cubic centimetre (1 cm^3 or 1 cc).* A cubic centimetre is shown here, its size being 1 cubic centimetre (cm^3), approximately that of a sugar cube. If a cube with edges of length 10 cm (1 dm) is formed, the result is 1000 cubic centimetres (1 cubic decimetre).

The unit that is used as the metric unit of liquid volume is the *litre* (l). One litre is defined as 1000 cubic centimetres. The large cube has a volume of 1 litre. Compared with the U.S. customary system, the litre is slightly larger than a quart ($1 \text{ l} \doteq 1.06 \text{ qt}$).

*The International System of Units (SI) symbol for cubic centimetre is cm^3. The symbol "cc" has also been used in the health professions to represent cubic centimetres.

Q1   Answer true or false:

    a. A litre is larger than a quart. _____

    b. $1 \text{ l} = 1000 \text{ cm}^3$ _____

    c. $1 \text{ l} = 1 \text{ dm}^3$ _____

    d. $1 \text{ cm}^3 = 1 \text{ cc}$ _____

\# \# \# • \# \# \# • \# \# \# • \# \# \# • \# \# \# • \# \# \# • \# \# \# • \# \# \# • \# \# \#

A1   **a.** true   **b.** true   **c.** true   **d.** true

---

2   The metric units of volume are defined using prefixes in the same way as the metric units of length. The volume units and their symbols are as follows:

1 kilolitre (kl)   = 1000 litres (l)
1 hectolitre (hl) =   100 litres
1 dekalitre (dal) =   10 litres
1 litre (l)   =   1 litre
1 decilitre (dl)   =   0.1 litre
1 centilitre (cl) =   0.01 litre
1 millilitre (ml) = 0.001 litre

Q2   Complete each equation using the information of Frames 1 and 2:

    a. $1 \text{ l} =$ _____ ml   **b.** $1 \text{ ml} =$ _____ l

    c. _____ $\text{cm}^3 = 1 \text{ cc}$ **d.** $1 \text{ l} =$ _____ dm^3

\# \# \# • \# \# \# • \# \# \# • \# \# \# • \# \# \# • \# \# \# • \# \# \# • \# \# \# • \# \# \#

A2   **a.** 1000   **b.** 0.001 or $\dfrac{1}{1000}$ **c.** 1   **d.** 1

---

3   In Frame 1 a litre was defined as 1000 cubic centimetres. Thus,

$1 \text{ cm}^3 = 0.001 \text{ l}$

In Frame 2 it was also given that

$1 \text{ ml} = 0.001 \text{ l}$

Since both 1 cm^3 and 1 ml are equal to 0.001 l, the two units must be equal to each other. That is,

$1 \text{ cm}^3 \text{ (cc)} = 1 \text{ ml}$

Therefore, it is possible to interchange the units millilitre and cubic centimetre. That is,

$1 \text{ ml} = 1 \text{ cm}^3 = 1 \text{ cc}$

Q3   The volume of a cube measuring 1 cm on a side can be named in what three ways?

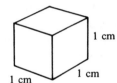

a. _____

b. _____

c. _____

• # # # • # # # • # # # • # # # • # # # • # # # • # # # • # #

A3   **a.** 1 cm^3 **b.** 1 ml   **c.** 1 cc   (any order)

Q4   Complete each of the equations:

a. $1 \, l = $ _____ ml   **b.** $1 \, l = $ _____ cm^3

c. $1 \, l = $ _____ cc   **d.** $1 \text{ cm}^3 \text{ (cc)} = $ _____ l

• # # # • # # # • # # # • # # # • # # # • # # # • # # # • # #

A4   **a.** 1000   **b.** 1000   **c.** 1000   **d.** 0.001 or $\dfrac{1}{1000}$

---

4   The millilitre is the division of a litre that is most commonly used in hospitals. The approximate size of some millilitre measures can be seen from the actual-size medicine glass illustrated. The approximate size of a millilitre can also be gained by comparing it with some common household system units. There are about 4–5 ml in one teaspoon and about 240 ml in an 8 ounce glass.

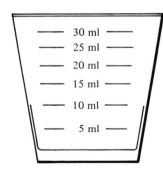

Fractional parts of a litre in hospital use are expressed in either millilitres or cubic centimetres. Common fractional parts of a litre are:

$\dfrac{1}{4} l = 250 \text{ ml (cm}^3 \text{ or cc)}$

$\dfrac{1}{2} l = 500 \text{ ml}$

$\dfrac{3}{4} l = 750 \text{ ml}$

Q5   Complete each of the following equations:

a. $1 \, l = $ _____ ml   **b.** $750 \text{ cc} = $ _____ l

c. $1\dfrac{1}{2} l = $ _____ ml   **d.** $250 \text{ ml} = $ _____ l

• # # # • # # # • # # # • # # # • # # # • # # # • # # # • # #

A5   **a.** 1000   **b.** $\dfrac{3}{4}$ **c.** 1500   **d.** $\dfrac{1}{4}$

Q6   A medication bottle contains one litre. If the bottle is full, how many 125 ml doses can be administered from it?

\# \# \#   •   \# \# \#   •   \# \# \#   •   \# \# \#   •   \# \# \#   •   \# \# \#   •   \# \# \#   •   \# \# \#   •   \# \# \#

A6   8 doses: $1000 \div 125 = 8$

---

5   The metric units of volume can be arranged in order from largest to smallest for use in conversion.

$$kl \xrightarrow{10} hl \xrightarrow{10} dal \xrightarrow{10} l \xrightarrow{10} dl \xrightarrow{10} cl \xrightarrow{10} ml \ (cm^3)$$

Example: $3.8 \, l = $ _____ ml

Solution: $kl \xrightarrow{10} hl \xrightarrow{10} dal \xrightarrow{10} l \xrightarrow{10} dl \xrightarrow{10} cl \xrightarrow{10} ml \ (cm^3)$

"ml" is *three* 10's to the *right* of "l" on the chart. Move the decimal point *three* places to the *right* (3.800). Thus, $3.8 \, l = 3800$ ml.

Q7 $25 \, l = $ _____ dal

\# \# \#   •   \# \# \#   •   \# \# \#   •   \# \# \#   •   \# \# \#   •   \# \# \#   •   \# \# \#   •   \# \# \#   •   \# \# \#

A7   2.5:   "dal" is *one* 10 to the *left* of "l" on the chart. Move the decimal point *one* place to the *left* (2.5.). Thus, $25 \, l = 2.5$ dal.

Q8 $200 \, ml = $ _____ cm^3

\# \# \#   •   \# \# \#   •   \# \# \#   •   \# \# \#   •   \# \# \#   •   \# \# \#   •   \# \# \#   •   \# \# \#   •   \# \# \#

A8   200: $1 \, ml = 1 \, cm^3$, therefore $200 \, ml = 200 \, cm^3$

Q9   Perform each conversion:

a. $750 \, ml = $ _____ l   **b.** $1.5 \, kl = $ _____ l

\# \# \#   •   \# \# \#   •   \# \# \#   •   \# \# \#   •   \# \# \#   •   \# \# \#   •   \# \# \#   •   \# \# \#   •   \# \# \#

A9   **a.** 0.75   **b.** 1500

Q10   The amount of air moved when a person inhales maximally, and then exhales maximally is called the vital capacity of his/her lungs. Normal vital capacity is between 3 litres and 5 litres. What is normal vital capacity in cubic centimetres?

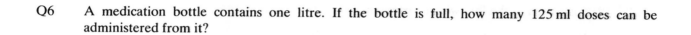

\# \# \#   •   \# \# \#   •   \# \# \#   •   \# \# \#   •   \# \# \#   •   \# \# \#   •   \# \# \#   •   \# \# \#   •   \# \# \#

A10   Between $3000 \, cm^3$ (cc) and $5000 \, cm^3$ (cc):   "cm^3" is *three* 10's to the *right* of "l" on the chart. Move the decimal point *three* places to the *right* (3.000 and 5.000).

Q11 Perform each of the following conversions:

a. 50 ml = _____ cc

b. 1500 ml = _____ l

c. $1\frac{3}{4}$ l = _____ ml

d. 1 kl = _____ l

⌗ ⌗ ⌗ • ⌗ ⌗ ⌗ • ⌗ ⌗ ⌗ • ⌗ ⌗ ⌗ • ⌗ ⌗ ⌗ • ⌗ ⌗ ⌗ • ⌗ ⌗ ⌗ • ⌗ ⌗ ⌗ • ⌗ ⌗ ⌗

A11 **a.** 50   **b.** 1.5   **c.** 1750: $1\frac{3}{4} = 1.75$ **d.** 1000

This completes the instruction for this section.

4.2 EXERCISE

1. The unit for liquid volume in the metric system is the _____.

2. The metric unit for liquid volume is approximately equal to what U.S. customary system unit?

3. Write symbols for each of the following:

   a. litre   **b.** millilitre   **c.** kilolitre

4. Complete each of the following equations:

   a. 1 ml = _____ l   **b.** 1 cm^3 = _____ ml   **c.** 1 l = _____ dm^3

   d. 1 kl = _____ l   **e.** $1\frac{3}{4}$ l = _____ ml   **f.** 500 ml = _____ l

5. Perform each of the following conversions:

   a. 250 ml = _____ l   **b.** 0.5 kl = _____ l

   c. 800 cc = _____ ml   **d.** 100 ml = _____ l

6. Which of the following most closely approximates 1 ml: $\frac{1}{4}$ teaspoon, $\frac{1}{2}$ litre, 1 quart

7. Which of the following most closely approximates 1 litre: 1 quart, 5 teaspoons, 1 gallon

4.2 EXERCISE ANSWERS

1. litre   **2.** quart

3. a. l   **b.** ml   **c.** kl

4. a. 0.001   **b.** 1   **c.** 1

    d. 1000   **e.** 1750   **f.** 0.5 $\left(\frac{1}{2}\right)$

5. a. 0.25   **b.** 500   **c.** 800   **d.** 0.1

6. $\frac{1}{4}$ teaspoon   **7.** 1 quart

4.3 UNITS OF MASS (WEIGHT)

1   The base unit of mass* (weight) in the metric system is the *kilogram*. The kilogram is defined as the mass of a cylinder of platinum–iridium alloy kept by the International Bureau of Weights and Measures in Sèvres, France. A duplicate of this cylinder is present in the National Bureau of

    *Mass is the quantity of matter that a body possesses; *weight* is force, the earth's attraction for a given mass. Technically, mass and weight are two different things. In commercial and everyday use, the term weight nearly always means mass.

Standards in the United States. When compared with a unit of the English system, 1 kilogram is approximately 2.2 pounds. The units of mass, their symbols and equivalents, are:

1 kilogram (kg)   = 1000 grams
1 hectogram (hg) = 100 grams
1 dekagram (dag) =   10 grams
1 gram (g)   =   1 gram
1 decigram (dg)   =   0.1 gram
1 centigram (cg) = 0.01 gram
1 milligram (mg) = 0.001 gram

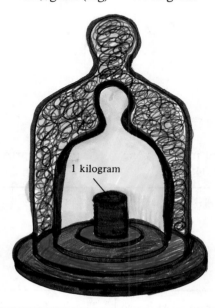

1 kilogram

Q1   Fill in the blanks:

   a. The _____ is the base unit of mass in the metric system.

   b. The approximate mass (weight) of 1 kg is _____ pounds.

\# \# \#   •   \# \# \#   •   \# \# \#   •   \# \# \#   •   \# \# \#   •   \# \# \#   •   \# \# \#   •   \# \# \#   •   \# \# \#

A1   **a.** kilogram   **b.** 2.2

Q2   Write the correct symbol for each unit:

   a. milligram _____   **b.** gram _____

   c. kilogram _____   **d.** centigram _____

\# \# \#   •   \# \# \#   •   \# \# \#   •   \# \# \#   •   \# \# \#   •   \# \# \#   •   \# \# \#   •   \# \# \#   •   \# \# \#

A2   **a.** mg   **b.** g   **c.** kg   **d.** cg

Q3   Complete each of the equations using the information of Frame 1:

   a. 1 kg =_____ g   **b.** 1 mg =_____ g

   c. 1 g =_____ kg   **d.** 1 g =_____ mg

\# \# \#   •   \# \# \#   •   \# \# \#   •   \# \# \#   •   \# \# \#   •   \# \# \#   •   \# \# \#   •   \# \# \#   •   \# \# \#

A3   **a.** 1000   **b.** 0.001   **c.** 0.001   **d.** 1000

2   Of the units listed in Frame 1, the most commonly used are the kilogram, the gram, and the milligram. Some common comparisons with the gram and the milligram are the mass (weight) of a large paper clip (1 g), the mass of a nickel (5 g), the mass of a piece of hair (1 mg), and the mass of a straight pin (500 mg).

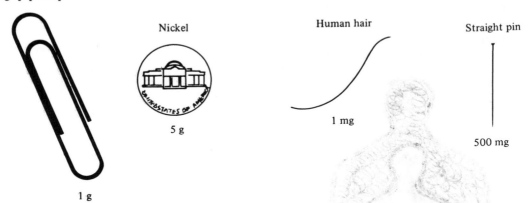

Large paper clip

Nickel

Human hair

Straight pin

5 g

1 mg

500 mg

1 g

Some common comparisons with the kilogram are the mass of a newborn baby (approximately 3–4 kg) and the mass of an adult male (approximately 80 kg).

Q4   Write the following units in order from largest to smallest:

gram, kilogram, milligram _____

\# \# \#   •   \# \# \#   •   \# \# \#   •   \# \# \#   •   \# \# \#   •   \# \# \#   •   \# \# \#   •   \# \# \#   •   \# \# \#

A4   kilogram, gram, milligram

3   To measure very small amounts of a drug, the microgram (μg) is used.* The symbol "μ" means micro or $\dfrac{1}{1\,000\,000}$.† The microgram is related to the gram and milligram as follows:

$1\,\mu g = 0.000\,001\,g$ or $1\,000\,000\,\mu g = 1\,g$
$1\,\mu g = 0.001\,mg$ or $1000\,\mu g = 1\,mg$

* The symbol mcg is also used for microgram.
† In the metric system when there are more than four digits to the right or left of the decimal point, the numerals are separated by a space into groups of three digits, starting at the decimal point. No commas are inserted.

Q5   Circle the smaller unit:

a. milligram, microgram   **b.** kilogram, gram

c. kilogram, milligram   **d.** microgram, gram

\# \# \#   •   \# \# \#   •   \# \# \#   •   \# \# \#   •   \# \# \#   •   \# \# \#   •   \# \# \#   •   \# \# \#   •   \# \# \#

A5   **a.** microgram   **b.** gram   **c.** milligram   **d.** microgram

Q6   Complete each equation:

a. 1 g = _____ mg   **b.** 1 mg = _____ μg

c. 1 g = _____ kg   **d.** 1 μg = _____ mg

\# \# \#   •   \# \# \#   •   \# \# \#   •   \# \# \#   •   \# \# \#   •   \# \# \#   •   \# \# \#   •   \# \# \#   •   \# \# \#

A6   **a.** 1000   **b.** 1000   **c.** 0.001   **d.** 0.001

4   Conversions between metric units of mass are possible using the procedures of the previous two sections. The metric units of mass are listed from largest to smallest as follows:

$$kg \xrightarrow{10} hg \xrightarrow{10} dag \xrightarrow{10} g \xrightarrow{10} dg \xrightarrow{10} cg \xrightarrow{10} mg \xrightarrow{1000} \mu g$$

Notice that "mg" and "μg" are not related by 10. Rather "mg" and "μg" are related by 1000. Thus, conversion between these two units will involve a movement of the decimal point three places right or left.

Example 1: 1250 g = _____ kg

Solution: $kg \xrightarrow{10} hg \xrightarrow{10} dag \xrightarrow{10} g \xrightarrow{10} dg \xrightarrow{10} cg \xrightarrow{10} mg$

"kg" is *three* 10's to the *left* of "g." Move the decimal point *three* places to the *left* (1250.). Thus, 1250 g = 1.25 kg.

Example 2: 42.5 g = _____ cg

Solution $kg \xrightarrow{10} hg \xrightarrow{10} dag \xrightarrow{10} g \xrightarrow{10} dg \xrightarrow{10} cg \xrightarrow{10} mg$

"cg" is *two* 10's to the *right* of "g." Move the decimal point *two* places to the *right* (42.50.). Thus 42.5 g = 4250 cg.

Q7   0.5 kg = _____ g

\# \# \# • \# \# \# • \# \# \# • \# \# \# • \# \# \# • \# \# \# • \# \# \# • \# \# \# • \# \# \#

A7   500: "g" is *three* 10's to the *right* of "kg." Move the decimal point *three* placed to the *right* (0.500).

Q8   Perform each conversion.

    a. 250 mg = _____ g   **b.** 0.03 g = _____ mg

\# \# \# • \# \# \# • \# \# \# • \# \# \# • \# \# \# • \# \# \# • \# \# \# • \# \# \# • \# \# \#

A8   **a.** 0.25   **b.** 30

Q9   You are to give 1.5 g of ascorbic acid. How many milligrams are you giving?

\# \# \# • \# \# \# • \# \# \# • \# \# \# • \# \# \# • \# \# \# • \# \# \# • \# \# \# • \# \# \#

A9   1500 mg: 1.5 g = _____ mg
    "mg" is *three* 10's to the *right* of "g." Move the decimal point *three* places to the *right* (1.500).

Q10   The doctor orders 10 mg of morphine sulphate. How many grams would you administer?

\# \# \# • \# \# \# • \# \# \# • \# \# \# • \# \# \# • \# \# \# • \# \# \# • \# \# \# • \# \# \#

A10   0.01 g: 10 mg = _____ g
    "g" is *three* 10's to the *left* of "mg." Move the decimal point *three* places to the *left* (010.).

5   Recall from Frame 3 that the units microgram and milligram are related by a factor of 1000. Thus, when using the diagram of Frame 4 for conversions between microgram and milligram, it is necessary to move the decimal point *three* places to the right or left.

Example: 750 μg = _____ mg

Solution: "mg" is to the *left* of "μg" and is related by 1000. Move the decimal point three places to the *left* (750.). Thus, 750 μg = 0.75 mg.

Q11   Complete the equations:

    a. 625 μg = _____ mg   **b.** 0.3 mg = _____ μg

\# \# \# • \# \# \# • \# \# \# • \# \# \# • \# \# \# • \# \# \# • \# \# \# • \# \# \# • \# \# \# • \# \# \#

A11   **a.** 0.625
    b. 300:   "μg" is to the *right* of "mg" and is related by 1000. Move the decimal point three places to the *right* (.300).

Q12   A physician orders 500 μg of vitamin B-12. What is the dosage in milligrams?

\# \# \# • \# \# \# • \# \# \# • \# \# \# • \# \# \# • \# \# \# • \# \# \# • \# \# \# • \# \# \# • \# \# \#

A12   0.5 mg

Q13   The order reads 0.25 g of tetracycline. How many milligrams would you administer?

\# \# \# • \# \# \# • \# \# \# • \# \# \# • \# \# \# • \# \# \# • \# \# \# • \# \# \# • \# \# \# • \# \# \#

A13   250 mg

Q14   A physician orders 750 micrograms of a drug. What is the equivalent of the drug in milligrams?

\# \# \# • \# \# \# • \# \# \# • \# \# \# • \# \# \# • \# \# \# • \# \# \# • \# \# \# • \# \# \# • \# \# \#

A14   0.75 mg

This completes the instruction for this section.

4.3   EXERCISE

1. The base unit for mass (weight) in the metric system is the _____.

2. What is the approximate English system weight of the metric base unit for mass? _____
3. Write symbols for each of the following:

    a. gram _____   **b.** kilogram _____   **c.** microgram _____   **d.** milligram _____
    4. Complete each of the following equations:

    a. 1 kg = _____ g   **b.** 1 mg = _____ g   **c.** 1 μg = _____ mg   **d.** 1 mg = _____ μg

5. Perform each of the following conversions:

a. 2.5 g = _____ mg   **b.** 500 mg = _____ g   **c.** 750 μg = _____ mg

d. 0.03 kg = _____ g   **e.** 1500 mg = _____ g   **f.** 2.5 mg = _____ μg

4.3   EXERCISE ANSWERS

1. kilogram   **2.** 2.2 pounds
3. a. g   **b.** kg   **c.** μg   **d.** mg
4. a. 1000   **b.** 0.001   **c.** 0.001   **d.** 1000
5. a. 2500   **b.** 0.5   **c.** 0.75   **d.** 30
     e. 1.5   **f.** 2500

4.4   TEMPERATURE AND TIME

1   The ability to accurately measure temperature is an essential skill for persons in health science professions. Not only is temperature an indication of body normality or abnormality, but it is used to destroy microorganisms, bacteria, and spores in the process of sterilization.

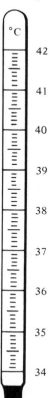

The most common device for measuring temperature is a thermometer. It consists of a graduated glass tube with a sealed, capillary bore in which mercury rises or falls as it expands or contracts from changes in temperature. Thus, when the thermometer bulb is immersed in liquid or placed in the patient's mouth under the tongue, or in the rectum, the heat present causes the mercury to rise in the tube until the temperature level present is registered. Clinical thermometers, used to measure body temperatures, differ from other thermometers in that they have a constriction above the bulb in the capillary bore which causes the mercury to remain at a given level. Thus, when a patient's temperature is taken there is adequate time to read the thermometer since the reading remains unchanged until a gentle shake causes the mercury to return to the bulb.

Q1   Answer true or false:

a. Temperature is an indicator of body normalcy. _____
b. The thermometer is a common temperature measuring device. _____
c. Thermometers for measuring body temperatures should be shaken following a reading to return the mercury to the bulb. _____

•   # # #   •   # # #   •   # # #   •   # # #   •   # # #   •   # # #   •   # # #   •   # #

A1   **a.** true   **b.** true   **c.** true

---

2   In countries using the metric system, two scales are used to measure temperature. The *Kelvin* scale is used for calculations involving gases, while the *Celsius* (formerly centigrade) scale is used for such things as laboratory work, the air and body temperature measurement.

The Kelvin scale, named after the British physicist Lord Kelvin (1878–1955), has its starting point at absolute zero (the temperature at which all molecular activity ceases) and a fixed point of 273.15 K at the triple point of water (the temperature at which water exists in all three states—vapor, liquid, and solid). The triple point of water is slightly above what we call the freezing point. The Celsius scale is named after the Swedish astronomer, Anders Celsius (1701–1744), who invented it.

The symbols for Kelvin (K) and Celsius (°C) temperatures are written without periods and with one space separating them from the numerical reading.

Examples:

310.15 K   not   310.15K
0 °C   not   0°C
100 °C   not   100°C.

Q2   Circle the temperature readings below which are written correctly.

310.15 °K   25 °C   10°C   200 K   30 °C.

•   # # #   •   # # #   •   # # #   •   # # #   •   # # #   •   # # #   •   # # #   •   # #

A2   25 °C, 200 K: 310.15 °K (degree symbol not used on K)
10°C (no space between 10 and °C)
30 °C. (period not used)

---

3   The Celsius scale is used for recording the temperature of the human body. Normal oral body temperature is 37 °C while normal rectal body temperature is 37.6 °C. The following details a range of oral body temperatures on the Celsius scale and the corresponding condition of the body.

Temperature	Condition
40 °C	Dangerous
39 °C	Very feverish
38 °C	Feverish
37 °C	Normal

Other important Celsius temperatures are the freezing point of water (0 °C), and the boiling point of water (100 °C). A comfortable room temperature is 20 °C.

The Kelvin and Celsius temperature scales are compared:

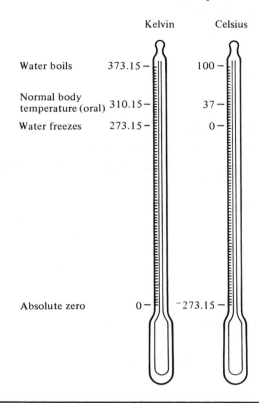

Q3   Complete each of the following:

    a. Write the freezing point of water in the Celsius and Kelvin temperature scales. _____ _____

    b. Write the boiling point of water in the Celsius and Kelvin scales. _____ _____

    c. Write the normal oral body temperature in the Celsius scale. _____

    d. Write the normal body rectal temperature in the Celsius scale. _____

\# \# \# • \# \# \# • \# \# \# • \# \# \# • \# \# \# • \# \# \# • \# \# \# • \# \# \# • \# \# \#

A3   **a.** 0 °C, 273.15 K   **b.** 100 °C, 373.15 K   **c.** 37 °C   **d.** 37.6 °C

---

4   Notice that the difference between the freezing and boiling points is 100 on both the Celsius and Kelvin scales. The only difference between the two scales is that each Kelvin temperature is 273.15 units more than each Celsius temperature. Thus, to find the Kelvin temperature, add 273.15 to the Celsius temperature. The procedure in symbols is: $K = C + 273.15$.

Example: What is the Kelvin temperature for 25 °C?

Solution: $K = C + 273.15$
           $K = 25 + 273.15$
           $K = 298.15$

Thus, 25 °C = 298.15 K

Q4   Find the Kelvin temperature:

a. $50\,°C =$ _____   **b.** $110\,°C =$ _____

\# \# \#   •   \# \# \#   •   \# \# \#   •   \# \# \#   •   \# \# \#   •   \# \# \#   •   \# \# \#   •   \# \# \#   •   \# \# \#

A4   **a.** 323.15 K   **b.** 383.15 K

---

5   To find the Celsius temperature given the Kelvin temperature, subtract 273.15 from the Kelvin temperature. The procedure in symbols is: $C = K - 273.15$.

Example: What is the Celsius temperature for 300 K?

Solution: $C = K - 273.15$
$C = 300 - 273.15$
$C = 300.00 - 273.15$
$C = 26.85$

Thus, $300\,K = 26.85\,°C$

Q5   Find the Celsius temperature:

a. $350.15\,K =$ _____   **b.** $273.15 K =$ _____

\# \# \#   •   \# \# \#   •   \# \# \#   •   \# \# \#   •   \# \# \#   •   \# \# \#   •   \# \# \#   •   \# \# \#   •   \# \# \#

A5   **a.** $77\,°C$ **b.** $0\,°C$

---

6   The 24-hour time system is not a part of the metric system. It is presented here, because it has been found useful for scheduling purposes in our country as well as in most foreign countries. The use of a 24 hour clock avoids the confusion of A.M. and P.M. and simplifies record keeping. In the 24-hour time system the first twelve hours (midnight to noon) are named the same as in the familiar 12-hour system. The latter twelve hours (noon to midnight) are named with the numbers from 13 to 24.

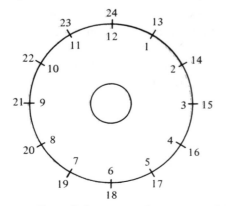

Four digits are used to express 24-hour time. The first two digits tell the hour, the last two digits indicate the minutes. The "h" following a 24-hour clock time stands for "hours."

24-Hour Clock System

Conventional Time System	24-Hour Clock System
12:01 A.M.	0001 h
1:00 A.M.	0100 h
2:00 A.M.	0200 h
3:00 A.M.	0300 h
4:00 A.M.	0400 h
5:00 A.M.	0500 h
6:00 A.M.	0600 h
7:00 A.M.	0700 h
8:00 A.M.	0800 h
9:00 A.M.	0900 h
10:00 A.M.	1000 h
11:00 A.M.	1100 h
12:00 noon	1200 h
1:00 P.M.	1300 h
2:00 P.M.	1400 h
3:00 P.M.	1500 h
4:00 P.M.	1600 h
5:00 P.M.	1700 h
6:00 P.M.	1800 h
7:00 P.M.	1900 h
8:00 P.M.	2000 h
9:00 P.M.	2100 h
10:00 P.M.	2200 h
11:00 P.M.	2300 h
12:00 midnight	2400 h

Q7 Change to 24-hour time:

a. 9:15 A.M. _____　　　　**b.** 8:20 P.M. _____

c. 10:30 P.M. _____　　　　**d.** 10:30 A.M. _____

• # # # • # # # • # # # • # # # • # # # • # # # • # # # • # #

A7　**a.** 0915 h　　　**b.** 2020 h　　　**c.** 2230 h　　　**d.** 1030 h

Q8 Change to 12-hour time:

a. 1245 h _____　　　　**b.** 1750 h _____

c. 0230 h _____　　　　**d.** 2110 h _____

• # # # • # # # • # # # • # # # • # # # • # # # • # # # • # #

A8　**a.** 12:45 P.M.　　**b.** 5:50 P.M.　　**c.** 2:30 A.M.　　**d.** 9:10 P.M.

7　In the 24-hour clock system, times preceded by zeros are read with "zero" or "oh." Times for each of the 24 hours are read with the word "hundred."

Examples:

Time	Correctly read
0530 h	"zero five thirty hours" or "oh five thirty hours"
0800 h	"zero eight hundred hours" or "oh eight hundred hours"
1600 h	"sixteen hundred hours"
2250 h	"twenty-two fifty hours"

Q9   Write the correct reading for each time:

   a. 0100 h _____   **b.** 1245 h _____

   c. 0700 h _____   **d.** 2330 h _____

•   # # #   •   # # #   •   # # #   •   # # #   •   # # #   •   # # #   •   # # #   •   # #

A9   **a.** zero one hundred hours or oh one hundred hours
     b. twelve forty-five hours
     c. zero seven hundred hours
     d. twenty-three thirty hours

Q10   Circle the time which is earlier in the day:

   a. 1100 h or 11:00 P.M.   **b.** 2100 h or 9:15 P.M.

   c. 1730 h or 5:20 P.M.   **d.** 0115 h or 1:00 P.M.

•   # # #   •   # # #   •   # # #   •   # # #   •   # # #   •   # # #   •   # # #   •   # #

A10   **a.** 1100 h   **b.** 2100 h   **c.** 5:20 P.M.   **d.** 0115 h

This completes the instruction for this section.

4.4   EXERCISE

1. Complete the table:

	Celsius	Kelvin
a. Freezing point of water	_____	_____
b. Normal body temperature	_____	_____
c. Boiling point of water	_____	_____

2. Circle the temperatures which are written correctly.

   42 °C.   42°C   273 K   20 °C   150K.

3. Complete each of the following:

   a. 345.15 K = _____ °C   **b.** 20 °C = _____ K   **c.** 85 °C = _____ K

   d. 273.15 K = _____ °C   **e.** 0 °C = _____ K   **f.** 310.15 K = _____ °C

4. Write the 24-hour clock time:
   a. 3:45 A.M.   **b.** 3:45 P.M.   **c.** 1:00 A.M.   **d.** 11:30 P.M.

5. Write the 12-hour clock time:
   a. 0910 h   **b.** 2400 h   **c.** 2300 h   **d.** 1530 h

6. Write the correct reading for each time:
   a. 1200 h   **b.** 0230 h   **c.** 0700 h   **d.** 2345 h

4.4   EXERCISE ANSWERS

1. a. 0 °C, 273.15 K   **b.** 37 °C, 310.15 K   **c.** 100 °C, 373.15 K
2. 273 K, 20 °C
3. a. 72   **b.** 293.15   **c.** 358.15
    d. 0   **e.** 273.15   **f.** 37

4. a. 0345 h   **b.** 1545 h   **c.** 0100 h   **d.** 2330 h
5. a. 9:10 A.M.   **b.** 12 midnight   **c.** 11:00 P.M.   **d.** 3:30 P.M.
6. a. twelve hundred hours   **b.** zero two thirty-hours
    c. zero seven hundred hours   **d.** twenty-three forty-five hours

4.5 METRIC–ENGLISH CONVERSION

1 During the period of gradual change from an English system of measurement to a metric system there will initially be, for some, confusion as to what a given measurement in one system means in terms of the other. Although, ideally, everyone will quickly learn to "think metric," most likely this will not happen overnight. The purpose of this section, therefore, is to develop the ability to perform conversions between units of the two systems. Recall from Section 4.1 the scale drawing comparing 1 metre and 1 yard.

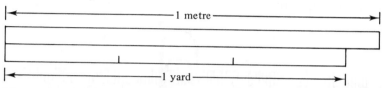

More precisely, the approximate conversion factors between the metre, yard, and foot are:

To Convert	Into	Multiply by	Conversion Fact
metres (m)	yards (yd)	1.1	1 m = 1.1 yd*
metres (m)	feet (ft)	3.3	1 m = 3.3 ft
yards (yd)	metres (m)	0.9	1 yd = 0.9 m

Example 1: Complete the equation. 12 m = _____ yd

Solution: To convert m to yd, multiply by 1.1. Thus, since 12(1.1) = 13.2, 12 m = 13.2 yd.

Example 2: Complete the equation. 440 yd = _____ m

Solution: To convert yd to m, multiply by 0.9. Thus, since 440(0.9) = 396, 440 yd = 396 m.

*In this text, the use of the "=" sign between a customary and a metric measurement will be understood to mean "is approximately equal to."

Q1 **a.** Which is longer, a metre or a yard? _____
    b. If a person is 2 m tall, is he taller or shorter than 6 ft (2 yd)? _____
    c. Write the following in order from smallest to largest:

       yard, foot, metre _____

• # # # • # # # • # # # • # # # • # # # • # # # • # # # • # #

A1   **a.** metre   **b.** taller   **c.** foot, yard, metre

Q2 Complete the equation:

    a. 42 yd = _____ m   **b.** 25.6 m = _____ yd

c. 800 m = _____ ft

d. 36 yd = _____ m

\# \# \# • \# \# \# • \# \# \# • \# \# \# • \# \# \# • \# \# \# • \# \# \# • \# \# \# • \# \# \#

A2   **a.** 37.8   **b.** 28.16   **c.** 2640   **d.** 32.4

---

2   The relationship among the inch, centimetre, and millimetre can be seen in a comparison of the metric and English rulers. Notice that a large paper clip approximates the metric units centimetre and millimetre quite closely. That is

1 centimetre = width of a large paper clip
1 millimetre = diameter of a paper-clip wire

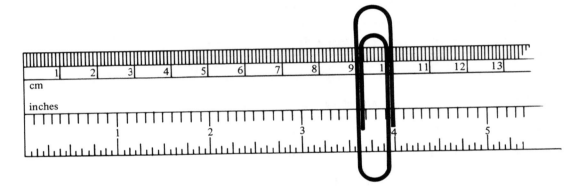

For conversion purposes, the approximations are:

To convert	Into	Multiply by	Conversion Fact
millimetres (mm)	inches (in.)	0.04	1 mm = 0.04 in.
centimetres (cm)	inches (in.)	0.4	1 cm = 0.4 in.
inches (in.)	centimetres (cm)	2.5	1 in. = 2.5 cm
feet (ft)	centimetres (cm)	30	1 ft = 30 cm

Example 1: Complete the equation. 175 cm = _____ in.

Solution: To convert cm to in., multiply by 0.4. Thus, since 175(0.4) = 70, 175 cm = 70 in.

Example 2: Complete the equation. 9.5 ft = _____ cm

Solution: To convert ft to cm, multiply by 30. Thus, since 9.5(30) = 285, 9.5 ft = 285 cm.

Q3   **a.** Which is larger, 1 cm or 1 in.? _____

b. Which is larger, 1 cm or 1 mm? _____
c. Write the following in order from smallest to largest:

mm, in., ft, yd, cm, m _____

\# \# \# • \# \# \# • \# \# \# • \# \# \# • \# \# \# • \# \# \# • \# \# \# • \# \# \# • \# \# \#

A3   **a.** 1 in.   **b.** 1 cm   **c.** mm, cm, in., ft, yd, m

Q4   Complete the equation:

   a. 25.4 cm = _____ in.

   b. 50 mm = _____ in.

   c. 48 ft = _____ cm

   d. 6 cm = _____ in.

•   # # #   •   # # #   •   # # #   •   # # #   •   # # #   •   # # #   •   # # #   •   # #

A4   **a.** 10.16   **b.** 2   **c.** 1440   **d.** 2.4

---

3   Charts are often used in medical facilities for rapid conversion between the metric and customary systems. The table that follows is a metric conversion table for use with the measurement of newborn infants:

Inch–centimetre Conversion Table

Inches	0	10	20	30	40	50
0	0	25.4	50.8	76.2	101.6	127.0
1	2.5	27.9	53.3	78.7	104.1	129.5
2	5.0	30.4	55.8	81.2	106.6	132.0
3	7.6	33.0	58.4	83.8	109.2	134.6
4	10.1	35.5	60.9	86.3	111.7	137.1
5	12.7	38.1	63.5	88.9	114.3	139.7
6	15.2	40.6	66.0	91.4	116.8	142.2
7	17.7	43.1	68.5	93.9	119.3	144.7
8	20.3	45.7	71.1	96.5	121.9	147.3
9	22.8	48.2	73.6	99.0	124.4	149.8

Example: Find the length in centimetres of a newborn infant 22 inches in length.

Solution: Locate 20 on the top scale and 2 on the side scale. The intersection of the 20 column and the 2 row is the equivalent of 22 inches in centimetres. Thus, 22 inches = 55.8 cm.

Q5   Find the length in centimetres of the following using the chart of Frame 3.

   a. 32 in. = _____   **b.** 46 in. = _____

•   # # #   •   # # #   •   # # #   •   # # #   •   # # #   •   # # #   •   # # #   •   # #

   a. 81.2 cm   **b.** 116.8 cm

---

4   The metric unit of measure for long distances is the kilometre. It is comparable to the U.S. customary unit the mile. Since 1 metre is approximately 3 feet, 1 kilometre is 1000 metres or 1000 (3 feet) = 3000 ft. Recall that 5280 ft = 1 mile. Thus 1 kilometre is a little longer than $\frac{1}{2}$ mile. For conversion purposes, the mile and kilometre are approximately related as follows:

To Convert	Into	Multiply by	Conversion Fact
kilometres (km)	miles (mi)	0.6	1 km = 0.6 mi
miles (mi)	kilometres (km)	1.6	1 mi = 1.6 km

Q6　**a.** Which is larger, a kilometre or a mile? _____
　　b. Write the following in order from smallest to largest:

　　in., cm, mm, yd, ft, mi, m, km _____

#　•　# # #　•　# # #　•　# # #　•　# # #　•　# # #　•　# # #　•　# # #　•　# #

A6　**a.** mile　　**b.** mm, cm, in., ft, yd, m, km, mi

Q7　Perform each conversion:

　　a. 10 mi = _____ km　　　　**b.** 50 km = _____ mi

#　•　# # #　•　# # #　•　# # #　•　# # #　•　# # #　•　# # #　•　# # #　•　# #

A7　**a.** 16　　　　　　　　　　**b.** 30

5　The following is a scale that gives approximate relationships between kilometres and miles. It can be used to check answers to conversion problems or to quickly estimate one reading in terms of the other.

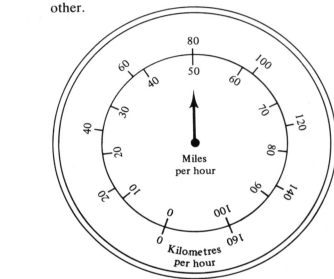

Q8　What is the approximate speed limit, in miles per hour, indicated by each of the following metric speed-limit signs (kilometres per hour):

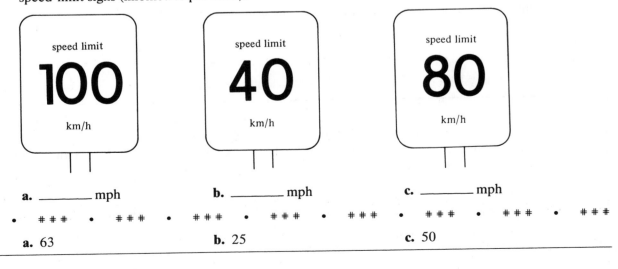

a. _____ mph　　　**b.** _____ mph　　　**c.** _____ mph

#　•　# # #　•　# # #　•　# # #　•　# # #　•　# # #　•　# # #　•　# # #　•　# #

A8　**a.** 63　　　　　　　**b.** 25　　　　　　　**c.** 50

Q9   Use the scale from Frame 5 to approximate the distance in miles to each of the following cities:

     a. Detroit, 70 kilometres _____

     b. Lansing, 105 kilometres _____

     c. Mackinac Bridge, 450 kilometres _____

\# \# \# • \# \# \# • \# \# \# • \# \# \# • \# \# \# • \# \# \# • \# \# \# • \# \# \# • \# \# \#

A9   **a.** 42 mi   **b.** 63 mi   **c.** 270 mi

     (*Note*: Answers may vary slightly.)

---

6   Units of area in the metric and U.S. customary systems are related in the same way as their corresponding linear (length) units. Thus, since 1 metre is larger than 1 yd, 1 square metre is larger than 1 square yard. Similarly, just as 1 inch is larger than 1 cm, 1 square inch is larger than 1 square centimetre.

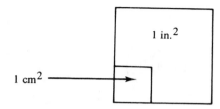

Some of the approximate relationships for units of area are:

To Convert	Into	Multiply by	Conversion Fact
square centimetres (cm^2)	square inches ($in.^2$)	0.16	$1\ cm^2 = 0.16\ in.^2$
square metres (m^2)	square yards (yd^2)	1.2	$1\ m^2 = 1.2\ yd^2$
square inches ($in.^2$)	square centimetres (cm^2)	6.5	$1\ in.^2 = 6.5\ cm^2$
square feet (ft^2)	square metres (m^2)	0.09	$1\ ft^2 = 0.09\ m^2$
square yards (yd^2)	square metres (m^2)	0.8	$1\ yd^2 = 0.8\ m^2$

Q10   The burn area of a patient was 15 square inches. What is the burn area in square centimetres?

\# \# \# • \# \# \# • \# \# \# • \# \# \# • \# \# \# • \# \# \# • \# \# \# • \# \# \# • \# \# \#

A10   97.5 cm^2

Q11   The barometer pressure recorded was 92 pounds per square centimetre. What is the pressure in pounds per square inch?

\# \# \# • \# \# \# • \# \# \# • \# \# \# • \# \# \# • \# \# \# • \# \# \# • \# \# \# • \# \# \#

A11   14.72

---

7   The metric units gram and kilogram are used in the same way as the U.S. customary units ounce and pound. The approximate relationships between these units are:

To Convert	Into	Multiply by	Conversion Fact
grams (g)	ounces (oz)	0.035	1 g = 0.035 oz
kilograms (kg)	pounds (lb)	2.2	1 kg = 2.2 lb
ounces (oz)	grams (g)	28	1 oz = 28 g
pounds (lb)	grams (g)	454	1 lb = 454 g
pounds (lb)	kilograms (kg)	0.454	1 lb = 0.454 kg

To help yourself think metric, notice that a kilogram is more than twice as large as a pound, while a gram is only approximately $\frac{1}{28}$ of an ounce. Some common comparisons with the gram are the weight of a large paper clip (1 g), the weight of a nickel (5 g), and of a pound of butter (454 g).

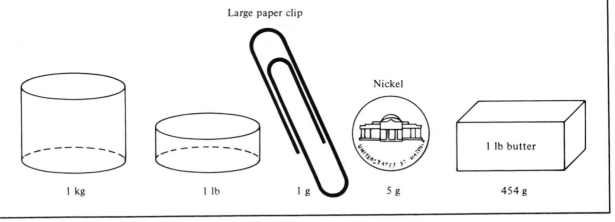

Large paper clip

Nickel

1 lb butter

1 kg   1 lb   1 g   5 g   454 g

Q12   Write the following in order from smallest to largest:

g, lb, kg, oz, mg _____

\# \# \# • \# \# \# • \# \# \# • \# \# \# • \# \# \# • \# \# \# • \# \# \# • \# \# \# • \# \# \#

A12   mg, g, oz, lb, kg

Q13   A patient's admittance weight is 180 lb. What is the patient's weight in kilograms?

\# \# \# • \# \# \# • \# \# \# • \# \# \# • \# \# \# • \# \# \# • \# \# \# • \# \# \# • \# \# \#

A13   81.72 kilograms

Q14   A 6-ounce sample has been taken. What is the weight of the sample in grams?

\# \# \# • \# \# \# • \# \# \# • \# \# \# • \# \# \# • \# \# \# • \# \# \# • \# \# \# • \# \# \#

A14   168 grams

Q15   Complete the equation. 20 g = _____ oz

\# \# \# • \# \# \# • \# \# \# • \# \# \# • \# \# \# • \# \# \# • \# \# \# • \# \# \# • \# \# \#

A15   0.7

8   The following table converts mass (weight) in pounds to kilograms.

Pound–Kilogram Conversion Table

Pounds	0	1	2	3	4	5	6	7	8	9
0	0.00	0.45	0.91	1.36	1.81	2.27	2.72	3.18	3.63	4.08
10	4.54	4.99	5.44	5.90	6.35	6.80	7.26	7.71	8.16	8.62
20	9.07	9.53	9.98	10.43	10.89	11.34	11.79	12.25	12.70	13.15
30	13.61	14.06	14.51	14.97	15.42	15.88	16.33	16.78	17.24	17.69
40	18.14	18.60	19.05	19.50	19.96	20.41	20.87	21.32	21.77	22.23
50	22.68	23.13	23.59	24.04	24.49	24.95	25.40	25.85	26.31	26.76
60	27.22	27.67	28.12	28.58	29.03	29.48	29.94	30.39	30.84	31.30
70	31.75	32.21	32.66	33.11	33.57	34.02	34.47	34.93	35.38	35.83
80	36.29	36.74	37.19	37.65	38.10	38.56	39.01	39.46	39.92	40.37
90	40.82	41.28	41.73	42.18	42.64	43.09	43.54	44.00	44.45	44.91
100	45.36	45.81	46.27	46.72	47.17	47.63	48.08	48.53	48.99	49.44
110	49.90	50.35	50.80	51.26	51.71	52.16	52.62	53.07	53.52	53.98
120	54.43	54.88	55.34	55.79	56.25	56.70	57.15	57.61	58.06	58.51
130	58.97	59.42	59.87	60.33	60.78	61.23	61.69	62.14	62.60	63.05
140	63.50	63.96	64.41	64.86	65.32	65.77	66.22	66.68	67.13	67.59
150	68.04	68.49	68.95	69.40	69.85	70.31	70.76	71.21	71.67	72.12
160	72.57	73.03	73.48	73.94	74.39	74.84	75.30	75.75	76.20	76.66
170	77.11	77.56	78.02	78.47	78.93	79.38	79.83	80.29	80.74	81.19
180	81.65	82.10	82.55	83.01	83.46	83.91	84.37	84.82	85.28	85.73
190	86.18	86.64	87.09	87.54	88.00	88.45	88.90	89.36	89.81	90.26
200	90.72	91.17	91.63	92.08	92.53	92.99	93.44	93.89	94.35	94.80

Example: Find the mass (weight) in kilograms of a patient with a mass of 125 pounds.

Solution: Locate 120 on the side scale and 5 on the top scale. The intersection of the 120 row and the 5 column is the equivalent of 125 pounds in kilograms. Thus, 125 lb = 56.7 kg.

Q16   Find the equivalent of each of the following in kilograms:

  a. 198 lb = _____   **b.** 9 lb = _____

•   # # #   •   # # #   •   # # #   •   # # #   •   # # #   •   # # #   •   # # #   •   # #

A16   **a.** 89.81 kg   **b.** 4.08 kg

9   Comparable units of liquid volume in the metric and U.S. customary systems are the litre and quart. Recall from Section 4.2 that a litre is slightly larger than a quart. Since the quart and litre so closely approximate each other, they are considered equal unless the situation requires a high degree of accuracy. Thus, useful approximations are:

1 quart = 1000 ml
1 pint = 500 ml
1 cup   = 250 ml

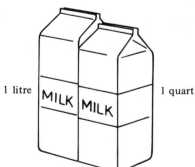

1 litre   1 quart

For small amounts of liquid the millilitre and ounce are comparable units. As can be seen from the actual size medicine cup shown at the left on the next page,

1 oz = 30 ml

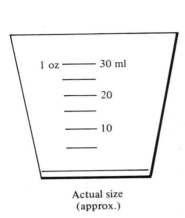

Actual size
(approx.)

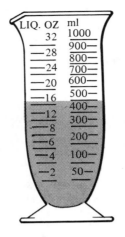

Scale drawing of 1 litre

The approximate conversion factors for metric and U.S. customary liquid volume units are:

To Convert	Into	Multiply by	Conversion Fact
millilitres (ml)	fluid ounces (oz)	0.03	1 ml = 0.03 oz
litres (l)	pints (pt)	2.1	1 l = 2.1 pt
litres (l)	quarts (qt)	1.06	1 l = 1.06 qt
litres (l)	gallons (gal)	0.26	1 l = 0.26 gal
fluid ounces (oz)	millilitres (ml)	30	1 oz = 30 ml
pints (pt)	litres (l)	0.47	1 pt = 0.47 l
quarts (qt)	litres (l)	0.95	1 qt = 0.95 l
gallons (gal)	litres (l)	3.8	1 gal = 3.8 l

Q17   The solution remaining in a container measured 12 oz. How many millilitres were in the container?

• # # # • # # # • # # # • # # # • # # # • # # # • # # # • # #

A17   360 ml

Q18   Write the approximate number of millilitres in each of the following:

a. 1 quart = _____   **b.** 1 pint = _____   **c.** 1 cup = _____

• # # # • # # # • # # # • # # # • # # # • # # # • # # # • # #

A18   **a.** 1000 ml   **b.** 500 ml   **c.** 250 ml

Q19   Use conversion factors to complete each equation:

a. 5 gal = _____ l   **b.** 240 ml = _____ oz

c. 18 oz = _____ ml   **d.** 7 pt = _____ l

• # # # • # # # • # # # • # # # • # # # • # # # • # # # • # #

A18   **a.** 19   **b.** 7.2   **c.** 540   **d.** 3.29

10   Volume measures in cubic units are approximately related in the metric and U.S. customary systems as follows:

To Convert	Into	Multiply by	Conversion Fact
cubic centimetres (cm^3)	cubic inches (in.^{3})	0.06	$1\ cm^3 = 0.06\ in.^3$
cubic metres (m^3)	cubic feet (ft^3)	35	$1\ m^3 = 35\ ft^3$
cubic metres (m^3)	cubic yards (yd^3)	1.3	$1\ m^3 = 1.3\ yd^3$
cubic inches (in.^{3})	cubic centimetres (cm^3)	16	$1\ in.^3 = 16.39\ cm^3$
cubic feet (ft^3)	cubic metres (m^3)	0.03	$1\ ft^3 = 0.03\ m^3$
cubic yards (yd^3)	cubic metres (m^3)	0.76	$1\ yd^3 = 0.76\ m^3$

Q20   A laboratory container has a volume of 3280 cubic centimetres. What is the volume in cubic inches?

\# \# \#   •   \# \# \#   •   \# \# \#   •   \# \# \#   •   \# \# \#   •   \# \# \#   •   \# \# \#   •   \# \# \#   •   \# \# \#

A20 $196.8\ in.^3$

Q21   A pharmacy storage area has a volume of 6 cubic metres. What is the volume in cubic feet?

\# \# \#   •   \# \# \#   •   \# \# \#   •   \# \# \#   •   \# \# \#   •   \# \# \#   •   \# \# \#   •   \# \# \#   •   \# \# \#

A21 $210\ ft^3$

11   Temperature in the metric system is measured on the Kelvin and the Celsius scales. The U.S. customary system uses the Fahrenheit scale for temperature measurement. The Fahrenheit scale was named in honor of its designer, Gabriel Fahrenheit, 1686–1736, a German physicist. The three scales are compared below. Important temperatures on the Fahrenheit scale are the freezing (32 °F) and boiling (212 °F) points of water and normal oral body temperature (98.6 °F).

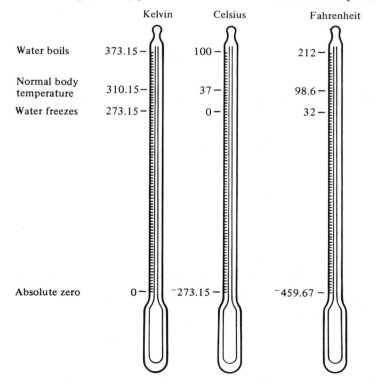

Q22   Complete the table:

	Normal body temperature	Freezing point	Boiling point
a. Celsius	_____	_____	_____
b. Fahrenheit	_____	_____	_____

\# \# \# • \# \# \# • \# \# \# • \# \# \# • \# \# \# • \# \# \# • \# \# \# • \# \# \# • \# \# \#

A22   **a.** 37 °C, 0 °C, 100 °C   **b.** 98.6 °F, 32 °F, 212 °F

---

12   The conversion formulas for Celsius (C) and Fahrenheit (F) temperatures are as follows:

$$C = \frac{F-32}{1.8} \quad \text{and} \quad F = 1.8C + 32$$

To change 75 °F to its corresponding Celsius temperature, we use the formula $C = \frac{F-32}{1.8}$ as follows:

$$C = \frac{F-32}{1.8}$$
$$C = \frac{75-32}{1.8}$$
$$C = \frac{43}{1.8}$$
C = 23.9   Hence, 75 °F = 23.9 °C.

All temperatures will be rounded off to the nearest tenth.

Q23   50 °F = _____ °C

\# \# \# • \# \# \# • \# \# \# • \# \# \# • \# \# \# • \# \# \# • \# \# \# • \# \# \# • \# \# \#

A23   10: $C = \frac{F-32}{1.8}$
$$C = \frac{50-32}{1.8}$$
$$C = \frac{18}{1.8}$$
C = 10

---

13   To change 25 °C to its corresponding Fahrenheit temperature, we use the formula F = 1.8C + 32 as follows:

F = 1.8C + 32
F = 1.8(25) + 32
F = 45 + 32
F = 77   Hence, 25 °C = 77 °F

Q24   80 °C = _____ °F

• # # # • # # # • # # # • # # # • # # # • # # # • # # # • # # # • # #

A24   176: $F = 1.8C + 32$
$$F = 1.8(80) + 32$$
$$F = 144 + 32$$
$$F = 176$$

Q25   Complete each of the following:

a. 95 °F = _____ °C   **b.** 0 °C = _____ °F

c. 68 °F = _____ °C   **d.** 10 °C = _____ °F

• # # # • # # # • # # # • # # # • # # # • # # # • # # # • # # # • # #

A25   **a.** 35   **b.** 32   **c.** 20   **d.** 50

---

14   The following chart is a comparison of the Celsius and Fahrenheit scales. It can be used for quick approximations between the two scales. Body temperature records, however, should be read directly from a °C clinical thermometer.

Approximate Body Temperature Equivalents (Fahrenheit to Celsius)

°F	°C	°F	°C	°F	°C	°F	°C
92.0	33.3	95.8	35.4	99.6	37.6	103.4	39.7
92.2	33.4	96.0	35.6	99.8	37.7	103.6	39.8
92.4	33.6	96.2	35.7	100.0	37.8	103.8	39.9
92.6	33.7	96.4	35.8	100.2	37.9	104.0	40.0
92.8	33.8	96.6	35.9	100.4	38.0	104.2	40.1
93.0	33.9	96.8	36.0	100.6	38.1	104.4	40.2
93.2	34.0	97.0	36.1	100.8	38.2	104.6	40.3
93.4	34.1	97.2	36.2	101.0	38.3	104.8	40.4
93.6	34.2	97.4	36.3	101.2	38.4	105.0	40.6
93.8	34.3	97.6	36.4	101.4	38.6	105.2	40.7
94.0	34.4	97.8	36.6	101.6	38.7	105.4	40.8
94.2	34.6	98.0	36.7	101.8	38.8	105.6	40.9
94.4	34.7	98.2	36.8	102.0	38.9	105.8	41.0
94.6	34.8	98.4	36.9	102.2	39.0	106.0	41.2
94.8	34.9	98.6	37.0	102.4	39.1	106.2	41.3
95.0	35.0	98.8	37.1	102.6	39.2	106.4	41.4
95.2	35.1	99.0	37.2	102.8	39.3	106.6	41.5
95.4	35.2	99.2	37.3	103.0	39.4	106.8	41.6
95.6	35.3	99.4	37.4	103.2	39.6	107.0	41.7

Example: 99.4 °F = _____ °C

Solution: Locate 99.4 in the °F column and read its corresponding Celsius temperature. Thus, 99.4 °F = 37.4 °C.

Q26 Use the chart of Frame 14 to complete the following:

    a. 102 °F = _____ °C   **b.** 38.6 °C = _____ °F

• # # # • # # # • # # # • # # # • # # # • # # # • # # # • # #

A26   **a.** 38.9   **b.** 101.4

Q27 Match the Celsius temperature with the appropriate descriptions:

    a. 19 °C _____   1. The temperature of a patient with a slight fever.

    b.   0 °C _____   2. The temperature of an air-conditioned room.

    c. 38 °C _____   3. The freezing point of water.

    d. 100 °C _____   4. The boiling point of water.

• # # # • # # # • # # # • # # # • # # # • # # # • # # # • # #

A27   **a.** 2   **b.** 3   **c.** 1   **d.** 4

This completes the instruction for this section.

Summary of Approximate Conversion Factors—Customary to Metric Conversion

To Convert	Into	Multiply by	Conversion Fact
	Length		
inches (in.)	centimetres (cm)	2.5	1 in = 2.5 cm
feet (ft)	centimetres (cm)	30	1 ft = 30 cm
yards (yd)	metres (m)	0.9	1 yd = 0.9 m
miles (mi)	kilometres (km)	1.6	1 mi = 1.6 km
	Area		
square inches (in.^{2})	square centimetres (cm^2)	6.5	1 in.^{2} = 6.5 cm^2
square feet (ft^2)	square metres (m^2)	0.09	1 ft^2 = 0.09 m^2
square yards (yd^2)	square metres (m^2)	0.8	1 yd^2 = 0.8 m^2
	Mass (weight)		
ounces (oz)	grams (g)	28	1 oz = 28 g
pounds (lb)	kilograms (kg)	0.454	1 lb = 0.454 kg
	Volume		
ounces (oz)	millilitres (ml)	30	1 oz = 30 ml
pints (pt)	litres (l)	0.47	1 pt = 0.47 l
quarts (qt)	litres (l)	0.95	1 qt = 0.95 l
gallons (gal)	litres (l)	3.8	1 gal = 3.8 l
cubic inches (in.^{3})	cubic centimetres (cm^3)	16.39	1 in.^{3} = 16.39 cm^3
cubic feet (ft^3)	cubic metres (m^3)	0.03	1 ft^3 = 0.03 m^3
cubic yards (yd^3)	cubic metres (m^3)	0.76	1 yd^3 = 0.76 m^3
	Temperature		
Fahrenheit	Celsius		$C = \dfrac{F - 32}{1.8}$

Summary of Approximate Conversion Factors—Metric to Customary Conversion

To Convert	Into	Multiply by	Conversion Fact
	Length		
millimetres (mm)	inches (in.)	0.04	1 mm = 0.04 in.
centimetres (cm)	inches (in.)	0.4	1 cm = 0.4 in.
metres (m)	feet (ft)	3.3	1 m = 3.3 ft

Summary of Approximate Conversion Factors—Metric to Customary Conversion (*Continued*)

metres (m)	yards (yd)	1.1	1 m = 1.1 yd
kilometres (km)	miles (mi)	0.6	1 km = 0.6 mi
	Area		
square centimetres (cm^2)	square inches (in.^{2})	0.16	1 cm^2 = 0.16 in.^{2}
square metres (m^2)	square yards (yd^2)	1.2	1 m^2 = 1.2 yd^2
	Mass (weight)		
grams (g)	ounces (oz)	0.035	1 g = 0.035 oz
kilograms (kg)	pounds (lb)	2.2	1 kg = 2.2 lb
	Volume		
millilitres (ml)	fluid ounces (oz)	0.03	1 ml = 0.03 oz
litres (l)	pints (pt)	2.1	1 l = 2.1 pt
litres (l)	quarts (qt)	1.06	1 l = 1.06 qt
litres (l)	gallons (gal)	0.26	1 l = 0.26 gal
cubic centimetres (cm^3)	cubic inches (in.^{3})	0.06	1 cm^3 = 0.06 in.^{3}
cubic metres (m^3)	cubic feet (ft^3)	35	1 m^3 = 35 ft^3
cubic metres (m^3)	cubic yards (yd^3)	1.3	1 m^3 = 1.3 yd^3
	Temperature		
Celsius	Fahrenheit		$F = 1.8C + 32$

4.5   EXERCISE

(Use the conversion charts on the preceding pages, where necessary, when completing this exercise.)

1. Circle the longer unit:

   a. metre, yard   **b.** inch, centimetre

   c. mile, kilometre   **d.** centimetre, millimetre

2. Complete each of the following equations:

   a. 50 mi = _____ km   **b.** 67 in. = _____ cm

   c. 30.7 mm = _____ in.   **d.** 150 km = _____ mi

3. A patient's height is recorded as 5 feet 10 inches (70 inches). What is the patient's height in centimetres?

4. A newborn baby's length is 45 centimetres. What is the length in inches?

5. The area on which a skin graft is to be performed is 12 square inches. What is the area in square centimetres?

6. Complete each of the following equations:

   a. 108 yd^2 = _____ m^2 **b.** 10 cm^2 = _____ in.^{2}

7. Circle the heavier unit:

   a. kg, lb   **b.** g, oz   **c.** g, lb   **d.** kg, g

8. A man weighs 180 pounds. What is his weight in kilograms?

9. Complete each of the following equations:

   a. 12 oz = _____ g   **b.** 5 lb = _____ kg

10. Circle the larger unit:

   a. l, qt   **b.** ml, oz   **c.** pt, l   **d.** gal, l

11. The amount of solution to be prepared was 500 ml. What is the amount in ounces?

12. Give the approximate equivalent of each of the following in millilitres:

   a. 1 cup   **b.** 1 qt   **c.** 1 pt

13. Perform each of the following conversions:

   a. 15 cm^3 = _____ in.^{3} **b.** 25 yd^3 = _____ m^3

14. Complete the table:

	Celsius	Fahrenheit
a. Boiling point of water	_____	_____
b. Normal body temperature (oral)	_____	_____
c. Freezing point of water	_____	_____

15. Determine the corresponding Fahrenheit or Celsius temperature equivalents:
   a. 20 °C   **b.** 85 °F   **c.** 5 °C   **d.** 37 °F

4.5   EXERCISE ANSWERS

1. a. metre	**b.** inch	**c.** mile	**d.** centimetre
2. a. 80	**b.** 167.5	**c.** 1.228	**d.** 90
3. 175 cm	**4.** 18 in.	**5.** 78 cm^2	
6. a. 86.4	**b.** 1.6		
7. a. kg	**b.** oz	**c.** lb	**d.** kg
8. 81 kg	**9. a.** 336	**b.** 2.27	
10. a. l	**b.** oz	**c.** l	**d.** gal
11. 15	**12. a.** 250 ml	**b.** 1000 ml	**c.** 500 ml
13. a. 0.9	**b.** 19		
14. a. 100 °C, 212 °F	**b.** 37 °F, 98.6 °F	**c.** 0 °C, 32 °F	
15. a. 68 °F	**b.** 29.4 °C	**c.** 41 °F	**d.** 2.8 °C

CHAPTER 4 SAMPLE TEST

At the completion of Chapter 4 you should be able to work the following problems.

4.1   UNITS OF LENGTH AND AREA

1. The base unit of length in the metric system is the _____ .

2. The base metric unit of length is slightly _____ than a yard.
                                                        (longer/shorter)

3. Fill in the correct multiple or division of ten:

   a. 1 km = _____ m   **b.** 1 mm = _____ m

   c. 1 cm = _____ mm   **d.** 1 cm = _____ m

4. Perform each of the following conversions:

   a. 45 cm = _____ m   **b.** 2.5 m = _____ cm

   c. 850 cm = _____ dm   **d.** 5 km = _____ m

5. A patient's height is 167 centimetres. What is the patient's height in metres?

6. Perform each of the following conversions:

   a. 25 cm^2 = _____ mm^2 **b.** 750 mm^2 = _____ cm^2

7. The burn area on a patient's body is 5 dm^2. What is the burn area in square centimetres?

4.2   UNITS OF VOLUME

8. The unit for liquid volume in the metric system is the _____.

9. The metric unit for liquid volume is slightly _____ than a quart.
(larger/smaller)

10. Perform each of the following conversions:

    a. 250 ml = _____ l   **b.** 50 ml = _____ cm^3

    c. 1.5 l = _____ ml   **d.** 1 l = _____ cm^3

11. Which of the following most closely approximates 1 millilitre?

1 quart, $\frac{1}{4}$ teaspoon, $\frac{1}{3}$ litre

4.3   UNITS OF MASS (WEIGHT)

12. The base unit for mass in the metric system is the _____.

13. The base metric unit for mass is _____ than a pound.
(larger/smaller)

14. Perform each of the following conversions:

    a. 250 mg = _____ g   **b.** 2.5 kg = _____ g

    c. 0.5 g = _____ mg   **d.** 750 mg = _____ g

15. The physician orders 0.5 mg of a drug. What is the dosage in micrograms?

4.4   TEMPERATURE AND TIME

16. What is the Celsius temperature for each of the following:
    a. Normal body temperature (oral)
    b. Freezing point of water
    c. Boiling point of water

17. What is the normal rectal body temperature in Celsius?

18. Perform the following conversions:

    a. 273.15 K = _____ °C   **b.** 50 °C = _____ K

19. Write the 24-hour clock time:
    a. 2:15 A.M.   **b.** 2:15 P.M.
    c. 12:30 A.M.   **d.** 11:00 P.M.

20. Write the 12-hour clock time:
    a. 0200 h   **b.** 1830 h
    c. 0015 h   **d.** 2000 h

21. Write the correct reading for each time:
    a. 0500 h
    b. 1530 h

4.5   METRIC–ENGLISH CONVERSION

(Use the conversion charts which precede 4.5 Exercise.)

22. Arrange the following from smallest to largest: ft, yd, m, mi, km, mm, cm

23. Circle the smaller unit:

    a. pound, kilogram   **b.** litre, quart

    c. millilitre, ounce   **d.** metre, foot

24. Perform each of the following conversions:

    a. 88 km = _____ mi   **b.** 55 in. = _____ cm

    c. 250 cm = _____ in.   **d.** 250 ml = _____ oz

    e. 350 g = _____ oz   **f.** 150 lb = _____ kg

    g. 50 cm^3 = _____ in.^{3} **h.** 12 m^2 = _____ yd^2

25. Complete the table:

	Fahrenheit	Celsius
a. Boiling point of water	_____	_____
b. Normal body temperature (oral)	_____	_____
c. Freezing point of water	_____	_____

26. Perform each conversion:

    a. 13 °C = _____ °F   **b.** 59 °F = _____ °C

    c. 32 °F = _____ °C   **d.** 95 °F = _____ °C

CHAPTER 4 SAMPLE TEST ANSWERS

1. metre   **2.** longer

3. a. 1000   **b.** 0.001   **c.** 10   **d.** 0.01

4. a. 0.45   **b.** 250   **c.** 85   **d.** 5000

5. a. 1.67   **6. a.** 2500   **b.** 7.5

7. 500   **8.** litre   **9.** larger

10. a. 0.25   **b.** 50   **c.** 1500   **d.** 1000

11. $\frac{1}{4}$ teaspoon   **12.** kilogram   **13.** larger

14. a. 0.25   **b.** 2500   **c.** 500   **d.** 0.75

15. 500   **16. a.** 37 °C   **b.** 0 °C   **c.** 100 °C

17. 37.6 °C   **18. a.** 0   **b.** 323.15

19. a. 0215 h   **b.** 1415 h   **c.** 0030 h   **d.** 2300 h

20. a. 2:00 A.M.   **b.** 6:30 P.M.   **c.** 12:15 A.M.   **d.** 8:00 P.M.

21. a. zero five hundred or oh five hundred hours

    b. fifteen thirty hours

22. mm, cm, ft, yd, m, km, mi

23. a. pound   **b.** quart   **c.** millilitre   **d.** foot

24. a. 52.8   **b.** 137.5   **c.** 100   **d.** 7.5

    e. 12.25   **f.** 68.1   **g.** 3   **h.** 14.4

25. a. 212 °F, 100 °C   **b.** 98.6 °F, 37 °C   **c.** 32 °F, 0 °C

26. a. 55.4   **b.** 15   **c.** 0   **d.** 35

CHAPTER 5

THE APOTHECARIES' AND HOUSEHOLD SYSTEMS

The trend in the United States today is toward using the metric system as the only system for weighing and measuring drugs. Some health personnel still use the apothecaries' system however, and thus it is important to know this system as well as its relationship to the metric and household systems.

5.1 THE APOTHECARIES' SYSTEM: WEIGHT

1   The apothecaries' system is a system of ancient derivation which is used exclusively in the medical field. It includes only units for weight and volume. The smallest unit of weight in the apothecaries' system is the *grain*. It is named after the millet grain which was used in ancient times to balance material that was being weighed on a scale. In common terms one grain is the weight of one drop of water. The abbreviation for grain (gr) uses lowercase letters.

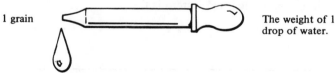

1 grain   The weight of 1 drop of water.

Q1   **a.** The smallest unit of weight in the apothecaries' system is the _____.

b. The abbreviation for grain is _____.

c. One grain is the weight of _____.

\# \# \#   •   \# \# \#   •   \# \# \#   •   \# \# \#   •   \# \# \#   •   \# \# \#   •   \# \# \#   •   \# \# \#   •   \# \# \#

A1   **a.** grain   **b.** gr   **c.** one drop of water

2   A grain is a very small unit of weight. So small, that it takes 15 grains to equal 1 gram. Recall from Chapter 4 that 1 gram is approximately the weight of a large paper clip. Thus, the weight of a large paper clip is about 15 grains.

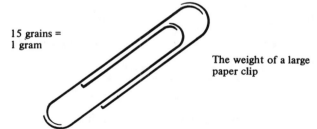

15 grains = 1 gram

The weight of a large paper clip

Since 1 gram is 15 times heavier than 1 grain, mistaking the two when giving medication could be serious. Thus, it is important to keep the relationship between the two straight. Likewise, do not confuse their symbols. 15 grains (gr) = 1 gram (g)

Q2 Circle the larger unit: grain, gram

• ### • ### • ### • ### • ### • ### • ### •

A2 gram

Q3 Write the abbreviation for each unit:

  a. gram_____ **b.** grain_____

• ### • ### • ### • ### • ### • ### • ### •

A3 **a.** g **b.** gr

Q4 Complete each of the following:

  a. _____gr = 1 g **b.** 1 gr = _____g

• ### • ### • ### • ### • ### • ### • ### •

A4 **a.** 15 **b.** $\dfrac{1}{15}$

---

3 The next largest unit of weight in the apothecaries' system is the *scruple*. One scruple is equal to 20 grains. The scruple is rarely used as a unit of weight; thus, you need not learn this relationship.

Q5 **a.** The smallest unit of weight in the apothecaries' system is the _____.

  b. The next largest unit of weight in the apothecaries' system is the _____.

• ### • ### • ### • ### • ### • ### • ### •

A5 **a.** grain **b.** scruple

---

4 A second often-used unit of weight in the apothecaries' system is the *dram*. It is named after the Greek drachma, an ancient silver coin which was supposed to have weighed the same amount. In common terms, one dram is the weight of one teaspoon of water. More precisely, one dram is equal to sixty grains. The symbol for dram is ʒ. The relationship which should be learned is:

60 grains (gr) = 1 dram (ʒ)

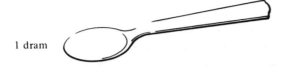

1 dram   The weight of 1 teaspoon of water

Q6 Write the abbreviation or symbol:

  a. grain_____ **b.** dram_____ **c.** gram_____

• ### • ### • ### • ### • ### • ### • ### •

A6 **a.** gr **b.** ʒ **c.** g

Q7 Complete each of the following:

  a. _____grains = 1 gram **b.** 1 dram = _____grains

• ### • ### • ### • ### • ### • ### • ### •

A7   **a.** 15   **b.** 60

Q8   Complete each of the following:

        a. Circle the largest unit: grain, dram, gram

        b. One dram is the weight of _____ .

•   # # #   •   # # #   •   # # #   •   # # #   •   # # #   •   # # #   •   # # #   •   # #

A8   **a.** dram   **b.** one teaspoon of water

---

5   The ounce and pound are the final units of weight in the apothecaries' system. The important relationships involving them are as follows:

    8 drams (ʒ) = 1 ounce (ℨ or oz)
      12 ounces = 1 pound (lb)

Notice that the symbol for ounce may be either ℨ or oz. The symbol ℨ is similar to that for dram (ʒ) except that it has one more zigzag on top. When using drug amounts larger than the ounce, the apothecaries', or 12-ounce pound is used. The apothecaries' pound is rarely needed, but when it is you should be aware that it is four ounces less than the standard, avoirdupois, 16-ounce pound.

Q9   Write the abbreviation or symbol:

        a. dram _____   **b.** ounce _____ or _____

        c. grain _____   **d.** pound _____

•   # # #   •   # # #   •   # # #   •   # # #   •   # # #   •   # # #   •   # # #   •   # #

A9   **a.** ʒ   **b.** ℨ or oz   **c.** gr   **d.** lb

Q10   Complete each of the following:

        a. 1 ounce = _____drams   **b.** 1 pound = _____ounces

        c. 1 gram = _____grains   **d.** 1 dram = _____grains

•   # # #   •   # # #   •   # # #   •   # # #   •   # # #   •   # # #   •   # # #   •   # #

A10   **a.** 8   **b.** 12   **c.** 15   **d.** 60

---

6   When drug amounts are recorded in the apothecaries' system, using abbreviations, the following procedures are used:

    1. Drug amounts are written following drug abbreviations or symbols.
    2. Small Roman numerals are used to express drug quantities unless the quantity is a fraction or a number containing a fraction (fractions other than 1/2).

                gr ix   9 grains
                lb vii   7 pounds

    3. Drug quantities involving a fraction or a number containing a fraction (fractions other than 1/2) are expressed in Arabic numerals following the unit.

$$ℨ\frac{1}{4} \qquad \frac{1}{4}\ \text{ounce}$$

$$\text{gr}\ 7\frac{1}{6} \qquad 7\frac{1}{6}\ \text{grains}$$

4. The symbol ss* is used for the fraction $\frac{1}{2}$.

$$\text{3 iiss} \qquad 2\frac{1}{2} \text{ drams}$$

If apothecaries' system units are not abbreviated, the amounts are written in ordinary Arabic numbers.

Examples: 12 ounces

$5\frac{1}{2}$ grains

*The symbol ss is derived from the word semi, meaning one-half.

Q11 Write abbreviations for each of the following:

a. 4 grains _____   b. 12 drams _____   c. 19 ounces _____

d. 20 pounds _____   e. $\frac{1}{3}$ dram _____   f. $6\frac{1}{2}$ ounces _____

• ### • ### • ### • ### • ### • ### • ### • ### •

A11 a. gr iv   b. ʒ xii   c. ʒ xix or oz xix

d. lb xx   e. ʒ $\frac{1}{3}$ f. ʒ viss or oz viss

Q12 Translate each of the following:

a. gr $\frac{1}{3}$ _____   b. ʒ xiv _____

c. ʒ xss _____   d. oz $5\frac{1}{7}$ _____

e. ʒ lxiv _____   f. lb viss _____

• ### • ### • ### • ### • ### • ### • ### • ### •

A12 a. $\frac{1}{3}$ grain   b. 14 drams   c. $10\frac{1}{2}$ ounces

d. $5\frac{1}{7}$ ounces   e. 64 drams   f. $6\frac{1}{2}$ pounds

7   It is important for health personnel to be able to perform conversions between apothecaries' system units of weight. One method for conversion uses multiplication and the arithmetic principle that something divided by itself is equal to 1. For example, $\frac{5}{5} = 1$, and since 1 foot is the same as 12 inches, $\frac{1 \text{ foot}}{12 \text{ inches}} = 1$. Some additional examples are:

1. $\frac{1 \text{ yard}}{3 \text{ feet}} = 1$ 2. $\frac{1 \text{ dram}}{60 \text{ grains}} = 1$ 3. $\frac{60 \text{ grains}}{1 \text{ dram}} = 1$

Q13 Fill in the missing numerator or denominator to make each of the following quotients equal to 1:

a. $\dfrac{\rule{1cm}{0.4pt}\text{grains}}{1 \text{ gram}} = 1$ b. $\dfrac{1 \text{ yd}}{\rule{1cm}{0.4pt}\text{in.}} = 1$

• ### • ### • ### • ### • ### • ### • ### • ### •

A13   **a.** 15   **b.** 36

---

8   The important equations relating apothecaries' system units of weight are:

gr	grain
ʒ	dram
℥	ounce
lb	pound

1 dram = 60 grains
1 ounce = 8 drams
1 pound = 12 ounces

The equal sign means that the amounts on opposite sides are the same.

Q14   Use the equations of Frame 8 to complete each of the following:

a. $\dfrac{1 \text{ dram}}{\underline{\hspace{1cm}}\text{grains}} = 1$

b. $\dfrac{1 \text{ pound}}{\underline{\hspace{1cm}}\text{ounces}} = 1$

c. $\dfrac{\underline{\hspace{1cm}}\text{drams}}{1 \text{ ounce}} = 1$

d. $\dfrac{1 \text{ ounce}}{\underline{\hspace{1cm}}\text{drams}} = 1$

\# \# \#   •   \# \# \#   •   \# \# \#   •   \# \# \#   •   \# \# \#   •   \# \# \#   •   \# \# \#   •   \# \# \#   •   \# \# \#

A14   **a.** 60   **b.** 12   **c.** 8   **d.** 8

---

9   Consider the following conversion between two apothecaries' system units of weight.

Example: Change 7 drams to grains.

Solution: To convert 7 drams to grains, we first choose a fraction equal to 1 which involves drams and grains. The fraction is either $\dfrac{1 \text{ dram}}{60 \text{ grains}} = 1$ or $\dfrac{60 \text{ grains}}{1 \text{ dram}} = 1$. Since we are *converting to grains*, use the fraction with *grains in the numerator*, and multiply this times 7 drams.

$$7 \text{ drams} \times \dfrac{60 \text{ grains}}{1 \text{ dram}} = 420 \text{ grains}$$

Notice that multiplying 7 drams by this fraction does not change its amount because the fraction is equal to 1. Notice also that if the conversion is set up correctly, the unit in the denominator cancels with the unit being converted.

Q15   **a.** Which fraction should be used to change 3 ounces to drams, $\dfrac{8 \text{ drams}}{1 \text{ ounce}}$ or $\dfrac{1 \text{ ounce}}{8 \text{ drams}}$?

b. Change 3 ounces to drams.

\# \# \#   •   \# \# \#   •   \# \# \#   •   \# \# \#   •   \# \# \#   •   \# \# \#   •   \# \# \#   •   \# \# \#   •   \# \# \#

A15   **a.** $\dfrac{8 \text{ drams}}{1 \text{ ounce}}$ **b.** 24 drams: $3 \text{ ounces} \times \dfrac{8 \text{ drams}}{1 \text{ ounce}} = 24 \text{ drams}$

Q16   Change 30 grains to drams.

\# \# \#   •   \# \# \#   •   \# \# \#   •   \# \# \#   •   \# \# \#   •   \# \# \#   •   \# \# \#   •   \# \# \#   •   \# \# \#

A16 $\frac{1}{2}$ dram: $30\ \text{grains} \times \dfrac{1\ \text{dram}}{60\ \text{grains}} = \dfrac{1}{2}\ \text{dram}$

Q17   Change 18 ounces to pounds.

\# \# \#   •   \# \# \#   •   \# \# \#   •   \# \# \#   •   \# \# \#   •   \# \# \#   •   \# \# \#   •   \# \# \#   •   \# \# \#

A17 $1\frac{1}{2}$ pounds: $18\ \text{ounces} \times \dfrac{1\ \text{pound}}{12\ \text{ounces}} = \dfrac{3}{2} = 1\frac{1}{2}\ \text{pounds}$

---

10   Many times the units to be converted are given in abbreviated form.

Example: Change ℥ xi to ʒ.

Solution: To perform the conversion, write the translation of the problem and proceed as before. Change 11 ounces to drams.

$$11\ \text{ounces} \times \dfrac{8\ \text{drams}}{1\ \text{ounce}} = 88\ \text{drams}$$

The answer should now be returned to abbreviated form. Thus, since 88 is lxxxviii in Roman numerals, the answer is ʒ lxxxviii.

Q18   Change ℥ ivss to ʒ.

\# \# \#   •   \# \# \#   •   \# \# \#   •   \# \# \#   •   \# \# \#   •   \# \# \#   •   \# \# \#   •   \# \# \#   •   \# \# \#

A18   ʒ xxxvi: $4\frac{1}{2}\ \text{ounces} \times \dfrac{8\ \text{drams}}{1\ \text{ounce}} = 36\ \text{drams}$

Q19   Change gr lx to ʒ.

\# \# \#   •   \# \# \#   •   \# \# \#   •   \# \# \#   •   \# \# \#   •   \# \# \#   •   \# \# \#   •   \# \# \#   •   \# \# \#

A19   ʒ i: $60\ \text{grains} \times \dfrac{1\ \text{dram}}{60\ \text{grains}} = 1\ \text{dram}$

Q20   Change ℥ lxxii to lb.

\# \# \#   •   \# \# \#   •   \# \# \#   •   \# \# \#   •   \# \# \#   •   \# \# \#   •   \# \# \#   •   \# \# \#   •   \# \# \#

A20   lb vi: $72\ \text{ounces} \times \dfrac{1\ \text{pound}}{12\ \text{ounces}} = 6\ \text{pounds}$

11   The important equations relating apothecaries' system units of weight are summarized as follows:

gr	grain
ʒ	dram
℥	ounce
lb	pound

1 dram = 60 grains
1 ounce = 8 drams
1 pound = 12 ounces

In some instances it is necessary to perform conversions between apothecaries' units which are not related directly by the three equations above.

Example: Change ℥ ii to gr.

Solution: To convert 2 ounces to grains, it is necessary to first convert ounces to drams.

$$2 \text{ ounces} \times \frac{8 \text{ drams}}{1 \text{ ounce}} = 16 \text{ drams}$$

The 16 drams can now be converted to grains.

$$16 \text{ drams} \times \frac{60 \text{ grains}}{1 \text{ dram}} = 960 \text{ grains}$$

Thus, ℥ ii = gr cmlx.

Q21   Change lb ii to ʒ by completing the following:
a. Change pounds to ounces.

b. Change ounces to drams.

c. Write the final anwer in Roman numerals.

•   # # #   •   # # #   •   # # #   •   # # #   •   # # #   •   # # #   •   # # #   •   # #

A21   **a.** 24 ounces: $2 \text{ pounds} \times \dfrac{12 \text{ ounces}}{1 \text{ pound}} = 24 \text{ ounces}$

b. 192 drams: $24 \text{ ounces} \times \dfrac{8 \text{ drams}}{1 \text{ ounce}} = 192 \text{ drams}$
c. ʒ cxcii

Q22   Change gr cdlxxx to ʒ by completing the following:
a. Change grains to drams.

b. Change drams to ounces.

c. Write the final answer in Roman numerals.

•   # # #   •   # # #   •   # # #   •   # # #   •   # # #   •   # # #   •   # # #   •   # #

A22   **a.** 8 drams: $480 \text{ grains} \times \dfrac{1 \text{ dram}}{60 \text{ grains}} = 8 \text{ drams}$

b. 1 ounce: $8 \text{ drams} \times \dfrac{1 \text{ ounce}}{8 \text{ drams}} = 1 \text{ ounce}$

c. ℥ i

---

12   Conversions similar to the previous two questions can be completed in just one process.

Example: Change ℥ lxxx to lb.

Solution: $80 \text{ drams} \times \dfrac{1 \text{ ounce}}{8 \text{ drams}} \times \dfrac{1 \text{ pound}}{12 \text{ ounces}} = \dfrac{80}{96} = \dfrac{5}{6} \text{ pound}$

Thus, ℥ lxxx $= \text{lb} \dfrac{5}{6}$. Notice that the units dram and ounce are canceled leaving the desired unit pound.

Q23   Change lb ss to ℥.

•   # # #   •   # # #   •   # # #   •   # # #   •   # # #   •   # # #   •   # # #   •   # #

A23   ℥ xlviii: $\dfrac{1}{2} \text{ pound} \times \dfrac{12 \text{ ounces}}{1 \text{ pound}} \times \dfrac{8 \text{ drams}}{1 \text{ ounce}} = \dfrac{96}{2} = 48 \text{ drams}$

Q24   Change gr cxx to ℥.

•   # # #   •   # # #   •   # # #   •   # # #   •   # # #   •   # # #   •   # # #   •   # #

A24   ℥ $\dfrac{1}{4}$: $120 \text{ grains} \times \dfrac{1 \text{ dram}}{60 \text{ grains}} \times \dfrac{1 \text{ ounce}}{8 \text{ drams}} = \dfrac{120}{480} = \dfrac{1}{4} \text{ ounce}$

This completes the instruction for this section.

5.1   EXERCISE

1. One _____ is the weight of one teaspoon of water.

2. One _____ is the weight of one drop of water.

3. Write an abbreviation or symbol for each of the following:
   a. grain   **b.** dram   **c.** ounce   **d.** pound

4. Complete each equation:

   a. 1 dram = _____ grains   **b.** 1 ounce = _____ drams

   c. 1 pound = _____ ounces   **d.** 1 gram = _____ grains

5. Write using symbols and Roman numerals:

   a. 24 grains   **b.** $9\dfrac{1}{2}$ ounces   **c.** 49 pounds   **d.** 19 drams

6. Perform each of the following conversions:

    a. Change gr cxx to ℨ.   **b.** Change lb iss to ℨ.   **c.** Change ℨ xii to oz.

    d. Change $3\frac{1}{5}$ to gr.   **e.** Change ℨ xxxvi to lb.   **f.** Change oz xii to ℨ.

7. Complete each of the following:

    a. ℨ viii = ℨ_____   **b.** ℨ ss = ℨ_____   **c.** gr xx = ℨ_____

    d. lb$\frac{1}{6}$ = ℨ_____   **e.** oz xviii = lb_____   **f.** ℨ ivss = gr_____

    g. lb iii = ℨ_____   **h.** gr cdlxxx = ℨ_____

5.1 EXERCISE ANSWERS

1. dram   **2.** grain

3. a. gr   **b.** ℨ   **c.** oz or ℨ   **d.** lb

4. a. 60   **b.** 8   **c.** 12   **d.** 15

5. a. gr xxiv   **b.** ℨ ixss   **c.** lb xlix   **d.** ℨ xix

6. a. ℨ ii   **b.** ℨ xviii   **c.** oz iss   **d.** gr xii

    e. lb iii   **f.** ℨ xcvi

7. a. ℨ i   **b.** ℨ iv   **c.** $3\frac{1}{3}$ **d.** ℨ ii

    e. lb iss   **f.** gr cclxx   **g.** cclxxxviii   **h.** ℨ i

5.2 THE APOTHECARIES' SYSTEM: VOLUME

1   The apothecaries' system units for liquid volume are related in the same way as the weight units. The smallest unit of liquid volume is the *minim*. It is considered the liquid equivalent of the grain. In common terms, the minim is the volume of one drop of water. The abbreviation for minim (m) is a lower case letter.*

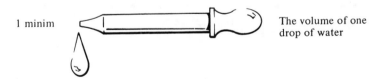

1 minim   The volume of one
drop of water

*The symbol for minim (m) is the same as that for metre (m). The unit desired will always be clear from the context of the work one is involved with.

Q1   The smallest unit of weight in the apothecaries' system is the _____.

    b. The smallest unit of liquid volume in the apothecaries' system is the _____.

    c. One minim is the volume of _____.

    d. The abbreviation for minim is _____.

• # # # • # # # • # # # • # # # • # # # • # # # • # # # • # #

A1   **a.** grain   **b.** minim   **c.** one drop of water   **d.** m

2 One fluidram (fluid dram) is the volume of one teaspoon of water. The symbol for fluidram is f℥. It is related to the minim by the following equation:

1 fluidram (f℥) = 60 minims (m)

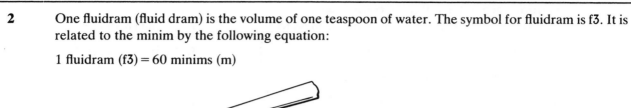

1 fluidram   The volume of 1 teaspoon of water

Q2   **a.** The symbol for fluidram is _____.

      b. The abbreviation for minim is _____.

      c. One fluidram is equal to _____ minims.

• # # # • # # # • # # # • # # # • # # # • # # # • # # # • # #

A2   **a.** f℥   **b.** m   **c.** 60

3 The apothecaries' system weight units dram and ounce are related by the equation:

8 drams = 1 ounce

The liquid volume units fluidram and fluidounce are similarly related. That is,

8 fluidrams = 1 fluidounce

In symbols, f℥ viii = f℥ i. Notice that the symbol for fluidounce is f℥.

Q3   Write the symbol or abbreviation:

      a. fluidram_____   **b.** dram_____   **c.** minim_____

      d. ounce_____   **e.** grain_____   **f.** fluidounce_____

• # # # • # # # • # # # • # # # • # # # • # # # • # # # • # #

A3   **a.** f℥   **b.** ℥   **c.** m   **d.** ℥ or oz   **e.** gr   **f.** f℥

Q4   Complete each equation:

      a. f℥ i = m_____   **b.** f℥ i = f℥_____

      c. ℥ i = gr_____   **d.** ℥ i = ℥_____

• # # # • # # # • # # # • # # # • # # # • # # # • # # # • # #

A4   **a.** lx   **b.** viii   **c.** lx   **d.** viii

4 Liquid volumes larger than fluidounces are often used. Since these are also used commonly in the home they are familiar to most everyone. The units and their relationships are as follows:

      1 pint (pt or O) = 16 fluidounces (f℥)
         1 quart (qt) = 2 pints
     1 gallon (gal or C) = 4 quarts

Q5   Write the symbol or abbreviation:

    a. quart_____

    b. pint_____ or _____

    c. gallon_____ or _____

\# \# \# • \# \# \# • \# \# \# • \# \# \# • \# \# \# • \# \# \# • \# \# \# • \# \# \# • \# \# \#

A5   **a.** qt   **b.** pt or O   **c.** gal or C

Q6   Complete each equation:

    a. C i = qt_____

    b. O i = f℥_____

    c. qt i = O_____

    d. f℥ i = f℈_____

\# \# \# • \# \# \# • \# \# \# • \# \# \# • \# \# \# • \# \# \# • \# \# \# • \# \# \# • \# \# \#

A6   **a.** iv   **b.** xvi   **c.** ii   **d.** viii

---

5   Conversions between apothecaries' system units of liquid volume are done as with units of weight.

Example 1: Change f℈ vi to m.

Solution: Change 6 fluidrams to minims.

$$6 \text{ fluidrams} \times \frac{60 \text{ minims}}{1 \text{ fluidram}} = 360 \text{ minims}$$

Thus, f℈ vi = m ccclx.

Example 2: Change O xxiv to qt.

Solution: Change 24 pints to quarts.

$$24 \text{ pints} \times \frac{1 \text{ quart}}{2 \text{ pints}} = \frac{24}{2} = 12 \text{ quarts}$$

Thus, O xxiv = qt xii.

Q7   Change f℈ iv to f℥.

\# \# \# • \# \# \# • \# \# \# • \# \# \# • \# \# \# • \# \# \# • \# \# \# • \# \# \# • \# \# \#

A7   f℥ ss: $4 \text{ fluidrams} \times \dfrac{1 \text{ fluidounce}}{8 \text{ fluidrams}} = \dfrac{4}{8} = \dfrac{1}{2} \text{ fluidounce}$

Q8   Change O ii to f℥.

\# \# \# • \# \# \# • \# \# \# • \# \# \# • \# \# \# • \# \# \# • \# \# \# • \# \# \# • \# \# \#

A8   f℥ xxxii: $2 \text{ pints} \times \dfrac{16 \text{ fluidounces}}{1 \text{ pint}} = 32 \text{ fluidounces}$

Q9   Change m xx to f℥.

• # # # • # # # • # # # • # # # • # # # • # # # • # # # • # # # • # #

A9   f℥ $\frac{1}{3}$:   20 minims $\times \dfrac{1\ \text{fluidram}}{60\ \text{minims}} = \dfrac{20}{60} = \dfrac{1}{3}$ fluidram

Q10   Complete each of the following:
  a. Change f℥ ii to m.   **b.** Change f℥ viii to O.

  c. Change gr xv to ℨ.   **d.** Change ℨ ss to ℨ.

  e. Change qt vi to C.   **f.** Change f℥ xxxii to f℥.

• # # # • # # # • # # # • # # # • # # # • # # # • # # # • # # # • # #

A10   **a.** m cxx   **b.** O ss   **c.** ℨ $\frac{1}{4}$ **d.** ℨ iv   **e.** C iss   **f.** f℥ iv

---

6   The important equations relating apothecaries' system units of weight and liquid volume are summarized as follows:

gr	grain
ℨ	dram
℥	ounce
lb	pound

Weight
1 dram = 60 grains
1 ounce = 8 drams
1 pound = 12 ounces

m	minim
f℥	fluidram
f℥	fluidounce
pt / O	pint
qt	quart
gal / C	gallon

Liquid Volume
1 fluidram = 60 minims
1 fluidounce = 8 fluidrams
1 pint = 16 fluidounces
1 quart = 2 pints
1 gallon = 4 quarts

Q11 Complete each of the following:

a. 1 fluidounce = _____ fluidrams

b. 1 dram = _____ minims

c. 1 quart = _____ pints

d. 1 gallon = _____ quarts

e. 1 pint = _____ fluidounces

f. 1 pound = _____ ounces

\# \# \# • \# \# \# • \# \# \# • \# \# \# • \# \# \# • \# \# \# • \# \# \# • \# \# \# • \# \# \#

A11 a. 8 b. 60 c. 2 d. 4 e. 16 f. 12

---

7 In some instances it is necessary to perform conversions between apothecaries' units which are not related directly by the equations of Frame 6.

Example 1: Change qt ii to f℥.

Solution: Change 2 quarts to fluidounces.

$$2 \text{ quarts} \times \frac{2 \text{ pints}}{1 \text{ quart}} \times \frac{16 \text{ fluidounces}}{1 \text{ pint}} = 64 \text{ fluidounces}$$

Thus, qt ii = f℥ lxiv.

Example 2: Change f℥ ss to m.

Solution: Change $\frac{1}{2}$ fluidounce to minims.

$$\frac{1}{2} \text{ fluidounce} \times \frac{8 \text{ fluidrams}}{1 \text{ fluidounce}} \times \frac{60 \text{ minims}}{1 \text{ fluidram}} = \frac{480}{2} = 240 \text{ minims}$$

Thus, f℥ ss = m ccxl.

Q12 Change f℥ xxxii to qt.

\# \# \# • \# \# \# • \# \# \# • \# \# \# • \# \# \# • \# \# \# • \# \# \# • \# \# \# • \# \# \#

A12 qt i: $32 \text{ fluidounces} \times \frac{1 \text{ pint}}{16 \text{ fluidounces}} \times \frac{1 \text{ quart}}{2 \text{ pints}} = 1 \text{ quart}$

Q13 Change O ii to f℥.

\# \# \# • \# \# \# • \# \# \# • \# \# \# • \# \# \# • \# \# \# • \# \# \# • \# \# \# • \# \# \#

A13 f℥ cclvi: $2 \text{ pints} \times \frac{16 \text{ fluidounces}}{1 \text{ pint}} \times \frac{8 \text{ fluidrams}}{1 \text{ fluidounce}} = 256 \text{ fluidrams}$

Q14 Change m cccxx to f℥.

\# \# \# • \# \# \# • \# \# \# • \# \# \# • \# \# \# • \# \# \# • \# \# \# • \# \# \# • \# \# \#

A14 $f\text{ʒ}\dfrac{2}{3}$: $320 \, \text{minims} \times \dfrac{1 \, \text{fluidram}}{60 \, \text{minims}} \times \dfrac{1 \, \text{fluidounce}}{8 \, \text{fluidrams}} = \dfrac{2}{3} \, \text{fluidounce}$

This completes the instruction for this section.

5.2   EXERCISE

1. One _____ is the volume of one teaspoon of water.
2. One _____ is the volume of one drop of water.
3. Write an abbreviation or symbol for each of the following:

a. minim   b. fluidounce   c. quart
d. fluidram   e. pint   f. gallon

4. Write using symbols and Roman numerals:

a. $15\dfrac{1}{2}$ minims   b. 19 quarts   c. 3 fluidounces

d. $\dfrac{2}{3}$ gallon   e. 14 fluidrams   f. 24 pints

5. Perform each of the following conversions:

a. Change fʒ lxiv to fᴣ.   b. Change m xxx to fᴣ.   c. Change C iii to qt.

d. Change fᴣ xxiv to O.   e. Change fʒ $\dfrac{1}{4}$ to m.   f. Change qt x to C.

g. Change O $\dfrac{3}{4}$ to fʒ.   h. Change m cdlxxx to fᴣ.

5.2   EXERCISE ANSWERS

1. fluidram   2. minim
3. a. m   b. fᴣ   c. qt
   d. fʒ   e. O or pt   f. C or gal
4. a. m xvss   b. qt xix   c. fᴣ iii
   d. C $\dfrac{2}{3}$ e. fᴣ xiv   f. O xxiv
5. a. fᴣ viii   b. fᴣ ss   c. qt xii   d. O iss
   e. m xv   f. C iiss   g. fᴣ xcvi   h. fᴣ i

5.3   HOUSEHOLD–APOTHECARY CONVERSION

1   The system of measurement that is commonly used in the home for cooking is the household system. It is, therefore, a convenient system for use by those who must take medication while at home. Since household system measures are not accurate, they should be avoided when administering drugs. Health sciences people may be called upon to convert apothecaries' system units into the household system, however, and so it is important to compare the two measurement systems.

The smallest unit in the household system is the *drop*. The abbreviation for drop (gtt) is written with lowercase letters. Although other household system measures are avoided in hospital drug administration, the drop is used for calculating intravenous (IV) fluid flow, as well as for certain x-ray and nuclear medicine preparations.

Q1   **a.** The smallest unit in the household system is the _____.

b. The abbreviation for drop is _____.

\# \# \#   •   \# \# \#   •   \# \# \#   •   \# \# \#   •   \# \# \#   •   \# \# \#   •   \# \# \#   •   \# \# \#   •   \# \# \#

A1   **a.** drop   **b.** gtt

Q2   Answer true or false:

a. Household system units are to be avoided in the administration of drugs. _____

b. The drop, although a household system unit, is used in calculating hospital IV fluid flow.

_____

\# \# \#   •   \# \# \#   •   \# \# \#   •   \# \# \#   •   \# \# \#   •   \# \# \#   •   \# \# \#   •   \# \# \#   •   \# \# \#

A2   **a.** true   **b.** true

---

2   Two other common household system units are the teaspoon (tsp) and the tablespoon (tbsp). The important equations relating drop, teaspoon and tablespoon are:

gtt	drop
tsp	teaspoon
tbsp	tablespoon

60 drops = 1 teaspoon
3 teaspoons = 1 tablespoon

Q3   Write abbreviations for each of the following:

a. drop _____   **b.** teaspoon _____

c. tablespoon _____   **d.** minim _____

\# \# \#   •   \# \# \#   •   \# \# \#   •   \# \# \#   •   \# \# \#   •   \# \# \#   •   \# \# \#   •   \# \# \#   •   \# \# \#

A3   **a.** gtt   **b.** tsp   **c.** tbsp   **d.** m

Q4   Complete each equation:

a. 1 tbsp = _____tsp   **b.** 1 tsp = _____gtt

\# \# \#   •   \# \# \#   •   \# \# \#   •   \# \# \#   •   \# \# \#   •   \# \# \#   •   \# \# \#   •   \# \# \#   •   \# \# \#

A4   **a.** 3   **b.** 60

---

3   Often drugs given in the home involve measuring the amount of fluid a patient should drink. The household system units used for this purpose are the ounce, glass, or teacup. They are related as follows:

2 tablespoons = 1 ounce
6 ounces = 1 teacup
8 ounces = 1 glass

Since household units are used with utensils which vary in size and accuracy, the above equivalents are only approximate.

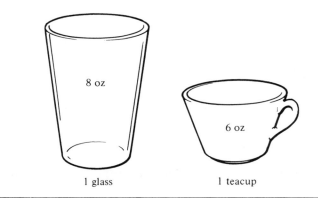

1 glass   1 teacup

Q5   Complete each of the following equations:

a. 1 oz = _____tbsp   **b.** 1 glass = _____oz

c. 1 teacup = _____oz   **d.** 1 tsp = _____gtt

\# \# \#   •   \# \# \#   •   \# \# \#   •   \# \# \#   •   \# \# \#   •   \# \# \#   •   \# \# \#   •   \# \# \#   •   \# \# \#

A5   **a.** 2   **b.** 8   **c.** 6   **d.** 60

---

4   Recall from Section 5.2, that one minim was approximately the volume of a drop of water. Similarly, one dram was the volume of a teaspoon of water. These approximations provide for the following relationships:

Household System	*Apothecaries' System*
1 drop (gtt) = 1 minim (m)	
1 teaspoon (tsp) = 1 fluidram (f℈)*	
1 tablespoon (tbsp) = 4 fluidrams	
1 glass = 8 fluidounces (f℥ or oz)	
1 teacup = 6 fluidounces	

*A scant teaspoon is generally accepted as being equivalent to 1 fluidram; a standard teaspoon, as accepted by the United States Pharmacopeia, contains $1\frac{1}{3}$ fluidrams.

Q6   Complete each of the following:

a. One minim is the volume of a _____ of water.

b. One fluidram is the volume of a _____ of water.

\# \# \#   •   \# \# \#   •   \# \# \#   •   \# \# \#   •   \# \# \#   •   \# \# \#   •   \# \# \#   •   \# \# \#   •   \# \# \#

A6   **a.** drop   **b.** teaspoon

Q7   Complete each of the following equations:

a. 1 tbsp = _____tsp   **b.** 1 tbsp = _____fluidrams

c. 1 glass = _____oz   **d.** 1 teacup = _____oz

\# \# \#   •   \# \# \#   •   \# \# \#   •   \# \# \#   •   \# \# \#   •   \# \# \#   •   \# \# \#   •   \# \# \#   •   \# \# \#

A7   **a.** 3   **b.** 4   **c.** 8   **d.** 6

Q8   The doctor orders 3 fluidrams of a medication. What is the corresponding order in the household system? _____

\# \# \#   •   \# \# \#   •   \# \# \#   •   \# \# \#   •   \# \# \#   •   \# \# \#   •   \# \# \#   •   \# \# \#   •   \# \# \#

A8   3 teaspoons

Q9   The doctor prescribes 5 minims of a medication in a glass of milk. What is the corresponding order in household units? _____

\# \# \#   •   \# \# \#   •   \# \# \#   •   \# \# \#   •   \# \# \#   •   \# \# \#   •   \# \# \#   •   \# \# \#   •   \# \# \#

A9   5 drops in a glass of milk

---

5   Conversions between the household and apothecaries' systems are completed as conversions in the previous section. When household system quantities are written in abbreviated form, the procedures are the same as when writing metric system quantities. That is, use Arabic numbers followed by the appropriate abbreviation.

Example: How many tablespoons in 8 fluidrams?

Solution: $8 \text{ fluidrams} \times \dfrac{1 \text{ tablespoon}}{4 \text{ fluidrams}} = \dfrac{8}{4} = 2 \text{ tablespoons}$

Thus, 8 fluidrams = 2 tbsp.

Q10   How many glasses in 24 fluidounces?

\# \# \#   •   \# \# \#   •   \# \# \#   •   \# \# \#   •   \# \# \#   •   \# \# \#   •   \# \# \#   •   \# \# \#   •   \# \# \#

A10   3 glasses: $24 \text{ fluidounces} \times \dfrac{1 \text{ glass}}{8 \text{ fluidounces}} = 3 \text{ glasses}$

Q11   Change 3 fluidrams to teaspoons.

\# \# \#   •   \# \# \#   •   \# \# \#   •   \# \# \#   •   \# \# \#   •   \# \# \#   •   \# \# \#   •   \# \# \#   •   \# \# \#

A11   3 teaspoons: 1 fluidram = 1 teaspoon

---

6   Consider the following example:

Example: Change 30 minims to teaspoons.

Solution: First change the minims to fluidrams.

$30 \text{ minims} \times \dfrac{1 \text{ fluidram}}{60 \text{ minims}} = \dfrac{30}{60} = \dfrac{1}{2} \text{ fluidram}$

Since 1 fluidram = 1 teaspoon, $\dfrac{1}{2}$ fluidram = $\dfrac{1}{2}$ teaspoon. Thus, 30 minims = $\dfrac{1}{2}$ tsp. Notice that this conversion could also have been made by first changing 30 minims to 30 drops, and then converting 30 drops to teaspoons. Either procedure is acceptable.

Q12   Change m cxx to tsp.

•   # # #   •   # # #   •   # # #   •   # # #   •   # # #   •   # # #   •   # # #   •   # #

A12   2 tsp: $120 \text{ minims} \times \dfrac{1 \text{ fluidram}}{60 \text{ minims}} = 2 \text{ fluidrams}$

2 fluidrams = 2 teaspoons

Q13   Change f℥ $\frac{1}{3}$ to gtt.

•   # # #   •   # # #   •   # # #   •   # # #   •   # # #   •   # # #   •   # # #   •   # #

A13   20 gtt: $\dfrac{1}{3} \text{ fluidram} \times \dfrac{60 \text{ minims}}{1 \text{ fluidram}} = \dfrac{60}{3} = 20 \text{ minims}$

20 minims = 20 drops

This completes the instruction for this section.

5.3   EXERCISE

1. The smallest unit in the household system is the _____.

2. One fluidram is the volume of one _____ of water.

3. One minim is the volume of one _____ of water.

4. Write abbreviations for each of the following:
   - **a.** teaspoon
   - **b.** minim
   - **c.** fluidram
   - **d.** drop
   - **e.** tablespoon
   - **f.** ounce

5. Complete each equation:
   - **a.** f℥ i = _____tsp
   - **b.** m i = _____gtt
   - **c.** 1 tbsp = _____tsp
   - **d.** 1 oz = _____tbsp
   - **e.** 1 glass = _____oz
   - **f.** 1 teacup = _____oz

6. Complete each of the following:
   - **a.** Change m cl to tsp.
   - **b.** Change f℥ xvi to glasses
   - **c.** Change f℥ ss to gtt.
   - **d.** Change f℥ iv to tsp.
   - **e.** Change f℥ ix to teacups.
   - **f.** Change f℥ x to tbsp.

7. The doctor orders m x. What is the corresponding household equivalent?

8. The doctor prescribes f℥ ii. What is the corresponding household equivalent?

5.3   EXERCISE ANSWERS

1. drop   2. teaspoon   3. drop

4. **a.** tsp   **b.** m   **c.** f℥   **d.** gtt   **e.** tbsp   **f.** oz

5. a. 1   **b.** 1   **c.** 3   **d.** 2   **e.** 8   **f.** 6

6. a. $2\frac{1}{2}$ tsp   **b.** 2 glasses   **c.** 30 gtt   **d.** 4 tsp

    e. $1\frac{1}{2}$ teacups   **f.** $2\frac{1}{2}$ tbsp

7. 10 drops   **8.** 2 teaspoons

5.4 APOTHECARY–METRIC CONVERSION

1

Health science professionals have occasion to use both the apothecaries' and metric systems in computing dosage of medications and in the preparation of solutions for external use. It is therefore important to be able to perform conversions between the two systems. Although conversions between the systems involve approximate equivalents, drug prescriptions given in the metric system may be safely converted to the apothecaries' system before being filled and vice versa.

Recall from Section 5.1 that the weight of one gram was equivalent to fifteen grains. Thus, conversions between the units grain and gram may be completed using the equation

15 grains(gr) = 1 gram(g)

Example: Change 20 g to gr.

Solution: $20 \text{ grams} \times \dfrac{15 \text{ grains}}{1 \text{ gram}} = 300 \text{ grains}$

Thus, 20 g = gr ccc.

Q1   Answer true or false:

   a. When dosages are prescribed in the metric system, it is acceptable to administer the apothecaries'

    approximate equivalent. _____

   b. 15 grains = 1 gram _____

   c. One gram is fifteen times as heavy as one grain. _____

\# \# \# • \# \# \# • \# \# \# • \# \# \# • \# \# \# • \# \# \# • \# \# \# • \# \# \# • \# \# \#

A1   **a.** true   **b.** true   **c.** true

Q2   Change gr clxxx to g.

\# \# \# • \# \# \# • \# \# \# • \# \# \# • \# \# \# • \# \# \# • \# \# \# • \# \# \# • \# \# \#

A2   12 g: $180 \text{ grains} \times \dfrac{1 \text{ gram}}{15 \text{ grains}} = \dfrac{180}{15} = 12 \text{ grams}$

Q3   Change 1.5 g to gr.

\# \# \# • \# \# \# • \# \# \# • \# \# \# • \# \# \# • \# \# \# • \# \# \# • \# \# \# • \# \# \#

A3   gr xxiiss: $1.5 \text{ grams} \times \dfrac{15 \text{ grains}}{1 \text{ gram}} = 22.5 \text{ grains}$

---

2   Recall from Section 5.1 that

60 grains = 1 dram

Recall also from Frame 1 the fact that

15 grains = 1 gram

Multiplying both sides of the above equation by 4 we have

60 grains = 4 grams

Hence, equating the right-hand sides of the first and third equations, we have

4 grams(g) = 1 dram(3)

Thus, one dram is approximately four times as large as one gram.

Q4   Complete each of the following:

a. _____grams = 1 dram   **b.** _____grains = 1 gram

c. _____grains = 1 dram   **d.** _____dram = 1 teaspoon

\# \# \# • \# \# \# • \# \# \# • \# \# \# • \# \# \# • \# \# \# • \# \# \# • \# \# \# • \# \# \#

A4   **a.** 4   **b.** 15   **c.** 60   **d.** 1

Q5   Circle the larger of the two units:
a. grain, gram   **b.** dram, gram

\# \# \# • \# \# \# • \# \# \# • \# \# \# • \# \# \# • \# \# \# • \# \# \# • \# \# \# • \# \# \#

A5   **a.** gram   **b.** dram

Q6   Change 3 xv to g.

\# \# \# • \# \# \# • \# \# \# • \# \# \# • \# \# \# • \# \# \# • \# \# \# • \# \# \# • \# \# \#

A6   60 g: $15 \text{ drams} \times \dfrac{4 \text{ grams}}{1 \text{ dram}} = 60 \text{ grams}$

Q7   Change 10 g to 3.

\# \# \# • \# \# \# • \# \# \# • \# \# \# • \# \# \# • \# \# \# • \# \# \# • \# \# \# • \# \# \#

A7   3 iiss: $10 \text{ grams} \times \dfrac{1 \text{ dram}}{4 \text{ grams}} = \dfrac{10}{4} = 2\dfrac{1}{2} \text{ drams}$

Q8   Change $3\frac{1}{4}$ to g.

\# \# \# • \# \# \# • \# \# \# • \# \# \# • \# \# \# • \# \# \# • \# \# \# • \# \# \# • \# \# \#

A8   1 g: $\frac{1}{4}\,\text{dram}\times\frac{4\text{ grams}}{1\text{ dram}}=1\text{ gram}$

Q9   Complete each of the following:
   a. Change 2 g to gr.   **b.** Change gr viiss to g.

   c. Change 56 g to ℨ.   **d.** Change ℨ vi to g.

\# \# \# • \# \# \# • \# \# \# • \# \# \# • \# \# \# • \# \# \# • \# \# \# • \# \# \# • \# \# \#

A9   **a.** gr xxx: $2\text{ grams}\times\frac{15\text{ grains}}{1\text{ gram}}=30\text{ grains}$

    b. 0.5 g*: $7\frac{1}{2}\text{ grains}\times\frac{1\text{ gram}}{15\text{ grains}}=\frac{15}{2}\times\frac{1}{15}=\frac{1}{2}\text{ gram}$

    c. ℨ xiv: $56\text{ grams}\times\frac{1\text{ dram}}{4\text{ grams}}=\frac{56}{4}=14\text{ drams}$

    d. 24 g: $6\text{ drams}\times\frac{4\text{ grams}}{1\text{ dram}}=24\text{ grams}$

* Metric quantities should be given in decimal rather than fraction form.

---

3   From the previous frame we have the equation

4 grams = 1 dram

In Section 5.1 it was stated that

8 drams = 1 ounce

Thus, it would appear that there are 4×8 or 32 grams in 1 ounce. However, since the equations above are not exact, the number of grams in an ounce is approximated as 30. That is,

30 grams (g) = 1 ounce (℥ or oz)

Thus, one ounce is approximately 30 times larger than one gram.

Q10   Circle the smaller unit:
   a. gram, dram   **b.** ounce, gram   **c.** grain, gram   **d.** ounce, dram

\# \# \# • \# \# \# • \# \# \# • \# \# \# • \# \# \# • \# \# \# • \# \# \# • \# \# \# • \# \# \#

A10   **a.** gram   **b.** gram   **c.** grain   **d.** dram

Q11   Complete each equation:

    a. ____ grains = 1 gram   **b.** ____ grams = 1 dram

    c. ____ grams = 1 ounce   **d.** ____ drams = 1 ounce

\# \# \# • \# \# \# • \# \# \# • \# \# \# • \# \# \# • \# \# \# • \# \# \# • \# \# \# • \# \# \#

A11   **a.** 15   **b.** 4   **c.** 30   **d.** 8

Q12   Change 50 g to ℥.

\# \# \# • \# \# \# • \# \# \# • \# \# \# • \# \# \# • \# \# \# • \# \# \# • \# \# \# • \# \# \#

A12   ℥ $1\frac{2}{3}$: $50 \text{ grams} \times \dfrac{1 \text{ ounce}}{30 \text{ grams}} = \dfrac{50}{30} = 1\frac{2}{3} \text{ ounces}$

Q13   Change ℥ xii to g.

\# \# \# • \# \# \# • \# \# \# • \# \# \# • \# \# \# • \# \# \# • \# \# \# • \# \# \# • \# \# \#

A13   360 g: $12 \text{ ounces} \times \dfrac{30 \text{ grams}}{1 \text{ ounce}} = 360 \text{ grams}$

Q14   Change 15 g to ℥.

\# \# \# • \# \# \# • \# \# \# • \# \# \# • \# \# \# • \# \# \# • \# \# \# • \# \# \# • \# \# \#

A14   ℥ ss: $15 \text{ grams} \times \dfrac{1 \text{ ounce}}{30 \text{ grams}} = \dfrac{15}{30} = \dfrac{1}{2} \text{ ounce}$

Q15   Complete each of the following:

    a. Change gr ccxxv to g.   **b.** Change 18 g to ℥.

    c. Change ℥ iii to g.   **d.** Change ʒ v to g.

\# \# \# • \# \# \# • \# \# \# • \# \# \# • \# \# \# • \# \# \# • \# \# \# • \# \# \# • \# \# \#

A15   **a.** 15 g   **b.** ℥ ivss   **c.** 90 g   **d.** 20 g

4   A final approximate equivalent between metric and apothecary units of weight relates milligrams and grains. The relationship is

60 milligrams (mg) = 1 grain (gr)*

Example: Change 300 mg to gr.

Solution: $300 \text{ milligrams} \times \dfrac{1 \text{ grain}}{60 \text{ milligrams}} = \dfrac{300}{60} = 5 \text{ grains}$

Thus, 300 mg = gr v.

*All metric–apothecary equivalents given in this section are approximate and represent quantities usually prescribed by physicians using one of these systems.

For situations requiring more precision such as prescriptions that require compounding, or when converting a pharmaceutical formula from one system to another, the United States Pharmacopeia lists the equivalent at 1 grain = 65 milligrams.

Q16   Change gr vi to mg.

•   # # #   •   # # #   •   # # #   •   # # #   •   # # #   •   # # #   •   # # #   •   # #

A16   360 mg: $6 \text{ grains} \times \dfrac{60 \text{ milligrams}}{1 \text{ grain}} = 360 \text{ milligrams}$

Q17   Change 150 mg to gr.

•   # # #   •   # # #   •   # # #   •   # # #   •   # # #   •   # # #   •   # # #   •   # #

A17   gr iiss: $150 \text{ milligrams} \times \dfrac{1 \text{ grain}}{60 \text{ milligrams}} = \dfrac{150}{60} = 2\dfrac{1}{2} \text{ grains}$

Q18   Change gr $\dfrac{1}{100}$ to mg.

•   # # #   •   # # #   •   # # #   •   # # #   •   # # #   •   # # #   •   # # #   •   # #

A18   0.6 mg: $\dfrac{1}{100} \text{ grain} \times \dfrac{60 \text{ milligrams}}{1 \text{ grain}} = \dfrac{3}{5} = 0.6 \text{ milligram}$

5   Following is a summary of the metric–apothecary approximation equations for units of weight:

Units of Weight

Metric System	*Apothecaries' System*
1 gram (g) = 15 grains (gr)	
4 grams = 1 dram (ʒ)	
30 grams = 1 ounce (ʒ or oz)	
60 milligrams (mg) = 1 grain	

Q19   Complete each of the following:
    a. Change 18 g to ℥.
                                            b. Change ℥ viii to g.

    c. Change gr $\dfrac{1}{150}$ to mg.
                                            d. Change gr ccxxv to g.

\# \# \#   •   \# \# \#   •   \# \# \#   •   \# \# \#   •   \# \# \#   •   \# \# \#   •   \# \# \#   •   \# \# \#   •   \# \# \#

A19   **a.** ℥ ivss   **b.** 240 g   **c.** 0.4 mg   **d.** 15 g

---

6   Recall from Sections 5.1 and 5.2 that in the apothecaries' system the units of volume and weight parallel each other. This is now helpful since the equations relating metric and apothecary units of weight can now be restated easily for units of volume.
    For example, just as grain and gram are related by the equation

1 gram = 15 grains

the comparable volume units millilitre and minim are related by the equation

1 millilitre (ml) = 15 or 16 minims (m)

    Notice that 1 millilitre is equal to either 15 or 16 minims. The millilitre is usually considered equal to 15 minims, although it is sometimes used equal to 16 minims in measuring injectable medications. Recall that 1 millilitre is the same as 1 cubic centimetre and thus the above equation is also correctly written

1 cubic centimetre (cm^3 or cc) = 15 or 16 minims (m)

Q20   Complete each equation:

    a. 1 ml = _____ cm^3
                                              b. 1 ml = _____ cc

    c. 1 ml = _____ m
                                              d. 1 cm^3 = _____ m

\# \# \#   •   \# \# \#   •   \# \# \#   •   \# \# \#   •   \# \# \#   •   \#.\# \#   •   \# \# \#   •   \# \# \#   •   \# \# \#

A20   **a.** 1   **b.** 1   **c.** 15 or 16   **d.** 15 or 16

Q21   Change 4 ml to m.

\# \# \#   •   \# \# \#   •   \# \# \#   •   \# \# \#   •   \# \# \#   •   \# \# \#   •   \# \# \#   •   \# \# \#   •   \# \# \#

A21   m lx: $4 \text{ millilitres} \times \dfrac{15 \text{ minims}}{1 \text{ millilitre}} = 60 \text{ minims}$

Q22   Change m lxxv to ml.

• # # # • # # # • # # # • # # # • # # # • # # # • # # # • # # # • # #

A22   5 ml: $75 \, \text{minims} \times \dfrac{1 \text{ millilitre}}{15 \text{ minims}} = \dfrac{75}{15} = 5 \text{ millilitres}$

Q23   Complete each of the following:

a. Change 15 ml to cm^3.   **b.** Change $\dfrac{1}{2}$ cc to m.

• # # # • # # # • # # # • # # # • # # # • # # # • # # # • # # # • # #

A23   **a.** $15 \, \text{cm}^3$ **b.** m viiss

---

7   The conversion of cubic centimetres to minims is frequently used to figure out how many minims remain in a bottle of intravenous (IV) fluid. It is, thus, an important conversion.

Example: $125 \, \text{cm}^3$ remain in a bottle of IV fluid. How many minims are left?

Solution: $125 \, \text{cm}^3 \times \dfrac{15 \text{ minims}}{1 \text{ millilitre}} = 1875 \text{ minims}$

Thus, $125 \, \text{cm}^3 = 1875$ minims.

Q24   250 cc were left in a bottle of IV fluid. How many minims were left?

• # # # • # # # • # # # • # # # • # # # • # # # • # # # • # # # • # #

A24   3750 minims: $250 \, \text{cc} \times \dfrac{15 \text{ minims}}{1 \text{ millilitre}} = 3750 \text{ minims}$

---

8   Recall that the relationship between the gram and dram is

4 grams = 1 dram

The parallel relationship for volume units is

4 millilitres (ml) = 1 fluidram (f3)

Q25   Change 24 ml to f3.

• # # # • # # # • # # # • # # # • # # # • # # # • # # # • # # # • # #

A25   f℥ vi: $24 \text{ millilitres} \times \dfrac{1 \text{ fluidram}}{4 \text{ millilitres}} = 6 \text{ fluidrams}$

Q26   Change f℥ xvi to cc.

\# \# \# • \# \# \# • \# \# \# • \# \# \# • \# \# \# • \# \# \# • \# \# \# • \# \# \# • \# \# \#

A26   64 cc: $16 \text{ fluidrams} \times \dfrac{4 \text{ cc}}{1 \text{ fluidrams}} = 64 \text{ cc}$

Q27   Complete each of the following:
   a. Change 30 ml to f℥.   **b.** Change 10 cm³ to f℥.

   c. Change m cv to ml.   **d.** Change f℥ x to ml.

\# \# \# • \# \# \# • \# \# \# • \# \# \# • \# \# \# • \# \# \# • \# \# \# • \# \# \# • \# \# \#

A27   **a.** f℥ viiss   **b.** f℥ iiss   **c.** 7 ml   **d.** 40 ml

---

9

The medicine cup shown demonstrates the approximate relationship between the ounce and cc or millilitre. The approximate relationship is

1 fluidounce (f℥ or oz) = 30 millilitres (ml)

(cup shown: 1 oz — 30 ml; ½ — 15 ml)

Notice that fractional equivalents are also shown on the graduations of the container. If not available, these are easily found using our conversion technique.

Example: Change f℥ ss to ml.

Solution: Change $\dfrac{1}{2}$ fluidounce to millilitres.

$\dfrac{1}{2} \text{ fluidounce} \times \dfrac{30 \text{ millilitres}}{1 \text{ fluidounce}} = 15 \text{ millilitres}$

Thus, f℥ ss = 15 ml.

Q28   Change oz $\frac{3}{4}$ to ml.

•   # # #   •   # # #   •   # # #   •   # # #   •   # # #   •   # # #   •   # # #   •   # #

A28   22.5 ml: $\frac{3}{4}$ fluidounce $\times \dfrac{30 \text{ millilitres}}{1 \text{ fluidounce}} = \dfrac{90}{4} = 22.5$ millilitres

Q29   Change f℥ iii to cc.

•   # # #   •   # # #   •   # # #   •   # # #   •   # # #   •   # # #   •   # # #   •   # #

A29   90 cc: 3 fluidounces $\times \dfrac{30 \text{ cc}}{1 \text{ fluidounce}} = 90$ cc

Q30   Change 25 ml to f℥.

•   # # #   •   # # #   •   # # #   •   # # #   •   # # #   •   # # #   •   # # #   •   # #

A30   f℥ $\frac{5}{6}$: 25 millilitres $\times \dfrac{1 \text{ fluidounce}}{30 \text{ millilitres}} = \dfrac{5}{6}$ fluidounces

Q31   Change 240 cc to f℥.

•   # # #   •   # # #   •   # # #   •   # # #   •   # # #   •   # # #   •   # # #   •   # #

A31   f℥ viii: 240 cc $\times \dfrac{1 \text{ fluidounce}}{30 \text{ cc}} = \dfrac{240}{30} = 8$ fluidounces

---

10   Recall from Chapter 4 that one litre is approximately equal to one quart. This provides the following approximate relationships:

1 litre (l) = 1 quart (qt)
1000 ml = 1 quart
500 ml = 1 pint (pt or O)

Q32   Use the relationships of Frame 10 to complete each of the following:
   a. Change pt vi to ml.   **b.** Change 1500 cc to O.

c. Change qt iv to ml.

d. Change 2500 ml to qt.

\# \# \# • \# \# \# • \# \# \# • \# \# \# • \# \# \# • \# \# \# • \# \# \# • \# \# \# • \# \# \#

A32   **a.** 3000 m: $6\ pints \times \dfrac{500\ millilitres}{1\ pint} = 3000\ millilitres$

b. O iii: $1500\ cc \times \dfrac{1\ pint}{500\ cc} = 3\ pints$

c. 4000 ml: $4\ quarts \times \dfrac{1000\ millilitres}{1\ quart} = 4000\ millilitres$

d. qt iiss: $2500\ millilitres \times \dfrac{1\ quart}{1000\ millilitres} = 2\dfrac{1}{2}\ quarts$

---

11   Following is a summary of the metric–apothecary approximation equations for units of volume:

Units of Volume

Metric System	Apothecaries' System
1 millilitre (ml)* = 15 or 16 minims (m)	
4 millilitres = 1 fluidram (f℥)	
30 millilitres = 1 fluidounce (f℥)	
500 millilitres = 1 pint (pt or O)	
1000 millilitres = 1 quart (qt)	
1 litre (l) = 1 quart	

*1 ml = 1 cm^3 = 1 cc

Q33   Complete each of the following:
a. Change 15 cc to f℥.

b. Change pt iiss to ml.

c. Change f℥ xxxii to ml.

d. Change m ccc to ml.

e. Change 25 ml to m.

f. Change 45 ml to cc.

\# \# \# • \# \# \# • \# \# \# • \# \# \# • \# \# \# • \# \# \# • \# \# \# • \# \# \# • \# \# \#

A33   **a.** f℥ ss   **b.** 1250 ml   **c.** 960 ml
d. 20 ml   **e.** m ccclxxv   **f.** 45 cc

This completes the instruction for this section.

**Summary of Metric–Apothecary
Approximation Equations**

Units of Weight

Metric System	*Apothecaries' System*

1 gram (g) = 15 grains (gr)
4 grams = 1 dram (ʒ)
30 grams = 1 ounce (ʒ)
60 milligrams (mg) = 1 grain

Units of Volume

Metric System	*Apothecaries' System*

1 millilitre (ml)* = 15 or 16 minims (m)
4 millilitres = 1 fluidram (fʒ)
30 millilitres = 1 fluidounce (fʒ)
500 millilitres = 1 pint (pt or O)
1000 millilitres = 1 quart (qt)
1 litre (l) = 1 quart

*1 ml = 1 cm^3 = 1 cc

5.4 EXERCISE

1. Complete each of the following equations:

a. _____grains = 1 gram   **b.** _____ml = 1 fluidram   **c.** _____mg = 1 grain

d. _____ml = 1 fluidounce **e.** _____ml = 1 quart   **f.** _____g = 1 ounce

2. Perform each of the following conversions:

a. Change 2 g to gr.	**b.** Change gr ss to mg.	**c.** Change 64 cc to fʒ.
d. Change 30 cc to m.	**e.** Change O iss to ml.	**f.** Change 120 g to ʒ.
g. Change fʒ xvi to ml.	**h.** Change 100 cm^3 to m.	**i.** Change gr ccx to g.
j. Change 10 g to ʒ.	**k.** Change 8 cc to fʒ.	**l.** Change 15 ml to fʒ.
m. Change 45 cc to ml.	**n.** Change m xv to cc.	

5.4 EXERCISE ANSWERS

1. a. 15	**b.** 4	**c.** 60	**d.** 30	**e.** 1000	**f.** 30

2. a. gr xxx	**b.** 30 mg	**c.** fʒ xvi	**d.** m cdl
e. 750 ml	**f.** ʒ xxx	**g.** 480 ml	**h.** m md
i. 14 g	**j.** ʒ $\frac{1}{3}$	**k.** fʒ ii	**l.** fʒ ss
m. 45 ml	**n.** 1 cc		

5.5 HOUSEHOLD–METRIC CONVERSION

1 The increasing use of the metric system will require that health sciences personnel be able to perform approximate conversions between the metric and household systems. Recall from preceding sections that all household system utensils are not identical. Thus, conversion factors involving the household system are only approximations. They can be used, however, in some situations outside of the hospital.

> The smallest unit of volume in the household system is the drop. One drop is approximately equal to 0.06 millilitres. That is,
>
> 1 drop (gtt) = 0.06 millilitres (ml)

Q1   Change 45 gtt to ml.

•   # # #   •   # # #   •   # # #   •   # # #   •   # # #   •   # # #   •   # # #   •   # #

A1   2.7 ml: $45 \, \text{drops} \times \dfrac{0.06 \text{ millilitres}}{1 \text{ drop}} = 2.7 \text{ millilitres}$

Q2   Change 120 ml to gtt.

•   # # #   •   # # #   •   # # #   •   # # #   •   # # #   •   # # #   •   # # #   •   # #

A2   2000 gtt: $120 \, \text{millilitres} \times \dfrac{1 \text{ drop}}{0.06 \text{ ml}} = \dfrac{120}{0.06} = 2000 \text{ drops}$

---

2   The approximate metric equivalents for the teaspoon and tablespoon are given by the following equations:

   1 teaspoon (tsp) = 5 millilitres (ml)
   1 tablespoon (tbsp) = 15 millilitres

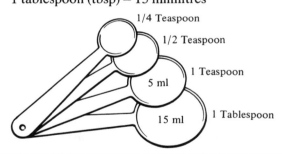

Q3   Complete each of the following:

   a. 1 tsp = _____ml   **b.** 1 gtt = _____ml   **c.** 1 tbsp = _____ml

•   # # #   •   # # #   •   # # #   •   # # #   •   # # #   •   # # #   •   # # #   •   # #

A3   **a.** 5   **b.** 0.06   **c.** 15

Q4   Change 60 ml to tbsp.

•   # # #   •   # # #   •   # # #   •   # # #   •   # # #   •   # # #   •   # # #   •   # #

A4   4 tbsp: $60 \, \cancel{\text{millilitres}} \times \dfrac{1 \text{ tablespoon}}{15 \, \cancel{\text{millilitres}}} = \dfrac{60}{15} = 4 \text{ tablespoon}$

Q5   Change 3 tsp to ml.

•   # # #   •   # # #   •   # # #   •   # # #   •   # # #   •   # # #   •   # # #   •   # #

A5   15 ml: $3 \, \cancel{\text{teaspoons}} \times \dfrac{5 \text{ millilitres}}{1 \, \cancel{\text{teaspoon}}} = 15 \text{ millilitres}$

Q6   Change 75 ml to tsp.

•   # # #   •   # # #   •   # # #   •   # # #   •   # # #   •   # # #   •   # # #   •   # #

A6   15 tsp: $75 \, \cancel{\text{millilitres}} \times \dfrac{1 \text{ teaspoon}}{5 \, \cancel{\text{millilitres}}} = \dfrac{75}{5} = 15 \text{ teaspoons}$

---

3   The containers that follow demonstrate the approximate relationship between the fluidounce and the millilitre. The relationship is

1 fluidounce (f℥ or oz) = 30 millilitres (ml)

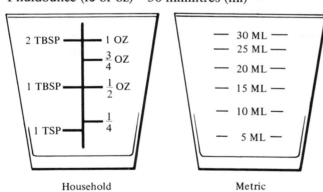

Household   Metric

Q7   Use the graduated containers of Frame 3 to complete the following:

     a. 1 tsp = _____ml   **b.** 1 oz = _____ml

     c. $\dfrac{1}{2}$ oz = _____ml   **d.** 1 tbsp = _____ml

•   # # #   •   # # #   •   # # #   •   # # #   •   # # #   •   # # #   •   # # #   •   # #

A7   **a.** 5   **b.** 30   **c.** 15   **d.** 15

Q8   Change 16 oz to ml.

•   # # #   •   # # #   •   # # #   •   # # #   •   # # #   •   # # #   •   # # #   •   # #

A8   480 ml: $16 \, \cancel{\text{fluidounces}} \times \dfrac{30 \text{ millilitres}}{1 \, \cancel{\text{fluidounce}}} = 480 \text{ millilitres}$

Q9   A graduated cylinder reads 240 ml. How many ounces does it contain?

\# \# \#   •   \# \# \#   •   \# \# \#   •   \# \# \#   •   \# \# \#   •   \# \# \#   •   \# \# \#   •   \# \# \#   •   \# \# \#

A9   8 oz: $240 \, \cancel{\text{millilitres}} \times \dfrac{1 \text{ fluidounce}}{30 \, \cancel{\text{millilitres}}} = \dfrac{240}{30} = 8 \text{ fluidounce}$

Q10   Complete each of the following:

   a. Change 25 ml to tsp.   **b.** Change 3 oz to ml.

   c. Change 45 ml to tbsp.   **d.** Change 750 ml to oz.

\# \# \#   •   \# \# \#   •   \# \# \#   •   \# \# \#   •   \# \# \#   •   \# \# \#   •   \# \# \#   •   \# \# \#   •   \# \# \#

A10   **a.** 5 tsp   **b.** 90 ml   **c.** 3 tbsp   **d.** 25 oz

---

4   The household system units glass and teacup are related to the metric system unit millilitre as follows:

1 teacup = 180 millilitres (ml)
  1 glass = 240 millilitres

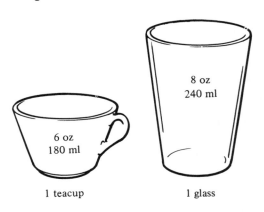

1 teacup   1 glass

Q11   Use the information of Frame 4 to complete each of the following:

   a. 1 teacup = _____oz   **b.** 1 teacup = _____ml

   c. 1 glass = _____oz   **d.** 1 glass = _____ml

\# \# \#   •   \# \# \#   •   \# \# \#   •   \# \# \#   •   \# \# \#   •   \# \# \#   •   \# \# \#   •   \# \# \#   •   \# \# \#

A11   **a.** 6   **b.** 180   **c.** 8   **d.** 240

Q12   Complete each of the following:
    a. Change 32 oz to glasses.   **b.** Change 60 ml to glasses.

    c. Change 3 teacups to ml.   **d.** Change 4 glasses to ml.

\# \# \# • \# \# \# • \# \# \# • \# \# \# • \# \# \# • \# \# \# • \# \# \# • \# \# \# • \# \# \#

A12   **a.** 4 glasses   **b.** $\frac{1}{4}$ glass   **c.** 540 ml   **d.** 960 ml

This completes the instruction for this section.

5.5   EXERCISE

1. Complete each of the following equations:
    a. 1 gtt = _____ml   **b.** 1 tbsp = _____ml
    c. 1 tsp = _____ml   **d.** 1 glass = _____ml

2. Perform each of the following conversions:
    a. Change 250 gtt to ml.   **b.** Change 5 tbsp to ml.
    c. Change 40 ml to tsp.   **d.** Change 600 ml to glasses.
    e. Change $1\frac{1}{2}$ glasses to ml.   **f.** Change 150 ml to gtt.

3. The doctor orders 3 glasses of water for a patient. How many millilitres are ordered for the patient?

4. A graduated cylinder reads 150 millilitres. How many tablespoons does the cylinder contain?

5. The doctor orders a patient to drink 2000 ml of fluids a day. Approximately how many glasses is this?

5.5   EXERCISE ANSWERS

1. a. 0.06   **b.** 15   **c.** 5   **d.** 240
2. a. 15 ml   **b.** 75 ml   **c.** 8 tsp
    d. 2.5 glasses   **e.** 360 ml   **f.** 2500 gtt
3. 720 millilitres   **4.** 10 tablespoons
5. approximately 8 glasses $\left(8\frac{1}{3}\right)$

Summary of Approximate Conversion Equations

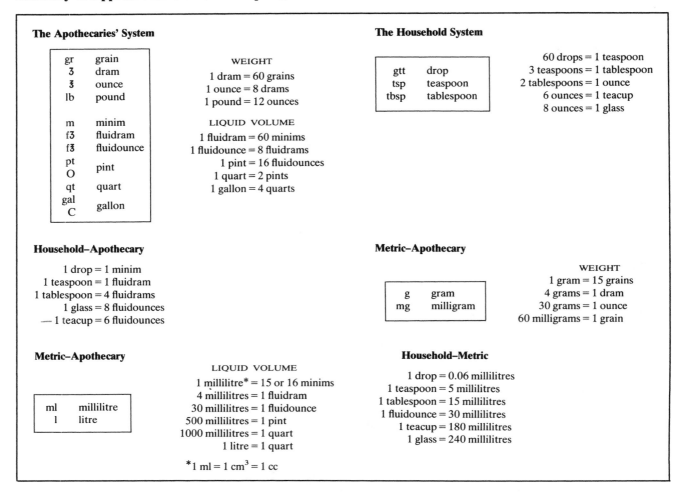

The Apothecaries' System

gr	grain
ʒ	dram
ʒ	ounce
lb	pound
m	minim
fʒ	fluidram
fʒ	fluidounce
pt / O	pint
qt	quart
gal / C	gallon

WEIGHT
1 dram = 60 grains
1 ounce = 8 drams
1 pound = 12 ounces

LIQUID VOLUME
1 fluidram = 60 minims
1 fluidounce = 8 fluidrams
1 pint = 16 fluidounces
1 quart = 2 pints
1 gallon = 4 quarts

The Household System

gtt	drop
tsp	teaspoon
tbsp	tablespoon

60 drops = 1 teaspoon
3 teaspoons = 1 tablespoon
2 tablespoons = 1 ounce
6 ounces = 1 teacup
8 ounces = 1 glass

Household–Apothecary

1 drop = 1 minim
1 teaspoon = 1 fluidram
1 tablespoon = 4 fluidrams
1 glass = 8 fluidounces
— 1 teacup = 6 fluidounces

Metric–Apothecary

g	gram
mg	milligram

WEIGHT
1 gram = 15 grains
4 grams = 1 dram
30 grams = 1 ounce
60 milligrams = 1 grain

Metric–Apothecary

ml	millilitre
l	litre

LIQUID VOLUME
1 millilitre* = 15 or 16 minims
4 millilitres = 1 fluidram
30 millilitres = 1 fluidounce
500 millilitres = 1 pint
1000 millilitres = 1 quart
1 litre = 1 quart

*1 ml = 1 cm^3 = 1 cc

Household–Metric

1 drop = 0.06 millilitres
1 teaspoon = 5 millilitres
1 tablespoon = 15 millilitres
1 fluidounce = 30 millilitres
1 teacup = 180 millilitres
1 glass = 240 millilitres

CHAPTER 5 SAMPLE TEST

At the completion of Chapter 5 you should be able to work the following problems.

5.1 THE APOTHECARIES' SYSTEM: WEIGHT

1. Fill in the correct unit of measure:

    a. One _____ is the weight of one drop of water.

    b. One _____ is the weight of one teaspoon of water.

2. Complete each equation:

    a. _____grains = 1 dram   **b.** _____grains = 1 gram

    c. _____ounces = 1 pound   **d.** _____drams = 1 ounce

3. Perform each of the following conversions:

    a. Change ʒ xx to ʒ.   **b.** Change oz viii to lb.

    c. Change gr cl to ʒ.   **d.** Change ʒ ss to gr.

5.2   THE APOTHECARIES' SYSTEM: VOLUME

4. Fill in the correct unit of measure:

  a. One _____ is the volume of a teaspoon of water.

  b. One _____ is the volume of a drop of water.

5. Complete each equation:

  a. 1 pint = _____fluidounces

  b. 1 fluidram = _____minims

  c. 1 fluidounce = _____fluidrams

  d. 1 gallon = _____quarts

6. Perform each of the following conversions:
  a. Change f℥ xcvi to O.
  b. Change f℈ iv to m.
  c. Change C ss to qt.
  d. Change pt xiv to oz.

5.3   HOUSEHOLD–APOTHECARY CONVERSION

7. Complete each equation:

  a. _____gtt = m i
  b. _____tsp = f℈ i
  c. 1 tbsp = f℈_____

  d. 1 glass = f℥_____
  e. _____gtt = 1 tsp
  f. _____tbsp = f℥ i

8. Perform each of the following conversions:
  a. Change f℥ xxviii to glasses.
  b. Change f℈ x to tsp.
  c. Change f℥ xiv to gtt.
  d. Change f℈ xx to tbsp.
  e. Change m xv to tsp.
  f. Change 5 glasses to oz.

5.4   APOTHECARY–METRIC CONVERSION

9. Complete each equation:

  a. 1 grain = _____mg
  b. 1 fluidram = _____ml
  c. 1 ounce = _____g

  d. 1 g = _____grains
  e. 1 quart = _____ml
  f. 1 fluidounce = _____ml

10. Perform each of the following conversions:
  a. Change gr cxiiss to g.
  b. Change f℈ ix to ml.
  c. Change 720 mg to gr.
  d. Change 110 ml to f℈.
  e. Change pt iv to ml.
  f. Change m ccclxxv to cc.

5.5   HOUSEHOLD–METRIC CONVERSION

11. Complete each equation:

  a. 1 tsp = _____ml

  b. 1 tbsp = _____ml

  c. 1 gtt = _____ml

  d. 1 teacup = _____ml

12. Perform each of the following conversions:
  a. Change 3 glasses to ml.
  b. Change 225 ml to gtt.
  c. Change 7 tsp to ml.
  d. Change 1200 cc to glasses.

CHAPTER 5 SAMPLE TEST ANSWERS

1. a. grain   **b.** dram

2. a. 60   **b.** 15   **c.** 12   **d.** 8

3. a. ℈ iiss   **b.** lb $\frac{2}{3}$ **c.** ℨ iiss   **d.** gr ccxl

4. a. fluidram   **b.** minim

5. a. 16   **b.** 60   **c.** 8   **d.** 4

6. a. O vi   **b.** m ccxl   **c.** qt ii   **d.** oz ccxxiv

7. a. 1   **b.** 1   **c.** iv   **d.** viii   **e.** 60   **f.** 2

8. a. $3\frac{1}{2}$ glasses   **b.** 10 tsp   **c.** 840 gtt

     d. 5 tbsp   **e.** $\frac{1}{4}$ tsp   **f.** oz xl

9. a. 60   **b.** 4   **c.** 30   **d.** 15   **e.** 1000   **f.** 30

10. a. 7.5 g   **b.** 270 ml   **c.** gr xii

     d. fℨ xxviiss   **e.** 2000 ml   **f.** 25 cc

11. a. 5   **b.** 15   **c.** 0.06   **d.** 180

12. a. 720 ml   **b.** 3750 gtt   **c.** 35 ml   **d.** 5 glasses

CHAPTER 6

SIGNED NUMBERS

6.1 INTRODUCTION

1   The whole numbers can be pictured using what is called a *number line* as follows:

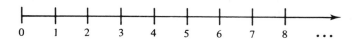

Each dot on the number line indicates the point where a specific number occurs and is called the *graph* of the number. The number that corresponds with each dot is called the *coordinate* of the point. The arrow on the end of the number line and the three dots that follow the last number shown both serve to indicate that the whole numbers are infinite or unending.

Q1   Graph the following whole numbers by placing dots at the appropriate points on the number line:
       a. 7   **b.** 2   **c.** 0

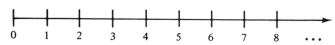

* * *   •   * * *   •   * * *   •   * * *   •   * * *   •   * * *   •   * * *   •   * * *   •   * * *

A1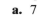

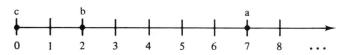

2   The number line of Frame 1 pictures the whole numbers spaced an equal distance apart, with each number indicating the *number of units that it is to the right of zero*. That is, the number 2 indicates the point that is 2 units to the right of zero. A new collection of numbers will now be defined by extending the number line to the *left* of zero and again marking off points an equal distance apart. This collection is named the *negative integers* and is written $^-1, ^-2, ^-3, \ldots$ (read "negative one," "negative two," "negative three," etc.). In the same way that 2 represents 2 units to the *right of zero*, the negative integer $^-2$ (negative two) will represent a distance of 2 units to the *left of zero*. To emphasize the difference in direction between the negative integers ($^-1, ^-2, ^-3, \ldots$) and the natural numbers ($1, 2, 3, \ldots$), the natural numbers are sometimes written $^+1, ^+2, ^+3, \ldots$ (read "positive one," "positive two," "positive three," etc.). The natural numbers are also correctly referred to as the *positive integers*. Thus, any positive integer can be written either with or without the positive sign. The positive integer $^+7$, for example, is also correctly represented as 7.

Q2 Graph each of the following numbers by placing dots at the appropriate points on the number line:
a. ⁻5 **b.** ⁺3 **c.** 0 **d.** ⁻1 **e.** 6

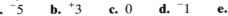

• # # # • # # # • # # # • # # # • # # # • # # # • # # # • # #

A2

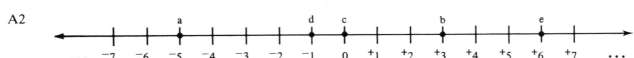

---

3 The collection that contains the negative integers, zero, and the positive integers is called the *integers*. The integers are pictured on the number line as follows:

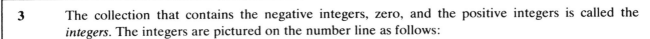

Each of the integers can be thought of as having two parts, *distance* and *direction*. The integer ⁺5, for example, represents a distance of 5 units to the *right* of zero. Similarly, the integer ⁻9 represents a distance of 9 units to the *left* of zero.

Q3 Write the distance and direction represented by each of the following integers:

	Distance	*Direction*
a. ⁻6	6 units	left of zero
b. ⁺42	_____	_____
c. ⁻42	_____	_____
d. 0	_____	_____

• # # # • # # # • # # # • # # # • # # # • # # # • # # # • # #

A3 **b.** 42 units, right of zero
c. 42 units, left of zero
d. 0 units, neither direction

---

4 The integers, . . . , ⁻3, ⁻2, ⁻1, 0, ⁺1, ⁺2, ⁺3, . . . , are also referred to as *signed numbers* because each one (except zero) has a direction designated by either a "⁻" or a "⁺" sign. Zero is an integer but is considered neither positive nor negative since its coordinate is neither to the right nor to the left of the zero point. Notice that the positive and negative signs are raised so that they will not be confused with addition and subtraction signs.

Q4 What is the sign of each of the following integers?

a. ⁺7 _____   **b.** 6 _____

c. ⁻3 _____   **d.** 0 _____

• # # # • # # # • # # # • # # # • # # # • # # # • # # # • # #

A4 **a.** positive   **b.** positive   **c.** negative
d. none: Zero has no sign.

---

5 As a result of the definition of the integers, each integer can be paired with a second integer that is the same distance from zero but in a different direction. The paired integers are called *opposites* and

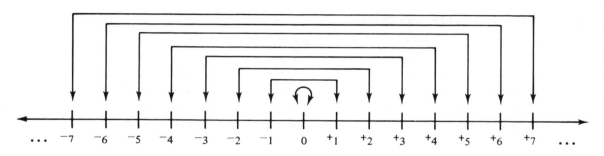

are shown in the accompanying drawing. Notice that each of the integers has a unique opposite. The opposite of ⁺4 is ⁻4. The opposite of ⁻6 is ⁺6. The opposite of 0 is 0. That is, zero is the only integer that is its own opposite.

Q5   Write the opposite of each of the following integers:

a. 5 _____   b. ⁻7 _____   c. 0 _____

d. ⁺1 _____   e. ⁻95 _____   f. 125 _____

• # # # • # # # • # # # • # # # • # # # • # # # • # # # • # #

A5   a. ⁻5   b. ⁺7   c. 0   d. ⁻1   e. ⁺95   f. ⁻125

This completes the instruction for this section.

6.1   EXERCISE

1. The collection . . . ⁻2, ⁻1, 0, 1, 2, . . . is called the _____.
2. Each integer is thought of as as having what two parts?
3. Write the distance and direction represented by each of the following integers:
    a. 15   b. ⁻3   c. 0   d. ⁺7
4. Graph each of the following integers: a. ⁻2   b. 4   c. 0   d. ⁺3

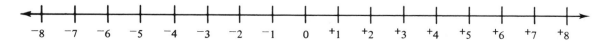

5. Write the opposite of each of the following integers:
    a. ⁺2   b. ⁻3   c. 11   d. 0

6.1   EXERCISE ANSWERS

1. integers
2. direction, distance
3. a. 15 units, right of zero
    b. 3 units, left of zero
    c. 0 units, neither right nor left
    d. 7 units, right of zero
4.

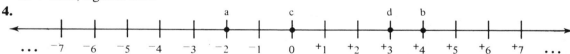

5. a. ⁻2   b. ⁺3   c. ⁻11   d. 0

6.2   ADDITION OF INTEGERS

1   In Section 6.1 each integer was shown to have associated with it both a distance and a direction. For example, ⁻5 denotes a distance of 5 units to the left of zero, and ⁺3 denotes a distance of 3 units and a direction right of zero. To develop a procedure for the addition of integers it will be helpful to associate with each integer an arrow that pictures its distance and direction. For example, the integer ⁺3 can be represented by any of the arrows above the following number line:

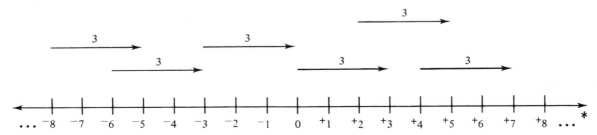

In this and the following sections the integer ⁺3 will be represented by any arrow that is *3 units long* and *points to the right*.

*When drawing the number line, it is common to omit the · · ·'s. It is understood that the line extends infinitely in both directions.

Q1   **a.** What is the length of each arrow on the following number line?   _____

b. What direction is indicated by each of the arrows?   _____

c. What integer is represented by each of the arrows?   _____

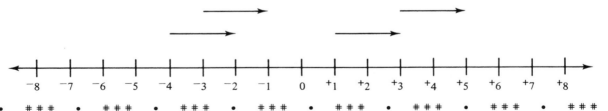

\# \# \#   •   \# \# \#   •   \# \# \#   •   \# \# \#   •   \# \# \#   •   \# \# \#   •   \# \# \#   •   \# \# \#   •   \# \# \#

A1   **a.** 2 units   **b.** right   **c.** ⁺2

2   The integer ⁻5 is represented by each of the arrows above the following number line:

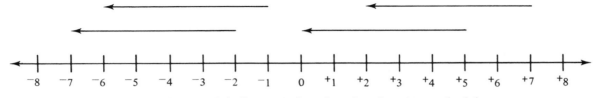

Each arrow represents ⁻5 since each is 5 *units in length* and each *points to the left*.

Q2   What integer is represented by each of the following arrows?   _____

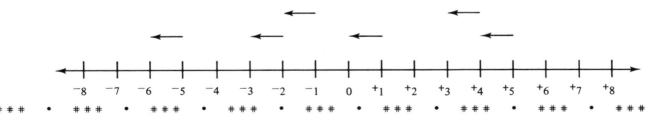

\# \# \#   •   \# \# \#   •   \# \# \#   •   \# \# \#   •   \# \# \#   •   \# \# \#   •   \# \# \#   •   \# \# \#   •   \# \# \#

A2   ⁻1: Each is 1 unit long and each points to the left.

Q3   Draw three arrows which each represent the integer ⁻4.

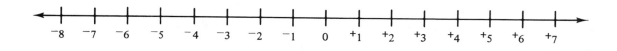

•   # # #   •   # # #   •   # # #   •   # # #   •   # # #   •   # # #   •   # # #   •   # #

A3   The arrows shown must each be 4 units in length and point to the left. For example,

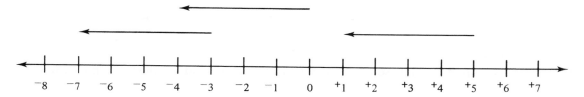

---

3   To add any two integers on the number line, use the following procedure:

Step 1: Represent the first addend* by an arrow that starts at zero.

Step 2: From the end of the first arrow, draw a second arrow to represent the second addend.

Step 3: Read the coordinate of the point at the end of the second arrow.

Examples:

1. $^{+}5 + ^{-}3$

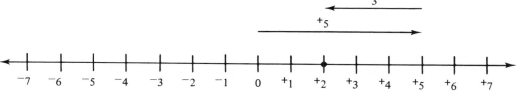

Dot denotes answer

Therefore, $^{+}5 + ^{-}3 = ^{+}2$.

2. $^{-}4 + ^{-}3$

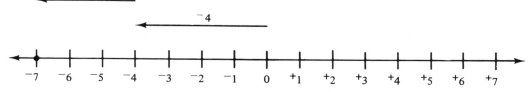

Therefore, $^{-}4 + ^{-}3 = ^{-}7$.

3. $^{+}2 + ^{-}8$

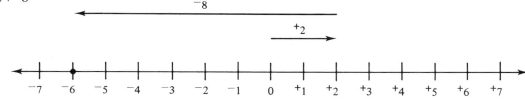

Therefore, $^{+}2 + ^{-}8 = ^{-}6$.

*An addend is a value that is being added to another value.

Q4   Find the sum $^-3 + ^+4$ by use of arrows for each of the addends on the following number line:

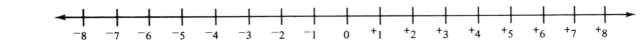

• # # # • # # # • # # # • # # # • # # # • # # # • # # # • # #

A4 $^+1$:

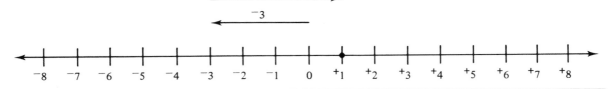

Q5   Find the sum $^+5 + ^-7$ by use of arrows for each of the addends on the following number line:

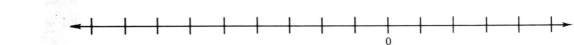

• # # # • # # # • # # # • # # # • # # # • # # # • # # # • # #

A5 $^-2$:

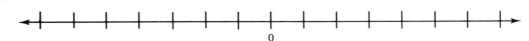
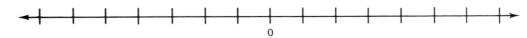
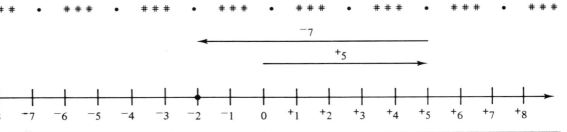

Q6   Find each of the following sums by use of the number line provided:

a. $^-4 + ^-5 =$ _____

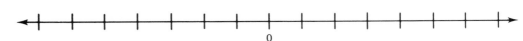

b. $^+3 + ^+2 =$ _____

c. $^-6 + 4 =$ _____

d. $^-5 + ^+9 =$ _____

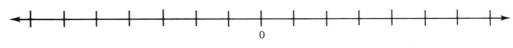

e. $^-6 + ^+6 =$ _____

• # # # • # # # • # # # • # # # • # # # • # # # • # # # • # #

A6   **a.** $^-9$ **b.** $^+5$ **c.** $^-2$ **d.** $^+4$ **e.** 0

---

4   It is sometimes helpful to notice certain facts about the sum of two integers. Study each of the following three example sets to see if you can discover the three facts demonstrated.

Sum of two positives	Sum of two negatives	Sum of a positive and a negative
$^+5+^+3=^+8$	$^-5+^-3=^-8$	$^-5+^+3=^-2$
$^+7+^+6=^+13$	$^-7+^-6=^-13$	$^+7+^-6=^+1$
$^+2+^+9=^+11$	$^-2+^-9=^-11$	$^+2+^-2=0$

The three facts that correspond with the preceding examples are:

1. The sum of two positive integers is a positive integer.
2. The sum of two negative integers is a negative integer.
3. The sum of a positive integer and a negative integer is sometimes positive, sometimes negative, and sometimes zero.

Q7   Use the facts of Frame 4 or a number line to find each of the following sums:

a. $^-3+^-6=$ _____   **b.** $^+5+^+8=$ _____

c. $^+4+^-1=$ _____   **d.** $^+2+^-7=$ _____

e. $^+3+^-3=$ _____   **f.** $^-5+^+5=$ _____

\# \# \#   •   \# \# \#   •   \# \# \#   •   \# \# \#   •   \# \# \#   •   \# \# \#   •   \# \# \#   •   \# \# \#   •   \# \# \#

A7   **a.** $^-9$ (fact 2)   **b.** $^+13$ (fact 1)   **c.** $^+3$ (fact 3)   **d.** $^-5$ (fact 3)
        e. 0 (fact 3)   **f.** 0

---

5   Recall from Section 6.1 that every integer has a unique opposite, and that opposites represent the same distance but different directions. Consider the sum of $^-7$ and its opposite, $^+7$, shown on the following number line:

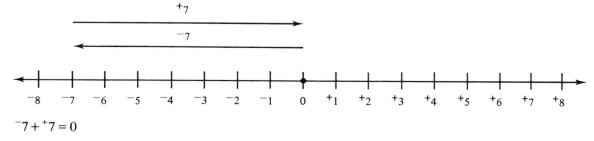

$^-7+^+7=0$

If the order of the addends is reversed, the sum remains unchanged:

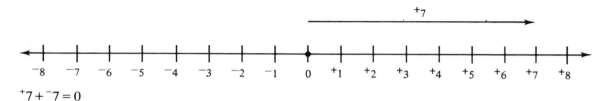

$^+7+^-7=0$

Thus, regardless of the order of the addends, the sum of $^+7$ and its opposite, $^-7$, is 0:

$^+7+^-7=^-7+^+7=0$

Q8 **a.** Find the sum $^-5 + {}^+5$.

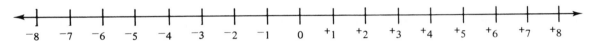

b. Find the sum $^+5 + {}^-5$.

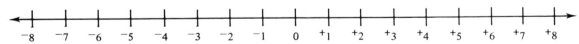

c. Is the sum in part **a** the same as the sum in part **b**? _____

• # # # • # # # • # # # • # # # • # # # • # # # • # # # • # #

A8 **a.** 0 **b.** 0 **c.** yes: $^-5 + {}^+5 = {}^+5 + {}^-5 = 0$

---

6 Because of the distance and direction relationships between opposites, the sum of any integer and its opposite is zero. This fact is generalized $a + {}^-a = {}^-a + a = 0.$*

Examples:

Opposites   Sum

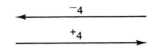

$^+4, {}^-4$ $^+4 + {}^-4 = 0$

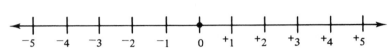

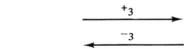

$^-3, {}^+3$ $^-3 + {}^+3 = 0$

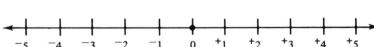

$0, 0$ $0 + 0 = 0$

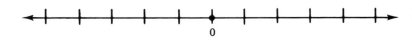

(Notice that the arrow representing zero is simply a dot at 0, because the integer zero has no length or direction.)

*The symbol ^-a means "the opposite of a."

Q9 **a.** What is the opposite of $^+6$? _____

b. What is the opposite of $^-9$? _____

• # # # • # # # • # # # • # # # • # # # • # # # • # # # • # #

A9 **a.** $^-6$ **b.** $^+9$

Q10 The sum of any integer and its opposite is _____.

• # # # • # # # • # # # • # # # • # # # • # # # • # # # • # #

A10 zero

Q11   Find each of the following sums:

    a. $^-3 + ^-3 =$ _____

    b. $^+5 + ^-5 =$ _____

    c. $^+7 + ^+7 =$ _____

    d. $^-6 + ^+6 =$ _____

    e. $^-8 + ^+8 =$ _____

    f. $0 + 0 =$ _____

\# \# \# • \# \# \# • \# \# \# • \# \# \# • \# \# \# • \# \# \# • \# \# \# • \# \# \# • \# \# \#

A11   **a.** $^-6$:   The sum of two negatives is a negative.
      b. 0:   The sum of two opposites is zero.
      c. $^+14$:   The sum of two positives is a positive.
      d. 0 **e.** 0 **f.** 0

Q12   Write a number in the blank to make each of the following a true statement:

    a. $^+2 + ^-2 =$ _____

    b. _____ $+ ^+7 = 0$

    c. $^-15 +$ _____ $= 0$

    d. $^+13 + ^-13 =$ _____

\# \# \# • \# \# \# • \# \# \# • \# \# \# • \# \# \# • \# \# \# • \# \# \# • \# \# \# • \# \# \#

A12   **a.** 0 **b.** $^-7$ **c.** $^+15$ **d.** 0

---

7   The sum of any natural number and zero is the natural number: for example, $0 + 2 = 2$ and $8 + 0 = 8$. The same is true of any integer and zero.

Examples: $^-3 + 0 = ^-3$
                $0 + ^+12 = ^+12$

This fact is called the *addition property of zero* and is generalized $a + 0 = 0 + a = a$ for any integer a.

Q13   Find each of the following sums:

    a. $0 + ^-5 =$ _____

    b. $^-4 + ^-9 =$ _____

    c. $^+4 + ^-4 =$ _____

    d. $^+11 + 0 =$ _____

    e. $^+5 + ^+7 =$ _____

    f. $^-7 + ^+3 =$ _____

\# \# \# • \# \# \# • \# \# \# • \# \# \# • \# \# \# • \# \# \# • \# \# \# • \# \# \# • \# \# \#

A13   **a.** $^-5$ **b.** $^-13$ **c.** 0 **d.** $^+11$ **e.** $^+12$ **f.** $^-4$

---

8   To find the sum of more than two integers, use the methods presented earlier to add the integers two at a time. For example, the sum $^-3 + ^+7 + ^-6$ is found:

$$^-3 + ^+7 + ^-6 = (^-3 + ^+7) + ^-6$$
$$= ^+4 + ^-6 \qquad \text{[Note: Read } (^-3 + ^+7) \text{ as "the quantity } ^-3 + ^+7\text{."]}$$
$$= ^-2$$

Notice that each sum of two integers can be found by starting at zero and using the number-line procedure if necessary.

Q14   Find the sum $^+3 + ^-2 + ^+5$.

\# \# \# • \# \# \# • \# \# \# • \# \# \# • \# \# \# • \# \# \# • \# \# \# • \# \# \# • \# \# \#

A14 $^+6$: $^+3 + ^-2 + ^+5 = (^+3 + ^-2) + ^+5$
$$= ^+1 + ^+5$$
$$= ^+6$$

Q15   Find the sum $^-4 + ^-7 + ^+3$.

\# \# \# • \# \# \# • \# \# \# • \# \# \# • \# \# \# • \# \# \# • \# \# \# • \# \# \# • \# \# \#

A15 $^-8$: $^-4 + ^-7 + ^+3 = (^-4 + ^-7) + ^+3$
$$= ^-11 + ^+3$$
$$= ^-8$$

---

9   The sum $^-3 + ^+5 + ^-6 + ^-2$ is found as follows:

$$^-3 + ^+5 + ^-6 + ^-2 = (^-3 + ^+5) + ^-6 + ^-2$$
$$= ^+2 + ^-6 + ^-2$$
$$= (^+2 + ^-6) + ^-2$$
$$= ^-4 + ^-2$$
$$= ^-6$$

Q16   Find each of the following sums:
     a. $^-3 + ^-5 + ^+8$ **b.** $^-4 + ^+5 + ^-1 + ^-3$

     c. $^-2 + ^-3 + ^-6$ **d.** $^+1 + ^+5 + ^+7$

\# \# \# • \# \# \# • \# \# \# • \# \# \# • \# \# \# • \# \# \# • \# \# \# • \# \# \# • \# \# \#

A16   **a.** 0   **b.** $^-3$ **c.** $^-11$ **d.** $^+13$

---

10   An important property of mathematics is the *commutative property of addition*. The commutative property of addition states that regardless of the *order* in which two numbers are added, the sum is the same. Many examples can be used to demonstrate this fact for the integers.

     Examples: $^-1 + ^+2 = ^+2 + ^-1$ (both sums are $^+1$)
                      $^-7 + ^-4 = ^-4 + ^-7$ (both sums are $^-11$)
                      $^+9 + ^-2 = ^-2 + ^+9$ (both sums are $^+7$)

     The commutative property of addition is generalized $a + b = b + a$ for any integers a and b.

Q17   Verify that $a + b = b + a$ is true for $a = ^-5$ and $b = ^+8$.

\# \# \# • \# \# \# • \# \# \# • \# \# \# • \# \# \# • \# \# \# • \# \# \# • \# \# \# • \# \# \#

A17 $^-5 + ^+8 = ^+8 + ^-5$ (both sums are $^+3$)

---

11   A second important mathematical property is the *associative property of addition*. It states that regardless of the grouping of addends, when three or more numbers are being added the sums are the same. Two examples using integers are as follows:

1. $(^-3 + {}^+4) + {}^-5 = {}^-3 + ({}^+4 + {}^-5)$
$\qquad {}^+1 + {}^-5 = {}^-3 + {}^-1$
$\qquad\quad {}^-4 = {}^-4$

2. $(^+7 + {}^+5) + {}^-10 = {}^+7 + ({}^+5 + {}^-10)$
$\qquad {}^+12 + {}^-10 = {}^+7 + {}^-5$
$\qquad\quad {}^+2 = {}^+2$

The associative property of addition is generalized $(a + b) + c = a + (b + c)$ for any integers a, b, and c.

Q18   Verify that $(a + b) + c = a + (b + c)$ is true for $a = {}^-2$, $b = {}^-7$, and $c = {}^+3$.

\# \# \#   •   \# \# \#   •   \# \# \#   •   \# \# \#   •   \# \# \#   •   \# \# \#   •   \# \# \#   •   \# \# \#   •   \# \# \#

A18 $(^-2 + {}^-7) + {}^+3 = {}^-2 + ({}^-7 + {}^+3)$
$\qquad {}^-9 + {}^+3 = {}^-2 + {}^-4$
$\qquad\quad {}^-6 = {}^-6$

12   Integers may be used in a discussion of respiration. A person's respiration takes place because of various pressures created by muscles of the thorax wall, the diaphragm, and the natural elasticity of the lung itself. These pressures cause air to flow into the lung during inspiration and out of the lung during expiration. The pressure is measured in cm of water and can be measured by a tube of water attached to the cavity containing the pressure as in Figure 1. The figure represents the lung

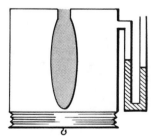

Figure 1

suspended in the thorax. The tube on the side indicates that there is less pressure inside the box than outside, causing the water to rise higher on the inside portion of the tube. We will call such a pressure "negative." The figure also represents the lung at rest where there remains a slight vacuum within the thorax of $^-4$ cm of water. This keeps the lung partially filled with air.

As the box expands by expanding the "bellows-like" bottom, the pressure becomes more negative and the balloon expands much as the lung does (see Figure 2). The tube indicates that the

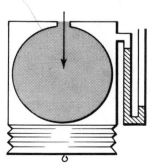

Figure 2

pressure is negative. As the muscles of the thorax relax, inside space contracts and the lung returns to its resting position as in the first figure of Frame 12.

If the floor of the box were pushed higher than its resting position, as in Figure 3, a positive pressure results and additional air is expelled from the balloon. When this is done in the human body, more air leaves the lungs but they are never emptied.

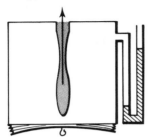

Figure 3

Q19   To the resting pressure of ⁻4 cm of water an additional pressure of ⁻22 cm of water is added. What is the total pressure in the thorax?

• # # # • # # # • # # # • # # # • # # # • # # # • # # # • # #

A19   ⁻26 cm: ⁻4 + ⁻22 = ⁻26

Q20   A patient was going through his normal inspiration with a pressure of ⁻6 cm of water when an obstruction closed his windpipe. His thorax muscles then provided an additional pressure of ⁻38 cm of water. What was the total pressure?

• # # # • # # # • # # # • # # # • # # # • # # # • # # # • # #

A20   ⁻44 cm: ⁻6 + ⁻38 = ⁻44

This completes the instruction for this section.

6.2   EXERCISE

1. Find each of the following sums:
   a. ⁻3 + ⁻5
   b. ⁺5 + ⁺9
   c. ⁺7 + ⁻6
   d. ⁻6 + ⁺6
   e. ⁻9 + 0
   f. ⁻3 + ⁺4 + ⁻3
   g. ⁻7 + ⁺6 + ⁺1
   h. 0 + ⁺4
   i. ⁻4 + ⁻3 + ⁺7 + ⁺4
   j. ⁻1 + ⁺6 + ⁻6 + ⁺1

2. Write a number in the blank to make each of the following a true statement:
   a. _____ + ⁻2 = 0
   b. ⁻8 + ⁺8 = _____
   c. ⁻12 + _____ = ⁻12
   d. ⁻12 + _____ = 0

3. The commutative and associative properties of addition are true for all integers. Identify each of the following as demonstrating the commutative or the associative property of addition.
   a. 4 + ⁻5 = ⁻5 + 4
   b. (⁻3 + 6) + ⁻4 = ⁻3 + (6 + ⁻4)
   c. ⁻1 + ⁻2 = ⁻2 + ⁻1
   d. (⁻5 + 0) + 5 = ⁻5 + (0 + 5)

6.2 EXERCISE ANSWERS

1. a. $^-8$ **b.** $^+14$ **c.** $^+1$ **d.** 0
   e. $^-9$ **f.** $^-2$ **g.** 0   **h.** $^+4$
   i. $^+4$ **j.** 0
2. a. $^+2$ **b.** 0   **c.** 0   **d.** $^+12$
3. a. commutative property of addition
   b. associative property of addition
   c. commutative property of addition
   d. associative property of addition

6.3 SUBTRACTION OF INTEGERS

1   Subtraction and addition can be thought of as opposite operations.* Consider, for example, the effect on any number x of first adding 5 and then performing the opposite operation of subtracting 5.

x
$x+5$ add 5
$x+5-5$ subtract 5
x

Notice that the operation of subtraction undoes what the operation of addition does, and the result is again the number x. The operation of addition also undoes an equal subtraction.

x
$x-5$ subtract 5
$x-5+5$ add 5
x

Thus, regardless of the order in which they are done, the operations of addition and subtraction are opposites. One operation undoes the other operation.

* Some mathematicians refer to addition and subtraction as "inverse operations."

Q1   **a.** What is the opposite operation of addition? _____

b. What is the opposite of adding 7 to any number? _____

• # # # • # # # • # # # • # # # • # # # • # # # • # # # • # #

A1   **a.** subtraction   **b.** subtracting 7

Q2   **a.** What is the opposite operation of subtraction? _____

b. What is the opposite of subtracting 3 from any number? _____

• # # # • # # # • # # # • # # # • ·# # # • # # # • # # # • # #

A2   **a.** addition   **b.** adding 3

2   Using the idea of addition and subtraction as opposite operations, the procedure for adding integers on the number line is easily modified for subtracting any two integers. Recall the procedure for finding the sum of any two integers on the number line.

$^-5+^+7$:

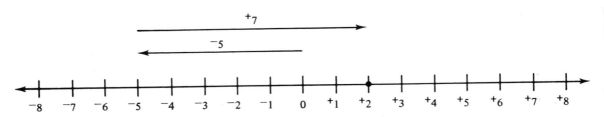

Step 1: Draw the arrow for the first addend (⁻5) from zero.

Step 2: From the tip of the first arrow, draw the arrow for the second addend (⁺7).

Step 3: Read the answer below the tip of the arrow for the second addend.

Thus, ⁻5 + ⁺7 = ⁺2.

Q3   Find the sum ⁺3 + ⁻9 using the number line given.

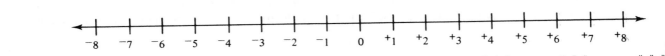

•   # # #   •   # # #   •   # # #   •   # # #   •   # # #   •   # # #   •   # # #   •   # #

A3   ⁻6:

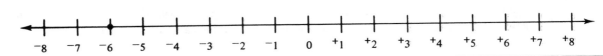

---

3   To find the difference ⁻3 − ⁻5, the following steps can be used:

Minuend   Subtrahend
   ↘   ↙
     ⁻3 − ⁻5

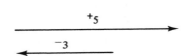

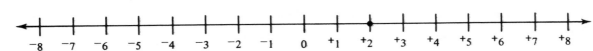

Step 1: Draw the arrow for the minuend (⁻3).

Step 2: Since subtraction is the opposite of addition, draw the arrow for the *opposite* of the subtrahend (⁺5) from the tip of the first arrow.

Step 3: Read the answer below the tip of the second arrow.

Thus, ⁻3 − ⁻5 = ⁺2.

Q4   Use the following number line to find the difference ⁻7 − ⁻4:

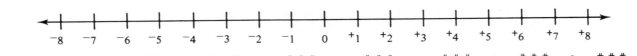

•   # # #   •   # # #   •   # # #   •   # # #   •   # # #   •   # # #   •   # # #   •   # #

A4 ⁻3:

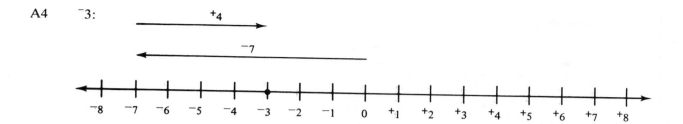

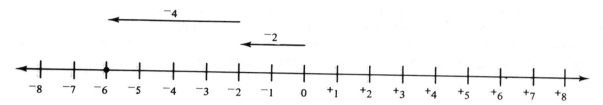

4 The difference ⁻2 − ⁺4 can be found as follows:

Step 1: Draw the arrow for the minuend (⁻2).

Step 2: Since subtraction is the opposite of addition, draw the arrow for the *opposite* of the subtrahend (⁻4).

Step 3: Read the answer below the tip of the second arrow.

Thus, ⁻2 − ⁺4 = ⁻6.

Q5 Use the number line provided to find the difference ⁺3 − ⁺10.

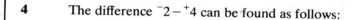

•   # # #   •   # # #   •   # # #   •   # # #   •   # # #   •   # # #   •   # # #   •   # #

A5 ⁻7:

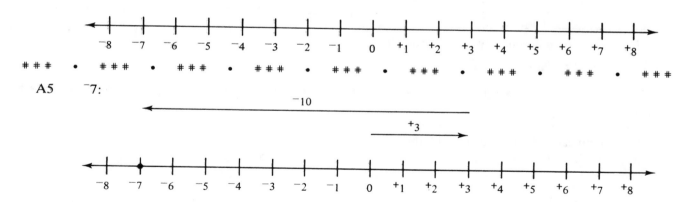

5 We repeat here the examples of Frames 3 and 4:

Minuend		Subtrahend		Difference
⁻3	−	⁻5	=	⁺2
⁻2	−	⁺4	=	⁻6

In each case the difference was found by first drawing the arrow for the minuend and then drawing the arrow for the *opposite* of the subtrahend.

This procedure is the basis for defining subtraction in terms of addition: *To find the difference of two integers, add the minuend to the opposite of the subtrahend.* That is, $a - b = a + {}^-b$ for any integers *a* and *b*.

Examples:

	Minuend		Subtrahend				Opposite of Subtrahend		Difference
1.	$^+7$	$-$	$\boxed{^+4}$	$=^+7$	$+$	$\boxed{^-4}$	$=$		$^+3$
2.	$^-3$	$-$	$\boxed{^+5}$	$=^-3$	$+$	$\boxed{^-5}$	$=$		$^-8$
3.	$^-4$	$-$	$\boxed{^-6}$	$=^-4$	$+$	$\boxed{^+6}$	$=$		$^+2$
4.	$^+2$	$-$	$\boxed{^+6}$	$=^+2$	$+$	$\boxed{^-6}$	$=$		$^-4$

Notice that in each example, two changes are involved: The operation sign for subtraction is changed to addition, and the subtrahend is changed to its opposite.

Q6   Find the difference $^-3-^+1$ using the number line provided.

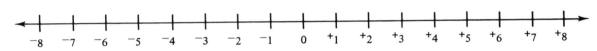

A6 $^-4$: $^-3-^+1=^-3+^-1$

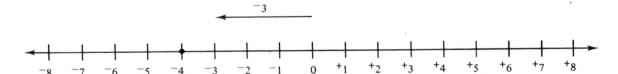

Q7   Find the difference by rewriting as a sum.

$^-4-^+7=^-4+$_____$=$_____

A7 $^-7, ^-11$

Q8   Find each of the following differences:

a. $^-2-^+5$ **b.** $^+7-^-5$

c. $^+1-^+9$ **d.** $^-5-^-3$

A8   **a.** $^-7$: $^-2-^+5=^-2+^-5=^-7$
   b. $^+12$: $^+7-^-5=^+7+^+5=^+12$
   c. $^-8$: $^+1-^+9=^+1+^-9=^-8$
   d. $^-2$: $^-5-^-3=^-5+^+3=^-2$

6   It is important to realize that the procedure of "adding the opposite" is done only with *subtraction*.

   1. To find a *sum*, follow the procedure for adding integers directly.
   2. To find a *difference*, *rewrite the problem as a sum* (by adding the opposite of the subtrahend to the minuend) and follow the procedure for adding integers.

Examples:

$$^-4-{}^+6={}^-4+{}^-6={}^-10$$
$$^+5+{}^-6={}^-1$$
$$^-7+{}^-4={}^-11$$
$$^-4-{}^-3={}^-4+{}^+3={}^-1$$

Q9 Which of the following problems must be rewritten?

   a. $^-4-{}^-5$ **b.** $^-2+{}^-1$

   c. $^+6+{}^-9$ **d.** $^+6-{}^+15$ _____

\# \# \# • \# \# \# • \# \# \# • \# \# \# • \# \# \# • \# \# \# • \# \# \# • \# \# \# • \# \# \#

A9 **a** and **d**: Subtraction problems must be rewritten (**b** and **c** are addition problems and thus can be answered directly).

Q10 Complete the problems of Q9.

\# \# \# • \# \# \# • \# \# \# • \# \# \# • \# \# \# • \# \# \# • \# \# \# • \# \# \# • \# \# \#

A10   **a.** $^-4-{}^-5={}^-4+{}^+5={}^+1$ **b.** $^-3$

      c. $^-3$ **d.** $^+6-{}^+15={}^+6+{}^-15={}^-9$

Q11 Complete each of the following as a sum or difference as indicated:

   a. $^-4+{}^-8$ **b.** $^+7-{}^+4$ **c.** $^-6-{}^+4$ **d.** $^-6+{}^+7$

   e. $^+2-{}^+5$ **f.** $^-4-{}^+8$ **g.** $^+4+{}^+7$ **h.** $^-1-{}^-1$

   i. $^+11+{}^-9$ **j.** $0-{}^-5$ **k.** $^-4+0$ **l.** $^+1-{}^+1$

   m. $^+5+{}^-5$ **n.** $^-2+{}^-3$ **o.** $^-3-{}^-3$ **p.** $^+5+{}^-7$

   q. $^+5-{}^+9$ **r.** $^-1+{}^+7$ **s.** $^-2-0$ **t.** $0-{}^+1$

\# \# \# • \# \# \# • \# \# \# • \# \# \# • \# \# \# • \# \# \# • \# \# \# • \# \# \# • \# \# \#

A11   **a.** $^-12$ **b.** $^+3$ **c.** $^-10$ **d.** $^+1$

      e. $^-3$ **f.** $^-12$ **g.** $^+11$ **h.** 0

      i. $^+2$ **j.** $^+5$ **k.** $^-4$ **l.** 0

      m. 0 **n.** $^-5$ **o.** 0 **p.** $^-2$

      q. $^-4$ **r.** $^+6$ **s.** $^-2$ **t.** $^-1$

7   When evaluating number sentences involving a combination of sums and differences, rewrite each of the differences as a sum and proceed as in Section 7.2, Frame 8. For example, the expression

$$^+3+{}^-7-{}^+5$$

    sum

    difference

involves a sum and a difference. First rewrite the difference as

$^+3 + {}^-7 + {}^-5$

The problem is now completed:

$^-4 + {}^-5$
$^-9$

Study the following examples:

1. $^-4 - {}^-2 + {}^+3$ **2.** $^-3 - {}^+4 - {}^+6 + {}^+7$
    $^-4 + {}^+2 + {}^+3$ $^-3 + {}^-4 + {}^-6 + 7$
    $^-2 + {}^+3$ $^-13 + 7$
    $^+1$ $^-6$

Q12   Evaluate $^-3 + {}^+5 - {}^+7$.

\# \# \# • \# \# \# • \# \# \# • \# \# \# • \# \# \# • \# \# \# • \# \# \# • \# \# \# • \# \# \#

A12 $^-5$: $^-3 + {}^+5 - {}^+7 = {}^-3 + {}^+5 + {}^-7 = {}^+2 + {}^-7 = {}^-5$

Q13   Evaluate $^+1 - {}^+5 - {}^+6$.

\# \# \# • \# \# \# • \# \# \# • \# \# \# • \# \# \# • \# \# \# • \# \# \# • \# \# \# • \# \# \#

A13 $^-10$: $^+1 - {}^+5 - {}^+6 = {}^+1 + {}^-5 + {}^-6 = {}^-4 + {}^-6 = {}^-10$

Q14   Evaluate $^+4 + {}^-3 - {}^+7 - {}^-6$.

\# \# \# • \# \# \# • \# \# \# • \# \# \# • \# \# \# • \# \# \# • \# \# \# • \# \# \# • \# \# \#

A14   0: $^+4 + {}^-3 - {}^+7 - {}^-6 = {}^+4 + {}^-3 + {}^-7 + {}^+6 = {}^+1 + {}^-7 + {}^+6 = {}^-6 + {}^+6 = 0$

Q15   Evaluate:

     a. $^-2 - {}^+5 + {}^+3$ **b.** $^+3 + {}^-5 + {}^-4$

     c. $^+4 - {}^-6 + {}^+7$ **d.** $^-6 - {}^+2 + {}^-7$

     e. $^-2 - {}^+3 - {}^+4$ **f.** $^+7 + {}^-2 - {}^+8 + {}^+3$

     g. $^+4 - 0 + {}^-4$ **h.** $0 - {}^+4 - {}^+3 + {}^+2$

     i. $^+6 - {}^+3 - {}^+5$ **j.** $^-6 + {}^-3 - {}^+10$

\# \# \# • \# \# \# • \# \# \# • \# \# \# • \# \# \# • \# \# \# • \# \# \# • \# \# \# • \# \# \#

A15   **a.** $^-4$: $^-2-^+5+^+3=^-2+^-5+^+3=^-7+^+3=^-4$

b. $^-6$

c. $^+17$

d. $^-15$: $^-6-^+2+^-7=^-6+^-2+^-7=^-15$

e. $^-9$

f. 0: $^+7+^-2-^+8+^+3=^+7+^-2+^-8+^+3=0$

g. 0

h. $^-5$: $0-^+4-^+3+^+2=0+^-4+^-3+^+2=^-7+^+2=^-5$

i. $^-2$: $^+6-^+3-^+5=^+6+^-3+^-5=^+3+^-5=^-2$

j. $^-19$

---

8   Consider the following examples:

$$^+3-^+4=^+3+^-4=^-1$$
$$^+4-^+3=^+1$$

The expressions $^+3-^+4$ and $^+4-^+3$ are not equivalent since they have different evaluations. Thus, $^+3-^+4=^+4-^+3$ is a false statement. $^+3-^+4\neq^+4-^+3$ is a true statement. ("$\neq$" means "is not equal to.")

Q16   **a.** Are $^-2-^+3$ and $^+3-^-2$ equivalent expressions?   _____

b. Is $^-2-^+3=^+3-^-2$ a true statement?   _____

\# \# \#   •   \# \# \#   •   \# \# \#   •   \# \# \#   •   \# \# \#   •   \# \# \#   •   \# \# \#   •   \# \# \#   •   \# \# \#

A16   **a.** no: $^-2-^+3=^-5$, whereas $^+3-^-2=^+5$

b. no

---

9   Frame 8 demonstrates that when the *order* of the numbers in a subtraction problem is changed the answers are not always the same. Thus, it is said that subtraction is *not* a commutative operation.

Q17   **a.** Are $^-5-4$ and $4-^-5$ equivalent expressions?   _____

b. Is subtraction a commutative operation?   _____

c. Is addition a commutative operation?   _____

\# \# \#   •   \# \# \#   •   \# \# \#   •   \# \# \#   •   \# \# \#   •   \# \# \#   •   \# \# \#   •   \# \# \#   •   \# \# \#

A17   **a.** no: $^-5-4=^-9$, whereas $4-^-5=^+9$

b. no   **c.** yes

Q18   Verify that $(^+3-^+5)-^+7$ and $^+3-(^+5-^+7)$ do not have the same evaluation.

\# \# \#   •   \# \# \#   •   \# \# \#   •   \# \# \#   •   \# \# \#   •   \# \# \#   •   \# \# \#   •   \# \# \#   •   \# \# \#

A18 $(^+3-^+5)-^+7=(^+3+^-5)+^-7=^-2+^-7=^-9$

$^+3-(^+5-^+7)=^+3-(^+5+^-7)=^+3-^-2=^+3+^+2=^+5$

Q19 $(^+3-^+5)-^+7=^+3-(^+5-^+7)$ is a _____ statement.
true/false

\# \# \# • \# \# \# • \# \# \# • \# \# \# • \# \# \# • \# \# \# • \# \# \# • \# \# \# • \# \# \#

A19 false

---

10 Question 19 demonstrates that when the *grouping* of three or more numbers in a subtraction problem is changed the answers are not always the same. Thus, it is said that subtraction is *not* an associative operation.

Q20 **a.** Are $(^+5-^+2)-^+1$ and $^+5-(^+2-^+1)$ equivalent expressions? _____

b. Is subtraction an associative operation? _____

c. Is addition an associative operation? _____

\# \# \# • \# \# \# • \# \# \# • \# \# \# • \# \# \# • \# \# \# • \# \# \# • \# \# \# • \# \# \#

A20 **a.** no: $(^+5-^+2)-^+1=^+2$ whereas $^+5-(^+2-^+1)=^+4$.
b. no **c.** yes

---

11 Recall from the previous section that the various pressures causing a person's respiration can be measured in centimetres of water by a tube of water attached to the cavity containing the pressure. Subtraction of integers is also applicable in this area.

Example: A patient in a weakened condition of health can only provide a pressure of $^-25$ cm of water. Due to constricted bronchi, she must be able to measure a pressure of $^-42$ cm of water. What additional pressure must a ventilating machine provide to assist her in breathing?

Solution: The difference between the two pressures is required.

$$^-42-^-25=^-42+25$$
$$=^-17 \text{ cm of water}$$

Q21 A patient is suffering from asthma which has constricted his bronchi so that he needs a pressure of $^-40$ cm of water to supply his lungs with air. If he can provide a pressure of $^-27$ cm of water, how much additional pressure must a ventilating machine provide?

\# \# \# • \# \# \# • \# \# \# • \# \# \# • \# \# \# • \# \# \# • \# \# \# • \# \# \# • \# \# \#

A21 $^-13$ cm of water: $^-40-^-27=^-40+27=^-13$

Q22 Suppose that the muscles of the chest are so weakened by disease that they can only provide a pressure of $^-5$ cm of water on inspiration and $^+7$ on expiration. If $^-30$ cm of water on inspiration and $^+25$ cm of water on expiration are needed for normal function of the lung, what additional pressures must an artificial ventilator provide?

\# \# \# • \# \# \# • \# \# \# • \# \# \# • \# \# \# • \# \# \# • \# \# \# • \# \# \# • \# \# \#

A22 $^-25$ cm of water for inspiration: $^-30-^-5=^-30+5=^-25$
$^+18$ cm of water for expiration: $^+25-^+7=^+25+^-7=^+18$

This completes the instruction for this section.

6.3   EXERCISE

1. Find the following sums:
   a. $^+3+^-7$ **b.** $^+12+^-9$ **c.** $^-5+^-6$ **d.** $^-9+^+12$
   e. $^-4+^+11$ **f.** $^+6+^-6$ **g.** $^-2+^+2$ **h.** $^+4+0$
   i. $0+^-7$ **j.** $^-3+^-4$

2. Write the opposite for each of the following integers:
   a. $^-5$ **b.** 0   **c.** $^+6$ **d.** $^-4$ **e.** 2   **f.** $^-1$

3. Find the following differences:
   a. $^-2-4$ **b.** $^-5-^-2$ **c.** $^-7-^-5$ **d.** $^-3-0$
   e. $^+6-^+9$ **f.** $^-4-^-4$ **g.** $^+3-^+2$ **h.** $0-^-1$
   i. $0-^+3$ **j.** $^-2-^-8$

4. Complete each of the following:
   a. $^+7+^-3$ **b.** $^-3+0$ **c.** $^-6-^+4$ **d.** $^+7-^+5$
   e. $^-5+^-9$ **f.** $^+7+^-7$ **g.** $0+^-4$ **h.** $^-6-^-7$
   i. $^-1-^+1$ **j.** $0+^+3$ **k.** $^-3-^+4$ **l.** $^-4+^+9$
   m. $^-5-0$ **n.** $0-^-5$ **o.** $^+6+^-9$ **p.** $^+4-^+5$
   q. $^-3+^+12$ **r.** $0+^-4$ **s.** $^-5+^+5$ **t.** $0-^-2$

5. Complete each of the following:
   a. $^+4-^+3+^-7$ **b.** $^-2-^-5-^-6$ **c.** $^-6+^+7+^-3$
   d. $^-4+^+6+^+4-^+6$ **e.** $^+2+^-2-0$ **f.** $^+3-^+2-^+4$
   g. $^+4+^-7-^+3$ **h.** $0-^+4+^+7$ **i.** $^-2-^+5-^+6$
   j. $^+6-0+^-3$

6.3   EXERCISE ANSWERS

1. a. $^-4$ **b.** $^+3$ **c.** $^-11$ **d.** $^+3$ **e.** $^+7$ **f.** 0   **g.** 0
   h. $^+4$ **i.** $^-7$ **j.** $^-7$

2. a. $^+5$ **b.** 0   **c.** $^-6$ **d.** $^+4$ **e.** $^-2$ **f.** $^+1$

3. a. $^-6$ **b.** $^-3$ **c.** $^-2$ **d.** $^-3$ **e.** $^-3$ **f.** 0   **g.** $^+1$
   h. $^+1$ **i.** $^-3$ **j.** $^+6$

4. a. $^+4$ **b.** $^-3$ **c.** $^-10$ **d.** $^+2$ **e.** $^-14$ **f.** 0   **g.** $^-4$
   h. $^+1$ **i.** $^-2$ **j.** $^+3$ **k.** $^-7$ **l.** $^+5$ **m.** $^-5$ **n.** $^+5$
   o. $^-3$ **p.** $^-1$ **q.** $^+9$ **r.** $^-4$ **s.** 0   **t.** $^+2$

5. a. $^-6$ **b.** $^+9$ **c.** $^-2$ **d.** 0   **e.** 0   **f.** $^-3$ **g.** $^-6$
   h. $^+3$ **i.** $^-13$ **j.** $^+3$

6.4   MULTIPLICATION OF INTEGERS

1   The operation of multiplication was developed as a shortcut procedure for addition. For example, the product $2 \cdot 3$ can be represented either as the sum of 2 threes or as the sum of 3 twos:

$$2 \cdot 3 = \underbrace{3+3} = 6$$
$$\qquad\quad \text{2 addends of 3}$$

or

$$3 \cdot 2 = \underbrace{2+2+2} = 6$$
$$\qquad\qquad \text{3 addends of 2}$$

Similarly, the product $^+7 \cdot {}^+4$ can be represented as either 7 positive fours or 4 positive sevens.

$^+7 \cdot {}^+4 = {}^+4 + {}^+4 + {}^+4 + {}^+4 + {}^+4 + {}^+4 + {}^+4 = {}^+28$

or

$^+4 \cdot {}^+7 = {}^+7 + {}^+7 + {}^+7 + {}^+7 = {}^+28$

Q1   Write $^+5 \cdot {}^+6$ as a sum in two ways.

\# \# \# • \# \# \# • \# \# \# • \# \# \# • \# \# \# • \# \# \# • \# \# \# • \# \# \# • \# \# \#

A1 $^+5 \cdot {}^+6 = {}^+6 + {}^+6 + {}^+6 + {}^+6 + {}^+6 = {}^+30$

or

$^+6 \cdot {}^+5 = {}^+5 + {}^+5 + {}^+5 + {}^+5 + {}^+5 + {}^+5 = {}^+30$

Q2   Write $^+3 \cdot {}^+9$ as a sum in two ways.

\# \# \# • \# \# \# • \# \# \# • \# \# \# • \# \# \# • \# \# \# • \# \# \# • \# \# \# • \# \# \#

A2 $^+3 \cdot {}^+9 = {}^+9 + {}^+9 + {}^+9 = {}^+27$

or

$^+9 \cdot {}^+3 = {}^+3 + {}^+3 + {}^+3 + {}^+3 + {}^+3 + {}^+3 + {}^+3 + {}^+3 + {}^+3 = {}^+27$

2   The procedure of writing a product as a sum can also be used to find the product of two integers. For example, the product $^+4 \cdot {}^-2$ can be written as the sum of 4 negative twos:

$$^+4 \cdot {}^-2 = \underbrace{{}^-2 + {}^-2 + {}^-2 + {}^-2}_{\text{4 addends of } {}^-2}$$

Since the sum on the right is equal to $^-8$ the product $^+4 \cdot {}^-2$ is $^-8$:

$^+4 \cdot {}^-2 = {}^-8$

Similarly, the product $^+3 \cdot {}^-7$ is $^-21$, because

$^+3 \cdot {}^-7 = {}^-7 + {}^-7 + {}^-7$
        $= {}^-21$

Q3   Write $^+2 \cdot {}^-6$ as a sum. _____

\# \# \# • \# \# \# • \# \# \# • \# \# \# • \# \# \# • \# \# \# • \# \# \# • \# \# \# • \# \# \#

A3 $^+2 \cdot {}^-6 = {}^-6 + {}^-6$

Q4   Find the product $^+2 \cdot {}^-6$

\# \# \# • \# \# \# • \# \# \# • \# \# \# • \# \# \# • \# \# \# • \# \# \# • \# \# \# • \# \# \#

A4 $^-12$

Q5   Find the product $^+3 \cdot {}^-5$ by writing it as a sum.

\# \# \# • \# \# \# • \# \# \# • \# \# \# • \# \# \# • \# \# \# • \# \# \# • \# \# \# • \# \# \#

A5 $^-15$: $^+3 \cdot {^-5} = {^-5} + {^-5} + {^-5} = {^-15}$

Q6   Find the product $^+7 \cdot {^-1}$ by writing it as a sum.

\# \# \# • \# \# \# • \# \# \# • \# \# \# • \# \# \# • \# \# \# • \# \# \# • \# \# \# • \# \# \#

A6 $^-7$: $^+7 \cdot {^-1} = {^-1} + {^-1} + {^-1} + {^-1} + {^-1} + {^-1} + {^-1} = {^-7}$

Q7   Find each of the following products:

  a. $^+5 \cdot {^-2} =$ _____   **b.** $^+6 \cdot {^-9} =$ _____   **c.** $^+1 \cdot {^-4} =$ _____

  d. $0 \cdot {^+4} =$ _____   **e.** $^+3 \cdot {^+3} =$ _____   **f.** $^+2 \cdot {^-8} =$ _____

\# \# \# • \# \# \# • \# \# \# • \# \# \# • \# \# \# • \# \# \# • \# \# \# • \# \# \# • \# \# \#

A7   **a.** $^-10$ **b.** $^-54$ **c.** $^-4$ **d.** 0 **e.** $^+9$ **f.** $^-16$

---

3   The product $^-5 \cdot {^+4}$ can be found by computing the sum of 4 negative fives:

$$^-5 \cdot {^+4} = \underbrace{{^-5} + {^-5} + {^-5} + {^-5}}_{\text{4 addends of } ^-5}$$

$$= {^-20}$$

Q8   Find the product $^-7 \cdot {^+5}$ by writing it as a sum.

\# \# \# • \# \# \# • \# \# \# • \# \# \# • \# \# \# • \# \# \# • \# \# \# • \# \# \# • \# \# \#

A8 $^-35$: $^-7 \cdot {^+5} = {^-7} + {^-7} + {^-7} + {^-7} + {^-7} = {^-35}$

Q9   Find the product $^+5 \cdot {^-7}$.

\# \# \# • \# \# \# • \# \# \# • \# \# \# • \# \# \# • \# \# \# • \# \# \# • \# \# \# • \# \# \#

A9 $^-35$: $^+5 \cdot {^-7} = {^-7} + {^-7} + {^-7} + {^-7} + {^-7} = {^-35}$

Q10   Find the product $^-4 \cdot {^+6}$.

\# \# \# • \# \# \# • \# \# \# • \# \# \# • \# \# \# • \# \# \# • \# \# \# • \# \# \# • \# \# \#

A10 $^-24$: $^-4 \cdot {^+6} = {^-4} + {^-4} + {^-4} + {^-4} + {^-4} + {^-4} = {^-24}$

Q11   Find the product $^-7 \cdot {^+9}$.

\# \# \# • \# \# \# • \# \# \# • \# \# \# • \# \# \# • \# \# \# • \# \# \# • \# \# \# • \# \# \#

A11 $^-63$

---

4   In each of the preceding products where the two factors had different signs (one positive and one negative), the product was negative. For example,

$$\underbrace{{}^{+}5 \cdot {}^{-}9}_{\substack{\text{different} \\ \text{signs}}} = {}^{-}45 \quad\quad \underbrace{{}^{-}7 \cdot {}^{+}8}_{\substack{\text{different} \\ \text{signs}}} = {}^{-}56$$

different negative different negative
signs   product   signs   product

These examples demonstrate the following rule for multiplying integers with different signs: *The product of two integers with different signs (one positive and one negative) is a negative integer.*

To make the multiplication of integers consistent with the multiplication of natural numbers, the rule for multiplying two positive integers is as follows: *The product of two positive integers is a positive integer.* For example,

$${}^{+}2 \cdot {}^{+}7 = {}^{+}14 \quad\quad 5 \cdot 8 = 40$$

The "+" sign is frequently omitted from positive numbers such as in the second example above. A number written without a sign is assumed to be positive.

Q12   Find the product in each of the following:

a. ${}^{-}2 \cdot {}^{+}3 =$ _____   b. ${}^{+}6 \cdot {}^{-}3 =$ _____   c. $4 \cdot 7 =$ _____

d. ${}^{+}1 \cdot {}^{-}5 =$ _____   e. ${}^{+}10 \cdot {}^{-}8 =$ _____   f. ${}^{+}5 \cdot {}^{+}3 =$ _____

g. ${}^{-}7 \cdot {}^{+}7 =$ _____   h. ${}^{-}8 \cdot {}^{+}6 =$ _____

\# \# \# • \# \# \# • \# \# \# • \# \# \# • \# \# \# • \# \# \# • \# \# \# • \# \# \# • \# \# \# .

A12   a. ${}^{-}6$ b. ${}^{-}18$ c. 28 d. ${}^{-}5$
      e. ${}^{-}80$ f. 15 g. ${}^{-}49$ h. ${}^{-}48$

5   Two important properties of whole numbers are also true for the integers. These are the *multiplication property of zero* and the *multiplication property of one*. The multiplication property of zero states that the product of any number and zero is zero.

Examples: $0 \cdot {}^{-}5 = 0$
                $8 \cdot 0 = 0$

In general, $a \cdot 0 = 0 \cdot a = 0$ for any integer a.

The multiplication property of one states that the product of any number and one is the identical number.

Examples: $1 \cdot {}^{-}7 = {}^{-}7$
                $2 \cdot 1 = 2$

In general, $a \cdot 1 = 1 \cdot a = a$ for any integer a.

Q13   Find each of the following products:

a. ${}^{-}4 \cdot 0 =$ _____   b. ${}^{+}8 \cdot 1 =$ _____

c. ${}^{-}3 \cdot {}^{+}4 =$ _____   d. $0 \cdot {}^{+}5 =$ _____

e. $6 \cdot 7 =$ _____   f. ${}^{+}9 \cdot {}^{-}9 =$ _____

\# \# \# • \# \# \# • \# \# \# • \# \# \# • \# \# \# • \# \# \# • \# \# \# • \# \# \# • \# \# \#

A13   a. 0 b. 8 c. ${}^{-}12$ d. 0 e. 42 f. ${}^{-}81$

6   The product of two integers with *different signs* is *negative*. The product of *two positive integers* is a *positive* integer. To discover the product of *two negative integers*, study the following series of products and notice the pattern that is present in the answers on the right.

$$^-2 \cdot {}^+4 = {}^-8$$
$$^-2 \cdot {}^+3 = {}^-6$$
$$^-2 \cdot {}^+2 = {}^-4$$
$$^-2 \cdot {}^+1 = {}^-2$$
$$^-2 \cdot 0 = 0$$
$$^-2 \cdot {}^-1 = ?$$
$$^-2 \cdot {}^-2 = ?$$

The pattern in the products on the right is that each answer increases by 2. Hence, to complete the pattern, the products are:

$$^-2 \cdot {}^-1 = {}^+2$$
$$^-2 \cdot {}^-2 = {}^+4$$

It is, thus, appropriate to state the rule for the product of two negative integers as follows: *The product of two negative integers is a positive integer.* For example,

$$^-7 \cdot {}^-4 = {}^+28 \qquad {}^-11 \cdot {}^-5 = {}^+55$$

Q14   Find the product $^-4 \cdot {}^-6$.

\# \# \# • \# \# \# • \# \# \# • \# \# \# • \# \# \# • \# \# \# • \# \# \# • \# \# \# • \# \# \#

A14 $^+24$ (or simply 24)

Q15 $^-3 \cdot 5 = $ _____

\# \# \# • \# \# \# • \# \# \# • \# \# \# • \# \# \# • \# \# \# • \# \# \# • \# \# \# • \# \# \#

A15 $^-15$

Q16 $^-9 \cdot {}^-6 = $ _____

\# \# \# • \# \# \# • \# \# \# • \# \# \# • \# \# \# • \# \# \# • \# \# \# • \# \# \# • \# \# \#

A16   54

Q17   Find the following products:

a. $^-3 \cdot 4 = $ _____   **b.** $^-4 \cdot {}^-9 = $ _____

c. $^-2 \cdot {}^-5 = $ _____   **d.** $9 \cdot {}^-8 = $ _____

e. $0 \cdot {}^-6 = $ _____   **f.** $^-12 \cdot 0 = $ _____

g. $5 \cdot {}^-1 = $ _____   **h.** $^-7 \cdot {}^-5 = $ _____

\# \# \# • \# \# \# • \# \# \# • \# \# \# • \# \# \# • \# \# \# • \# \# \# • \# \# \# • \# \# \#

A17   **a.** $^-12$ **b.** 36   **c.** 10   **d.** $^-72$
      e. 0   **f.** 0   **g.** $^-5$ **h.** 35

7   Study the effect of multiplying any integer by $^-1$ in the following examples:

$$^-1 \cdot 4 = {}^-4 \qquad {}^-1 \cdot {}^-5 = {}^+5$$

In the first example, multiplying 4 by negative one changes it to $^-4$, its opposite. In the second example, the product of $^-5$ and negative one changes $^-5$ to $^+5$, its opposite. The fact that negative one times a number is the opposite of the number is often called the *multiplication property of* $^-1$. In general, $^-1 \cdot a = a \cdot {}^-1 = {}^-a$ for any integer a. (Note: ^-a is read "the opposite of a.")

Q18 Find each of the following products:

    a. $^-1 \cdot {}^-7 =$ _____

    b. $1 \cdot {}^-7 =$ _____

    c. $^-1 \cdot 9 =$ _____

    d. $^-1 \cdot 0 =$ _____

\# \# \#　•　\# \# \#　•　\# \# \#　•　\# \# \#　•　\# \# \#　•　\# \# \#　•　\# \# \#　•　\# \# \#　•　\# \# \#

A18　**a.** 7　　　　**b.** $^-7$　　　　**c.** $^-9$　　　　**d.** 0

8　It is important for later work that the student be able to read the multiplication property of $^-1$ both from left to right and from right to left. Reading from left to right it says that multiplying by $^-1$ gives the opposite of the integer involved:

The integer		Its opposite
$^-1 \cdot$	$^+6 =$	$^-6$
$^-1 \cdot$	$^-9 =$	$^+9$

Reading from right to left it says that any integer can be expressed as a product of $^-1$ and its opposite.

The integer		Its opposite
$^-5$	$= {}^-1 \cdot$	$^+5$
$^-7$	$= {}^-1 \cdot$	$^+7$
$^+6$	$= {}^-1 \cdot$	$^-6$
$^+3$	$= {}^-1 \cdot$	$^-3$

Q19 Complete the following statements using the multiplication property of $^-1$:

    a. $^-1 \cdot {}^+7 =$ _____

    b. $^-1 \cdot$ _____ $= {}^+5$

    c. $^-3 = {}^-1 \cdot$ _____

    d. _____ $\cdot {}^-8 = {}^+8$

\# \# \#　•　\# \# \#　•　\# \# \#　•　\# \# \#　•　\# \# \#　•　\# \# \#　•　\# \# \#　•　\# \# \#　•　\# \# \#

A19　**a.** $^-7$　**b.** $^-5$　**c.** $^+3$　**d.** $^-1$

Q20 Find the product:

    a. $^-3 \cdot {}^+2 =$ _____

    b. $^+2 \cdot {}^-3 =$ _____

\# \# \#　•　\# \# \#　•　\# \# \#　•　\# \# \#　•　\# \# \#　•　\# \# \#　•　\# \# \#　•　\# \# \#　•　\# \# \#

A20　**a.** $^-6$　　　　　　　　**b.** $^-6$

Q21　**a.** Evaluate $^-7 \cdot {}^-8$. _____

    b. Evaluate $^-8 \cdot {}^-7$. _____

\# \# \#　•　\# \# \#　•　\# \# \#　•　\# \# \#　•　\# \# \#　•　\# \# \#　•　\# \# \#　•　\# \# \#　•　\# \# \#

A21　**a.** 56　　　　　　　　**b.** 56

Q22　**a.** Evaluate $3 \cdot {}^-5$. _____

    b. Evaluate $^-5 \cdot 3$. _____

\# \# \#　•　\# \# \#　•　\# \# \#　•　\# \# \#　•　\# \# \#　•　\# \# \#　•　\# \# \#　•　\# \# \#　•　\# \# \#　•　\# \# \#

A22　**a.** $^-15$　　　　　　　　**b.** $^-15$

9   Questions 21 and 22 demonstrate that the integers are commutative with respect to the operation of multiplication. The *commutative property of multiplication* states that regardless of the order in which two or more numbers are multiplied, the products are the same.

Examples: 1. $^-3 \cdot {^+9} = {^+9} \cdot {^-3}$ **2.** $^-12 \cdot {^-5} = {^-5} \cdot {^-12}$
$^-27 = {^-27}$ $^+60 = {^+60}$

In general, $a \cdot b = b \cdot a$ for any integers a and b.
    Another important property of the integers is the *associative property of multiplication*. It states that the grouping of factors in a product does not affect the answer.

Example: $7(^-3 \cdot 2) = (7 \cdot {^-3})2$
$7(^-6) = (^-21)2$
$^-42 = {^-42}$

In general, $a(b \cdot c) = (a \cdot b)c$ for any integers a, b, and c.

Q23   **a.** Is $^-253 \cdot 479 = 479 \cdot {^-253}$ a true statement?   _____

    b. Is $^-6(7 \cdot {^-3}) = (^-6 \cdot 7) \cdot {^-3}$ a true statement?   _____

•   # # #   •   # # #   •   # # #   •   # # #   •   # # #   •   # # #   •   # # #   •   # #

A23   **a.** yes: The commutative property of multiplication is true for all integers.
    b. yes: The associative property of multiplication is true for all integers.

10   Frame 9 makes it possible to state the following procedure for finding a product of more than two numbers. To find the product of more than two numbers:

Step 1: Do all work within parentheses first.

Step 2: Find the product of two numbers at a time in *any order desired*.

Examples:

1. $^-2 \cdot {^+4} \cdot {^-5}$
$^+10 \cdot {^+4}$ (since there are no parentheses, follow step 2)
40

2. $^+3(^-6 \cdot {^-5}) \cdot {^+9}$
$^+3(^+30) \cdot {^+9}$ (since parentheses are involved,
$^+90 \cdot {^+9}$ use step 1 and then step 2)
810

Q24   Find the product $^-2 \cdot {^-3} \cdot {^+5}$.

•   # # #   •   # # #   •   # # #   •   # # #   •   # # #   •   # # #   •   # # #   •   # #

A24   30

Q25   Find the product $(^-1 \cdot {^+3})(^-4 \cdot {^-7})$.

•   # # #   •   # # #   •   # # #   •   # # #   •   # # #   •   # # #   •   # # #   •   # #

A25 $^-84$: $(^-1 \cdot {^+3})(^-4 \cdot {^-7}) = {^-3} \cdot {^+28} = {^-84}$

Q26   Find each of the following products:

a. $^-2 \cdot {}^-4 \cdot 0$

b. $(^-3 \cdot {}^+4) \cdot {}^-5$

c. $^-6 \cdot {}^+11 \cdot {}^+10$

d. $^-1(^+3 \cdot {}^-5)$

e. $(^+4 \cdot 0)(^-7 \cdot {}^-6)$

f. $(^-2 \cdot {}^+3)(^-4 \cdot {}^-6)$

\# \# \# • \# \# \# • \# \# \# • \# \# \# • \# \# \# • \# \# \# • \# \# \# • \# \# \# • \# \# \#

A26   **a.** 0   **b.** 60   **c.** $^-660$ **d.** 15   **e.** 0   **f.** $^-144$

---

11   It has been established that the integers are commutative and associative with respect to addition and multiplication. Two additional properties of the integers are the *distributive property of multiplication over addition* and the *distributive property of multiplication over subtraction*. Examples of each are shown below:

(Distributive property of multiplication over addition) $2(^-5+7) = 2 \cdot {}^-5 + 2 \cdot 7$

(Distributive property of multiplication over subtraction) $3(^-4-6) = 3 \cdot {}^-4 - 3 \cdot 6$

The distributive properties state that the evaluations of the expressions on opposite sides of the equal sign are the same.

Q27   **a.** Evaluate $2(^-5+7)$ by working within the parentheses first.

b. Evaluate $2 \cdot {}^-5 + 2 \cdot 7$

\# \# \# • \# \# \# • \# \# \# • \# \# \# • \# \# \# • \# \# \# • \# \# \# • \# \# \# • \# \# \#

A27   **a.** 4: $2(^-5+7) = 2(2) = 4$
       b. 4: $2 \cdot {}^-5 + 2 \cdot 7 = {}^-10 + 14 = 4$

Q28   **a.** Evaluate $3(^-4-6)$ by working within the parentheses first.

b. Evaluate $3 \cdot {}^-4 - 3 \cdot 6$

\# \# \# • \# \# \# • \# \# \# • \# \# \# • \# \# \# • \# \# \# • \# \# \# • \# \# \# • \# \# \#

A28   **a.** $^-30$: $3(^-4-6) = 3(^-4 + {}^-6) = 3(^-10) = {}^-30$
       b. $^-30$: $3 \cdot {}^-4 - 3 \cdot 6 = {}^-12 - 18 = {}^-12 + {}^-18 = {}^-30$

Q29   Use the examples of Frame 11 to complete the following (without evaluating):

$8(^-2+5)=8\cdot\underline{\hspace{1cm}}+8\cdot\underline{\hspace{1cm}}$

\# \# \#   •   \# \# \#   •   \# \# \#   •   \# \# \#   •   \# \# \#   •   \# \# \#   •   \# \# \#   •   \# \# \#   •   \# \# \#

A29 $8(^-2+5)=8\cdot{}^-2+8\cdot5$

Q30   Complete the following (without evaluating):

$7(^-3-{}^-4)=7\cdot\underline{\hspace{1cm}}-7\cdot\underline{\hspace{1cm}}$

\# \# \#   •   \# \# \#   •   \# \# \#   •   \# \# \#   •   \# \# \#   •   \# \# \#   •   \# \# \#   •   \# \# \#   •   \# \# \#

A30 $7(^-3-{}^-4)=7\cdot{}^-3-7\cdot{}^-4$

---

12   The distributive properties are often classified as right or left depending on which side of the parentheses the number lies.

Examples:

1. Left distributive property of multiplication over addition

$5(2+{}^-6)=5\cdot2+5\cdot{}^-6$

2. Right distributive property of multiplication over addition

$(2+{}^-6)5=2\cdot5+{}^-6\cdot5$

3. Left distributive property of multiplication over subtraction

$3(2-7)=3\cdot2-3\cdot7$

4. Right distributive property of multiplication over subtraction

$(2-7)3=2\cdot3-7\cdot3$

Q31   **a.** Evaluate $5(2+{}^-6)$ by working within parentheses first.

b. Evaluate $5\cdot2+5\cdot{}^-6$

\# \# \#   •   \# \# \#   •   \# \# \#   •   \# \# \#   •   \# \# \#   •   \# \# \#   •   \# \# \#   •   \# \# \#   •   \# \# \#

A31   **a.** $^-20$: $5(2+{}^-6)=5({}^-4)={}^-20$
      b. $^-20$: $5\cdot2+5\cdot{}^-6=10+{}^-30={}^-20$

Q32 $3(5+{}^-7)=3\cdot5+3\cdot{}^-7$ is an example of the _____ distributive property of _____ over _____.

\# \# \#   •   \# \# \#   •   \# \# \#   •   \# \# \#   •   \# \# \#   •   \# \# \#   •   \# \# \#   •   \# \# \#   •   \# \# \#

A32   left, multiplication, addition

This completes the instruction for this section.

6.4   EXERCISE

1. The product of two integers with different signs is a _____ integer.
2. The product of any integer and zero is _____.

3. The product of any two integers with the same sign is a _____ integer.

4. Fill in the blanks so that a true statement results:

   a. _____ · 5 = 0

   b. ⁻1 · 7 = _____

   c. ⁺8 = _____ · ⁻8

   d. ⁻1 · ⁻5 = _____

5. Find each of the following products:

   a. ⁺4 · ⁻9

   b. ⁻3 · ⁻4

   c. ⁻2 · 0

   d. ⁻1 · ⁺9

   e. ⁻1 · ⁺7

   f. 5 · ⁻7

   g. 0 · ⁻9

   h. ⁻6 · ⁻9

   i. 11 · ⁻5

   j. 7 · ⁻8

6. Find each of the following products:

   a. ⁺2 · ⁻3 · ⁻4

   b. (⁺7 · ⁻1) · ⁻7

   c. ⁻1 · ⁻7 · ⁻8

   d. ⁻1 · ⁻1 · 0

   e. ⁻5 · 0 · ⁻6 · ⁺3

   f. 4 · 3 · ⁻5

   g. (⁻4 · ⁻4)(⁻2 · ⁺2)

   h. ⁻7(9 · ⁻3) · ⁺2

   i. ⁺6(⁻3 · ⁺2)

   j. (⁻2 · 4)(3 · ⁻3)

   k. (⁺6 · ⁻3) · ⁺2

   l. ⁻4 · 5(⁻6 · 0)

   m. ⁻2(⁻3 + ⁻5)

   n. (⁻7 − ⁻4)4

6.4   EXERCISE ANSWERS

1. negative

2. zero

3. positive

4. a. 0   **b.** ⁻7   **c.** ⁻1   **d.** 5

5. a. ⁻36   **b.** 12   **c.** 0   **d.** ⁻9   **e.** ⁻7

   f. ⁻35   **g.** 0   **h.** 54   **i.** ⁻55   **j.** ⁻56

6. a. 24   **b.** 49   **c.** ⁻56   **d.** 0   **e.** 0   **f.** ⁻60   **g.** ⁻64

   h. 378   **i.** ⁻36   **j.** 72   **k.** ⁻36   **l.** 0   **m.** 16   **n.** ⁻12

6.5   DIVISION OF INTEGERS

1   The operation of division is closely related to that of multiplication. A division problem is often checked using the multiplication operation. As was the case with addition and subtraction, multiplication and division are also opposite or inverse operations; that is, one undoes the effect of the other. For example,

$$10 \div 2 = 5 \quad \text{because} \quad 5 \cdot 2 = 10 \quad \text{or} \quad 8\overline{)56}^{\,7} \quad \text{because} \quad 7 \cdot 8 = 56$$

Q1   12 ÷ 3 = 4, because _____ · _____ = _____.

\# \# \#   •   \# \# \#   •   \# \# \#   •   \# \# \#   •   \# \# \#   •   \# \# \#   •   \# \# \#   •   \# \# \#   •   \# \# \#

A1   4 · 3 = 12

Q2 $7\overline{)63}^{\,9}$, because _____ · _____ = _____.

\# \# \#   •   \# \# \#   •   \# \# \#   •   \# \# \#   •   \# \# \#   •   \# \# \#   •   \# \# \#   •   \# \# \#   •   \# \# \#

A2   9 · 7 = 63

Q3   Use multiplication to find the quotient and write the check: $45 \div 9 =$ _____, because
_____ .

\# \# \# • \# \# \# • \# \# \# • \# \# \# • \# \# \# • \# \# \# • \# \# \# • \# \# \# • \# \# \#

A3 $45 \div 9 = \underline{5}$, because $\underline{5 \cdot 9 = 45}$

Q4   Use multiplication to find the quotient and check the result: $82 \div 2 =$ _____, because
_____ .

\# \# \# • \# \# \# • \# \# \# • \# \# \# • \# \# \# • \# \# \# • \# \# \# • \# \# \# • \# \# \#

A4 $82 \div 2 = \underline{41}$, because $\underline{41 \cdot 2 = 82}$

2	Consider the following quotient and check:

$^-27 \div {^+9} = \square$ because $\square \cdot {^+9} = {^-27}$

Since $^-3$ makes the product statement true, it also satisfies the quotient statement:

$^-27 \div {^+9} = \boxed{^-3}$ because $\boxed{^-3} \cdot {^+9} = {^-27}$

Q5   Place an integer in the $\square$ to form a true statement: $^+12 \div {^-3} = \square$ because $\square \cdot {^-3} = {^+12}$

\# \# \# • \# \# \# • \# \# \# • \# \# \# • \# \# \# • \# \# \# • \# \# \# • \# \# \# • \# \# \#

A5 $^+12 \div {^-3} = \boxed{^-4}$, because $\boxed{^-4} \cdot {^-3} = {^+12}$

Q6   Place an integer in the $\square$ to form a true statement: $^-16 \div {^+2} = \square$ because $\square \cdot {^+2} = {^-16}$

\# \# \# • \# \# \# • \# \# \# • \# \# \# • \# \# \# • \# \# \# • \# \# \# • \# \# \# • \# \# \#

A6 $^-16 \div {^+2} = \boxed{^-8}$, because $\boxed{^-8} \cdot {^+2} = {^-16}$

Q7   Find the quotient and write the check as a multiplication problem: $^+56 \div {^-8} =$ _____ because
_____ $\cdot {^-8} = {^+56}$

\# \# \# • \# \# \# • \# \# \# • \# \# \# • \# \# \# • \# \# \# • \# \# \# • \# \# \# • \# \# \#

A7 $^+56 \div {^-8} = \underline{^-7}$, because $\underline{^-7} \cdot {^-8} = {^+56}$

Q8   Find the quotient and write the check as a multiplication problem: $^-30 \div {^+10} =$ _____ because
_____ .

\# \# \# • \# \# \# • \# \# \# • \# \# \# • \# \# \# • \# \# \# • \# \# \# • \# \# \# • \# \# \#

A8 $\underline{^-3}$, because $\underline{^-3} \cdot {^+10} = {^-30}$

Q9 $^+15 \div {^-3} =$ _____

\# \# \# • \# \# \# • \# \# \# • \# \# \# • \# \# \# • \# \# \# • \# \# \# • \# \# \# • \# \# \#

A9 $^-5$

3	Each of the problems in Q5 through Q9 involved the quotient of two integers with different signs. Study the problems and their answers below:

$^+12 \div {^-3} = {^-4}$
$^-16 \div {^+2} = {^-8}$
$^+56 \div {^-8} = {^-7}$
$^-30 \div {^+10} = {^-3}$
$^+15 \div {^-3} = {^-5}$

Q10   What is true of all the answers in Frame 3? _____

\# \# \#   •   \# \# \#   •   \# \# \#   •   \# \# \#   •   \# \# \#   •   \# \# \#   •   \# \# \#   •   \# \# \#   •   \# \# \#

A10   Each answer is a negative integer.

---

4   The examples of Frame 3 demonstrate the following definition for the division of two integers with different signs: *The quotient of two integers with different signs is a negative integer.*

A division problem is also correctly written as a fraction. Thus, $20 \div 4 = 5$ can also be written $\dfrac{20}{4} = 5$. Study the following examples:

$$\frac{^-36}{^+4} = ^-9 \qquad ^+27 \div ^+9 = ^+3$$

$$48 \div ^-6 = ^-8 \qquad \frac{^+14}{^-2} = ^-7$$

Q11   Find the following quotients:

    a. $\dfrac{^-25}{^+5} = $ _____   **b.** $^-25 \div ^+5 = $ _____

    c. $\dfrac{^-90}{^+10} = $ _____   **d.** $^+12 \div ^-2 = $ _____

    e. $^+1 \div ^-1 = $ _____   **f.** $\dfrac{^+45}{^-9} = $ _____

\# \# \#   •   \# \# \#   •   \# \# \#   •   \# \# \#   •   \# \# \#   •   \# \# \#   •   \# \# \#   •   \# \# \#   •   \# \# \#

A11   **a.** $^-5$ **b.** $^-5$ **c.** $^-9$ **d.** $^-6$ **e.** $^-1$ **f.** $^-5$

---

5   To determine the sign of the *quotient* of two *integers* with the *same sign*, consider the integer that converts the following open sentence into a true statement.

$^-20 \div ^-5 = \square$ because $\square \cdot ^-5 = ^-20$

The correct integer replacement is $^+4$. That is, $^-20 \div ^-5 = ^+4$, because $^+4 \cdot ^-5 = ^-20$.

Q12   Place an integer in the $\square$ to form a true statement: $^-15 \div ^-3 = \square$ because $\square \cdot ^-3 = ^-15$

\# \# \#   •   \# \# \#   •   \# \# \#   •   \# \# \#   •   \# \# \#   •   \# \# \#   •   \# \# \#   •   \# \# \#   •   \# \# \#

A12 $^+5$: $^-15 \div ^-3 = \boxed{^+5}$, because $\boxed{^+5} \cdot ^-3 = ^-15$.

Q13   Find the quotient and write the check as a multiplication problem: $^-63 \div ^-7 = $ _____ because _____ $\cdot ^-7 = ^-63$

\# \# \#   •   \# \# \#   •   \# \# \#   •   \# \# \#   •   \# \# \#   •   \# \# \#   •   \# \# \#   •   \# \# \#   •   \# \# \#

A13 $^+9$: $^-63 \div ^-7 = \underline{^+9}$, because $\underline{^+9} \cdot ^-7 = ^-63$

Q14 $^-81 \div ^-9 = $ _____

\# \# \#   •   \# \# \#   •   \# \# \#   •   \# \# \#   •   \# \# \#   •   \# \# \#   •   \# \# \#   •   \# \# \#   •   \# \# \#

A14 $^+9$ (or simply 9)

---

6   The quotient of Q12 through Q14 involved integers with the same sign. The answer in each case was a positive integer. The rule suggested for quotients of this type is as follows: *The quotient of two* *integers with the same sign is a positive integer.* Some examples of the above rule are:

1. $\dfrac{^-36}{^-4} = {}^+9$ **2.** $^-26 \div {}^-2 = {}^+13$

3. $^+42 \div {}^+21 = {}^+2$ **4.** $\dfrac{18}{3} = 6$

Q15   Find the quotient of $^-24 \div {}^-6$.

\# \# \# • \# \# \# • \# \# \# • \# \# \# • \# \# \# • \# \# \# • \# \# \# • \# \# \# • \# \# \#

A15   4

Q16 $\dfrac{^-56}{^-7} = $ _____

\# \# \# • \# \# \# • \# \# \# • \# \# \# • \# \# \# • \# \# \# • \# \# \# • \# \# \# • \# \# \#

A16   8

Q17   Find each of the following quotients:

a. $\dfrac{^-12}{^-3} = $ _____   **b.** $^+72 \div {}^-6 = $ _____   **c.** $^+4 \div {}^-4 = $ _____

d. $^-93 \div {}^-3 = $ _____   **e.** $\dfrac{^-19}{^-19} = $ _____   **f.** $14 \div 7 = $ _____

g. $\dfrac{^+24}{^-6} = $ _____   **h.** $\dfrac{^-24}{^+6} = $ _____   **i.** $^-28 \div {}^-7 = $ _____

j. $^-1 \div {}^+1 = $ _____   **k.** $^-1 \div {}^-1 = $ _____   **l.** $\dfrac{^-2}{^-2} = $ _____

\# \# \# • \# \# \# • \# \# \# • \# \# \# • \# \# \# • \# \# \# • \# \# \# • \# \# \# • \# \# \#

A17   **a.** 4   **b.** $^-12$ **c.** $^-1$ **d.** 31   **e.** 1   **f.** 2   **g.** $^-4$
      h. $^-4$ **i.** 4   **j.** $^-1$ **k.** 1   **l.** 1

7   The *quotient* of two integers with *different signs* is a *negative* integer: for example, $^-12 \div {}^+6 = {}^-2$. The *product* of two integers with *different signs* is also a *negative* integer: for example, $^-4 \cdot {}^+6 = {}^-24$.

Q18   The quotient of two integers with the *same sign* is a _____ integer.

\# \# \# • \# \# \# • \# \# \# • \# \# \# • \# \# \# • \# \# \# • \# \# \# • \# \# \# • \# \# \#

A18   positive

Q19   The product of two integers with the *same sign* is a _____ integer.

\# \# \# • \# \# \# • \# \# \# • \# \# \# • \# \# \# • \# \# \# • \# \# \# • \# \# \# • \# \# \#

A19   positive

Q20   **a.** The quotient of two integers with *different signs* is a _____ integer.

      b. The product of two integers with *different signs* is a _____ integer.

\# \# \# • \# \# \# • \# \# \# • \# \# \# • \# \# \# • \# \# \# • \# \# \# • \# \# \# • \# \# \#

A20   **a.** negative   **b.** negative

---

8   The rules for multiplication and division are the same. They may be summarized:

1. *The product or quotient of two integers with the same sign is positive.*
2. *The product or quotient of two integers with different signs is negative.*

(*Note*: The above rules are sometimes abbreviated.)

   In multiplication or division of integers:

1. Same sign—positive.
2. Different signs—negative.

This gives a quick and easy means to remember the signs in a multiplication or division problem.

Q21   Find the following products and quotients:

a. $^-15 \div ^-3 = $ _____   **b.** $\dfrac{^+18}{^-3} = $ _____   **c.** $^-4 \cdot ^-8 = $ _____

d. $\dfrac{^-14}{^-7} = $ _____   **e.** $^+7 \cdot ^-3 = $ _____   **f.** $^-5 \cdot ^-9 = $ _____

g. $\dfrac{^-12}{^+3} = $ _____   **h.** $^+7 \cdot ^-6 = $ _____   **i.** $^-8 \cdot 0 = $ _____

j. $\dfrac{^+27}{^-9} = $ _____   **k.** $^+48 \div ^-12 = $ _____   **l.** $^-32 \div ^-4 = $ _____

• # # # • # # # • # # # • # # # • # # # • # # # • # # # • # #

A21   **a.** 5   **b.** $^-6$ **c.** 32   **d.** 2   **e.** $^-21$ **f.** 45   **g.** $^-4$
       h. $^-42$ **i.** 0   **j.** $^-3$ **k.** $^-4$ **l.** 8

---

9   In Section 6.4 the multiplication property of $^-1$ was stated. According to this property, *negative one times a number is the opposite of the number.* For example, $^-1 \cdot ^+5 = ^-5$ and $^-1 \cdot ^-3 = ^+3$. Consider the result of dividing an integer by $^-1$ in the following examples:

$$\frac{^+3}{^-1} = ^-3 \qquad \frac{^-5}{^-1} = ^+5$$

Q22   When $^+3$ is divided by $^-1$, the quotient is _____.

• # # # • # # # • # # # • # # # • # # # • # # # • # # # • # #

A22 $^-3$:   the opposite of $^+3$

Q23   When $^-5$ is divided by $^-1$, the quotient is _____.

• # # # • # # # • # # # • # # # • # # # • # # # • # # # • # #

A23 $^+5$:   the opposite of $^-5$

---

10   The preceding examples demonstrate that the result of dividing an integer by $^-1$ is the same as when multiplying an integer by $^-1$. In each case, the answer is the opposite of the integer being multiplied or divided. The *division property of* $^-1$ states that $\dfrac{a}{^-1} = ^-a$ is true for any integer a.

Q24 Complete each of the following:

a. $^-1 \cdot {^+7} =$ _____

b. $\dfrac{^+7}{^-1} =$ _____

c. $^-1 \cdot {^-5} =$ _____

d. $\dfrac{^-5}{^-1} =$ _____

e. $^-x = {^-1} \cdot$ _____

f. $\dfrac{x}{^-1} =$ _____

• # # # • # # # • # # # • # # # • # # # • # # # • # # # • # #

A24 a. $^-7$ b. $^-7$ c. 5 d. 5 e. $^-x = {^-1} \cdot x$ f. $\dfrac{x}{^-1} = {^-x}$

---

11 The number zero is frequently confusing when involved as a divisor or dividend in a division problem. Consider the open sentence

$0 \div 5 = \square$ because $\square \cdot 5 = 0$

The integer that converts the open sentence to a true statement is zero:

$0 \div 5 = \boxed{0}$ because $\boxed{0} \cdot 5 = 0$

Q25 What integer converts the open sentence to a true statement? $0 \div {^-9} = \square$ because $\square \cdot {^-9} = 0$

• # # # • # # # • # # # • # # # • # # # • # # # • # # # • # #

A25 0: $0 \div {^-9} = \boxed{0}$, because $\boxed{0} \cdot {^-9} = 0$

Q26 $0 \div {^+2} =$ _____, because _____

• # # # • # # # • # # # • # # # • # # # • # # # • # # # • # #

A26 <u>0</u>, because <u>$0 \cdot {^+2} = 0$</u>

Q27 $0 \div {^-8} =$ _____

• # # # • # # # • # # # • # # # • # # # • # # # • # # # • # #

A27 0

---

12 When zero is the divisor, the quotient is said to be *undefined*. To understand why, consider the open sentence

$4 \div 0 = \square$ because $\square \cdot 0 = 4$

There is no answer to the product $\square \cdot 0 = 4$, so there is no answer to the corresponding quotient $4 \div 0 = \square$. That is, $4 \div 0$ is undefined, because *no number* $\cdot\, 0 = 4$.

Q28 $7 \div 0 =$ _____, because _____

• # # # • # # # • # # # • # # # • # # # • # # # • # # # • # #

A28 <u>undefined</u>, because <u>no number $\cdot\, 0 = 7$</u>

Q29 $^-3 \div 0 =$ _____

• # # # • # # # • # # # • # # # • # # # • # # # • # # # • # #

A29 undefined

13 *When zero is the divisor* in a division problem, *the quotient is* said to be *undefined*. That is, $\frac{x}{0} =$ undefined. For example,

$$\frac{^-3}{0} = \text{undefined} \qquad ^+12 \div 0 = \text{undefined}$$

When zero is divided by any nonzero integer, the quotient is zero. That is, $\frac{0}{x} = 0$ for any nonzero integer x.

Examples:

1. $\frac{0}{7} = 0$ **2.** $0 \div 6 = 0$

Q30 Complete each of the following quotients:

a. $0 \div {}^-2 = \underline{\hspace{2cm}}$ **b.** ${}^-2 \div 0 = \underline{\hspace{2cm}}$

c. $\frac{0}{{}^+7} = \underline{\hspace{2cm}}$ **d.** $\frac{7}{0} = \underline{\hspace{2cm}}$

e. ${}^-3 \div 0 = \underline{\hspace{2cm}}$ **f.** $10 \div {}^-1 = \underline{\hspace{2cm}}$

g. $\frac{{}^-4}{{}^-2} = \underline{\hspace{2cm}}$ **h.** $0 \div {}^-4 = \underline{\hspace{2cm}}$

i. $\frac{42}{{}^-6} = \underline{\hspace{2cm}}$ **j.** $\frac{8}{0} = \underline{\hspace{2cm}}$

\# \# \# • \# \# \# • \# \# \# • \# \# \# • \# \# \# • \# \# \# • \# \# \# • \# \# \# • \# \# \#

A30 **a.** 0   **b.** undefined   **c.** 0
    d. undefined   **e.** undefined   **f.** ${}^-10$
    g. 2   **h.** 0   **i.** ${}^-7$
    j. undefined

Q31 Evaluate:

a. ${}^+4 \div {}^-2 = \underline{\hspace{1.5cm}}$ **b.** ${}^-2 \div 4 = \underline{\hspace{1.5cm}}$

\# \# \# • \# \# \# • \# \# \# • \# \# \# • \# \# \# • \# \# \# • \# \# \# • \# \# \# • \# \# \#

A31 **a.** ${}^-2$ **b.** $\frac{{}^-2}{4} = \frac{{}^-1}{2}$

Q32 Is ${}^+4 \div {}^-2 = {}^-2 \div {}^+4$ a true statement?   \underline{\hspace{2cm}}

\# \# \# • \# \# \# • \# \# \# • \# \# \# • \# \# \# • \# \# \# • \# \# \# • \# \# \# • \# \# \#

A32 no

14 The statement $a \div b = b \div a$ is false for most integers a and b. Therefore, the integers are not commutative with respect to the operation of division.

Q33   Evaluate:

a. $(^-20 \div ^-10) \div ^+2$ **b.** $^-20 \div (^-10 \div ^+2)$

\# \# \#   •   \# \# \#   •   \# \# \#   •   \# \# \#   •   \# \# \#   •   \# \# \#   •   \# \# \#   •   \# \# \#   •   \# \# \#

A33   **a.** 1: $(^-20 \div ^-10) \div ^+2 = ^+2 \div ^+2 = 1$
        b. 4: $^-20 \div (^-10 \div ^+2) = ^-20 \div ^-5 = 4$

Q34   Is $(^-20 \div ^-10) \div ^+2 = ^-20 \div (^-10 \div ^+2)$ a true statement?   _____

\# \# \#   •   \# \# \#   •   \# \# \#   •   \# \# \#   •   \# \# \#   •   \# \# \#   •   \# \# \#   •   \# \# \#   •   \# \# \#

A34   no

---

15   The statement $(a \div b) \div c = a \div (b \div c)$ is false for most integers a, b, and c. Therefore, the integers are not associative with respect to the operation of division.

Q35   Complete the following:

a. The integers _____ commutative with respect to multiplication.
        are/are not

b. The integers _____ commutative with respect to division.
        are/are not

c. $(^-16 \div ^+4) \div ^+2 = ^-16 \div (^+4 \div ^+2)$ _____ a true statement.
        is/is not

\# \# \#   •   \# \# \#   •   \# \# \#   •   \# \# \#   •   \# \# \#   •   \# \# \#   •   \# \# \#   •   \# \# \#   •   \# \# \#

A35   **a.** are   **b.** are not   **c.** is not

This completes the instruction for this section.

6.5   EXERCISE

1. Find each of the following quotients:

a. $72 \div ^-9$ **b.** $\dfrac{^-18}{2}$ **c.** $^-15 \div ^-5$ **d.** $^-5 \div ^-5$

e. $0 \div ^-7$ **f.** $\dfrac{^-24}{^-6}$ **g.** $\dfrac{10}{0}$ **h.** $\dfrac{0}{^-2}$

i. $^-13 \div ^-1$ **j.** $\dfrac{^-8}{8}$

2. Find each of the following products and quotients:

a. $\dfrac{^-51}{3}$ **b.** $\dfrac{0}{^-12}$ **c.** $^-12 \cdot ^-5$ $\dfrac{^-45}{^-3}$

e. $\dfrac{5}{^-1}$ **f.** $\dfrac{4}{0}$ **g.** $^-5 \cdot 0$ **h.** $^-4 \cdot 0$

i. $0 \div 3$ **j.** $^-1 \cdot 3$ **k.** $\dfrac{0}{^-5}$ **l.** $^-6 \cdot ^-7$

m. $\dfrac{^-75}{^-15}$ **n.** $7 \cdot ^-9$ **o.** $^-3 \cdot 0$ **p.** $\dfrac{^-8}{^-2}$

q. $^-1 \cdot 6$ **r.** $^-32 \div 4$ **s.** $^-8 \cdot ^-1$ **t.** $7 \cdot 0$

3. The product or quotient of two integers with the same sign is a _____ integer.

4. The product or quotient of two integers with different signs is a _____ integer.

5. Answer true or false: The integers are
   a. associative for division
   b. commutative for multiplication
   c. commutative for division
   d. associative for multiplication

6.5   EXERCISE ANSWERS

1. a. ⁻8	**b.** ⁻9	**c.** 3	**d.** 1
e. 0	**f.** 4	**g.** undefined	**h.** 0
i. 13	**j.** 1		
2. a. ⁻17	**b.** 0	**c.** 60	**d.** 15
e. ⁻5	**f.** undefined	**g.** 0	**h.** 0
i. 0	**j.** ⁻3	**k.** 0	**l.** 42
m. 5	**n.** ⁻63	**o.** 0	**p.** 4
q. ⁻6	**r.** ⁻8	**s.** 8	**t.** 0

3. positive
4. negative

5. a. false	**b.** true	**c.** false	**d.** true

6.6   OPERATIONS WITH RATIONAL NUMBERS

1   The rational numbers are an extension of the integers which are formed by including with the integers the positive and negative fractions. A rational number is defined as follows: *A rational number is any number which can be written in the form $\frac{p}{q}$, where p and q are integers and $q \neq 0$.*

Some examples of rational numbers are:

$$\frac{2}{3} \qquad \frac{^-5}{7} \qquad 4 \qquad ^-2 \qquad 0 \qquad 3\frac{1}{7}$$

$\frac{2}{3}$ and $\frac{^-5}{7}$ are rational numbers, because they are written in the form $\frac{p}{q}$ and their denominators (q) are not zero. Integers, such as 4, ⁻2, and 0, are rational numbers, because they can be written in the form $\frac{p}{q}$ by using 1 as their denominators. That is, $4 = \frac{4}{1}$, $^-2 = \frac{^-2}{1}$, and $0 = \frac{0}{1}$. $3\frac{1}{7}$ is a rational number, because it can be written in the form $\frac{p}{q}$ using its improper fraction equivalent. That is, $3\frac{1}{7} = \frac{22}{7}$.

*The symbol $\neq$ means "is not equal to."

Q1   Which of the following are rational numbers? $^-5, \frac{3}{0}, \frac{1}{2}, 2\frac{1}{6}$ _____

•   # # #   •   # # #   •   # # #   •   # # #   •   # # #   •   # # #   •   # # #   •   # #

A1 $^-5$, $\dfrac{1}{2}$, and $2\dfrac{1}{6}$: $\dfrac{3}{0}$ is not a rational number, because its denominator is zero and its value is thus undefined.

Q2   Write in the $\dfrac{p}{q}$ form:

     a. $^-5 = $ _____   **b.** $\dfrac{1}{2} = $ _____   **c.** $2\dfrac{1}{6} = $ _____

• # # # • # # # • # # # • # # # • # # # • # # # • # # # • # # # • # #

A2   **a.** $\dfrac{^-5}{1}$ **b.** $\dfrac{1}{2}$ **c.** $\dfrac{13}{6}$

---

2   By the definition, the rational numbers include many different types of numbers. They include positive and negative *fractions*, both proper and improper, because these are already in the required $\dfrac{p}{q}$ form. They include positive and negative *mixed numbers*, because any mixed number can be rewritten as an improper fraction in the required $\dfrac{p}{q}$ form. Finally, the rational numbers include the natural numbers, the whole numbers, and the integers, because each of these numbers can be written in the $\dfrac{p}{q}$ form using the number 1 as the denominator q. Just as the natural numbers, whole numbers, and integers, the rational numbers are an infinite or unending collection.

Q3   Write each rational number in the $\dfrac{p}{q}$ form:

     a. $^-3 = $ _____   **b.** $4\dfrac{2}{7} = $ _____   **c.** $0 = $ _____

• # # # • # # # • # # # • # # # • # # # • # # # • # # # • # # # • # #

     a. $\dfrac{^-3}{1}$ **b.** $\dfrac{30}{7}$ **c.** $\dfrac{0}{1}$

---

3   A positive mixed number can be written as the sum of its whole-number and fraction parts. For example, $3\dfrac{2}{5} = 3 + \dfrac{2}{5}$. The improper-fraction form is found:

$$3\dfrac{2}{5} = \frac{3 \cdot 5 + 2}{5}$$
$$= \frac{15 + 2}{5}$$
$$= \frac{17}{5}$$

    A similar procedure can be used with negative mixed numbers:

$$^-3\dfrac{1}{2} = {}^-\left(3\dfrac{1}{2}\right)$$
$$= {}^-\left(\frac{3 \cdot 2 + 1}{2}\right)$$
$$= {}^-\left(\frac{7}{2}\right) \quad \text{(read ``the opposite of seven halves'')}$$
$$= \frac{^-7}{2} \quad \text{(read ``negative seven halves'')}$$

Q4 Find the improper-fraction form:

a. $^{-}4\frac{1}{7}$

b. $^{-}2\frac{2}{9}$

• # # # • # # # • # # # • # # # • # # # • # # # • # # # • # #

A4 a. $\frac{^{-}29}{7}$: $^{-}4\frac{1}{7} = ^{-}\left(4\frac{1}{7}\right)$

$= ^{-}\left(\frac{4 \cdot 7 + 1}{7}\right)$

$= ^{-}\left(\frac{29}{7}\right)$

$= \frac{^{-}29}{7}$

b. $\frac{^{-}20}{9}$: $^{-}2\frac{2}{9} = ^{-}\left(2\frac{2}{9}\right)$

$= ^{-}\left(\frac{2 \cdot 9 + 2}{9}\right)$

$= ^{-}\left(\frac{20}{9}\right)$

$= \frac{^{-}20}{9}$

Q5 Write each of the rational numbers in the $\frac{p}{q}$ form:

a. $7 = $ _____

b. $^{-}5\frac{1}{4} = $ _____

c. $\frac{2}{3} = $ _____

d. $^{-}4 = $ _____

e. $4\frac{1}{2} = $ _____

f. $^{-}2\frac{4}{5} = $ _____

• # # # • # # # • # # # • # # # • # # # • # # # • # # # • # #

A5 a. $\frac{7}{1}$

b. $\frac{^{-}21}{4}$

c. $\frac{2}{3}$

d. $\frac{^{-}4}{1}$

e. $\frac{9}{2}$

f. $\frac{^{-}14}{5}$

---

4 The number line used to graph rational numbers in a manner similar to that used with integers. The rational numbers $\frac{3}{4}$ and $^{-}4\frac{2}{3}$ and their opposites are graphed on the following number line:

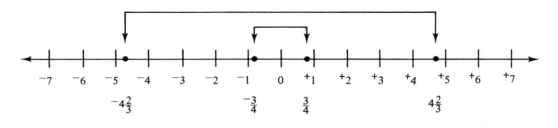

Q6 Graph the rational numbers and their opposites:

a. $^{-}2\frac{1}{2}$

b. $1\frac{2}{3}$

c. $^{-}4$

d. 0

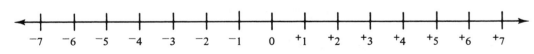

• # # # • # # # • # # # • # # # • # # # • # # # • # # # • # #

A6

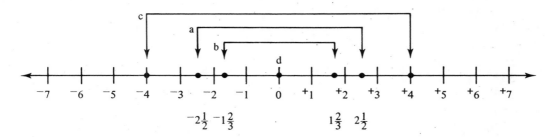

$$-2\tfrac{1}{2} \quad -1\tfrac{2}{3} \qquad\qquad\qquad 1\tfrac{2}{3} \quad 2\tfrac{1}{2}$$

Note that zero is its own opposite.

---

5   It is also possible to describe a *rational number* in terms of its decimal representation: *A rational number is any number whose decimal representation is either a terminating or a repeating decimal.*

Examples:

$\dfrac{1}{2} = 0.5$ terminating   (Note: Bar indicates that digit(s) under bar repeat endlessly.)

$\dfrac{1}{3} = 0.\overline{3}\ (0.3333\cdots)$ repeating

$\dfrac{^-5}{8} = {}^-0.625$ terminating

$\dfrac{2}{7} = 0.\overline{285714}\ (0.285714285714\cdots)$ repeating

$^-4 = {}^-4.0$ terminating

The decimal representation of a rational number in $\dfrac{p}{q}$ form is found by dividing the numerator (p) by the denominator (q) and then applying the sign, if the rational number is negative.

Example 1: Find the decimal representation of $\dfrac{^-3}{4}$.

Solution:

```
    0.75
4)3.00
    2 8
    ‾‾‾‾
      20
      20
      ‾‾
       0
```

Thus, $\dfrac{^-3}{4} = {}^-0.75$. The decimal is *terminating* since its division comes out evenly (0 remainder).

Example 2: Find the decimal representation of $2\dfrac{5}{33}$.

Solution:

$$2\dfrac{5}{33} = \dfrac{71}{33}$$

$$\begin{array}{r} 2.1515\cdots \text{ (repeating 15s)} \\ 33\overline{)71.0000} \\ 66 \\ \hline 50 \\ 33 \\ \hline 170 \\ 165 \\ \hline 50 \\ 33 \\ \hline 170 \\ 165 \\ \hline 5 \quad \text{etc.} \end{array}$$

Thus, $2\frac{5}{33} = 2.\overline{15}$. The decimal is infinite because its division does not come out evenly; it is *repeating* because it repeats itself in blocks of the digits 15. That is, $2.\overline{15} = 2.151515\cdots$ (repeating 15s).

Q7   Find the decimal representation and state whether each is terminating or repeating:

a. $\dfrac{^-2}{3} =$ _____ _____   **b.** $2\dfrac{1}{5} =$ _____ _____

c. $5 =$ _____ _____   **d.** $\dfrac{^-7}{9} =$ _____ _____

e. $^-3\dfrac{1}{7} =$ _____ _____   **f.** $\dfrac{5}{8} =$ _____ _____

g. $\dfrac{^-7}{11} =$ _____ _____

\# \# \#   •   \# \# \#   •   \# \# \#   •   \# \# \#   •   \# \# \#   •   \# \# \#   •   \# \# \#   •   \# \# \#   •   \# \# \#

A7   **a.** $^-0.\overline{6}$, repeating   **b.** 2.2, terminating
      c. 5.0, terminating   **d.** $^-0.\overline{7}$, repeating
      e. $^-3.\overline{142857}$, repeating   **f.** 0.625, terminating
      g. $^-0.\overline{63}$, repeating

6   Since the fractions are the same collection as the nonnegative rationals, the procedure used in the addition of rational numbers is much the same as that used for the addition of fractions.
       To add two rational numbers:

Step 1: If the denominators are different, find the least common denominator (LCD).

Step 2: Write the sum of the numerators over the common denominator.

Step 3: Apply the rules for the addition of integers to the numerator.

Step 4: If possible, reduce the rational number to lowest terms.

Examples:

1. $\dfrac{3}{32} + \dfrac{^-11}{32} = \dfrac{3 + ^-11}{32}$ Step 2   (step 1 is not necessary)

   $= \dfrac{^-8}{32}$ Step 3

   $= \dfrac{^-1}{4}$ Step 4

2. $\dfrac{^-5}{8}+\dfrac{3}{7}=\dfrac{^-35}{56}+\dfrac{24}{56}$ Step 1 $\left(\text{because } \dfrac{^-5\times7}{8\times7}=\dfrac{^-35}{56} \text{ and } \dfrac{3\times8}{7\times8}=\dfrac{24}{56}\right)$

$=\dfrac{^-35+24}{56}$ Step 2

$=\dfrac{^-11}{56}$ Step 3

Q8   Find the sum:

   a. $\dfrac{^-7}{8}+\dfrac{3}{8}$ b. $\dfrac{^-1}{6}+\dfrac{4}{5}$

\# \# \#   •   \# \# \#   •   \# \# \#   •   \# \# \#   •   \# \# \#   •   \# \# \#   •   \# \# \#   •   \# \# \#   •   \# \# \#

A8   a. $\dfrac{^-1}{2}$: $\dfrac{^-7}{8}+\dfrac{3}{8}=\dfrac{^-7+3}{8}$ b. $\dfrac{19}{30}$: $\dfrac{^-1}{6}+\dfrac{4}{5}$

$=\dfrac{^-4}{8}$ $\dfrac{^-5}{30}+\dfrac{24}{30}$

$=\dfrac{^-1}{2}$ $\dfrac{19}{30}$

Q9   Find the sum:

   a. $\dfrac{^-2}{3}+\dfrac{^-5}{9}$ b. $\dfrac{5}{6}+\dfrac{^-7}{6}$

   c. $\dfrac{^-2}{15}+\dfrac{19}{15}$ d. $\dfrac{7}{12}+\dfrac{4}{7}$

   e. $\dfrac{5}{14}+\dfrac{^-3}{4}$ f. $\dfrac{^-7}{16}+\dfrac{^-1}{4}$

   g. $\dfrac{7}{9}+\dfrac{^-4}{12}$ h. $\dfrac{^-1}{8}+\dfrac{^-4}{15}$

\# \#   •   \# \# \#   •   \# \# \#   •   \# \# \#   •   \# \# \#   •   \# \# \#   •   \# \# \#   •   \# \# \#   •   \# \# \#

A9   **a.** $^-1\frac{2}{9}$ **b.** $\frac{^-1}{3}$ **c.** $1\frac{2}{15}$ **d.** $1\frac{13}{84}$

e. $\frac{^-11}{28}$ **f.** $\frac{^-11}{16}$ **g.** $\frac{4}{9}$ **h.** $\frac{^-47}{120}$

---

7   To find a sum of two or more rational numbers where integers or mixed numbers are involved, the following procedures will be used:

1. Write all integers in $\frac{p}{q}$ form using a denominator of 1.

2. Write all mixed numbers as improper fractions in $\frac{p}{q}$ form.

3. Follow the rules for adding two rational numbers as previously stated, working from left to right.

Example 1: Find the sum $^-1\frac{1}{5}+3\frac{2}{5}$.

Solution:

$$^-1\frac{1}{5}+3\frac{2}{5}=\frac{^-6}{5}+\frac{17}{5}$$
$$=\frac{^-6+17}{5}$$
$$=\frac{11}{5}$$
$$=2\frac{1}{5}$$

Example 2: Find the sum $2\frac{4}{7}+^-5$.

Solution:

$$2\frac{4}{7}+^-5=\frac{18}{7}+\frac{^-5}{1}$$
$$=\frac{18}{7}+\frac{^-35}{7}$$
$$=\frac{18+^-35}{7}$$
$$=\frac{^-17}{7}$$
$$=^-2\frac{3}{7}$$

Q10   Find the sum:

a. $^-2\frac{3}{5}+8$

b. $^-5\frac{2}{7}+\frac{3}{5}$

•   # # #   •   # # #   •   # # #   •   # # #   •   # # #   •   # # #   •   # # #   •   # #

A10   **a.** $5\frac{2}{5}$: $^-2\frac{3}{5}+8=\frac{^-13}{5}+\frac{8}{1}$

$$=\frac{^-13}{5}+\frac{40}{5}$$
$$=\frac{27}{5}$$
$$=5\frac{2}{5}$$

b. $^-4\frac{24}{35}$: $^-5\frac{2}{7}+\frac{3}{5}=\frac{^-37}{7}+\frac{3}{5}$

$$=\frac{^-185}{35}+\frac{21}{35}$$
$$=\frac{^-185+21}{35}$$
$$=\frac{^-164}{35}$$
$$=^-4\frac{24}{35}$$

Q11   Find the sum:

    a. $2\frac{7}{8} + {}^-6\frac{3}{8}$ **b.** ${}^-7\frac{2}{3} + 4$

    c. $6\frac{1}{5} + {}^-3\frac{4}{7}$ **d.** ${}^-1\frac{2}{3} + {}^-4\frac{5}{6}$

    e. $\frac{5}{9} + {}^-3\frac{1}{2}$ **f.** $\frac{{}^-5}{7} + {}^-3$

    g. ${}^-8 + \frac{3}{11}$ **h.** ${}^-4\frac{3}{8} + 5$

    i. $\frac{2}{3} + \frac{{}^-5}{8} + \frac{{}^-5}{6}$ **j.** ${}^-3\frac{1}{7} + {}^-2\frac{5}{8}$

\# \# \# • \# \# \# • \# \# \# • \# \# \# • \# \# \# • \# \# \# • \# \# \# • \# \# \# • \# \# \#

A11   **a.** ${}^-3\frac{1}{2}$ **b.** ${}^-3\frac{2}{3}$ **c.** $2\frac{22}{35}$ **d.** ${}^-6\frac{1}{2}$

       e. ${}^-2\frac{17}{18}$ **f.** ${}^-3\frac{5}{7}$ **g.** ${}^-7\frac{8}{11}$ **h.** $\frac{5}{8}$

       i. $\frac{{}^-19}{24}$ **j.** ${}^-5\frac{43}{56}$

Q12   Write the opposite for each rational number:

    a. $\frac{2}{3}$ ____   **b.** $\frac{{}^-5}{8}$ ____   **c.** 7 ____

    d. ${}^-4$ ____   **e.** $1\frac{2}{3}$ ____   **f.** ${}^-5\frac{4}{7}$ ____

\# \# \# • \# \# \# • \# \# \# • \# \# \# • \# \# \# • \# \# \# • \# \# \# • \# \# \# • \# \# \#

A12   **a.** $\dfrac{^-2}{3}$ **b.** $\dfrac{5}{8}$ **c.** $^-7$ **d.** 4

e. $^-1\dfrac{2}{3}$ **f.** $5\dfrac{4}{7}$

---

8   The definition of subtraction for integers is also true for the set of rational numbers. That is, $x - y = x + {}^-y$ *for all rational-number replacements of x and y.*

To subtract any two rational numbers:

Step 1: Use the definition of subtraction to rewrite the difference as a sum.

Step 2: Apply the procedures previously developed to find the sum.

Example 1: Find the difference $\dfrac{4}{5} - \dfrac{7}{12}$.

Solution:

$$\dfrac{4}{5} - \dfrac{7}{12} = \dfrac{4}{5} + \dfrac{^-7}{12}$$
$$= \dfrac{48}{60} + \dfrac{^-35}{60}$$
$$= \dfrac{13}{60}$$

Example 2: Find the difference $\dfrac{^-4}{7} - \dfrac{^-5}{6}$.

Solution:

$$\dfrac{^-4}{7} - \dfrac{^-5}{6} = \dfrac{^-4}{7} + \dfrac{5}{6}$$
$$= \dfrac{^-24}{42} + \dfrac{35}{42}$$
$$= \dfrac{11}{42}$$

Example 3: Find the difference $^-7\dfrac{1}{3} - {}^-2$.

Solution:

$$^-7\dfrac{1}{3} - {}^-2 = {}^-7\dfrac{1}{3} + 2$$
$$= \dfrac{^-22}{3} + \dfrac{2}{1}$$
$$= \dfrac{^-22}{3} + \dfrac{6}{3}$$
$$= \dfrac{^-16}{3}$$
$$= {}^-5\dfrac{1}{3}$$

Q13   Rewrite each difference as a sum (do not evaluate):

a. $\dfrac{1}{3} - \dfrac{4}{9} =$ _____   **b.** $\dfrac{^-3}{5} - \dfrac{^-2}{3} =$ _____

    c. $^-4\frac{2}{3}-1\frac{2}{5}=$ _____   **d.** $3-{}^-1\frac{3}{10}=$ _____

\# \# \# • \# \# \# • \# \# \# • \# \# \# • \# \# \# • \# \# \# • \# \# \# • \# \# \# • \# \# \#

A13   **a.** $\frac{1}{3}+\frac{^-4}{9}$ **b.** $\frac{^-3}{5}+\frac{2}{3}$ **c.** $^-4\frac{2}{3}+{}^-1\frac{2}{5}$ **d.** $3+1\frac{3}{10}$

Q14   Find the difference:

    a. $\frac{1}{3}-\frac{4}{9}$ **b.** $\frac{^-3}{5}-\frac{^-2}{3}$

    c. $^-4\frac{2}{3}-1\frac{2}{7}$ **d.** $3-{}^-1\frac{3}{10}$

\# \# \# • \# \# \# • \# \# \# • \# \# \# • \# \# \# • \# \# \# • \# \# \# • \# \# \# • \# \# \#

A14   **a.** $\frac{^-1}{9}$: $\frac{1}{3}-\frac{4}{9}=\frac{1}{3}+\frac{^-4}{9}$ **b.** $\frac{1}{15}$: $\frac{^-3}{5}-\frac{^-2}{3}=\frac{^-3}{5}+\frac{2}{3}$

$$=\frac{3}{9}+\frac{^-4}{9} \qquad\qquad\qquad =\frac{^-9}{15}+\frac{10}{15}$$

$$=\frac{^-1}{9} \qquad\qquad\qquad\qquad =\frac{1}{15}$$

    c. $^-5\frac{20}{21}$: $^-4\frac{2}{3}-1\frac{2}{7}={}^-4\frac{2}{3}+{}^-1\frac{2}{7}$ **d.** $4\frac{3}{10}$: $3-{}^-1\frac{3}{10}=3+1\frac{3}{10}$

$$=\frac{^-14}{3}+\frac{^-9}{7} \qquad\qquad\qquad =\frac{3}{1}+\frac{13}{10}$$

$$=\frac{^-98}{21}+\frac{^-27}{21} \qquad\qquad\qquad =\frac{30}{10}+\frac{13}{10}$$

$$=\frac{^-125}{21} \qquad\qquad\qquad\qquad =\frac{43}{10}$$

$$={}^-5\frac{20}{21} \qquad\qquad\qquad\qquad =4\frac{3}{10}$$

Q15   Find the difference:

    a. $\frac{^-5}{24}-\frac{7}{24}$ **b.** $2\frac{3}{16}-1\frac{5}{16}$ **c.** $\frac{^-7}{21}-\frac{^-5}{7}$ **d.** $^-2\frac{1}{9}-3\frac{2}{5}$

e. $5\frac{3}{8}-7\frac{4}{9}$ **f.** $\frac{^-3}{16}-4$ **g.** $18-\frac{5}{17}$ **h.** $\frac{^-6}{13}-4\frac{1}{2}$

i. $16\frac{3}{10}-5\frac{7}{8}$ **j.** $^-15\frac{1}{6}-{}^-2\frac{7}{15}$

\# \# \#   •   \# \# \#   •   \# \# \#   •   \# \# \#   •   \# \# \#   •   \# \# \#   •   \# \# \#   •   \# \# \#   •   \# \# \#

A15   **a.** $\frac{^-1}{2}$ **b.** $\frac{7}{8}$ **c.** $\frac{8}{21}$ **d.** $^-5\frac{23}{45}$

   e. $^-2\frac{5}{72}$ **f.** $^-4\frac{3}{16}$ **g.** $17\frac{12}{17}$ **h.** $^-4\frac{25}{26}$

   i. $10\frac{17}{40}$ **j.** $^-12\frac{7}{10}$

---

9   Let $\frac{a}{b}$ and $\frac{c}{d}$ stand for any two rational numbers. The product of $\frac{a}{b}$ and $\frac{c}{d}$ is defined as:

$$\frac{a}{b}\cdot\frac{c}{d}=\frac{ac}{bd},\qquad bd\neq 0$$

where ac is the product of the numerators and bd is the product of the denominators.

Example 1: Find the product $\frac{^-3}{7}\cdot\frac{^-5}{4}$.

Solution:

$$\frac{^-3}{7}\cdot\frac{^-5}{4}=\frac{^-3\cdot{}^-5}{7\cdot4}=\frac{15}{28}$$

As with fractions, a common procedure when multiplying rational numbers is to divide any numerator and any denominator by a common factor. This procedure is called *reducing* (sometimes referred to as "canceling").

Example 2: Find the product $\frac{^-3}{5}\cdot\frac{5}{12}$.

Solution:

$$\frac{^-\overset{-1}{3}}{\underset{1}{5}}\cdot\frac{\overset{1}{5}}{\underset{4}{12}}=\frac{^-1}{4}$$

Example 3: Find the product $\frac{^-9}{12}\cdot\frac{^-5}{7}$.

Solution:

$$\frac{\overset{-3}{\cancel{9}}}{\underset{4}{\cancel{12}}} \cdot \frac{-5}{7} = \frac{15}{28}$$

As is the case with the sum and difference of two rational numbers, the product of two rational numbers is always reduced to lowest terms.

Q16   Find the product:

    a. $\dfrac{-6}{5} \cdot \dfrac{-2}{3}$
                                  b. $\dfrac{15}{16} \cdot \dfrac{-4}{25}$

\# \# \# • \# \# \# • \# \# \# • \# \# \# • \# \# \# • \# \# \# • \# \# \# • \# \# \# • \# \# \#

A16   **a.** $\dfrac{4}{5}$: $\dfrac{-6}{5} \cdot \dfrac{\overset{-2}{\cancel{-2}}}{\underset{1}{\cancel{3}}} = \dfrac{4}{5}$
                           b. $\dfrac{-3}{20}$: $\dfrac{\overset{3}{\cancel{15}}}{\underset{4}{\cancel{16}}} \cdot \dfrac{\overset{-1}{\cancel{-4}}}{\underset{5}{\cancel{25}}} = \dfrac{-3}{20}$

---

10 $\dfrac{-2}{3}$ and $\dfrac{2}{-3}$ are equivalent forms for the same rational number. Both represent a negative rational number since they involve a quotient of integers with unlike signs. When writing a negative rational number, it is customary to place the negative sign on the number in the numerator. For example, $\dfrac{5}{-8}$ is usually written $\dfrac{-5}{8}$.

Q17   Find the product:

    a. $\dfrac{-12}{15} \cdot \dfrac{3}{6}$
                                  b. $\dfrac{-4}{6} \cdot \dfrac{-13}{18}$

    c. $\dfrac{7}{12} \cdot \dfrac{9}{-11}$
                                  d. $\dfrac{-5}{7} \cdot \dfrac{6}{-13}$

    e. $\dfrac{5}{-28} \cdot \dfrac{-16}{17}$
                                  f. $\dfrac{4}{-7} \cdot \dfrac{7}{4}$

\# \# \# • \# \# \# • \# \# \# • \# \# \# • \# \# \# • \# \# \# • \# \# \# • \# \# \# • \# \# \#

A17   **a.** $\dfrac{-2}{5}$ **b.** $\dfrac{13}{27}$ **c.** $\dfrac{-21}{44}$ **d.** $\dfrac{30}{91}$ **e.** $\dfrac{20}{119}$ **f.** $^-1$

---

11   When finding a product of two or more rational numbers where integers or mixed numbers are involved:

    1. Write all integers in $\dfrac{p}{q}$ form with a denominator of 1.

2. Write all mixed numbers as improper fractions in $\frac{p}{q}$ form.

3. Use the rule of Frame 9 to find the product.

Example 1: Find the product $5\frac{2}{9} \cdot {}^-3$.

Solution:

$$5\frac{2}{9} \cdot {}^-3 = \frac{47}{\overset{}{\underset{3}{9}}} \cdot \frac{{}^-\overset{-1}{\cancel{3}}}{1} = \frac{{}^-47}{3} = {}^-15\frac{2}{3}$$

Example 2: Find the product ${}^-5\frac{1}{3} \cdot {}^-3\frac{9}{16}$.

Solution:

$$ {}^-5\frac{1}{3} \cdot {}^-3\frac{9}{16} = \frac{{}^-\overset{-1}{\cancel{16}}}{\underset{1}{\cancel{3}}} \cdot \frac{{}^-\overset{-19}{\cancel{57}}}{\underset{1}{\cancel{16}}} = 19 $$

Q18   Find the product:

a. $\dfrac{{}^-3}{11} \cdot 3$

b. $\dfrac{4}{{}^-5} \cdot \dfrac{{}^-10}{12}$

c. ${}^-5\frac{2}{9} \cdot {}^-12$

d. $2\frac{1}{3} \cdot {}^-1\frac{3}{4}$

e. ${}^-4 \cdot \dfrac{{}^-1}{4}$

f. $3\frac{1}{5} \cdot {}^-1\frac{1}{2}$

\# \# \# • \# \# \# • \# \# \# • \# \# \# • \# \# \# • \# \# \# • \# \# \# • \# \# \# • \# \# \# • \# \# \#

A18   **a.** $\dfrac{{}^-9}{11}$ **b.** $\dfrac{2}{3}$ **c.** $62\frac{2}{3}$ **d.** ${}^-4\frac{1}{12}$ **e.** 1   **f.** ${}^-4\frac{4}{5}$

---

12   Two rational numbers whose product is 1 are called *reciprocals*. Thus, 5 and $\frac{1}{5}$ are reciprocals,

because $5 \cdot \frac{1}{5} = \frac{\overset{1}{\cancel{5}}}{1} \cdot \frac{1}{\underset{1}{\cancel{5}}} = \frac{1}{1} = 1$. Similarly, $\frac{{}^-5}{8}$ and $\frac{8}{{}^-5}$ are reciprocals, because $\frac{{}^-\overset{1}{\cancel{5}}}{\underset{1}{\cancel{8}}} \cdot \frac{\overset{1}{\cancel{8}}}{\underset{1}{{}^-\cancel{5}}} = \frac{1}{1} = 1$

In general, to find the reciprocal of any nonzero rational number, write the number in $\frac{p}{q}$ form and

interchange the numerator and denominator to form $\frac{q}{p}$.

Example 1: Write the reciprocal for ${}^-2\frac{1}{3}$.

Solution:

$$-2\frac{1}{3} = \frac{-7}{3}; \quad \text{thus, the reciprocal of } -2\frac{1}{3} \text{ is } \frac{3}{-7}, \text{ which is written } \frac{-3}{7}$$

Example 2: Write the reciprocal for 3.

Solution:

$$3 = \frac{3}{1}: \quad \text{thus, the reciprocal of 3 is } \frac{1}{3}$$

Zero has no reciprocal, because $0 = \frac{0}{1}$ and $\frac{1}{0}$ is undefined.

Q19   Write the reciprocal:

a. $\frac{2}{3}$ _____   **b.** $-1\frac{5}{9}$ _____   **c.** 12 _____   **d.** $\frac{1}{13}$ _____

e. $7\frac{3}{8}$ _____   **f.** -2 _____

• # # # • # # # • # # # • # # # • # # # • # # # • # # # • # #

A19   **a.** $\frac{3}{2}$ **b.** $\frac{-9}{14}$ **c.** $\frac{1}{12}$ **d.** 13   **e.** $\frac{8}{59}$ **f.** $\frac{-1}{2}$

13   Let $\frac{a}{b}$ and $\frac{c}{d}$ stand for any two rational numbers with $\frac{c}{d} \neq 0$. Consider the simplification of the following quotient:

$$\frac{a}{b} \div \frac{c}{d} = \frac{\dfrac{a}{b}}{\dfrac{c}{d}} = \frac{\dfrac{a}{b} \cdot \dfrac{d}{c}}{\dfrac{c}{d} \cdot \dfrac{d}{c}} = \frac{\dfrac{a}{b} \cdot \dfrac{d}{c}}{1} = \frac{a}{b} \cdot \frac{d}{c}$$

Thus, the *definition of division for two rational numbers* (with a nonzero divisor) is stated:

$$\frac{a}{b} \div \frac{c}{d} = \frac{a}{b} \cdot \frac{d}{c} = \frac{ad}{bc}, \qquad \frac{c}{d} \neq 0$$

In words, the quotient of two rational numbers with a nonzero divisor is equal to the product of the first (dividend) times the reciprocal of the second (divisor).

Example 1: Find the quotient $\frac{2}{3} \div \frac{4}{9}$.

Solution:

$$\frac{2}{3} \div \frac{4}{9} = \frac{\overset{1}{2}}{\underset{1}{3}} \cdot \frac{\overset{3}{9}}{\underset{2}{4}} \qquad \left(\text{the reciprocal of } \frac{4}{9} \text{ is } \frac{9}{4}\right)$$

$$= \frac{3}{2}$$

$$= 1\frac{1}{2}$$

Example 2: Find the quotient $\dfrac{4}{5} \div \dfrac{^-6}{7}$.

Solution:

$$\frac{4}{5} \div \frac{^-6}{7} = \frac{\overset{2}{\cancel{4}}}{5} \cdot \frac{^-7}{\cancel{6}} \qquad \left(\text{the reciprocal of } \frac{^-6}{7} \text{ is } \frac{^-7}{6}\right)$$

$$= \frac{^-14}{15}^{\;3}$$

Q20 Find the quotient:

a. $\dfrac{4}{5} \div \dfrac{2}{3}$ b. $\dfrac{5}{6} \div \dfrac{^-15}{16}$

\# \# \# • \# \# \# • \# \# \# • \# \# \# • \# \# \# • \# \# \# • \# \# \# • \# \# \# • \# \# \#

A20   a. $1\dfrac{1}{5}$: $\dfrac{4}{5} \div \dfrac{2}{3} = \dfrac{\overset{2}{\cancel{4}}}{5} \cdot \dfrac{3}{\underset{1}{\cancel{2}}} = \dfrac{6}{5}$ b. $\dfrac{^-8}{9}$: $\dfrac{5}{6} \div \dfrac{^-15}{16} = \dfrac{\overset{1}{\cancel{5}}}{\underset{3}{\cancel{6}}} \cdot \dfrac{^-\overset{^-8}{\cancel{16}}}{\underset{3}{\cancel{15}}} = \dfrac{^-8}{9}$

---

14   When finding a quotient of two rational numbers where integers or mixed numbers are involved:

1. Write all integers in $\dfrac{p}{q}$ form with a denominator of 1.

2. Write all mixed numbers as improper fractions in $\dfrac{p}{q}$ form.

3. Use the rule of the previous frame to find the quotient.

Example 1: Find the quotient $\dfrac{^-5}{14} \div 3\dfrac{2}{7}$.

Solution:

$$\frac{^-5}{14} \div 3\frac{2}{7} = \frac{^-5}{14} \div \frac{23}{7} = \frac{^-5}{\underset{2}{\cancel{14}}} \cdot \frac{\overset{1}{\cancel{7}}}{23} = \frac{^-5}{46}$$

Example 2: Find the quotient $^-2\dfrac{5}{8} \div 12$.

Solution:

$$^-2\frac{5}{8} \div 12 = \frac{^-21}{8} \div \frac{12}{1} = \frac{^-\overset{^-7}{\cancel{21}}}{8} \cdot \frac{1}{\underset{4}{\cancel{12}}} = \frac{^-7}{32}$$

Q21 Find the quotient:

a. $\dfrac{^-11}{15} \div {^-4}\dfrac{2}{5}$ b. $^-8 \div 2\dfrac{2}{3}$

\# \# \# • \# \# \# • \# \# \# • \# \# \# • \# \# \# • \# \# \# • \# \# \# • \# \# \# • \# \# \#

A21 a. $\frac{1}{6}$: $\frac{^-11}{15} \div ^-4\frac{2}{5} = \frac{^-11}{15} \div \frac{^-22}{5} = \frac{^-\overset{1}{\cancel{11}}}{\underset{3}{\cancel{15}}} \cdot \frac{\overset{1}{\cancel{5}}}{\underset{2}{\cancel{22}}} = \frac{1}{6}$ b. $^-3$: $^-8 \div 2\frac{2}{3} = \frac{^-8}{1} \div \frac{8}{3} = \frac{^-\overset{1}{\cancel{8}}}{1} \cdot \frac{3}{\underset{1}{\cancel{8}}} = ^-3$

Q22 Find the quotient:

a. $\frac{^-29}{50} \div 3\frac{1}{10}$ b. $^-4\frac{1}{5} \div ^-3\frac{1}{3}$

c. $^-4\frac{1}{5} \div 3$ d. $\frac{1}{2} \div ^-2$

e. $4 \div 4\frac{5}{8}$ f. $^-8 \div \frac{^-1}{8}$

g. $0 \div 3\frac{4}{7}$ h. $^-15 \div ^-2\frac{5}{8}$

• # # # • # # # • # # # • # # # • # # # • # # # • # # # • # #

A22 a. $\frac{^-29}{155}$ b. $1\frac{13}{50}$ c. $^-1\frac{2}{5}$ d. $\frac{^-1}{4}$

e. $\frac{32}{37}$ f. 64 g. 0 h. $5\frac{5}{7}$

---

15 Certain properties of integers have been established in previous sections. The integers are commutative and associative with respect to the operations of addition and multiplication. The distributive properties hold for multiplication over addition and subtraction. These properties are also true for the rational numbers. In addition, the following statements are true for any rational number *a*.

1. Addition property of zero:

$a + 0 = 0 + a = a$

2. Multiplication property of zero:

$a \cdot 0 = 0a = 0$

3. Multiplication property of one:

$a \cdot 1 = 1a = a$

Q23   The associative property of addition states that $(a+b)+c = a+(b+c)$. Verify that $(a+b)+c$ and $a+(b+c)$ are equivalent when $a = \dfrac{3}{5}$, $b = \dfrac{7}{10}$, and $c = \dfrac{9}{20}$.

\# \# \#   •   \# \# \#   •   \# \# \#   •   \# \# \#   •   \# \# \#   •   \# \# \#   •   \# \# \#   •   \# \# \#   •   \# \# \#

A23 $(a+b)+c = \left(\dfrac{3}{5}+\dfrac{7}{10}\right)+\dfrac{9}{20}$ $a+(b+c) = \dfrac{3}{5}+\left(\dfrac{7}{10}+\dfrac{9}{20}\right)$

$\qquad\qquad = \left(\dfrac{6}{10}+\dfrac{7}{10}\right)+\dfrac{9}{20}$ $\qquad\quad = \dfrac{3}{5}+\left(\dfrac{14}{20}+\dfrac{9}{20}\right)$

$\qquad\qquad = \dfrac{13}{10}+\dfrac{9}{20}$ $\qquad\qquad = \dfrac{3}{5}+\dfrac{23}{20}$

$\qquad\qquad = \dfrac{26}{20}+\dfrac{9}{20}$ $\qquad\qquad = \dfrac{12}{20}+\dfrac{23}{20}$

$\qquad\qquad = \dfrac{35}{20}$ $\qquad\qquad = \dfrac{35}{20}$

$\qquad\qquad = 1\dfrac{3}{4}$ $\qquad\qquad = 1\dfrac{3}{4}$

Q24   The left distributive property of multiplication over subtraction states that $a(b-c) = ab - ac$. Verify that $a(b-c)$ and $ab - ac$ are equivalent when $a = \dfrac{2}{3}$, $b = \dfrac{4}{5}$, and $c = \dfrac{3}{7}$.

\# \# \#   •   \# \# \#   •   \# \# \#   •   \# \# \#   •   \# \# \#   •   \# \# \#   •   \# \# \#   •   \# \# \#   •   \# \# \#

A24 $a(b-c) = \dfrac{2}{3}\left(\dfrac{4}{5}-\dfrac{3}{7}\right)$ $ab - ac = \dfrac{2}{3}\cdot\dfrac{4}{5}-\dfrac{2}{3}\cdot\dfrac{3}{7}$

$\qquad\qquad = \dfrac{2}{3}\left(\dfrac{28}{35}-\dfrac{15}{35}\right)$ $\qquad\qquad = \dfrac{8}{15}-\dfrac{2}{7}$

$\qquad\qquad = \dfrac{2}{3}\left(\dfrac{13}{35}\right)$ $\qquad\qquad = \dfrac{56}{105}-\dfrac{30}{105}$

$\qquad\qquad = \dfrac{26}{105}$ $\qquad\qquad = \dfrac{26}{105}$

This completes the instruction for this section.

6.6   EXERCISE

1. Find the sum:

a. $\dfrac{2}{3} + \dfrac{^-5}{3}$

b. $\dfrac{^-4}{5} + \dfrac{3}{8}$

c. $\dfrac{^-1}{6} + \dfrac{^-4}{18}$

d. $\dfrac{^-6}{7} + 0$

e. $^-3\dfrac{3}{4} + 1\dfrac{1}{4}$

f. $15 + ^-2\dfrac{4}{11}$

g. $3\dfrac{2}{5} + \dfrac{^-17}{5}$

h. $^-1\dfrac{2}{3} + ^-7\dfrac{3}{5}$

i. $\dfrac{3}{10} + \dfrac{^-7}{6} + \dfrac{5}{12}$

j. $\dfrac{^-5}{24} + \dfrac{7}{8} + \dfrac{^-7}{12}$

2. Find the difference:

a. $\dfrac{2}{3} - \dfrac{5}{3}$

b. $\dfrac{3}{7} - \dfrac{7}{9}$

c. $4 - 2\dfrac{4}{7}$

d. $2\dfrac{1}{3} - 5\dfrac{1}{4}$

e. $^-3 - 2\dfrac{3}{7}$

f. $3\dfrac{2}{5} - 4\dfrac{1}{7}$

g. $\dfrac{^-5}{8} - \dfrac{^-1}{8}$

h. $^-6\dfrac{1}{5} - ^-1\dfrac{3}{7}$

i. $^-2\dfrac{1}{3} - ^-2\dfrac{1}{3}$

j. $12\dfrac{4}{9} - 3$

3. Find the product:

a. $\dfrac{^-4}{15} \cdot \dfrac{9}{16}$

b. $\dfrac{^-4}{5} \cdot \dfrac{^-2}{7}$

c. $\dfrac{^-3}{4} \cdot 1\dfrac{1}{3}$

d. $0 \cdot 5\dfrac{7}{17}$

e. $\dfrac{^-6}{17} \cdot \dfrac{^-17}{6}$

f. $^-1\dfrac{2}{5} \cdot \dfrac{^-5}{7}$

g. $5\dfrac{1}{4} \cdot 11\dfrac{1}{3}$

h. $\dfrac{1}{4} \cdot \dfrac{^-2}{3} \cdot \dfrac{6}{7}$

i. $^-2\dfrac{1}{3} \cdot \dfrac{6}{7} \cdot \dfrac{^-1}{2}$

j. $^-4\dfrac{2}{3} \cdot \dfrac{2}{5} \cdot \dfrac{^-3}{14}$

4. Find the quotient:

a. $\dfrac{^-4}{15} \div \dfrac{3}{2}$

b. $\dfrac{^-7}{8} \div \dfrac{^-3}{4}$

c. $^-2\dfrac{1}{2} \div 5$

d. $^-2 \div \dfrac{^-6}{11}$

e. $^-3\dfrac{2}{3} \div ^-3\dfrac{1}{3}$

f. $\dfrac{2}{3} \div \dfrac{5}{2}$

g. $\dfrac{3}{17} \div ^-1$

h. $0 \div 3$

i. $3 \div 0$

j. $\dfrac{^-5}{11} \div \dfrac{0}{1}$

5. Perform the indicated operation:

a. $1\dfrac{3}{7} + ^-2\dfrac{4}{7}$

b. $\dfrac{^-5}{8} - \dfrac{4}{5}$

c. $\dfrac{8}{45} \cdot \dfrac{^-5}{16}$

d. $^-3\dfrac{1}{3} \div \dfrac{^-9}{10}$

e. $1\dfrac{2}{11} + 3\dfrac{15}{11}$

f. $\dfrac{^-8}{15} \cdot 0 \cdot 8\dfrac{1}{4}$

g. $^-5 \div \dfrac{^-7}{5}$

h. $4\dfrac{2}{3} \div ^-8$

i. $2\dfrac{1}{3} + ^-4 + 1\dfrac{2}{5}$

j. $\left(\dfrac{3}{5} \div \dfrac{^-2}{7}\right) \div \dfrac{^-3}{5}$

6.6   EXERCISE ANSWERS

1. a. $^-1$
   b. $\dfrac{^-17}{40}$
   c. $\dfrac{^-7}{18}$
   d. $\dfrac{^-6}{7}$

   e. $^-2\dfrac{1}{2}$
   f. $12\dfrac{7}{11}$
   g. 0
   h. $^-9\dfrac{4}{15}$

   i. $\dfrac{^-9}{20}$
   j. $\dfrac{1}{12}$

2. a. $^-1$
   b. $\dfrac{^-22}{63}$
   c. $1\dfrac{3}{7}$
   d. $^-2\dfrac{11}{12}$

   e. $^-5\dfrac{3}{7}$
   f. $\dfrac{^-26}{35}$
   g. $\dfrac{^-1}{2}$
   h. $^-4\dfrac{27}{35}$

   i. 0
   j. $9\dfrac{4}{9}$

3. a. $\dfrac{^-3}{20}$
   b. $\dfrac{8}{35}$
   c. $^-1$
   d. 0

   e. 1
   f. 1
   g. $59\dfrac{1}{2}$
   h. $\dfrac{^-1}{7}$

   i. 1
   j. $\dfrac{2}{5}$

4. a. $\dfrac{^-8}{45}$
   b. $1\dfrac{1}{6}$
   c. $\dfrac{^-1}{2}$
   d. $3\dfrac{2}{3}$

   e. $1\dfrac{1}{10}$
   f. $\dfrac{4}{15}$
   g. $\dfrac{^-3}{17}$
   h. 0

   i. undefined
   j. undefined

5. a. $^-1\dfrac{1}{7}$
   b. $^-1\dfrac{17}{40}$
   c. $\dfrac{^-1}{18}$
   d. $3\dfrac{19}{27}$

   e. $5\dfrac{6}{11}$
   f. 0
   g. $3\dfrac{4}{7}$
   h. $\dfrac{^-7}{12}$

   i. $\dfrac{^-4}{15}$
   j. $3\dfrac{1}{2}$

CHAPTER 6 SAMPLE TEST

At the completion of Chapter 6 you should be able to work the following problems.

6.1   INTRODUCTION

1. The collection of numbers . . . $^-2, ^-1, 0, 1, 2, \ldots$ is called the _____.
2. Each integer is thought of as having what two parts?
3. Graph each of the following integers on the number line:
   a. 2   **b.** $^-7$ **c.** 5   **d.** 0

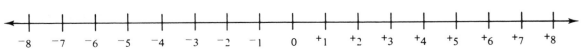

4. Write the opposite of each of the following integers:
   a. $^-5$ **b.** 3   **c.** 0   **d.** 7

6.2   ADDITION OF INTEGERS

5. Find the sum:
- **a.** $^-3 + ^-6$
- **b.** $^-5 + 8$
- **c.** $3 + ^-11$
- **d.** $0 + ^-2$
- **e.** $5 + ^-5$
- **f.** $^-2 + 7 + ^-5$
- **g.** $^-3 + ^-5 + 6$
- **h.** $9 + ^-3 + 6$

6.3   SUBTRACTION OF INTEGERS

6. Find the difference:
- **a.** $^-2 - 5$
- **b.** $3 - 7$
- **c.** $6 - ^-3$
- **d.** $^-1 - ^-2$
- **e.** $11 - 9$
- **f.** $5 - 7 - ^-3$

7. Complete each of the following:
- **a.** $^-5 + 7$
- **b.** $^-5 - 7$
- **c.** $0 - 5$
- **d.** $^-3 + 0$
- **e.** $^-4 + ^-9$
- **f.** $6 - ^-9$
- **g.** $^-4 + 7 - 6$
- **h.** $2 - 1 - ^-1$

6.4   MULTIPLICATION OF INTEGERS

8. Find the product:
- **a.** $^-2 \cdot 5$
- **b.** $^-4 \cdot ^-6$
- **c.** $^-3 \cdot 0$
- **d.** $5 \cdot ^-9$
- **e.** $^-1 \cdot 13$
- **f.** $0 \cdot ^-1$
- **g.** $^-2 \cdot 4 \cdot ^-5$
- **h.** $(6 \cdot ^-2)(^-3 \cdot ^-2)$
- **i.** $^-3(4 + ^-7)$
- **j.** $2(^-4 + 4)$

6.5   DIVISION OF INTEGERS

9. Find the quotient:
- **a.** $^-36 \div 9$
- **b.** $^-18 \div ^-6$
- **c.** $\dfrac{^-12}{4}$
- **d.** $\dfrac{^-25}{^-5}$
- **e.** $10 \div 0$
- **f.** $\dfrac{0}{^-6}$
- **g.** $0 \div ^-2$
- **h.** $\dfrac{4}{0}$

6.6   OPERATIONS WITH RATIONAL NUMBERS

10. Find the sum:
- **a.** $\dfrac{^-4}{7} + \dfrac{7}{12}$
- **b.** $\dfrac{^-2}{3} + \dfrac{^-5}{8}$
- **c.** $^-3\dfrac{1}{3} + 2\dfrac{7}{9}$
- **d.** $\dfrac{^-3}{16} + 3$

11. Find the difference:
- **a.** $\dfrac{5}{16} - \dfrac{3}{16}$
- **b.** $1\dfrac{4}{5} - \dfrac{^-2}{3}$
- **c.** $4\dfrac{1}{3} - 5\dfrac{2}{5}$
- **d.** $\dfrac{^-7}{9} - 2$

12. Find the product:
- **a.** $\dfrac{^-4}{15} \cdot \dfrac{^-5}{16}$
- **b.** $3 \cdot ^-4\dfrac{2}{3}$
- **c.** $^-2\dfrac{1}{3} \cdot 0$
- **d.** $^-5\dfrac{1}{3} \cdot ^-1\dfrac{2}{5}$

13. Find the quotient:

a. $\dfrac{^-9}{16} \div \dfrac{3}{8}$ b. $\dfrac{5}{12} \div 7$ c. $^-2\dfrac{1}{3} \div ^-4\dfrac{5}{16}$ d. $^-2 \div \dfrac{^-8}{9}$

14. Perform the indicated operation:

a. $\dfrac{^-2}{3} - \dfrac{4}{7}$ b. $^-1 \cdot \dfrac{3}{4}$ c. $\dfrac{^-2}{7} \div ^-1\dfrac{4}{21}$ d. $3\dfrac{1}{5} \cdot ^-4\dfrac{2}{5}$

e. $\dfrac{^-5}{12} - \dfrac{^-5}{12}$ f. $\dfrac{2}{7} \div \dfrac{24}{35}$ g. $\dfrac{^-6}{51} \cdot \dfrac{17}{18} \cdot \dfrac{^-1}{3}$ h. $^-1\dfrac{7}{8} + 9\dfrac{3}{5}$

CHAPTER 6 SAMPLE TEST ANSWERS

1. integers

2. distance, direction

3.

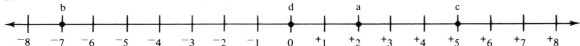

4. a. 5   **b.** $^-3$ **c.** 0   **d.** $^-7$

5. a. $^-9$ **b.** 3   **c.** $^-8$ **d.** $^-2$

e. 0   **f.** 0   **g.** $^-2$ **h.** 12

6. a. $^-7$ **b.** $^-4$ **c.** 9   **d.** 1

e. 2   **f.** 1

7. a. 2   **b.** $^-12$ **c.** $^-5$ **d.** $^-3$

e. $^-13$ **f.** 15   **g.** $^-3$ **h.** 2

8. a. $^-10$ **b.** 24   **c.** 0   **d.** $^-45$

e. $^-13$ **f.** 0   **g.** 40   **h.** $^-72$

i. 9   **j.** 0

9. a. $^-4$ **b.** 3   **c.** $^-3$ **d.** 5

e. undefined   **f.** 0   **g.** 0   **h.** undefined

10. a. $\dfrac{1}{84}$ **b.** $^-1\dfrac{7}{24}$ **c.** $\dfrac{^-5}{9}$ **d.** $2\dfrac{13}{16}$

11. a. $\dfrac{1}{8}$ **b.** $2\dfrac{7}{15}$ **c.** $^-1\dfrac{1}{15}$ **d.** $^-2\dfrac{7}{9}$

12. a. $\dfrac{1}{12}$ **b.** $^-14$ **c.** 0   **d.** $7\dfrac{7}{15}$

13. a. $^-1\dfrac{1}{2}$ **b.** $\dfrac{5}{84}$ **c.** $\dfrac{112}{207}$ **d.** $2\dfrac{1}{4}$

14. a. $^-1\dfrac{5}{21}$ **b.** $\dfrac{^-3}{4}$ **c.** $\dfrac{6}{25}$ **d.** $^-14\dfrac{2}{25}$

e. 0   **f.** $\dfrac{5}{12}$ **g.** $\dfrac{1}{27}$ **h.** $7\dfrac{29}{40}$

CHAPTER 7

ALGEBRAIC EXPRESSIONS AND EQUATION SOLVING

7.1 SIMPLIFYING ALGEBRAIC EXPRESSIONS

1 Expressions such as $a+3$, $5y-zx$, and $9(b+7)$ are referred to as "open expressions." These expressions are also correctly called algebraic expressions. Since letters (variables) in an algebraic expression can be replaced by rational numbers, all properties valid for the rational numbers can be used when simplifying algebraic expressions. The purpose of this section is to develop skill in the use of these properties for the simplification of algebraic expressions.

The building blocks or components of algebraic expressions are called terms. When an algebraic expression shows only additions, the *terms* are the parts separated by plus signs. Subtraction signs appearing in an algebraic expression can be converted to addition signs using the definition of subtraction.

Examples:	*Terms*
$8y+3$	$8y$ and 3
$\frac{1}{2}x-4+2y=\frac{1}{2}x+{}^-4+2y$	$\frac{1}{2}x$, ${}^-4$, and $2y$
$x-3y-6=x+{}^-3y+{}^-6$	x, ${}^-3y$, and ${}^-6$

Q1 Identify the terms in the algebraic expression $4a+7ab-12$. _____

\# \# \# • \# \# \# • \# \# \# • \# \# \# • \# \# \# • \# \# \# • \# \# \# • \# \# \# • \# \# \#

A1 $4a$, $7ab$, and ${}^-12$

2 The *like terms* of an algebraic expression are terms that have exactly the same literal coefficients (letter factors). The like terms of the algebraic expression $7x-3y-\frac{2}{3}x+6$ are $\frac{{}^-2}{3}x$ and $7x$, because each has the literal coefficient x.

In the expression $\frac{4}{5}y-3xy+\frac{2}{3}x-2y+8xy$ there are two sets of like terms. They are $\frac{4}{5}y$ and ${}^-2y$, with the letter factor y, and ${}^-3xy$ and $8xy$, with the letter factors x and y.

Numbers without a literal factor are called *constants* and are considered to be like terms. That is, 5, ${}^-7$, $\frac{7}{8}$, 3, and so on, are constants and like terms.

Q2 Identify the like terms in each of the following algebraic expressions:

a. $4x-2y+3-6x$ _____

b. $6 - 2y + \dfrac{5}{9}$ _____

c. $5r - 6s + 2rs - \dfrac{1}{2}s$ _____

d. $6a - 2b + 3ab$ _____

\# \# \#   •   \# \# \#   •   \# \# \#   •   \# \# \#   •   \# \# \#   •   \# \# \#   •   \# \# \#   •   \# \# \#   •   \# \# \#

A2   **a.** $4x, \; {}^-6x$ **b.** $6, \dfrac{5}{9}$ **c.** ${}^-6s, \dfrac{{}^-1}{2}s$

d. There are no like terms in part **d.**

---

3   Algebraic expressions are simplified by combining (by addition or subtraction) like terms. The justification for combining like terms is the distributive property of multiplication over addition or the distributive property of multiplication over subtraction. For example, $5x - 7x$ is simplified:

Justification

$5x - 7x$
$(5 - 7)x$ right distributive property of multiplication over subtraction
${}^-2x$ number fact: $5 - 7 = {}^-2$

Therefore, $5x - 7x$ simplifies to ${}^-2x$.

Q3   Use a distributive property to simplify the following expressions:

a. $4a - 7a$ **b.** $\dfrac{2}{3}x + \dfrac{1}{4}x$

\# \# \#   •   \# \# \#   •   \# \# \#   •   \# \# \#   •   \# \# \#   •   \# \# \#   •   \# \# \#   •   \# \# \#   •   \# \# \#

A3   **a.** ${}^-3a$: $4a - 7a = (4 - 7)a = {}^-3a$ **b.** $\dfrac{11}{12}x$: $\dfrac{2}{3}x + \dfrac{1}{4}x = \left(\dfrac{2}{3} + \dfrac{1}{4}\right)x = \dfrac{11}{12}x$

---

4   Consider the following simplification:

Justification

$4x - 3x$
$(4 - 3)x$ right distributive property of multiplication over subtraction
$1x$ number fact: $4 - 3 = 1$
x multiplication property of one

Therefore, $4x - 3x = x$.

Q4   Simplify $9y - 8y$.

\# \# \#   •   \# \# \#   •   \# \# \#   •   \# \# \#   •   \# \# \#   •   \# \# \#   •   \# \# \#   •   \# \# \#   •   \# \# \#

A4 y: $9y - 8y = (9 - 8)y = 1y = y$

Q5   Simplify $7b - 6b$.

\# \# \#   •   \# \# \#   •   \# \# \#   •   \# \# \#   •   \# \# \#   •   \# \# \#   •   \# \# \#   •   \# \# \#   •   \# \# \#

A5   *b*

---

5   By the multiplication property of one, *x* also equals 1*x*. This idea is used to simplify expressions such as $4x + x$ or $3b - b$.

Example 1: Simplify $4x + x$.

Solution:

Justification

$4x + x$
$4x + 1x$ multiplication property of one
$(4 + 1)x$ right distributive property of multiplication over addition
$5x$ number fact: $4 + 1 = 5$

Therefore, $4x + x = 5x$.

Example 2: Simplify $3b - b$.

Solution:
$3b - b$
$3b - 1b$ multiplication property of one
$(3 - 1)b$ right distributive property of multiplication over subtraction
$2b$ number fact: $3 - 1 = 2$

Therefore, $3b - b = 2b$.

Q6   Simplify:

a. $7y + y$ **b.** $x + 2x$ **c.** $b - 5b$ **d.** $a - \frac{2}{3}a$

\# \# \# • \# \# \# • \# \# \# • \# \# \# • \# \# \# • \# \# \# • \# \# \# • \# \# \# • \# \# \#

A6   **a.** $8y$: $7y + y$ **b.** $3x$: $x + 2x$ **c.** ^-4b: $b - 5b$ **d.** $\frac{1}{3}a$: $a - \frac{2}{3}a$
            $7y + 1y$ $1x + 2x$ $1b - 5b$ $1a - \frac{2}{3}a$
            $(7 + 1)y$ $(1 + 2)x$ $(1 - 5)b$ $\left(1 - \frac{2}{3}\right)a$
             $8y$ $3x$ ^-4b $\frac{1}{3}a$

---

6   By the multiplication property of negative one, $^-1x = {}^-x$. Consider its use in the simplification of $x - 2x$.

Justification

$x - 2x$
$1x - 2x$ multiplication property of one
$(1 - 2)x$ right distributive property of multiplication over subtraction
^-1x number fact: $1 - 2 = {}^-1$
^-x multiplication property of negative one

Therefore, $x - 2x = {}^-x$.

Q7 Simplify:
   a. $7x - 8x$ b. $12y - 13y$

\# \# \# • \# \# \# • \# \# \# • \# \# \# • \# \# \# • \# \# \# • \# \# \# • \# \# \# • \# \# \#

A7   a. ^-x: $7x - 8x = (7-8)x = {}^-1x = {}^-x$ b. ^-y

---

7   Notice that using a distributive property to simplify algebraic expressions is merely the process of combining the numerical coefficients of the like terms. Thus, the simplification process can be shortened as follows:

$$^-5b + 3b = {}^-2b \quad \text{because} \quad {}^-5 + 3 = {}^-2$$
$$\frac{^-1}{2}z - \frac{2}{3}z = \frac{^-7}{6}z \quad \text{because} \quad \frac{^-1}{2} - \frac{2}{3} = \frac{^-7}{6}$$

In algebra, numbers are usually written in $\frac{p}{q}$ form rather than as mixed numbers. Thus, in the preceding example, the answer is written as $\frac{^-7}{6}z$ rather than as $^-1\frac{1}{6}z$.

Q8   Simplify the following algebraic expressions by combining the numerical coefficients of the like terms:

    a. $7y - 12y = $ _____   b. $4b - b = $ _____

    c. $\frac{^-2}{3}x + \frac{4}{5}x = $ _____   d. $y - y = $ _____

\# \# \# • \# \# \# • \# \# \# • \# \# \# • \# \# \# • \# \# \# • \# \# \# • \# \# \# • \# \# \#

A8   a. ^-5y: Because $7 - 12 = {}^-5$ b. $3b$: Because $4 - 1 = 3$
       c. $\frac{2}{15}x$: Because $\frac{^-2}{3} + \frac{4}{5} = \frac{2}{15}$ d. 0: Because $1 - 1 = 0$

---

8   To simplify expressions involving more than two terms, a similar procedure is followed. Study the following examples:

   $3y - 12y + 7$ $^-8x - 3x + 9 - 12$
      $^-9y + 7$ $^-11x - 3$

Q9   Simplify each of the following expressions:
    a. $^-3m - 7m + 9$ b. $11 - 1 + 7x - 3x$

    c. $5y + 7y - 6 + 3$ d. $4 - 10 + 8y - \frac{3}{2}y$

\# \# \# • \# \# \# • \# \# \# • \# \# \# • \# \# \# • \# \# \# • \# \# \# • \# \# \# • \# \# \#

A9   a. $^-10m + 9$ b. $10 + 4x$ c. $12y - 3$ d. $^-6 + \frac{13}{2}y$

---

9   The expression $5x - 7$ may also be written $^-7 + 5x$. This fact is verified below:

Justification

$5x - 7$

$5x + {}^-7$ definition of subtraction

$^-7 + 5x$ commutative property of addition

Q10   Verify that $3x - 4 = {}^-4 + 3x$ by completing the following:

Justification

$3x - 4$

a. _____   definition of subtraction

b. _____   commutative property of addition

• # # # • # # # • # # # • # # # • # # # • # # # • # # # • # # # • # #

A10   **a.** $3x + {}^-4$ **b.** $^-4 + 3x$

---

10   The expression $^-8 - 7x$ may also be written $^-7x - 8$. The verification is as follows:

Justification

$^-7x - 8$

$^-7x + {}^-8$ definition of subtraction

$^-8 + {}^-7x$ commutative property of addition

$^-8 - 7x$ definition of subtraction

Q11   Verify that $^-2x - 9 = {}^-9 - 2x$ by completing the following:

Justification

$^-2x - 9$

a. _____   definition of subtraction

b. _____   commutative property of addition

c. _____   definition of subtraction

• # # # • # # # • # # # • # # # • # # # • # # # • # # # • # # # • # #

A11   **a.** $^-2x + {}^-9$ **b.** $^-9 + {}^-2x$ **c.** $^-9 - 2x$

---

11   Frame 9 showed that $5x - 7$ could be written $^-7 + 5x$. Frame 10 showed that $^-8 - 7x = {}^-7x - 8$. These frames demonstrate the following useful procedure: *In an algebraic expression, the terms may be rearranged in any order as long as the original sign of each term is left unchanged.*

Examples:

1. $5 - 2x = {}^-2x + 5$

2. $3x - \dfrac{4}{5} = \dfrac{^-4}{5} + 3x$

3. $\dfrac{^-3}{4}x - 5 = {}^-5 - \dfrac{3}{4}x$

4. $^-2x + 3 + 5x - 7 = {}^-2x + 5x + 3 - 7$

Notice in Example 4 that the terms are arranged so that the like terms are together.

Q12   Write equivalent expressions for each of the following:

a. $3x + 2 = $ _____   **b.** $^-5x - 4 = $ _____

c. $\dfrac{^-5}{8}x + 12 = $ _____   **d.** $^-4x + 3 - 2x = $ _____

e. $^-2x - 7 - 5x + 6 = $ _____

\# \# \# • \# \# \# • \# \# \# • \# \# \# • \# \# \# • \# \# \# • \# \# \# • \# \# \# • \# \# \#

A12   **a.** $2 + 3x$ **b.** $^-4 - 5x$ **c.** $12 - \dfrac{5}{8}x$

       d. $^-4x - 2x + 3$ **e.** $^-2x - 5x - 7 + 6$

---

12   The expression $5x - 2 - 3x - 9$ may be simplified by rearranging and combining the like terms as follows:

$5x - 2 - 3x - 9$

$5x - 3x - 2 - 9$

$2x - 11$

Q13   Simplify $7 - 3t + 9 - 6t$ by rearranging and combining the like terms.

\# \# \# • \# \# \# • \# \# \# • \# \# \# • \# \# \# • \# \# \# • \# \# \# • \# \# \# • \# \# \#

A13 $^-9t + 16$ or $16 - 9t$: $7 - 3t + 9 - 6t$

                                 $^-3t - 6t + 7 + 9$

                                 $^-9t + 16$

Q14   Simplify $4x - 3 - 5x + 6 - x$.

\# \# \# • \# \# \# • \# \# \# • \# \# \# • \# \# \# • \# \# \# • \# \# \# • \# \# \# • \# \# \#

A14 $^-2x + 3$ or $3 - 2x$: $4x - 3 - 5x + 6 - x$

                                 $4x - 5x - x - 3 + 6$

                                 $^-2x + 3$

Q15   Simplify the following algebraic expressions:

a. $^-3 + 5x + 7$ **b.** $5y - 6 + 2y$ **c.** $^-3x - 4 - x$

d. $x + 3x + 7 - 9$ **e.** $^-2z + 3 - 5z - 1$ **f.** $6t + 3 - 7t - 6 + t$

\# \# \# • \# \# \# • \# \# \# • \# \# \# • \# \# \# • \# \# \# • \# \# \# • \# \# \# • \# \# \#

A15   **a.** $5x + 4$ or $4 + 5x$ **b.** $7y - 6$ or $^-6 + 7y$ **c.** $^-4x - 4$ or $^-4 - 4x$

       d. $4x - 2$ or $^-2 + 4x$ **e.** $^-7z + 2$ or $2 - 7z$ **f.** $^-3$

13 The associative and commutative properties of multiplication are used whenever there is a need to change the grouping or order of multiplication as an aid in the simplification of algebraic expressions. The associative property of multiplication is used to simplify $3(4x)$ as follows:

Justification

$3(4x)$
$(3 \cdot 4)x$ associative property of multiplication
$12x$ number fact

Thus, $3(4x) = 12x$.

Q16 Use the associative property of multiplication to simplify $^-5(7y)$.

\# \# \# • \# \# \# • \# \# \# • \# \# \# • \# \# \# • \# \# \# • \# \# \# • \# \# \# • \# \# \#

A16 ^-35y: $^-5(7y) = (^-5 \cdot 7)y = ^-35y$

14 The expression $7\left(\dfrac{^-3}{7}t\right)$ is simplified:

Justification

$7\left(\dfrac{^-3}{7}t\right)$

$\left(7 \cdot \dfrac{^-3}{7}\right)t$ associative property of multiplication

^-3t number fact: $\dfrac{7}{1} \cdot \dfrac{^-3}{7} = ^-3$

Thus, $7\left(\dfrac{^-3}{7}t\right) = ^-3t$.

Q17 Simplify $^-9\left(\dfrac{^-1}{9}x\right)$.

\# \# \# • \# \# \# • \# \# \# • \# \# \# • \# \# \# • \# \# \# • \# \# \# • \# \# \# • \# \# \#

A17 x: $^-9\left(\dfrac{^-1}{9}x\right) = \left(^-9 \cdot \dfrac{^-1}{9}\right)x = 1x = x$

15 The expression $\dfrac{3}{5}\left(\dfrac{^-4}{9}y\right)$ is simplified:

Justification

$\dfrac{3}{5}\left(\dfrac{^-4}{9}y\right)$

$\left(\dfrac{3}{5} \cdot \dfrac{^-4}{9}\right)y$ associative property of multiplication

$\dfrac{^-4}{15}y$ number fact

Thus, $\dfrac{3}{5}\left(\dfrac{^-4}{9}y\right) = \dfrac{^-4}{15}y$.

Q18   Simplify $\dfrac{^-3}{4}\left(\dfrac{^-2}{7}z\right)$.

• # # # • # # # • # # # • # # # • # # # • # # # • # # # • # #

A18 $\dfrac{3}{14}z$: $\dfrac{^-3}{4}\left(\dfrac{^-2}{7}z\right)=\left(\dfrac{^-3}{4}\cdot\dfrac{^-2}{7}\right)z=\dfrac{3}{14}z$

Q19   Simplify each of the following algebraic expressions:

    a. $4\left(\dfrac{3}{4}x\right)$ **b.** $\dfrac{2}{3}\left(\dfrac{3}{2}y\right)$ **c.** $^-5\left(\dfrac{^-2}{15}z\right)$

    d. $\dfrac{^-6}{7}\left(\dfrac{5}{12}t\right)$ **e.** $\dfrac{^-5}{9}\left(\dfrac{^-9}{5}m\right)$ **f.** $\dfrac{1}{7}(7x)$

• # # # • # # # • # # # • # # # • # # # • # # # • # # # • # #

A19   **a.** $3x$ **b.** y **c.** $\dfrac{2}{3}z$ **d.** $\dfrac{^-5}{14}t$ **e.** m **f.** x

---

16   Both the commutative and associative properties of multiplication are used to simplify $\left(\dfrac{3}{4}x\right)\dfrac{2}{3}$ as follows:

Justification

$\left(\dfrac{3}{4}x\right)\dfrac{2}{3}$

$\dfrac{2}{3}\left(\dfrac{3}{4}x\right)$ commutative property of multiplication

$\left(\dfrac{2}{3}\cdot\dfrac{3}{4}\right)x$ associative property of multiplication

$\dfrac{1}{2}x$ number fact

Q20   Use the commutative and associative properties of multiplication to simplify $\left(\dfrac{2}{5}x\right)5$.

• # # # • # # # • # # # • # # # • # # # • # # # • # # # • # #

A20 $2x$: $\left(\dfrac{2}{5}x\right)5=5\left(\dfrac{2}{5}x\right)=\left(5\cdot\dfrac{2}{5}\right)x=2x$

Q21   Simplify $\left(\dfrac{^-3}{5}x\right)\cdot\dfrac{^-5}{3}$ by use of the commutative and associative properties.

• # # # • # # # • # # # • # # # • # # # • # # # • # # # • # #

A21 $x:\ \left(\dfrac{^-3}{5}x\right)\cdot\dfrac{^-5}{3}=\dfrac{^-5}{3}\left(\dfrac{^-3}{5}x\right)=\left(\dfrac{^-5}{3}\cdot\dfrac{^-3}{5}\right)x=1x=x$

---

17   The left distributive property of multiplication over addition and the left distributive property of multiplication over subtraction state that

$a(b+c)=ab+ac$

and

$a(b-c)=ab-ac$

for all rational-number replacements of a, b, and c.

Examples:

1. $3(7+5)=3\cdot7+3\cdot5$
2. $2(1-9)=2\cdot1-2\cdot9$

Q22   Use the left distributive property of multiplication over addition to fill in the blanks.

$5(2+9)=$ _____ $+$ _____

\# \# \#   •   \# \# \#   •   \# \# \#   •   \# \# \#   •   \# \# \#   •   \# \# \#   •   \# \# \#   •   \# \# \#   •   \# \# \#

A22 $5(2+9)=5\cdot2+5\cdot9$

---

18   When parentheses are removed from an algebraic expression, the same procedure is used. For example, to remove the parentheses from $3(x+2)$, proceed as follows:

$$3(x+2)=3\cdot x+3\cdot2$$
$$=3x+6$$

Q23   Use the left distributive property of multiplication over addition to remove the parentheses from $7(y+3)$.

\# \# \#   •   \# \# \#   •   \# \# \#   •   \# \# \#   •   \# \# \#   •   \# \# \#   •   \# \# \#   •   \# \# \#   •   \# \# \#

A23 $7y+21$: $7(y+3)=7\cdot y+7\cdot3=7y+21$

Q23   Use the left distributive property of multiplication over subtraction to remove the parentheses from $7(a-5)$.

\# \# \#   •   \# \# \#   •   \# \# \#   •   \# \# \#   •   \# \# \#   •   \# \# \#   •   \# \# \#   •   \# \# \#   •   \# \# \#

A24 $7a-35$: $7(a-5)=7\cdot a-7\cdot5=7a-35$

Q25   Remove the parentheses
    a. $2(x-9)$ **b.** $5(x+1)$

    c. $6(2-y)$ **d.** $8(2+c)$

\# \# \#   •   \# \# \#   •   \# \# \#   •   \# \# \#   •   \# \# \#   •   \# \# \#   •   \# \# \#   •   \# \# \#   •   \# \# \#

A25   **a.** $2x - 18$ **b.** $5x + 5$ **c.** $12 - 6y$ **d.** $16 + 8c$

---

19   To remove the parentheses from $(a + 3)$, recall that by the multiplication property of one:

$(a + 3) = 1 \cdot (a + 3)$

Thus,

$$(a + 3) = 1 \cdot (a + 3)$$
$$= 1 \cdot a + 1 \cdot 3$$
$$= a + 3$$

Notice that the result is exactly the expression within the parentheses.

Examples:

$(b + 2) = b + 2$
$(7 - y) = 7 - y$
$(2x - 3) = 2x - 3$

Q26   Remove the parentheses

a. $(x - 9) =$ _____   **b.** $(3 - x) =$ _____   **c.** $(5x + 6) =$ _____

\# \# \#   •   \# \# \#   •   \# \# \#   •   \# \# \#   •   \# \# \#   •   \# \# \#   •   \# \# \#   •   \# \# \#   •   \# \# \#

A26   **a.** $x - 9$ **b.** $3 - x$ **c.** $5x + 6$

---

20   The right distributive property of multiplication over addition and the right distributive property of multiplication over subtraction state that

$(a + b)c = ac + bc$

and

$(a - b)c = ac - bc$

for all rational numbers a, b, and c.

Examples:

1. $(3 + 5)2 = 3 \cdot 2 + 5 \cdot 2$

2. $(7 - 4)\dfrac{3}{8} = 7 \cdot \dfrac{3}{8} - 4 \cdot \dfrac{3}{8}$

Q27   Use the right distributive property of multiplication over addition to fill in the blanks.

$(4 + 9)7 =$ _____ $+$ _____

\# \# \#   •   \# \# \#   •   \# \# \#   •   \# \# \#   •   \# \# \#   •   \# \# \#   •   \# \# \#   •   \# \# \#   •   \# \# \#

A27 $(4 + 9)7 = 4 \cdot 7 + 9 \cdot 7$

Q28   Use the right distributive property of multiplication over subtraction to fill in the blanks.

$\left(\dfrac{5}{6} - 1\right)6 =$ _____ $-$ _____

\# \# \#   •   \# \# \#   •   \# \# \#   •   \# \# \#   •   \# \# \#   •   \# \# \#   •   \# \# \#   •   \# \# \#   •   \# \# \#

A28 $\left(\dfrac{5}{6} - 1\right)6 = \dfrac{5}{6} \cdot 6 - 1 \cdot 6$

21 The right distributive properties are also used to simplify algebraic expressions.

Examples:

1. $(x-2)3 = x \cdot 3 - 2 \cdot 3$
$= 3x - 6$ (it is customary to rewrite $x \cdot 3$ as $3x$)
2. $(5+r)3 = 5 \cdot 3 + r \cdot 3$
$= 15 + 3r$

Q29 Use the right distributive property of multiplication over addition to remove the parentheses from $(2+x)7$.

\# \# \# • \# \# \# • \# \# \# • \# \# \# • \# \# \# • \# \# \# • \# \# \# • \# \# \# • \# \# \#

A29 $14+7x$: $(2+x)7 = 2 \cdot 7 + x \cdot 7$
$= 14 + 7x$

Q30 Use the right distributive property of multiplication over subtraction to remove the parentheses from $(y-4)5$.

\# \# \# • \# \# \# • \# \# \# • \# \# \# • \# \# \# • \# \# \# • \# \# \# • \# \# \# • \# \# \#

A30 $5y-20$: $(y-4)5 = y \cdot 5 - 4 \cdot 5$
$= 5y - 20$

22 To remove the parentheses in the algebraic expression $3(4x-7)$, the following steps are used:

$3(4x-7) = 3 \cdot 4x - 3 \cdot 7$
$= 12x - 21$

Q31 Remove the parentheses from $7(6x-4)$.

\# \# \# • \# \# \# • \# \# \# • \# \# \# • \# \# \# • \# \# \# • \# \# \# • \# \# \# • \# \# \#

A31 $42x-28$: $7(6x-4) = 7 \cdot 6x - 7 \cdot 4$
$= 42x - 28$

Q32 Remove the parentheses from $4\left(12 - \dfrac{3}{4}x\right)$.

\# \# \# • \# \# \# • \# \# \# • \# \# \# • \# \# \# • \# \# \# • \# \# \# • \# \# \# • \# \# \#

A32 $48-3x$

23 To remove the parentheses from $(3x-2)5$, the procedure is as follows:

$(3x-2)5 = 3x \cdot 5 - 2 \cdot 5$
$= 5 \cdot 3x - 2 \cdot 5$
$= 15x - 10$

Q33   Remove the parentheses from $(7x - 4)9$.

•   # # #   •   # # #   •   # # #   •   # # #   •   # # #   •   # # #   •   # # #   •   # #

A33 $63x - 36$: $(7x - 4)9 = 7x \cdot 9 - 4 \cdot 9$
$$= 9 \cdot 7x - 4 \cdot 9$$
$$= 63x - 36$$

Q34   Remove the parentheses from $(5a + 7)2$.

•   # # #   •   # # #   •   # # #   •   # # #   •   # # #   •   # # #   •   # # #   •   # #

A34 $10a + 14$

24	To remove the parentheses from $4(^-x + 7)$, recall that ^-x means ^-1x (multiplication property of negative one). Thus,

$$4(^-x + 7) = 4(^-1x + 7)$$
$$= 4 \cdot ^-1x + 4 \cdot 7$$
$$= ^-4x + 28 \quad \text{or} \quad 28 - 4x$$

Q35   Remove the parentheses from $3(^-x - 5)$

•   # # #   •   # # #   •   # # #   •   # # #   •   # # #   •   # # #   •   # # #   •   # #

A35 $^-3x - 15$: $3(^-x - 5) = 3(^-1x - 5)$
$$= 3 \cdot ^-1x - 3 \cdot 5$$
$$= ^-3x - 15$$

25	When removing parentheses by use of the distributive properties, it is convenient to be able to find the result mentally (without showing work). For example, to remove parentheses from $5(3x - 6)$, write only $5(3x - 6) = 15x - 30$.

Q36   Mentally remove the parentheses from $2(8 - 5t)$.

•   # # #   •   # # #   •   # # #   •   # # #   •   # # #   •   # # #   •   # # #   •   # #

A36 $16 - 10t$

Q37   Mentally remove the parentheses from $3\left(7 - \dfrac{4}{3}y\right)$.

•   # # #   •   # # #   •   # # #   •   # # #   •   # # #   •   # # #   •   # # #   •   # #

A37 $21 - 4y$

Q38   Remove the parentheses from $(6z + 1)9$.

•   # # #   •   # # #   •   # # #   •   # # #   •   # # #   •   # # #   •   # # #   •   # #

A38 $54z + 9$

26 To remove the parentheses from $^-5(3x-4)$, the following steps can be used:

$$^-5(3x-4) = {}^-5 \cdot 3x - {}^-5 \cdot 4$$
$$= {}^-15x - {}^-20$$
$$= {}^-15x + 20$$

You should notice that $^-15x - {}^-20$ is equivalent to $^-15x + 20$ because of the definition of subtraction. The expression $^-15x + 20$ is considered to be in simplest form. The expression $20 - 15x$ may also be written.

Q39 Remove the parentheses from $^-4(7x-9)$ and write in simplest form.

• # # # • # # # • # # # • # # # • # # # • # # # • # # # • # #

A39 $^-28x + 36$ or $36 - 28x$:
$$^-4(7x-9) = {}^-4 \cdot 7x - {}^-4 \cdot 9$$
$$= {}^-28x - {}^-36$$
$$= {}^-28x + 36$$

Q40 Remove the parentheses from $^-5(^-3x+4)$ and write in simplest form.

• # # # • # # # • # # # • # # # • # # # • # # # • # # # • # #

A40 $15x - 20$:
$$^-5(^-3x+4) = {}^-5 \cdot {}^-3x + {}^-5 \cdot 4$$
$$= 15x + {}^-20$$
$$= 15x - 20$$

27 The expression $(^-4x-7) \cdot {}^-8$ is simplified:

$$(^-4x-7) \cdot {}^-8 = {}^-4x \cdot {}^-8 - 7 \cdot {}^-8$$
$$= 32x - {}^-56$$
$$= 32x + 56$$

Q41 Simplify $(3y+9) \cdot {}^-6$.

• # # # • # # # • # # # • # # # • # # # • # # # • # # # • # #

A41 $^-18y - 54$:
$$(3y+9) \cdot {}^-6 = 3y \cdot {}^-6 + 9 \cdot {}^-6$$
$$= {}^-18y + {}^-54$$
$$= {}^-18y - 54$$

Q42 Simplify $(^-a-5) \cdot {}^-2$.

• # # # • # # # • # # # • # # # • # # # • # # # • # # # • # #

A42 $2a + 10$:
$$(^-a-5) \cdot {}^-2 = {}^-a \cdot {}^-2 - 5 \cdot {}^-2$$
$$= 2a - {}^-10$$
$$= 2a + 10$$

28   By the multiplication property of negative one, the expression $^-(3x+7)$ is equivalent to $^-1(3x+7)$. Thus $^-(3x+7)$ is simplified:

$$^-(3x+7) = {}^-1(3x+7)$$
$$= {}^-1 \cdot 3x + {}^-1 \cdot 7$$
$$= {}^-3x + {}^-7$$
$$= {}^-3x - 7$$

An alternative method to the above is to notice that $^-(3x+7)$ means the *opposite of* $(3x+7)$, which can be found by taking the opposite of each term within the parentheses. Thus,

$$^-(3x+7) = {}^-3x + {}^-7$$
$$= {}^-3x - 7$$

Q43   Write an equivalent expression for $^-(5+2y)$ by forming the opposite of each term within the parentheses.

\# \# \#   •   \# \# \#   •   \# \# \#   •   \# \# \#   •   \# \# \#   •   \# \# \#   •   \# \# \#   •   \# \# \#   •   \# \# \#

A43 $^-5 - 2y$: $^-(5+2y) = {}^-5 + {}^-2y$

Q44   Simplify $^-1(5+2y)$ by removing the parentheses.

\# \# \#   •   \# \# \#   •   \# \# \#   •   \# \# \#   •   \# \# \#   •   \# \# \#   •   \# \# \#   •   \# \# \#   •   \# \# \#

A44 $^-5 - 2y$: $^-1(5+2y) = {}^-1 \cdot 5 + {}^-1 \cdot 2y$
$$= {}^-5 + {}^-2y$$
$$= {}^-5 - 2y$$

Q45   Simplify $^-(4b-5)$

\# \# \#   •   \# \# \#   •   \# \# \#   •   \# \# \#   •   \# \# \#   •   \# \# \#   •   \# \# \#   •   \# \# \#   •   \# \# \#

A45 $^-4b + 5$ or $5 - 4b$: $^-(4b-5) = {}^-1(4b-5)$
$$= {}^-1 \cdot 4b - {}^-1 \cdot 5$$
$$= {}^-4b - {}^-5$$
$$= {}^-4b + 5 \text{ or } 5 - 4b$$

or $^-(4b-5) = {}^-4b - {}^-5$
$$= {}^-4b + 5 \text{ or } 5 - 4b$$

Q46   Simplify $^-(x-7)$.

\# \# \#   •   \# \# \#   •   \# \# \#   •   \# \# \#   •   \# \# \#   •   \# \# \#   •   \# \# \#   •   \# \# \#   •   \# \# \#

A46 $^-x + 7$ or $7 - x$

29   An algebraic expression is said to be in "simplest" form when:

1. All parentheses have been removed.
2. All like terms have been combined.

3. The definition of subtraction has been applied to remove all of the "raised" negative signs that can be removed.

Examples: *Simplest Form?*
$3x + 5 - 2x$ no, like terms not combined
$7x - 3 + 2y$ yes
$4(x - 2) + 3x$ no, parentheses not removed and like terms not combined
$3 + {}^-5y$ no, raised negative sign can be removed by writing $3 - 5y$
$9t - {}^-4$ no, raised negative sign can be removed by writing $9t + 4$
${}^-5x - 2$ yes

Q47   Indicate whether each of the following expressions are in simplest form. If the expression is not in simplest form, briefly state why.

a. $4x - 2y + 9$ _____   _____

b. $3(2 - 4y) - 1$ _____   _____

c. $5t - 6 + 9t$ _____   _____

d. $8x - 5 + {}^-y$ _____   _____

e. $5x + 7y - 3xy$ _____   _____

\# \# \# • \# \# \# • \# \# \# • \# \# \# • \# \# \# • \# \# \# • \# \# \# • \# \# \# • \# \# \#

A47   **a.** yes
b. no, parentheses not removed and like terms not combined
c. no, like terms not combined
d. no, raised negative sign can be removed by writing $8x - 5 - y$
e. yes

Q48   Simplify $5 - 6t + 3 - 9t$ by rearranging and combining the like terms.

\# \# \# • \# \# \# • \# \# \# • \# \# \# • \# \# \# • \# \# \# • \# \# \# • \# \# \# • \# \# \#

A48 ${}^-15t + 8$ or $8 - 15t$: $5 - 6t + 3 - 9t$
${}^-6t - 9t + 5 + 3$
${}^-15t + 8$ or $8 - 15t$

Q49   Simplify ${}^-3x + 7x - 5 + x$.

\# \# \# • \# \# \# • \# \# \# • \# \# \# • \# \# \# • \# \# \# • \# \# \# • \# \# \# • \# \# \#

A49 $5x - 5$: ${}^-3x + 7x - 5 + x$
${}^-3x + 7x + x - 5$
$5x - 5$

30   To simplify expressions that involve parentheses:

1. Use the distributive properties to remove parentheses.
2. Rearrange and combine the like terms.

Examples:

1. $2(3y-7)+4$
$6y-14+4$
$6y-10$

2. $^-2x+\frac{4}{9}(x-4)$

$^-2x+\frac{4}{9}x-\frac{16}{9}$

$\frac{^-14}{9}x-\frac{16}{9}$ $\left(\text{Note: }^-2+\frac{4}{9}=\frac{^-14}{9}\right)$

Q50 Simplify $5(2x-1)+7$.

\# \# \# • \# \# \# • \# \# \# • \# \# \# • \# \# \# • \# \# \# • \# \# \# • \# \# \# • \# \# \#

A50 $10x+2$: $5(2x-1)+7$
$10x-5+7$
$10x+2$

Q51 Simplify $3x+7(^-x+4)$.

\# \# \# • \# \# \# • \# \# \# • \# \# \# • \# \# \# • \# \# \# • \# \# \# • \# \# \# • \# \# \#

A51 $^-4x+28$ or $28-4x$: $3x+7(^-x+4)$
$3x+^-7x+7\cdot4$
$^-4x+28$ or $28-4x$

Q52 Simplify each of the following:
a. $(7x+8)-3$ **b.** $3(2t-4)+7$ **c.** $8b+2(b-3)$

d. $(^-5+2x)-3x$ **e.** $(^-3x+4)-9$ **f.** $^-7(4-x)+3x$

\# \# \# • \# \# \# • \# \# \# • \# \# \# • \# \# \# • \# \# \# • \# \# \# • \# \# \# • \# \# \#

A52 **a.** $7x+5$ **b.** $6t-5$ **c.** $10b-6$
d. $^-x-5$ **e.** $^-3x-5$ **f.** $10x-28$

31 Recall that the expression $^-(x+3)$ could be simplified in either of two ways:

$^-(x+3)=^-1(x+3)$ *or* $^-(x+3)=^-x+^-3$
$=^-1\cdot x+^-1\cdot3$ $=^-x-3$
$=^-x+^-3$
$=^-x-3$

$[^-(x+3)$ means the opposite of $(x+3)$, which is the same as the opposite of each term within the parentheses]

Q53 Simplify:

a. $^-(y+9)=$ _____ **b.** $^-(2x+7)=$ _____

c. $^-\left(4z - \dfrac{4}{3}\right) =$ _____   **d.** $^-(b - 12) =$ _____

e. $^-(5y + 7) =$ _____

\# \# \# • \# \# \# • \# \# \# • \# \# \# • \# \# \# • \# \# \# • \# \# \# • \# \# \# • \# \# \#

A53 **a.** $^-y - 9$ **b.** $^-2x - 7$

c. $^-4z + \dfrac{4}{3}$ or $\dfrac{4}{3} - 4z$ **d.** $^-b + 12$ or $12 - b$

e. $^-5y - 7$

---

32 To simplify $4 - (x + 7)$ the following steps are used:

$$4 - (x + 7) = 4 + \,^-(x + 7)$$
$$= 4 + \,^-x + \,^-7$$
$$= \,^-x + \,^-3$$
$$= \,^-x - 3$$

Q54 Simplify $15 - (2x + 7)$.

\# \# \# • \# \# \# • \# \# \# • \# \# \# • \# \# \# • \# \# \# • \# \# \# • \# \# \# • \# \# \#

A54 $^-2x + 8$ or $8 - 2x$: $15 - (2x + 7) = 15 + \,^-(2x + 7)$
$$= 15 + \,^-2x + \,^-7$$
$$= \,^-2x + 8 \text{ or } 8 - 2x$$

Q55 Simplify $^-4 - (2b - 3)$.

\# \# \# • \# \# \# • \# \# \# • \# \# \# • \# \# \# • \# \# \# • \# \# \# • \# \# \# • \# \# \#

A55 $^-2b - 1$: $^-4 - (2b - 3) = \,^-4 + \,^-(2b - 3)$
$$= \,^-4 + \,^-2b - \,^-3$$
$$= \,^-4 + \,^-2b + 3$$
$$= \,^-2b - 1$$

Q56 Simplify each of the following:

a. $4 - (y + 3)$ **b.** $2z - (z - 5)$

c. $9 - (2a - 4)$ **d.** $6y - (2y + 7)$

\# \# \# • \# \# \# • \# \# \# • \# \# \# • \# \# \# • \# \# \# • \# \# \# • \# \# \# • \# \# \#

A56 **a.** $^-y + 1$ or $1 - y$ **b.** $z + 5$
     c. $^-2a + 13$ or $13 - 2a$ **d.** $4y - 7$

---

33 To simplify $(2x + 7) - (3x - 4)$, remove the parentheses and combine like terms as follows:

$$(2x + 7) - (3x - 4) = (2x + 7) + \,^-(3x - 4)$$
$$= (2x + 7) + \,^-3x - \,^-4$$
$$= 2x + 7 + \,^-3x + 4$$
$$= \,^-x + 11$$

Notice that parentheses preceded by no sign (or a "+" sign) are removed by just dropping them, whereas parentheses preceded by a "−" sign are removed by rewriting the subtraction problem as an addition problem and taking the opposite of the terms within the parentheses.

Q57　Remove the parentheses only (do not simplify):　$(x-5)-(2x+7)$

#　•　# # #　•　# # #　•　# # #　•　# # #　•　# # #　•　# # #　•　# # #　•　# #

A57　$x-5+{}^-2x+{}^-7$:　$(x-5)-(2x+7)=(x-5)+{}^-(2x+7)$
$$= x-5+{}^-2x+{}^-7$$

Q58　Simplify the result in A57.

#　•　# # #　•　# # #　•　# # #　•　# # #　•　# # #　•　# # #　•　# # #　•　# #

A58　${}^-x-12$

Q59　Remove the parentheses only (do not simplify):　$(1-3b)-(4b-7)$

#　•　# # #　•　# # #　•　# # #　•　# # #　•　# # #　•　# # #　•　# # #　•　# #

A59　$1-3b+{}^-4b-{}^-7$

Q60　Simplify the result in A59.

#　•　# # #　•　# # #　•　# # #　•　# # #　•　# # #　•　# # #　•　# # #　•　# #

A60　${}^-7b+8$ or $8-7b$

Q61　Simplify each of the following expressions:
　　a. $(5-4x)-(x+3)$　　　　**b.** $(2x-5)-(3-5x)$　　　　**c.** $({}^-5+b)-(b-5)$

　　d. ${}^-(4y+3)-(7y+3)$　　　**e.** $(z-9)-({}^-z-5)$　　　**f.** ${}^-(x+5)-(x-5)$

#　•　# # #　•　# # #　•　# # #　•　# # #　•　# # #　•　# # #　•　# # #　•　# #

A61　**a.** ${}^-5x+2$ or $2-5x$　　　**b.** $7x-8$　　　　　　**c.** 0
　　d. ${}^-11y-6$　　　　　　　**e.** $2z-4$　　　　　　　**f.** ${}^-2x$

34　To simplify expressions such as $3(x-2)-4(x+3)$, the following steps are used:

$$3(x-2)-4(x+3)=3(x-2)+{}^-4(x+3)$$
$$= 3x-6+{}^-4x+{}^-12$$
$$= 3x+{}^-6+{}^-4x+{}^-12$$
$$= {}^-x+{}^-18$$
$$= {}^-x-18$$

Note: The work is usually shortened to:

$$3(x-2)-4(x+3)=3x-6-4x-12$$
$$=~^-x-18$$

Q62   Remove the parentheses only (do not simplify): $5(y+7)-2(y-4)$

\# \# \#   •   \# \# \#   •   \# \# \#   •   \# \# \#   •   \# \# \#   •   \# \# \#   •   \# \# \#   •   \# \# \#   •   \# \# \#

A62 $5y+35-2y+8$

Q63   Complete the simplification of A62.

\# \# \#   •   \# \# \#   •   \# \# \#   •   \# \# \#   •   \# \# \#   •   \# \# \#   •   \# \# \#   •   \# \# \#   •   \# \# \#

A63 $3y+43$

Q64   Remove the parentheses only (do not simplify): $2(2x-3)-4(x+5)$

\# \# \#   •   \# \# \#   •   \# \# \#   •   \# \# \#   •   \# \# \#   •   \# \# \#   •   \# \# \#   •   \# \# \#   •   \# \# \#

A64 $4x-6-4x-20$

Q65   Complete the simplification of A64.

\# \# \#   •   \# \# \#   •   \# \# \#   •   \# \# \#   •   \# \# \#   •   \# \# \#   •   \# \# \#   •   \# \# \#   •   \# \# \#

A65 $^-26$

Q66   Simplify each of the following algebraic expressions:
   a. $(3x-4)-2(2x+5)$ **b.** $^-2(b+7)-(3b-5)$

   c. $2(y+3)+3(^-2y-7)$ **d.** $(y+7)-2(y+5)$

\# \# \#   •   \# \# \#   •   \# \# \#   •   \# \# \#   •   \# \# \#   •   \# \# \#   •   \# \# \#   •   \# \# \#   •   \# \# \#

A66   **a.** $^-x-14$ **b.** $^-5b-9$ **c.** $^-4y-15$ **d.** $^-y-3$

This completes the instruction for this section.

7.1   EXERCISE

1. Identify the like terms in each of the following algebraic expressions:
   a. $3x-5y-6x+4$ **b.** $3r-2+7s-6$
2. Simplify by combining like terms:
   a. $4x-2x$ **b.** $m-3-7m$
   c. $7-4y-6-3y$ **d.** $\frac{3}{5}x-\frac{4}{7}x-2$

3. Simplify by use of the commutative and/or associative properties of addition:
   a. $(3x - 2) + 5x$
   b. $^-15 + (7 - 8a)$
   c. $^-x + \left(7x - \dfrac{2}{5}x\right)$
   d. $\left(\dfrac{3}{5}b - \dfrac{2}{3}b\right) + b$

4. Simplify:
   a. $4y + {}^-9$
   b. $5 - 2r + 2s - 6r$
   c. $\dfrac{1}{3}x + y - 6xy - 4y$
   d. $4m + 7 - 3m + {}^-7 - m$

5. Simplify:
   a. $2\left(\dfrac{3}{4}x\right)$
   b. $\dfrac{^-1}{5}\left(\dfrac{^-4}{9}y\right)$
   c. $\dfrac{^-1}{7}(7m)$
   d. $\dfrac{5}{7}\left(\dfrac{7}{5}x\right)$
   e. $\left(\dfrac{^-1}{9}z\right) \cdot {}^-9$
   f. $\left(\dfrac{^-3}{5}x\right)\dfrac{2}{3}$
   g. $(4y)\dfrac{5}{4}$
   h. $\left(\dfrac{^-3}{5}x\right)20$

6. Simplify:
   a. $2(x - 3)$
   b. $(y + 7) \cdot {}^-3$
   c. $^-4(2x - 3)$
   d. $(4 - 2x)5$
   e. $(7x - 9)$
   f. $^-(7x - 9)$
   g. $^-(^-t + 2)$
   h. $^-5(^-7 - 3x)$
   i. $(6x - 5) \cdot {}^-8$
   j. $^-7(3y + {}^-9)$

7. Simplify:
   a. $^-4y + 9 + 2y + 5$
   b. $\dfrac{4}{5}x - \dfrac{2}{3}x + 2 - 9$
   c. $(7x + 8) - 8$
   d. $^-2(x + 7) - 3$
   e. $\dfrac{^-4}{5}(y + 10) + 7$
   f. $4 - (z + 7)$
   g. $3(x + 2) + 7(x - 5)$
   h. $(y - 6) - (4y + 7)$
   i. $^-7(x + 2) - 2(3x - 7)$
   j. $^-\left(\dfrac{1}{3}x + 5\right) - (5 - x)$

7.1   EXERCISE ANSWERS

1. a. $3x$ and ^-6x
   b. $^-2$ and $^-6$

2. a. $2x$
   b. $^-6m - 3$
   c. $^-7y + 1$ or $1 - 7y$
   d. $\dfrac{1}{35}x - 2$

3. a. $8x - 2$
   b. $^-8a - 8$
   c. $\dfrac{28}{5}x$
   d. $\dfrac{14}{15}b$

4. a. $4y - 9$
   b. $^-8r + 2s + 5$
   c. $\dfrac{1}{3}x - 3y - 6xy$
   d. 0

5. a. $\dfrac{3}{2}x$
   b. $\dfrac{4}{45}y$
   c. ^-m
   d. x
   e. z
   f. $\dfrac{^-2}{5}x$
   g. $5y$
   h. ^-12x

6. a. $2x - 6$
   b. $^-3y - 21$
   c. $^-8x + 12$ or $12 - 8x$
   d. $20 - 10x$
   e. $7x - 9$
   f. $^-7x + 9$ or $9 - 7x$
   g. $t - 2$
   h. $15x + 35$
   i. $^-48x + 40$ or $40 - 48x$
   j. $^-21y + 63$ or $63 - 21y$

7. a. $^-2y + 14$ or $14 - 2y$
   b. $\dfrac{2}{15}x - 7$
   c. $7x$

d. $^-2x - 17$

e. $\dfrac{^-4}{5}y - 1$

f. $^-z - 3$

g. $10x - 29$

h. $^-3y - 13$

i. ^-13x

j. $\dfrac{2}{3}x - 10$

7.2   EQUATIONS, FUNDAMENTAL PRINCIPLES OF EQUALITY

1   Section 7.1 dealt with the procedures involved in simplifying algebraic expressions. These skills will now be utilized in the study of equations. An equation is a statement in which the expressions on opposite sides of an equal sign represent the same number. Some examples of equations are

$3 + 4 = 9 - 2$
$15 = y + 4$
$x - 2 = 6$
$2x - 3 = 5x + 9$

The expressions on opposite sides of the equals sign are referred to as the left and right *sides* of the equation. For example,

$$\underbrace{4x - 7}_{\text{left side}} = \underbrace{2 - 6x}_{\text{right side}}$$

Q1   Identify the left and right sides of the following equations:

a. $14 - 9 = 5$ left side _____; right side _____

b. $3 = y + 1$ left side _____; right side _____

c. $3x - 7 = 8x + 13$ left side _____; right side _____

\# \# \#   •   \# \# \#   •   \# \# \#   •   \# \# \#   •   \# \# \#   •   \# \# \#   •   \# \# \#   •   \# \# \#   •   \# \# \#

A1   **a.** left side, $14 - 9$; right side, 5
b. left side, 3; right side, $y + 1$
c. left side, $3x - 7$; right side, $8x + 13$

2   Equations that do not contain enough information to be judged as either true or false are often referred to as *open sentences*. Thus,

$18 - y = 14$ and $x + 6 = 9$

are examples of open sentences, because they cannot be judged true or false until numbers are replaced for the unknown quantities y and x. If y is replaced by 10 in the open sentence $18 - y = 14$, the resulting statement $18 - 10 = 14$ is false. If x is replaced by 3 in the open sentence $x + 6 = 9$, the resulting statement $3 + 6 = 9$ is true.

Q2   **a.** If x is replaced by 7 in the open sentence $x - 2 = 5$, is the resulting statement true or false?   _____

b. If y is replaced by 4 in the open sentence $12 + y = 15$, is the resulting statement true or false?   _____

\# \# \#   •   \# \# \#   •   \# \# \#   •   \# \# \#   •   \# \# \#   •   \# \# \#   •   \# \# \#   •   \# \# \#   •   \# \# \#

A2   **a.** true: $7 - 2 = 5$
     b. false: $12 + 4 \neq 15$

---

3   Since it is not always possible to guess the solution to an equation, it is necessary to study some basic procedures that can be used to solve equations. Recall that an equation is a statement in which the expressions on opposite sides of the equal sign represent the same number. Since it is necessary to maintain this equality between sides, a basic rule in solving equations is that *whatever operation is performed on one side of an equation must also be performed on the other side of the equation.*

In general, solving an equation is like untying a knot, in that you always do the opposite of what has been done to form the equation. The equation has been solved when it has been changed to the form "a variable = a number" or "a number = a variable." If the variable is x, the form is "$x = a$ number" or "a number $= x$."

In the equation $x - 2 = 10$, for example, 2 has been subtracted from x to equal 10. Since *the opposite of subtracting 2 is adding 2,* the equation can be solved by adding 2 to both sides as follows:

$$x - 2 = 10 \quad \text{(add 2 to both sides)}$$
$$x - 2 + 2 = 10 + 2$$
$$x = 12$$

The solution can be checked by seeing if it converts the original open sentence into a true statement.

Check: $x - 2 = 10$
         $12 - 2 \overset{?}{=} 10$
         $10 = 10$

So 12 is the correct solution, because 12 converts $x - 2 = 10$ into the true statement $10 = 10$.

The solution of the preceding equation demonstrates the *addition principle of equality: If the same number is added to both sides of an equation, the result is another equation with the same solution.* In general, if $a = b$, then $a + c = b + c$ for any numbers a, b, and c.

Q3   Solve the following equations using the addition principle of equality and check the solutions:
     a. $x - 3 = 5$ **b.** $y - 12 = {}^{-}7$ **c.** $3 = x - 6$

•   # # #   •   # # #   •   # # #   •   # # #   •   # # #   •   # # #   •   # # #   •   # #

A3   **a.** $x - 3 = 5$ (3 was subtracted from x, so add 3 to both sides)
             $x - 3 + 3 = 5 + 3$
                    $x = 8$
     Check: $x - 3 = 5$
              $8 - 3 \overset{?}{=} 5$
                 $5 = 5$

     b. $y - 12 = {}^{-}7$ (12 was subtracted from x, so add 12 to both sides)
             $y - 12 + 12 = {}^{-}7 + 12$
                    $y = 5$
     Check: $y - 12 = {}^{-}7$
              $5 - 12 \overset{?}{=} {}^{-}7$
                 ${}^{-}7 = {}^{-}7$

c. $3 = x - 6$ (6 was subtracted from x, so add 6 to both sides)

$3 + 6 = x - 6 + 6$

$9 = x$

Check: $3 = x - 6$

$3 \stackrel{?}{=} 9 - 6$

$3 = 3$

---

4   Observe that in the equation $x + 4 = 13$, 4 has been added to x to equal 13. The opposite of adding 4 is subtracting 4, so the equation can be solved by subtracting 4 from both sides as follows:

$x + 4 = 13$

$x + 4 - 4 = 13 - 4$

$x = 9$

Check: $x + 4 = 13$

$9 + 4 \stackrel{?}{=} 13$

$13 = 13$

The solution of the preceding equation demonstrates a second principle useful in solving equations, the *subtraction principle of equality: If the same number is subtracted from both sides of an equation, the result is another equation with the same solution.* In general, if $a = b$, then $a - c = b - c$ for any numbers a, b, and c.

Q4   Solve the following equations using the subtraction principle of equality and check each of the solutions:

a. $y + 1 = 16$ **b.** $x + 14 = {}^-29$ **c.** $34 = x + 11$

\# \# \#   •   \# \# \#   •   \# \# \#   •   \# \# \#   •   \# \# \#   •   \# \# \#   •   \# \# \#   •   \# \# \#   •   \# \# \#   •   \# \# \#

A4   **a.** $y + 1 = 16$ (1 was added to y, so subtract 1 from both sides)

$y + 1 - 1 = 16 - 1$

$y = 15$

Check: $y + 1 = 16$

$15 + 1 \stackrel{?}{=} 16$

$16 = 16$

b. $x + 14 = {}^-29$ (14 was added to x, so subtract 14 from both sides)

$x + 14 - 14 = {}^-29 - 14$

$x = {}^-43$

Check: $x + 14 = {}^-29$

${}^-43 + 14 \stackrel{?}{=} {}^-29$

${}^-29 = {}^-29$

c. $34 = x + 11$ (11 was added to x, so subtract 11 from both sides)

$34 - 11 = x + 11 - 11$

$23 = x$

Check: $34 = x + 11$

$34 \stackrel{?}{=} 23 + 11$

$34 = 34$

---

5   It is often necessary to simplify one or both sides of an equation by combining like terms before proceeding with the solution. For example,

$$x - 5 = 15 - 2 \quad \text{(simplify by combining like terms)}$$
$$x - 5 = 13$$
$$x - 5 + 5 = 13 + 5$$
$$x = 18$$

Q5 Solve the equation by first combining like terms: $y - 7 + 2 = 13$

\# \# \# • \# \# \# • \# \# \# • \# \# \# • \# \# \# • \# \# \# • \# \# \# • \# \# \# • \# \# \#

A5 $y - 7 + 2 = 13$
$\quad y - 5 = 13$
$y - 5 + 5 = 13 + 5$
$\quad\quad y = 18$

Q6 Use the addition and subtraction principles of equality to solve the following equations and check each of the solutions:

a. $x - 2 = 5$ **b.** $y + 7 = 11$ **c.** $1 = x - 7$

d. $x + 3 = 3$ **e.** $12 = x + 8$ **f.** $x - 7 = {}^{-}5$

g. $11 + y = {}^{-}7$ **h.** $x + 6 = 5$ **i.** ${}^{-}3 = y + 9$

j. $7 + x = 2$ **k.** $y + 7 = 2 - 11$ **l.** ${}^{-}4 + x = 7 - 14$

\# \# \# • \# \# \# • \# \# \# • \# \# \# • \# \# \# • \# \# \# • \# \# \# • \# \# \# • \# \# \#

A6   **a.** $x = 7$ **b.** $y = 4$ **c.** $8 = x \ (x = 8)$ **d.** $x = 0$
     e. $4 = x \ (x = 4)$ **f.** $x = 2$ **g.** $y = {}^{-}18$ **h.** $x = {}^{-}1$
     i. ${}^{-}12 = y \ (y = {}^{-}12)$ **j.** $x = {}^{-}5$ **k.** $y = {}^{-}16$ **l.** $x = {}^{-}3$

6   In each of the equations solved so far the understood coefficient of the variable is 1. That is, x is understood to be the same as $1x$. We now turn to equations in which the coefficient of the variable is a number other than 1. Some examples of this type are ${}^{-}5x = 20$ and $\frac{3}{7}y = 27$. Consider, first, the equation

$$4x = 24$$

Recall that the term $4x$ means 4 times x. Since the variable x has been multiplied by 4 and the opposite of multiplying by 4 is dividing by 4, the equation can be solved by dividing both sides of the equation by 4 as follows:

$$4x = 24 \quad\quad \text{Check:} \quad 4x = 24$$
$$\frac{4x}{4} = \frac{24}{4} \quad\quad\quad\quad 4(6) \overset{?}{=} 24$$
$$1x = 6 \quad\quad\quad\quad\quad\quad 24 = 24$$
$$x = 6$$

The procedure used in the preceding equation demonstrates the *division principle of equality: If both sides of an equation are divided by the same nonzero number, the result is another equation with the same solution.* (Zero is excluded since division by zero is impossible.) In general, if $a = b$, then $\dfrac{a}{c} = \dfrac{b}{c}$ for any numbers a, b, and c, $c \neq 0$.

Examples:

1. $^-3x = 75$ (x was multiplied by $^-3$, so divide both sides by $^-3$)

    $\dfrac{^-3x}{^-3} = \dfrac{75}{^-3}$

    $1x = {}^-25$

    $x = {}^-25$

    Check: $^-3x = 75$

    $^-3(^-25) \overset{?}{=} 75$

    $75 = 75$

2. $^-17y = {}^-29$ (y was multiplied by $^-17$, so divide both sides by $^-17$)

    $\dfrac{^-17y}{^-17} = \dfrac{^-29}{^-17}$

    $1y = \dfrac{29}{17}$

    $y = \dfrac{29}{17}$

    Check: $^-17y = {}^-29$

    $^-17\left(\dfrac{29}{17}\right) \overset{?}{=} {}^-29$

    $^-29 = {}^-29$

Notice that the number used to divide both sides is exactly the same as the coefficient of the variable.

Q7   Solve the following equations using the division principle of equality and check each of the solutions:

a. $2x = 10$ **b.** $^-4y = 12$ **c.** $4y = {}^-8$ **d.** $^-3x = {}^-7$

•   # # #   •   # # #   •   # # #   •   # # #   •   # # #   •   # # #   •   # # #   •   # #

A7   **a.** $2x = 10$ Check: $2x = 10$

$\dfrac{2x}{2} = \dfrac{10}{2}$ $2(5) \overset{?}{=} 10$

$1x = 5$ $10 = 10$

$x = 5$

b. $^-4y = 12$ Check: $^-4y = 12$

$\dfrac{^-4y}{^-4} = \dfrac{12}{^-4}$ $^-4(^-3) \overset{?}{=} 12$

$1y = {}^-3$ $12 = 12$

$y = {}^-3$

c. $4y = {}^-8$ Check: $4y = {}^-8$

$\dfrac{4y}{4} = \dfrac{^-8}{4}$ $4(^-2) \overset{?}{=} {}^-8$

$1y = {}^-2$ $^-8 = {}^-8$

$y = {}^-2$

d. $^-3x = {}^-7$ Check: $^-3x = {}^-7$

$\dfrac{^-3x}{^-3} = \dfrac{^-7}{^-3}$ $\dfrac{^-3}{1}\left(\dfrac{7}{3}\right) \overset{?}{=} {}^-7$

$1x = \dfrac{7}{3}$ $^-7 = {}^-7$

$x = \dfrac{7}{3}$

7   When the coefficient of the variable in an equation is a fraction, a similar procedure can be followed. For example, in the equation $\frac{3}{4}x = 12$, because the variable x has been multiplied by $\frac{3}{4}$, the equation can be solved by dividing both sides by $\frac{3}{4}$.

$$\frac{3}{4}x = 12 \quad \left(\text{divide by } \frac{3}{4}\right)$$

$$\frac{\frac{3}{4}x}{\frac{3}{4}} = \frac{12}{\frac{3}{4}}$$

$$1x = 12 \div \frac{3}{4}$$

$$x = 12 \cdot \frac{4}{3}$$

$$x = 16$$

The above solution can be simplified if it is recalled by dividing by $\frac{3}{4}$ is the same as multiplying by its reciprocal, $\frac{4}{3}$. Thus, the value of $1x$ (or x) can be found by multiplying both sides of the equation by $\frac{4}{3}$ as follows:

$$\frac{3}{4}x = 12 \qquad \text{Check:} \qquad \frac{3}{4}x = 12$$

$$\frac{4}{3}\left(\frac{3}{4}x\right) = \frac{4}{3}(12) \qquad\qquad \frac{3}{4}(16) \stackrel{?}{=} 12$$

$$1x = \frac{4}{3}\left(\frac{12}{1}\right) \qquad\qquad\qquad 12 = 12$$

$$x = 16$$

The procedure used to solve the preceding equation demonstrates the fourth principle useful in solving equations, the *multiplication principle of equality: If both sides of an equation are multiplied by the same nonzero number, the result is another equation with the same solution.* In general, if $a = b$, then $ac = bc$ for any numbers a, b, and c, $c \neq 0$.

Study the following examples of the multiplication principle of equality before proceeding to the problems of Q8.

Examples:

1. $\frac{5}{7}y = 10$

$$\frac{7}{5}\left(\frac{5}{7}y\right) = \frac{7}{5}(10)$$

$$1y = \frac{7}{5} \cdot \frac{10}{1}$$

$$y = 14$$

Check: $\frac{5}{7}y = 10$

$$\frac{5}{7}(14) \stackrel{?}{=} 10$$

$$10 = 10$$

2. $\frac{^-2}{3}x = \frac{4}{5}$

$$\frac{^-3}{2}\left(\frac{^-2}{3}x\right) = \frac{^-3}{2}\left(\frac{4}{5}\right)$$

$$1x = \frac{^-6}{5}$$

$$x = \frac{^-6}{5} \text{ or } ^-1\frac{1}{5}$$

Check: $\frac{^-2}{3}x = \frac{4}{5}$

$$\frac{^-2}{3}\left(\frac{^-6}{5}\right) \stackrel{?}{=} \frac{4}{5}$$

$$\frac{4}{5} = \frac{4}{5}$$

Q8　Use the multiplication principle of equality to solve the following equations and check each of the solutions:

a. $\dfrac{1}{2}x = 12$　　　　**b.** $\dfrac{4}{5}y = {}^-40$　　　　**c.** $\dfrac{{}^-3}{7}x = \dfrac{5}{12}$　　　　**d.** $\dfrac{{}^-6}{7}y = {}^-3$

#　•　# # #　•　# # #　•　# # #　•　# # #　•　# # #　•　# # #　•　# # #　•　# #

A8　**a.**
$$\frac{1}{2}x = 12$$
$$\frac{2}{1}\left(\frac{1}{2}x\right) = \frac{2}{1}(12)$$
$$1x = \frac{2}{1}\left(\frac{12}{1}\right)$$
$$x = 24$$

Check:　$\dfrac{1}{2}x = 12$
$$\frac{1}{2}(24) \overset{?}{=} 12$$
$$12 = 12$$

b.
$$\frac{4}{5}y = {}^-40$$
$$\frac{5}{4}\left(\frac{4}{5}y\right) = \frac{5}{4}({}^-40)$$
$$1y = \frac{5}{4}\left(\frac{{}^-40}{1}\right)$$
$$y = {}^-50$$

Check:　$\dfrac{4}{5}y = {}^-40$
$$\frac{4}{5}({}^-50) \overset{?}{=} {}^-40$$
$${}^-40 = {}^-40$$

c.
$$\frac{{}^-3}{7}x = \frac{5}{12}$$
$$\frac{{}^-7}{3}\left(\frac{{}^-3}{7}x\right) = \frac{{}^-7}{3}\left(\frac{5}{12}\right)$$
$$1x = \frac{{}^-35}{36}$$
$$x = \frac{{}^-35}{36}$$

Check:　$\dfrac{{}^-3}{7}x = \dfrac{5}{12}$
$$\frac{{}^-3}{7}\left(\frac{{}^-35}{36}\right) \overset{?}{=} \frac{5}{12}$$
$$\frac{5}{12} = \frac{5}{12}$$

d.
$$\frac{{}^-6}{7}y = {}^-3$$
$$\frac{{}^-7}{6}\left(\frac{{}^-6}{7}y\right) = \frac{{}^-7}{6}({}^-3)$$
$$1y = \frac{7}{2}$$
$$y = \frac{7}{2}$$

Check:　$\dfrac{{}^-6}{7}y = {}^-3$
$$\frac{{}^-6}{7}\left(\frac{7}{2}\right) \overset{?}{=} {}^-3$$
$${}^-3 = {}^-3$$

8　The equation $\dfrac{x}{7} = 3$ can be solved in a manner similar to that used with the preceding equations. Using the understood coefficient 1 for x, the solution proceeds as follows:

$$\frac{x}{7} = 3$$
$$\frac{1x}{7} = 3$$
$$\frac{1}{7}x = 3$$
$$\frac{7}{1}\left(\frac{1}{7}x\right) = \frac{7}{1}(3)$$
$$1x = 21 \qquad \text{(this step is usually omitted)}$$
$$x = 21$$

Q9 Solve the following equations using the understood coefficient 1 for the variable:

a. $\dfrac{x}{5} = 2$

b. $\dfrac{^-y}{8} = 2$

• # # # • # # # • # # # • # # # • # # # • # # # • # # # • # #

A9 **a.** $\dfrac{x}{5} = 2$

$\dfrac{1x}{5} = 2$

$\dfrac{1}{5}x = 2$

$\dfrac{5}{1} \cdot \dfrac{1}{5}x = \dfrac{5}{1}(2)$

$x = 10$

b. $\dfrac{^-y}{8} = 2$

$\dfrac{^-1y}{8} = 2$

$\dfrac{^-1}{8}y = 2$

$\dfrac{^-8}{1} \cdot \dfrac{^-1}{8}y = \dfrac{^-8}{1}(2)$

$y = {}^-16$

---

9 It is often necessary to solve equations of the form $^-x = a$ for some number a, that is, equations with a coefficient of $^-1$ on the variable. These can be solved using the multiplication principle of equality. For example,

$^-x = 9$

$^-1x = 9$

$(^-1)(^-1x) = (^-1)(9)$

$x = {}^-9$

Q10 Use the procedure of Frame 9 to solve each of the following equations:

a. $^-x = 5$

b. $^-y = {}^-7$

• # # # • # # # • # # # • # # # • # # # • # # # • # # # • # #

A10 **a.** $^-x = 5$

$^-1x = 5$

$(^-1)(^-1x) = (^-1)(5)$

$x = {}^-5$

b. $^-y = {}^-7$

$^-1y = {}^-7$

$(^-1)(^-1y) = {}^-1(^-7)$

$y = 7$

Q11 Solve the following equations (do step 2 mentally):

a. $^-x = \dfrac{^-3}{5}$

b. $^-y = 0$

• # # # • # # # • # # # • # # # • # # # • # # # • # # # • # #

A11 **a.** $^-x = \dfrac{^-3}{5}$

$(^-1)(^-x) = (^-1)\left(\dfrac{^-3}{5}\right)$

$x = \dfrac{3}{5}$

b. $^-y = 0$

$(^-1)(^-y) = (^-1)(0)$

$y = 0$

This completes the instruction for this section.

7.2   EERCISE

1. Use the addition and subtraction principles of equality to solve the following equations, and check each of the solutions:

a. $x - 3 = {}^-5$ **b.** $y + 9 = 4$ **c.** $7 = y + 8$

d. $x - 9 = {}^-9$ **e.** ${}^-2 = 5 + y$ **f.** $3 + y = {}^-11$

g. $x - 3 = 14 - 23$ **h.** ${}^-5 - 3 = x + 8$

2. Use the multiplication and division principles of equality to solve the following equations, and check each of the solutions:

a. $2x = 10$ **b.** $\dfrac{2}{5}x = 20$ **c.** ${}^-4y = 12$ **d.** $\dfrac{3}{8}x = 24$

e. $\dfrac{x}{5} = {}^-3$ **f.** $5y = {}^-15$ **g.** ${}^-4x = {}^-8$ **h.** ${}^-y = 12$

i. $\dfrac{x}{4} = {}^-4$ **j.** $\dfrac{{}^-5}{7}y = 10$ **k.** $5y = {}^-6$ **l.** $\dfrac{{}^-3}{11}x = \dfrac{2}{3}$

m. ${}^-x = {}^-1$ **n.** $13x = {}^-26$ **o.** $\dfrac{x}{4} = \dfrac{3}{4}$ **p.** ${}^-7y = {}^-5$

q. $\dfrac{9}{16} = \dfrac{{}^-3}{4}x$ **r.** $12 = \dfrac{x}{2}$ **s.** $32y = {}^-4$ **t.** $\dfrac{7}{8}y = 0$

u. $\dfrac{x}{5} = \dfrac{1}{5}$ **v.** $\dfrac{{}^-5}{6}x = \dfrac{{}^-2}{3}$ **w.** $8 = {}^-y$ **x.** $3y = {}^-4$

y. ${}^-7x = \dfrac{3}{5}$ **z.** $\dfrac{{}^-4}{9} = {}^-3y$

3. Use the addition, subtraction, multiplication, and division principles of equality to solve the following equations, and check each of the solutions:

a. $x - 3 = 7$ **b.** $4y = {}^-12$ **c.** $\dfrac{{}^-2}{3}x = \dfrac{{}^-4}{5}$ **d.** $y + 9 = 2$

e. $3 + x = 5$ **f.** ${}^-5y = 25$ **g.** $\dfrac{1}{2}x = 7$ **h.** $\dfrac{3}{4}y = {}^-12$

i. $15 = x - 7$ **j.** $42 = {}^-6y$ **k.** $10 = \dfrac{{}^-2}{5}y$ **l.** $0 = \dfrac{4}{7}x$

m. $x - 3 = {}^-5$ **n.** ${}^-12 + x = 5$ **o.** $x + 7 = 11 - 5$ **p.** $\dfrac{{}^-4}{3}x = 2$

q. $5y = \dfrac{3}{7}$ **r.** $13 = 4 + x$ **s.** $5 + x = {}^-3$ **t.** ${}^-7y = \dfrac{14}{15}$

7.2   EXERCISE ANSWERS

1. a. $x = {}^-2$ **b.** $y = {}^-5$ **c.** ${}^-1 = y$ **d.** $x = 0$

  e. ${}^-7 = y$ **f.** $y = {}^-14$ **g.** $x = {}^-6$ **h.** ${}^-16 = x$

2. a. $x = 5$ **b.** $x = 50$ **c.** $y = {}^-3$ **d.** $x = 64$

  e. $x = {}^-15$ **f.** $y = {}^-3$ **g.** $x = 2$ **h.** $y = {}^-12$

  i. $x = {}^-16$ **j.** $y = {}^-14$ **k.** $y = \dfrac{{}^-6}{5}$ **l.** $x = \dfrac{{}^-22}{9}$

  m. $x = 1$ **n.** $y = {}^-2$ **o.** $x = 3$ **p.** $y = \dfrac{5}{7}$

  q. $x = \dfrac{{}^-3}{4}$ **r.** $x = 24$ **s.** $y = \dfrac{{}^-1}{8}$ **t.** $y = 0$

u. $x = 1$	**v.** $x = \dfrac{4}{5}$	**w.** $y = {}^-8$	**x.** $y = \dfrac{{}^-4}{3}$
y. $x = \dfrac{{}^-3}{35}$	**z.** $y = \dfrac{4}{27}$		

3. a. $x = 10$ **b.** $y = {}^-3$ **c.** $x = \dfrac{6}{5}$ **d.** $y = {}^-7$

e. $x = 2$ **f.** $x = {}^-5$ **g.** $x = 14$ **h.** $y = {}^-16$
i. $x = 22$ **j.** $y = {}^-7$ **k.** $y = {}^-25$ **l.** $x = 0$

m. $x = {}^-2$ **n.** $x = 17$ **o.** $x = {}^-1$ **p.** $x = \dfrac{{}^-3}{2}$

q. $y = \dfrac{3}{35}$ **r.** $x = 9$ **s.** $x = {}^-8$ **t.** $y = \dfrac{{}^-2}{15}$

7.3   SOLVING EQUATIONS BY THE USE OF TWO OR MORE STEPS

1   Frequently it is necessary to use more than one step in solving an equation. Recall that if the variable is x, an equation is solved when it is changed to the form "$x =$ a number" or "a number $= x$." Thus the aim is to *isolate all terms involving variables on one side of the equation and all numbers on the opposite side.* By "isolate" it is meant that *only* terms involving variables are alone on one side of the equation and *only* number terms are alone on the other side of the equation.

In the equation $3x - 4 = 11$ the objective is to isolate the x term on the left side. Since 4 has been subtracted from $3x$, add 4 (the opposite of subtracting 4) to both sides of the equation.

$$3x - 4 = 11$$
$$3x - 4 + 4 = 11 + 4$$
$$3x = 15$$

With the number and variable terms isolated on opposite sides, reduce the $3x$ to $1x$ by use of the division principle of equality.

$3x = 15$ Check: $3x - 4 = 11$
$\dfrac{3x}{3} = \dfrac{15}{3}$ $3(5) - 4 \overset{?}{=} 11$
$x = 5$ $11 = 11$

Q1   **a.** Solve the equation $5x - 3 = 7$ by first adding 3 to both sides.

b. Check the solution to the equation.

•   # # #   •   # # #   •   # # #   •   # # #   •   # # #   •   # # #   •   # # #   •   # #

A1   **a.** $5x - 3 = 7$ (3 was subtracted, so add 3 to both sides)
$5x - 3 + 3 = 7 + 3$
$5x = 10$ (x was multiplied by 5, so divide both sides by 5)
$\dfrac{5x}{5} = \dfrac{10}{5}$
$x = 2$

b. Check: $5x - 3 = 7$
$5(2) - 3 \overset{?}{=} 7$
$7 = 7$

2 In the equation $^-9 = 5x + 6$, since 6 has been added to $5x$, do the opposite and subtract 6 from both sides.

$$^-9 = 5x + 6$$
$$^-9 - 6 = 5x + 6 - 6$$
$$^-15 = 5x$$

With the number and variable terms isolated on opposite sides, reduce the $5x$ to $1x$ by use of the division principle of equality.

$$^-15 = 5x$$
$$\frac{^-15}{5} = \frac{5x}{5}$$
$$^-3 = x$$

Check: $^-9 = 5x + 6$
$^-9 \stackrel{?}{=} 5(^-3) + 6$
$^-9 \stackrel{?}{=} {}^-15 + 6$
$^-9 = {}^-9$

Q2 **a.** Solve $12 = {}^-4x + 8$. **b.** Check the solution to the equation.

• # # # • # # # • # # # • # # # • # # # • # # # • # # # • # #

A2 **a.**
$$12 = {}^-4x + 8$$
$$12 - 8 = {}^-4x + 8 - 8$$
$$4 = {}^-4x$$
$$\frac{4}{^-4} = \frac{^-4x}{^-4}$$
$$^-1 = x$$

b. Check: $12 = {}^-4x + 8$
$12 \stackrel{?}{=} {}^-4(^-1) + 8$
$12 \stackrel{?}{=} 4 + 8$
$12 = 12$

3 In the equation $3 + 2x = 7$, the variable term will be isolated on the left side if 3 is subtracted from both sides:

$$3 + 2x = 7$$
$$3 + 2x - 3 = 7 - 3$$
$$2x = 4$$

The solution can now be completed by use of the division principle of equality:

$$\frac{2x}{2} = \frac{4}{2}$$
$$x = 2$$

Q3 Solve $7 - 5x = 12$ by first isolating the variable term.

• # # # • # # # • # # # • # # # • # # # • # # # • # # # • # #

A3
$$7 - 5x = 12$$
$$7 - 5x - 7 = 12 - 7$$
$$^-5x = 5$$
$$\frac{^-5x}{^-5} = \frac{5}{^-5}$$
$$x = {}^-1$$

---

4 In the equation $^-17 = {}^-8 - 3x$, the variable term will be isolated on the right side if 8 is added to both sides:

$$^-17 = {}^-8 - 3x$$
$$^-17 + 8 = {}^-8 - 3x + 8$$
$$^-9 = {}^-3x$$

The solution can now be completed by use of the division principle of equality:

$$\frac{^-9}{^-3} = \frac{^-3x}{^-3}$$
$$3 = x$$

Q4 Solve $0 = {}^-5 + 7x$ by first isolating the variable term.

• # # # • # # # • # # # • # # # • # # # • # # # • # # # • # #

A4 $$0 = {}^-5 + 7x$$
$$0 + 5 = {}^-5 + 7x + 5$$
$$5 = 7x$$
$$\frac{5}{7} = \frac{7x}{7}$$
$$\frac{5}{7} = x$$

---

5 In the preceding equations, it is important to notice that the *addition or subtraction principles of equality* are used *first* with the *multiplication or division principles of equality* used in the *final step* of the problem. Study the following two examples before proceeding to Q5.

Examples:

1. $$\frac{^-2}{3}x + 7 = 1$$ Check: $$\frac{^-2}{3}x + 7 = 1$$

$$\frac{^-2}{3}x + 7 - 7 = 1 - 7$$ $$\frac{^-2}{3}(9) + 7 \overset{?}{=} 1$$

$$\frac{^-2}{3}x = {}^-6$$ $$^-6 + 7 = 1$$
$$1 = 1$$

$$\frac{^-3}{2} \cdot \frac{^-2}{3}x = \frac{^-3}{2}(^-6)$$

$$x = 9$$

2. $$^-3 = {}^-3 + 4x$$ Check: $$^-3 = {}^-3 + 4x$$
$$^-3 + 3 = {}^-3 + 4x + 3$$ $$^-3 \overset{?}{=} {}^-3 + 4(0)$$
$$0 = 4x$$ $$^-3 \overset{?}{=} {}^-3 + 0$$
$$\frac{0}{4} = \frac{4x}{4}$$ $$^-3 = {}^-3$$
$$0 = x$$

Q5 Solve the following equations by first applying the addition or subtraction principles of equality and then the multiplication or division principles of equality:

a. $3x - 7 = {}^-19$

b. $5 = \dfrac{4}{5}y - 3$

c. $0 = {}^-6 + 12x$

d. $25 = 7 - 2x$

\# \# \#   •   \# \# \#   •   \# \# \#   •   \# \# \#   •   \# \# \#   •   \# \# \#   •   \# \# \#   •   \# \# \#   •   \# \# \#

A5   **a.**
$$3x - 7 = {}^-19$$
$$3x - 7 + 7 = {}^-19 + 7$$
$$3x = {}^-12$$
$$\frac{3x}{3} = \frac{{}^-12}{3}$$
$$x = {}^-4$$

b.
$$5 = \frac{4}{5}y - 3$$
$$5 + 3 = \frac{4}{5}y - 3 + 3$$
$$8 = \frac{4}{5}y$$
$$\frac{5}{4}(8) = \frac{5}{4} \cdot \frac{4}{5}y$$
$$10 = y$$

c.
$$0 = {}^-6 + 12x$$
$$0 + 6 = {}^-6 + 12x + 6$$
$$6 = 12x$$
$$\frac{6}{12} = \frac{12x}{12}$$
$$\frac{1}{2} = x$$

d.
$$25 = 7 - 2x$$
$$25 - 7 = 7 - 2x - 7$$
$$18 = {}^-2x$$
$$\frac{18}{{}^-2} = \frac{{}^-2x}{{}^-2}$$
$${}^-9 = x$$

6   In the preceding equations a variable term occurred on only one side of the equation. If variable terms occur on both sides of the equation, the general procedure used in solving the equation is the same. That is, *isolate all terms involving variables on one side of the equation and all numbers on the opposite side.*

For example, consider the equation

$$3x - 2 = x + 6$$

To isolate the variable terms on the left side, subtract x from both sides:

$$3x - 2 - x = x + 6 - x$$
$$2x - 2 = 6$$

To isolate the numbers on the right, add 2 to both sides:

$$2x - 2 + 2 = 6 + 2$$
$$2x = 8$$

The final step involves the division principle of equality:

$$\frac{2x}{2} = \frac{8}{2}$$
$$x = 4$$

Q6 **a.** Solve $5x - 4 = 2x + 5$ by isolating the terms that involve the variables on the left side and the numbers on the right side.

b. Check the solution.

\# \# \#   •   \# \# \#   •   \# \# \#   •   \# \# \#   •   \# \# \#   •   \# \# \#   •   \# \# \#   •   \# \# \#   •   \# \# \#

A6 **a.**
$$5x - 4 = 2x + 5$$
$$5x - 4 - 2x = 2x + 5 - 2x$$
$$3x - 4 = 5$$
$$3x - 4 + 4 = 5 + 4$$
$$3x = 9$$
$$\frac{3x}{3} = \frac{9}{3}$$
$$x = 3$$

b.
$$5x - 4 = 2x + 5$$
$$5(3) - 4 \stackrel{?}{=} 2(3) + 5$$
$$15 - 4 \stackrel{?}{=} 6 + 5$$
$$11 = 11$$

---

7 Consider the equation $x + 3 = 15 - 5x$. If you decide to isolate the terms involving variables on the left side and the numbers on the right side, you must add $5x$ and subtract 3 from both sides.

$$x + 3 = 15 - 5x$$
$$x + 3 + 5x = 15 - 5x + 5x$$
$$6x + 3 = 15$$
$$6x + 3 - 3 = 15 - 3$$
$$6x = 12$$
$$\frac{6x}{6} = \frac{12}{6}$$
$$x = 2$$

Check:
$$x + 3 = 15 - 5x$$
$$2 + 3 \stackrel{?}{=} 15 - 5(2)$$
$$5 = 5$$

Q7 **a.** Solve $4x + 7 = 2x + 8$ by isolating the terms involving variables on the left and the numbers on the right.

b. Check the solution.

\# \# \#   •   \# \# \#   •   \# \# \#   •   \# \# \#   •   \# \# \#   •   \# \# \#   •   \# \# \#   •   \# \# \#   •   \# \# \#

A7 **a.**
$$4x + 7 = 2x + 8$$
$$4x + 7 - 2x = 2x + 8 - 2x$$
$$2x + 7 = 8$$
$$2x + 7 - 7 = 8 - 7$$
$$2x = 1$$
$$\frac{2x}{2} = \frac{1}{2}$$
$$x = \frac{1}{2}$$

b.
$$4x + 7 = 2x + 8$$
$$4 \cdot \frac{1}{2} + 7 \stackrel{?}{=} 2 \cdot \frac{1}{2} + 8$$
$$2 + 7 \stackrel{?}{=} 1 + 8$$
$$9 = 9$$

8   The preceding problems have been solved by isolating the terms that involve variables on the left side. However, equations can be solved by isolating the variable on either side. You may wish to isolate the variable on the side that makes the coefficient of the variable positive.

Example 1: Solve $3x - 1 = x + 5$ by isolating the variable on the left side.

Solution:
Subtract x from and add 1 to both sides:

$$3x - 1 = x + 5$$
$$3x - 1 - x = x + 5 - x$$
$$2x - 1 = 5$$
$$2x - 1 + 1 = 5 + 1$$
$$2x = 6$$
$$x = 3$$

Example 2: Solve $3x - 1 = x + 5$ by isolating the variable on the right side.

Solution:
Subtract $3x$ and 5 from both sides:

$$3x - 1 = x + 5$$
$$3x - 1 - 3x = x + 5 - 3x$$
$$^-1 = {}^-2x + 5$$
$$^-1 - 5 = {}^-2x + 5 - 5$$
$$^-6 = {}^-2x$$
$$3 = x$$

The same solution was obtained by isolating the variable on either side.

Q8   Solve $5x - 3 = 6x + 9$ by isolating the variable on the left side.

•   # # #   •   # # #   •   # # #   •   # # #   •   # # #   •   # # #   •   # # #   •   # #

A8 $$5x - 3 = 6x + 9$$
$$5x - 3 - 6x = 6x + 9 - 6x$$
$$^-x - 3 = 9$$
$$^-x - 3 + 3 = 9 + 3$$
$$^-x = 12$$
$$x = {}^-12$$

Q9   Solve $5x - 3 = 6x + 9$ by isolating the variable on the right side.

•   # # #   •   # # #   •   # # #   •   # # #   •   # # #   •   # # #   •   # # #   •   # #

A9
$$5x - 3 = 6x + 9$$
$$5x - 3 - 5x = 6x + 9 - 5x$$
$$^-3 = x + 9$$
$$^-3 - 9 = x + 9 - 9$$
$$^-12 = x$$

Q10   Solve by isolating the variable on the side that makes the coefficient of the variable positive:
 a. $2x + 1 = ^-x - 2$ **b.** $^-4x + 2 = 7x + 3$

\# \# \#   •   \# \# \#   •   \# \# \#   •   \# \# \#   •   \# \# \#   •   \# \# \#   •   \# \# \#   •   \# \# \#   •   \# \# \#

A10   **a.**
$$2x + 1 = ^-x - 2$$
$$2x + 1 + x = ^-x - 2 + x$$
$$3x + 1 = ^-2$$
$$3x + 1 - 1 = ^-2 - 1$$
$$3x = ^-3$$
$$x = ^-1$$

b.
$$^-4x + 2 = 7x + 3$$
$$^-4x + 2 + 4x = 7x + 3 + 4x$$
$$2 = 11x + 3$$
$$2 - 3 = 11x + 3 - 3$$
$$^-1 = 11x$$
$$\frac{^-1}{11} = x$$

---

9   To solve equations that involve parentheses, first simplify both sides of the equation wherever possible, and then proceed as before.

Examples:

1. $2x - (x + 2) = 7$
$$2x - x - 2 = 7 \qquad \text{(remove parentheses)}$$
$$x - 2 = 7 \qquad \text{(combine like terms)}$$
$$x - 2 + 2 = 7 + 2$$
$$x = 9$$

2. $x + 5 = x + (2x - 3)$
$$x + 5 = x + 2x - 3 \qquad \text{(remove parentheses)}$$
$$x + 5 = 3x - 3 \qquad \text{(combine like terms)}$$
$$x + 5 - x = 3x - 3 - x$$
$$5 = 2x - 3$$
$$5 + 3 = 2x - 3 + 3$$
$$8 = 2x$$
$$4 = x$$

Q11   Solve by first simplifying both sides of the equation:
 a. $5x - (2x + 7) = 8$ **b.** $6x = 8 + (2x - 4)$

\# \# \#   •   \# \# \#   •   \# \# \#   •   \# \# \#   •   \# \# \#   •   \# \# \#   •   \# \# \#   •   \# \# \#   •   \# \# \#

A11   **a.** $5x - (2x + 7) = 8$
$5x - 2x - 7 = 8$
$3x - 7 = 8$
$3x - 7 + 7 = 8 + 7$
$3x = 15$
$\dfrac{3x}{3} = \dfrac{15}{3}$
$x = 5$

b. $6x = 8 + (2x - 4)$
$6x = 8 + 2x - 4$
$6x = 4 + 2x$
$6x - 2x = 4 + 2x - 2x$
$4x = 4$
$\dfrac{4x}{4} = \dfrac{4}{4}$
$x = 1$

---

10   To solve $2(5x + 3) - 3(x - 5) = 7$, the following steps are used:

$2(5x + 3) - 3(x - 5) = 7$
$10x + 6 - 3x + 15 = 7$
$7x + 21 = 7$
$7x + 21 - 21 = 7 - 21$
$7x = {}^{-}14$
$\dfrac{7x}{7} = \dfrac{{}^{-}14}{7}$
$x = {}^{-}2$

Q12   Solve:
a. $5(x + 6) = 45$

b. $3(x - 2) = x - 2(3x - 1)$

\# \# \# • \# \# \# • \# \# \# • \# \# \# • \# \# \# • \# \# \# • \# \# \# • \# \# \# • \# \# \#

A12   **a.** $5(x + 6) = 45$
$5x + 30 = 45$
$5x + 30 - 30 = 45 - 30$
$5x = 15$
$\dfrac{5x}{5} = \dfrac{15}{5}$
$x = 3$

b. $3(x - 2) = x - 2(3x - 1)$
$3x - 6 = x - 6x + 2$
$3x - 6 = {}^{-}5x + 2$
$3x - 6 + 5x = {}^{-}5x + 2 + 5x$
$8x - 6 = 2$
$8x - 6 + 6 = 2 + 6$
$8x = 8$
$\dfrac{8x}{8} = \dfrac{8}{8}$
$x = 1$

---

11   When solving equations such as $5 - 4(x + 3) = 1$, it is again important to first simplify both sides of the equation by removing parentheses and combining like terms.

Example:

$5 - 4(x + 3) = 1$
$5 - 4x - 12 = 1$
${}^{-}4x - 7 = 1$
${}^{-}4x - 7 + 7 = 1 + 7$
${}^{-}4x = 8$
$\dfrac{{}^{-}4x}{{}^{-}4} = \dfrac{8}{{}^{-}4}$
$x = {}^{-}2$

Q13   Solve:

a. $5-3(x-2)=14$

b. $x+8={}^-10-6(2x-3)$

\# \# \# • \# \# \# • \# \# \# • \# \# \# • \# \# \# • \# \# \# • \# \# \# • \# \# \# • \# \# \#

A13   **a.**

$$5-3(x-2)=14$$
$$5-3x+6=14$$
$${}^-3x+11=14$$
$${}^-3x+11-11=14-11$$
$$\frac{{}^-3x}{{}^-3}=\frac{3}{{}^-3}$$
$$x={}^-1$$

b.

$$x+8={}^-10-6(2x-3)$$
$$x+8={}^-10-12x+18$$
$$x+8=8-12x$$
$$x+8+12x=8-12x+12x$$
$$13x+8=8$$
$$13x+8-8=8-8$$
$$13x=0$$
$$\frac{13x}{13}=\frac{0}{13}$$
$$x=0$$

12   Many times it is necessary to solve equations that involve several rational numbers (fractions). This is usually done by eliminating the fractions from the equation by use of the multiplication property of equality, and solving the resulting equation using the procedures of previous sections.

The fractions can be eliminated from the equation $\frac{x}{2}-4=\frac{x}{3}$ by multiplying both sides of the equation by each of the denominators, 2 and 3.

Example:

$$\frac{x}{2}-4=\frac{x}{3}$$
$$2\left(\frac{x}{2}-4\right)=2\left(\frac{x}{3}\right)$$
$$2\left(\frac{x}{2}\right)-2(4)=2\left(\frac{x}{3}\right)$$
$$x-8=\frac{2x}{3}$$

The first fraction has now been eliminated.

$$3(x-8)=3\left(\frac{2x}{3}\right)$$
$$3(x)-3(8)=3\left(\frac{2x}{3}\right)$$
$$3x-24=2x$$

All fractions have now been eliminated and the solution can be completed using the procedures already studied.

$$3x-24=2x$$
$$3x-24-2x=2x-2x$$
$$x-24=0$$
$$x-24+24=0+24$$
$$x=24$$

Check: $\frac{x}{2}-4=\frac{x}{3}$

$\frac{24}{2}-4\stackrel{?}{=}\frac{24}{3}$

$12-4\stackrel{?}{=}8$

$8=8$

Q14   **a.** Eliminate the fractions from the equation $\frac{x}{2}=5+\frac{x}{3}$ by first multiplying both sides of the equation by 2 and then by 3.

b. Solve the resulting equation   **c.** Check the solution.

\# \# \#   •   \# \# \#   •   \# \# \#   •   \# \# \#   •   \# \# \#   •   \# \# \#   •   \# \# \#   •   \# \# \#   •   \# \# \#

A14   **a.** $\dfrac{x}{2}=5+\dfrac{x}{3}$

$2\left(\dfrac{x}{2}\right)=2\left(5+\dfrac{x}{3}\right)$

$2\left(\dfrac{x}{2}\right)=2(5)+2\left(\dfrac{x}{3}\right)$

$x=10+\dfrac{2x}{3}$

$3(x)=3\left(10+\dfrac{2x}{3}\right)$

$3(x)=3(10)+3\cdot\dfrac{2x}{3}$

$3x=30+2x$

b. $3x-2x=30+2x-2x$

$x=30$

c. $\dfrac{x}{2}=5+\dfrac{x}{3}$

$\dfrac{30}{2}\overset{?}{=}5+\dfrac{30}{3}$

$15\overset{?}{=}5+10$

$15=15$

---

13   A much shorter procedure for eliminating several fractions from an equation is to multiply both sides by just *one* number. For example, rather than to multiply the equation $\frac{x}{4}-3=\frac{x}{5}$ by the two numbers 4 and 5, the fractions can be eliminated by multiplying both sides by *one* number which has both factors 4 and 5. The smallest number with both factors 4 and 5 is 20. Therefore, multiply both sides of the equation by 20.

$$20\left(\frac{x}{4}-3\right)=20\left(\frac{x}{5}\right)$$

$$20\left(\frac{x}{4}\right)-20(3)=20\left(\frac{x}{5}\right)$$

$$5x-60=4x$$

With the fractions eliminated, the solution of the equation can now be completed:

$5x-60=4x$ Check: $\dfrac{x}{4}-3=\dfrac{x}{5}$

$5x-60-4x=4x-4x$

$x-60=0$ $\dfrac{60}{4}-3\overset{?}{=}\dfrac{60}{5}$

$x-60+60=0+60$

$x=60$ $15-3\overset{?}{=}12$

$12=12$

Q15   **a.** Eliminate the fractions from the equation $\frac{x}{3} - 4 = \frac{x}{5}$ by multiplying both sides by the smallest number with the factors 3 and 5.

b. Solve the resulting equation.   **c.** Check the solution.

\# \# \#   •   \# \# \#   •   \# \# \#   •   \# \# \#   •   \# \# \#   •   \# \# \#   •   \# \# \#   •   \# \# \#   •   \# \# \#

A15   **a.** The smallest number is 15.

$$15\left(\frac{x}{3} - 4\right) = 15\left(\frac{x}{5}\right)$$

$$15\left(\frac{x}{3}\right) - 15(4) = 15\left(\frac{x}{5}\right)$$

$$5x - 60 = 3x$$

b. $5x - 60 - 3x = 3x - 3x$

$2x - 60 = 0$

$2x - 60 + 60 = 0 + 60$

$2x = 60$

$\dfrac{2x}{2} = \dfrac{60}{2}$

$x = 30$

c. Check: $\dfrac{x}{3} - 4 = \dfrac{x}{5}$

$\dfrac{30}{3} - 4 \overset{?}{=} \dfrac{30}{5}$

$10 - 4 \overset{?}{=} 6$

$6 = 6$

---

14   The procedure of eliminating the fractions from an equation is called "clearing an equation of fractions." An equation can be cleared of fractions by multiplying both sides by the smallest number that all the denominators in the equation will divide into evenly. This number is called the least common denominator (LCD) for the fractions in the equation.

Q16   Solve the following equations by first clearing them of fractions using the LCD.

a. $\dfrac{2x}{3} - 5 = \dfrac{x}{4}$ **b.** $\dfrac{2}{3}x - \dfrac{2}{5} = \dfrac{2}{5}x$ **c.** $\dfrac{x}{2} + \dfrac{5}{2} = \dfrac{2x}{3}$

\# \# \#   •   \# \# \#   •   \# \# \#   •   \# \# \#   •   \# \# \#   •   \# \# \#   •   \# \# \#   •   \# \# \#   •   \# \# \#

A16   **a.** The LCD is 12.

$$12\left(\frac{2x}{3} - 5\right) = 12\left(\frac{x}{4}\right)$$

$$12\left(\frac{2x}{3}\right) - 12(5) = 12\left(\frac{x}{4}\right)$$

$$8x - 60 = 3x$$

$$8x - 60 - 3x = 3x - 3x$$

$$5x - 60 = 0$$

$$5x - 60 + 60 = 0 + 60$$

$$5x = 60$$

$$\frac{5x}{5} = \frac{60}{5}$$

$$x = 12$$

b. The LCD is 15.

$$15\left(\frac{2}{3}x - \frac{2}{5}\right) = 15\left(\frac{2}{5}x\right)$$

$$15\left(\frac{2}{3}x\right) - 15\left(\frac{2}{5}\right) = 15\left(\frac{2}{5}x\right)$$

$$10x - 6 = 6x$$

$$10x - 6 - 6x = 6x - 6x$$

$$4x - 6 = 0$$

$$4x - 6 + 6 = 0 + 6$$

$$4x = 6$$

$$\frac{4x}{4} = \frac{6}{4}$$

$$x = \frac{3}{2}$$

c. The LCD is 6. The solution is $x = 15$.

15 The steps used when solving an equation with fractions are:

Step 1: Determine the LCD.

Step 2: Multiply both sides of the equation by the LCD. This step "clears" the equation of all fractions.

Step 3: Solve the resulting equation.

Step 4: Check the solution.

Q17 Solve each of the following equations using the preceding four-step procedure:

a. $\dfrac{x}{2} = 7 - \dfrac{2x}{3}$
   b. $\dfrac{7x}{8} + \dfrac{5}{6} = \dfrac{1}{12}$

c. $\dfrac{9}{10} = \dfrac{^-3}{4}x + \dfrac{2}{5}$
   d. $\dfrac{3y}{5} + \dfrac{5}{2} = \dfrac{^-y}{5} - \dfrac{3}{2}$

\# \# \# • \# \# \# • \# \# \# • \# \# \# • \# \# \# • \# \# \# • \# \# \# • \# \# \# • \# \# \#

A17 **a.** The LCD is 6.

$$6\left(\frac{x}{2}\right) = 6\left(7 - \frac{2x}{3}\right)$$

$$6\left(\frac{x}{2}\right) = 6(7) - 6\left(\frac{2x}{3}\right)$$

$$3x = 42 - 4x$$

$$3x + 4x = 42 - 4x + 4x$$

$$7x = 42$$

$$\frac{7x}{7} = \frac{42}{7}$$

$$x = 6$$

Check: $\dfrac{x}{2} = 7 - \dfrac{2x}{3}$

$$\frac{6}{2} \overset{?}{=} 7 - \frac{2(6)}{3}$$

$$3 \overset{?}{=} 7 - \frac{12}{3}$$

$$3 = 3$$

b. The LCD is 24. The solution is $x = \dfrac{^-6}{7}$.

c. The LCD is 20. The solution is $x = \dfrac{^-2}{3}$.

d. The LCD is 10.

$$10\left(\frac{3y}{5} + \frac{5}{2}\right) = 10\left(\frac{^-y}{5} - \frac{3}{2}\right)$$

$$10\left(\frac{3y}{5}\right) + 10\left(\frac{5}{2}\right) = 10\left(\frac{^-y}{5}\right) - 10\left(\frac{3}{2}\right)$$

$$6y + 25 = ^-2y - 15$$

$$6y + 25 + 2y = ^-2y - 15 + 2y$$

$$8y + 25 = ^-15$$

$$8y + 25 - 25 = ^-15 - 25$$

$$8y = ^-40$$

$$\frac{8y}{8} = \frac{^-40}{8}$$

$$y = ^-5$$

Check: $\dfrac{3y}{5} + \dfrac{5}{2} = \dfrac{^-y}{5} - \dfrac{3}{2}$

$$\frac{3(^-5)}{5} + \frac{5}{2} \overset{?}{=} \frac{^-(^-5)}{5} - \frac{3}{2}$$

$$^-3 + \frac{5}{2} \overset{?}{=} 1 - \frac{3}{2}$$

$$\frac{^-1}{2} = \frac{^-1}{2}$$

This completes the instruction for this section.

7.3   EXERCISE

1. Solve and check each of the following:

a. $2x - 3 = 9$ **b.** $15 = 4y + 7$ **c.** $6x + 11 = {}^-7$

d. ${}^-5y + 1 = {}^-4$ **e.** $\dfrac{2}{5}x - 3 = 11$ **f.** $6 = 6 - 7y$

g. $5 - y = 12$ **h.** $6 = 2x + 5$ **i.** $7 - \dfrac{1}{2}x = 3$

j. ${}^-3y = {}^-5$ **k.** $4 + 3y = 0$ **l.** $2 = {}^-3 + \dfrac{5}{7}y$

m. $6 = 9 - x$ **n.** $\dfrac{{}^-3}{4}x - 3 = 5$

2. Solve the following equations by isolating the terms that involve variables on one side and the numbers on the opposite side:

a. $2x + 3 = x + 4$ **b.** $7 + 3x = 4x - 2$
c. $12 + x = 2x + 3$ **d.** $5x + 3 = x - 1$
e. $4y = y + 9$ **f.** $2 - 3y = 2y + 2$
g. $x + 11 = {}^-x + 5$ **h.** ${}^-2y + 3 = {}^-5y + 5$
i. ${}^-7x + 3 - 5x = 0$ **j.** $9 = 3x - 15$
k. $4x - 11 = 2 - x$ **l.** $3 + 4y = {}^-2y + 1$

3. Solve:

a. $2(x - 4) = 10$ **b.** $2x + 3 = 4 + (x - 6)$
c. $6x - (x - 7) = 22$ **d.** $3(x - 5) = {}^-7 + 2(x - 4)$
e. $2(x - 3) - 3(2x + 5) = {}^-25$ **f.** $4 - 2(x + 1) = 2x + 4$
g. $3x + 10 = 7 - 5(2x + 15)$ **h.** $2(3x - 6) + 4 = 22 - 2(x - 1)$

4. Solve each of the following equations:

a. $\dfrac{4x}{5} - 2 = 10$ **b.** $\dfrac{2x}{3} + 3 = \dfrac{4}{5}$

c. $\dfrac{3y}{4} - \dfrac{2}{3} = \dfrac{5}{12}$ **d.** $\dfrac{x}{2} - 6 = \dfrac{x}{4}$

e. $\dfrac{1}{2}x - 7 = \dfrac{2}{3}x$ **f.** $\dfrac{3}{2} - \dfrac{x}{3} = 5 + \dfrac{x}{6}$

g. $\dfrac{3x}{4} - \dfrac{1}{2} = \dfrac{x}{4} + \dfrac{11}{2}$ **h.** $\dfrac{3}{4}x + \dfrac{5}{3} = \dfrac{1}{2}x - \dfrac{1}{3}$

7.3   EXERCISE ANSWERS

1. a. $x = 6$ **b.** $y = 2$ **c.** $x = {}^-3$ **d.** $y = 1$

e. $x = 35$ **f.** $y = 0$ **g.** $y = {}^-7$ **h.** $x = \dfrac{1}{2}$

i. $x = 8$ **j.** $y = \dfrac{5}{3}$ **k.** $y = \dfrac{{}^-4}{3}$ **l.** $y = 7$

m. $x = 3$ **n.** $x = \dfrac{{}^-32}{3}$

2. a. $x = 1$ **b.** $x = 9$ **c.** $x = 9$ **d.** $x = {}^-1$

e. $y = 3$ **f.** $y = 0$ **g.** $x = {}^-3$ **h.** $y = \dfrac{2}{3}$

i. $x = \dfrac{1}{4}$ **j.** $x = 8$ **k.** $x = \dfrac{13}{5}$ **l.** $y = \dfrac{{}^-1}{3}$

3. a. $x = 9$ **b.** $x = {}^-5$ **c.** $x = 3$ **d.** $x = 0$

  e. $x = 1$ **f.** $x = \dfrac{-1}{2}$ **g.** $x = {}^-6$ **h.** $x = 4$

4. a. $x = 15$ **b.** $x = \dfrac{-33}{10}$ **c.** $y = \dfrac{13}{9}$ **d.** $x = 24$

  e. $x = {}^-42$ **f.** $x = {}^-7$ **g.** $x = 12$ **h.** $x = {}^-8$

7.4 LITERAL EQUATIONS

1 An equation having more than one letter (variable) is sometimes called a *literal* equation. The literal equations most commonly used by technicians are *formulas*. Formulas are mathematical ways of representing the relationships between certain quantities. For example, $F = 1.8C + 32$ is the Celsius to Fahrenheit conversion formula studied in Chapter 4. It uses variables to represent that the sum of 1.8 times a given Celsius temperature (C) and 32 is equal to the corresponding Fahrenheit temperature (F).

Q1 **a.** The equation $F = 1.8C + 32$ is called a _____ equation.

  b. The literal equations most commonly used by technicians are called _____.

\# \# \# • \# \# \# • \# \# \# • \# \# \# • \# \# \# • \# \# \# • \# \# \# • \# \# \# • \# \# \#

A1 **a.** literal   **b.** formulas

2 Occasionally we wish to solve a literal equation for one variable in terms of the others. This formula "rearrangement" is done in order to make formula evaluations easier, or to write a given formula in an alternate way so that a different variable can be emphasized.

Example: Solve the literal equation $K = C + 273.15$ for C.

Solution: The equation can be solved using the *subtraction principle of equality*.

$K = C + 273.15$
$K - 273.15 = C + 273.15 - 273.15$ (subtract 273.15 from both sides)
$K - 273.15 = C$

Thus, $C = K - 273.15$. (Notice that this is the Kelvin–Celsius conversion formula of Section 4.4.)

Q2 The equation $R = F + 460$ relates the temperature on a Fahrenheit scale to the absolute temperature on the Rankine scale. Solve this equation for F.

\# \# \# • \# \# \# • \# \# \# • \# \# \# • \# \# \# • \# \# \# • \# \# \# • \# \# \# • \# \# \#

A2 $F = R - 460$: $R = F + 460$
    $R - 460 = F + 460 - 460$ (subtract 460 from both sides)
    $R - 460 = F$

3 Sometimes subscripts (smaller numbers or letters written to the right and below other letters) are used to distinguish between two different values of the same quantity. For example, in the formula $V_1 C_1 = V_2 C_2$ the subscripts are 1 and 2. Read V_1 as V sub-one, V_2 as V sub-two, etc.

The formula $V_1C_1 = V_2C_2$ can be solved for any given variable using the *division principle of equality*.

Example: Solve the literal equation $V_1C_1 = V_2C_2$ for V_2.

Solution: $V_1C_1 = V_2C_2$

$$\frac{V_1C_1}{C_2} = \frac{V_2C_2}{C_2} \quad \text{(divide both sides by } C_2\text{)}$$

$$\frac{V_1C_1}{C_2} = V_2$$

Thus, $V_2 = \dfrac{V_1C_1}{C_2}$.

Q3   Solve the literal equation $V_1C_1 = V_2C_2$ for C_1.

•   # # #   •   # # #   •   # # #   •   # # #   •   # # #   •   # # #   •   # # #   •   # #

A3 $C_1 = \dfrac{V_2C_2}{V_1}$: $V_1C_1 = V_2C_2$

$$\frac{V_1C_1}{V_1} = \frac{V_2C_2}{V_1}$$

$$C_1 = \frac{V_2C_2}{V_1}$$

Q4   Solve the literal equation $Pr = 2ST$ for P.

$$P = \frac{2ST}{R}$$

•   # # #   •   # # #   •   # # #   •   # # #   •   # # #   •   # # #   •   # # #   •   # #

A4 $P = \dfrac{2ST}{r}$: $Pr = 2ST$

$$\frac{Pr}{r} = \frac{2ST}{r}$$

$$P = \frac{2ST}{r}$$

---

4   The conversion formula for Celsius temperatures to Fahrenheit temperatures is $F = 1.8C + 32$. This formula can be solved for C using two principles of equality.

Example: Solve $F = 1.8C + 32$ for C.

Solution: In the equation $F = 1.8C + 32$, the term containing the C will be isolated on the right if 32 is subtracted from both sides.

$$F = 1.8C + 32$$
$$F - 32 = 1.8C + 32 - 32 \quad \text{(subtract 32 from both sides)}$$
$$F - 32 = 1.8C$$

The solution can now be completed using the division principle.

$$\frac{F-32}{1.8}=\frac{1.8C}{1.8} \quad \text{(divide both sides by 1.8)}$$

$$\frac{F-32}{1.8}=C$$

Thus, $C=\dfrac{F-32}{1.8}$.

Q5   Solve the literal equation $p=2l+2w$ for l.

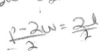

• # # # • # # # • # # # • # # # • # # # • # # # • # # # • # #

A5 $l=\dfrac{p-2w}{2}$: $p=2l+2w$

$$p-2w=2l+2w-2w$$
$$p-2w=2l$$
$$\frac{p-2w}{2}=\frac{2l}{2}$$
$$\frac{p-2w}{2}=l$$

Q6   Solve the literal equation $y=ax+b$ for x.

• # # # • # # # • # # # • # # # • # # # • # # # • # # # • # #

A6 $x=\dfrac{y-b}{a}$: $y=ax+b$

$$y-b=ax+b-b$$
$$y-b=ax$$
$$\frac{y-b}{a}=\frac{ax}{a}$$
$$\frac{y-b}{a}=x$$

5   The *multiplication principle of equality* is used to clear literal equations of fractions before solving for a specific variable.

Example: Solve Boyle's law $\dfrac{P_1}{P_2}=\dfrac{V_2}{V_1}$, for P_2.

Solution: The equation is first cleared of fractions by multiplying both sides by the LCD $P_2 V_1$.

$$\frac{P_1}{P_2} = \frac{V_2}{V_1}$$

$$P_2 V_1 \left(\frac{P_1}{P_2}\right) = P_2 V_1 \left(\frac{V_2}{V_1}\right)$$

$$V_1 P_1 = P_2 V_2$$

With the fractions eliminated, the solution of the equation can now be completed using the division principle of equality.

$$\frac{V_1 P_1}{V_2} = \frac{P_2 V_2}{V_2}$$

$$\frac{V_1 P_1}{V_2} = P_2$$

Thus, $P_2 = \dfrac{V_1 P_1}{V_2}$.

Q7 Solve Boyle's law, $\dfrac{P_1}{P_2} = \dfrac{V_2}{V_1}$, for V_1.

• # # # • # # # • # # # • # # # • # # # • # # # • # # # • # #

A7 $V_1 = \dfrac{P_2 V_2}{P_1}$:

$$\frac{P_1}{P_2} = \frac{V_2}{V_1}$$

$$P_2 V_1 \left(\frac{P_1}{P_2}\right) = P_2 V_1 \left(\frac{V_2}{V_1}\right)$$

$$V_1 P_1 = P_2 V_2$$

$$\frac{V_1 P_1}{P_1} = \frac{P_2 V_2}{P_1}$$

$$V_1 = \frac{P_2 V_2}{P_1}$$

Q8 Solve $\dfrac{C_1}{C_2} = \dfrac{V_2}{V_1}$ for C_1.

• # # # • # # # • # # # • # # # • # # # • # # # • # # # • # #

A8 $C_1 = \dfrac{C_2 V_2}{V_1}$:

$$\dfrac{C_1}{C_2} = \dfrac{V_2}{V_1}$$

$$C_2 V_1 \left(\dfrac{C_1}{C_2}\right) = C_2 V_1 \left(\dfrac{V_2}{V_1}\right)$$

$$V_1 C_1 = C_2 V_2$$

$$\dfrac{V_1 C_1}{V_1} = \dfrac{C_2 V_2}{V_1}$$

$$C_1 = \dfrac{C_2 V_2}{V_1}$$

Q9   Solve $P = \dfrac{2S}{R}$ for S.

\# \# \#   •   \# \# \#   •   \# \# \#   •   \# \# \#   •   \# \# \#   •   \# \# \#   •   \# \# \#   •   \# \# \#   •   \# \# \#

A9 $S = \dfrac{RP}{2}$: $P = \dfrac{2S}{R}$

$$R(P) = R\left(\dfrac{2S}{R}\right)$$

$$RP = 2S$$

$$\dfrac{RP}{2} = \dfrac{2S}{2}$$

$$\dfrac{RP}{2} = S$$

---

6   When variables are used in formulas to represent physical quantities, both capital and small letters may be used. The use of capital or small letters is usually arbitrary but once a formula has gained acceptance in a certain form among scientists or technicians it is necessary to follow it exactly. The formula, $A = \dfrac{1}{2}bh$, for example, has two small letters and one capital letter.

Q10   The formula $V = \pi r^2 h$ has been rewritten below in a number of ways. Circle the correct one.
      a. $V = \pi R^2 h$ **b.** $V = \pi r^2 h$ **c.** $v = \pi r^2 h$

\# \# \#   •   \# \# \#   •   \# \# \#   •   \# \# \#   •   \# \# \#   •   \# \# \#   •   \# \# \#   •   \# \# \#   •   \# \# \#

A10   **b.** $V = \pi r^2 h$

Q11   Solve $A = \dfrac{1}{2}bh$ for b.

\# \# \#   •   \# \# \#   •   \# \# \#   •   \# \# \#   •   \# \# \#   •   \# \# \#   •   \# \# \#   •   \# \# \#   •   \# \# \#

A11 $b = \dfrac{2A}{h}$: $A = \dfrac{1}{2}bh$

$$2(A) = 2\left(\dfrac{1}{2}bh\right)$$

$$2A = bh$$

$$\dfrac{2A}{h} = \dfrac{bh}{h}$$

$$\dfrac{2A}{h} = b$$

Q12   Solve $V = \dfrac{1}{3}bh$ for h.

• # # # • # # # • # # # • # # # • # # # • # # # • # # # • # #

A12 $h = \dfrac{3V}{b}$: $V = \dfrac{1}{3}bh$

$$3(V) = 3\left(\dfrac{1}{3}bh\right)$$

$$3V = bh$$

$$\dfrac{3V}{b} = \dfrac{bh}{b}$$

$$\dfrac{3V}{b} = h$$

---

7   Technicians are often involved with measuring the elasticity (ability to expand) of various parts of the body. A measurement of elasticity, called *compliance*, can be made to evaluate the work of breathing. It gives an estimate of the stiffness of the lungs and thorax. The total compliance is represented in the following formula by the variable C with a subscript of LT. The total compliance consists of the sum of the compliance of the lungs (C_L) and the compliance of the thorax (C_T). The formula is given as:

$$\dfrac{1}{C_{LT}} = \dfrac{1}{C_L} + \dfrac{1}{C_T}$$

Q13   Solve $\dfrac{1}{C_{LT}} = \dfrac{1}{C_L} + \dfrac{1}{C_T}$ for $\dfrac{1}{C_L}$.

• # # # • # # # • # # # • # # # • # # # • # # # • # # # • # #

A13 $\dfrac{1}{C_L} = \dfrac{1}{C_{LT}} - \dfrac{1}{C_T}$: $\qquad \dfrac{1}{C_{LT}} = \dfrac{1}{C_L} + \dfrac{1}{C_T}$

$$\dfrac{1}{C_{LT}} - \dfrac{1}{C_T} = \dfrac{1}{C_L} + \dfrac{1}{C_T} - \dfrac{1}{C_T}$$

$$\dfrac{1}{C_{LT}} - \dfrac{1}{C_T} = \dfrac{1}{C_L}$$

---

8 The conversion formula from Fahrenheit temperatures to Celsius temperatures, $C = \dfrac{F-32}{1.8}$, can be solved for F as follows:

$$C = \dfrac{F-32}{1.8} \qquad \text{The LCD is 1.8.}$$

$$1.8(C) = 1.8\left(\dfrac{F-32}{1.8}\right)$$

$$1.8C = F - 32$$

With the equation cleared of fractions the solution is now completed using the *addition property of equality*.

$$1.8C + 32 = F - 32 + 32 \quad \text{(adding 32 to both sides)}$$

$$1.8C + 32 = F$$

Thus, $F = 1.8C + 32$.

Chapter 4 presented two formulas for Celsius–Fahrenheit conversions. With the ability to solve literal equations, only one formula need be remembered.

Q14 Solve $l = \dfrac{p-2w}{2}$ for p.

•   # # #   •   # # #   •   # # #   •   # # #   •   # # #   •   # # #   •   # # #   •   # #

A14 $p = 2l + 2w$: $\qquad l = \dfrac{p-2w}{2}$

$$2(l) = 2\left(\dfrac{p-2w}{2}\right)$$

$$2l = p - 2w$$

$$2l + 2w = p - 2w + 2w$$

$$2l + 2w = p$$

---

9 The conversion formula from Fahrenheit to Celsius in fraction form is given as $C = \dfrac{5}{9}(F-32)$. It can be solved for F as follows:

$$C = \dfrac{5}{9}(F-32)$$

$$\frac{9}{5}C = \frac{9}{5}\left[\frac{5}{9}(F-32)\right] \qquad \left(\text{multiply both sides by } \frac{9}{5}\right)$$

$$\frac{9}{5}C = F - 32$$

$$\frac{9}{5}C + 32 = F - 32 + 32 \qquad \text{(add 32 to both sides)}$$

$$\frac{9}{5}C + 32 = F$$

Thus, $F = \frac{9}{5}C + 32$.

Q16   Use the subtraction and multiplication principles of equality to solve the equation $F = \frac{9}{5}C + 32$ for C.

•   # # #   •   # # #   •   # # #   •   # # #   •   # # #   •   # # #   •   # # #   •   # #

A16 $C = \frac{5}{9}(F-32):$ $F = \frac{9}{5}C + 32$

$$F - 32 = \frac{9}{5}C + 32 - 32$$

$$F - 32 = \frac{9}{5}C$$

$$\frac{5}{9}(F-32) = \frac{5}{9}\left(\frac{9}{5}C\right)$$

$$\frac{5}{9}(F-32) = C$$

This completes the instruction for this section.

7.4   EXERCISE

1. Use the addition, subtraction, multiplication, or division principles of equality to solve each of the following literal equations for the variable indicated.

a. $K = C + 273.15$, for C   **b.** $F = R + 460$, for R

c. $V_1 C_1 = V_2 C_2$, for C_2 **d.** $V_1 C_1 = V_2 C_2$, for V_1

e. $\frac{1}{C_{LT}} = \frac{1}{C_L} + \frac{1}{C_T}$, for $\frac{1}{C_T}$ **f.** $X = X_1 - X_2$, for X_1

2. Solve each literal equation for the variable indicated.

a. $F = 1.8C + 32$, for C   **b.** $p = 2l + 2w$, for l

c. $V = \frac{1}{3}bh$, for b **d.** $A = \frac{1}{2}bh$, for h

e. $C = \frac{F - 32}{1.8}$, for F   **f.** $l = \frac{p - 2w}{2}$, for w

7.4 EXERCISE ANSWERS

1. a. $C = K - 273.15$

b. $R = F - 460$

c. $C_2 = \dfrac{V_1 C_1}{V_2}$

d. $V_1 = \dfrac{V_2 C_2}{C_1}$

e. $\dfrac{1}{C_T} = \dfrac{1}{C_{LT}} - \dfrac{1}{C_L}$

f. $X_1 = X + X_2$

2. a. $C = \dfrac{F - 32}{1.8}$

b. $l = \dfrac{p - 2w}{2}$

c. $b = \dfrac{3V}{h}$

d. $h = \dfrac{2A}{b}$

e. $F = 1.8C + 32$

f. $w = \dfrac{2l - p}{^-2}$ or $w = \dfrac{^-2l + p}{2}$ or $w = \dfrac{p - 2l}{2}$

CHAPTER 7 SAMPLE TEST

At the completion of Chapter 7 you should be able to work the following problems.

7.1 SIMPLIFYING ALGEBRAIC EXPRESSIONS

1. Simplify by combining like terms:
   a. $3x - 5y - 6x + 4$
   b. $5 - 2r + 2s - 6r$
   c. $4x + {}^-9$
   d. $4m + 7 - 3m + {}^-7 - m$

2. Simplify using the associative, commutative, and distributive properties:
   a. $2\left(\dfrac{3}{4}x\right)$
   b. $\dfrac{^-5}{3}\left(\dfrac{^-3}{5}x\right)$
   c. $2(x - 3)$
   d. $^-4(2x - 8)$
   e. $^-({}^-t + 2)$
   f. $(4 - 2x)5$

3. Simplify:
   a. $(7x + 8) - 8$
   b. $^-2(x + 7) - 3$
   c. $4 - (z + 7)$
   d. $3(x + 2) + 7(x - 5)$
   e. $(y - 6) - (4y + 7)$
   f. $^-7(x + 2) - 2(3x - 7)$

7.2 EQUATIONS, FUNDAMENTAL PRINCIPLES OF EQUALITY

4. Solve using the addition and subtraction principles of equality:
   a. $x + 7 = {}^-11$
   b. $x - 7 = {}^-7$
   c. $12 = x - 3$
   d. $5 - 7 = x + 9$

5. Solve using the multiplication and division principles of equality:
   a. $5y = {}^-20$
   b. $\dfrac{2}{3}x = 12$
   c. $\dfrac{4}{5} = \dfrac{^-3}{5}x$
   d. $\dfrac{5}{9}y = 0$

7.3 SOLVING EQUATIONS BY THE USE OF TWO OR MORE STEPS

6. Solve each of the following equations:

a. $3x - 5 = 7$
b. $5 - y = 12$
c. $4 + 3y = 0$

d. $2x + 3 = x + 4$
e. $2 - 3y = 2y + 2$
f. $6x - (x - 7) = 22$

g. $\dfrac{2}{3}x - 2 = \dfrac{4}{9}x$
h. $\dfrac{3}{7}y + \dfrac{3}{2} = \dfrac{^-y}{7} + \dfrac{35}{2}$

7.4 LITERAL EQUATIONS

7. Solve each literal equation for the variable indicated.

a. $F = R + 460$, for R
b. $X = X_1 - X_2$, for X_1

c. $V_1 C_1 = V_2 C_2$, for C_1
d. $P_1 V_1 = P_2 V_2$, for V_2

e. $F = 1.8C + 32$, for C
f. $A = \dfrac{1}{2}bh$, for b

g. $\dfrac{P_1}{P_2} = \dfrac{V_2}{V_1}$, for P_2
h. $w = \dfrac{p - 2l}{2}$, for l

CHAPTER 7 SAMPLE TEST ANSWERS

1. a. $^-3x - 5y + 4$
b. $2s - 8r + 5$
c. $4x - 9$
d. 0

2. a. $\dfrac{3}{2}x$
b. x
c. $2x - 6$

d. $^-8x + 32$
e. $t - 2$
f. $20 - 10x$

3. a. $7x$
b. $^-2x - 17$
c. $^-3 - z$

d. $10x - 29$
e. $^-3y - 13$
f. ^-13x

4. a. $x = ^-18$
b. $x = 0$
c. $x = 15$
d. $x = ^-11$

5. a. $y = ^-4$
b. $x = 18$
c. $x = \dfrac{^-4}{3}$
d. $y = 0$

6. a. $x = 4$
b. $y = ^-7$
c. $y = \dfrac{^-4}{3}$
d. $x = 1$

e. $y = 0$
f. $x = 3$
g. $x = 9$
h. $y = 28$

7. a. $R = F - 460$
b. $X_1 = X + X_2$
c. $C_1 = \dfrac{V_2 C_2}{V_1}$

d. $V_2 = \dfrac{P_1 V_1}{P_2}$
e. $C = \dfrac{F - 32}{1.8}$
f. $b = \dfrac{2A}{h}$

g. $P_2 = \dfrac{P_1 V_1}{V_2}$
h. $l = \dfrac{2w - p}{^-2}$ or $l = \dfrac{^-2w + p}{2}$ or $l = \dfrac{p - 2w}{2}$

CHAPTER 8

RATIO AND PROPORTION

8.1 INTRODUCTION TO RATIO AND PROPORTION

1   A fraction can be used to compare two quantities or numbers. Suppose that Sally has $13 and Linda has $39. Sally then has $\frac{13}{39}$ or $\frac{1}{3}$ as much money as Linda. When a fraction is used in this way to compare two numbers, the fraction is called a ratio. A *ratio* is the quotient of two quantities or numbers. The ratio $\frac{1}{3}$ is read "one to three" and can be written using a colon as $1:3$.

Q1   **a.** 4 of 7 square regions are shaded. Write the ratio of the shaded regions to the total region. _____

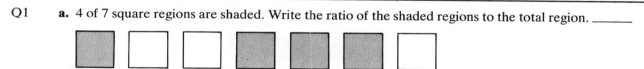

     b. Of the 12 rectangular regions, 5 are shaded. Write the ratio of shaded regions to the total region.

     _____

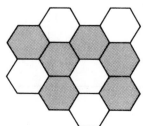

     c. 6 of the 11 hexagonal regions are shaded. Write the indicated ratio. _____

     d. 5 of the 11 hexagonal regions are *not* shaded. What ratio represents this statement? _____

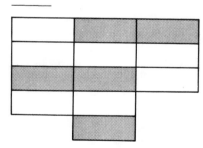

     e. _____ of 6 circular regions are shaded.

     f. Write the ratio. _____

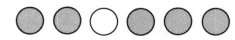

g. 4 of _____ squares are circled.

h. Write the ratio. _____

i. _____ of _____ triangular regions are shaded.

j. Write the indicated ratio. _____

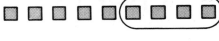

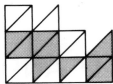

\# \# \# • \# \# \# • \# \# \# • \# \# \# • \# \# \# • \# \# \# • \# \# \# • \# \# \# • \# \# \# • \# \# \#

A1   **a.** $\frac{4}{7}$ or $4:7$ **b.** $\frac{5}{12}$ or $5:12$ **c.** $\frac{6}{11}$ or $6:11$ **d.** $\frac{5}{11}$ or $5:11$

e. 5   **f.** $\frac{5}{6}$ or $5:6$ **g.** 9   **h.** $\frac{4}{9}$ or $4:9$

i. 9, 18   **j.** $\frac{9}{18}$ or $9:18\left(\frac{1}{2}$ or $1:2\right)$

Q2   The comparison of one quantity to another by division is called a _____.

\# \# \# • \# \# \# • \# \# \# • \# \# \# • \# \# \# • \# \# \# • \# \# \# • \# \# \# • \# \# \# • \# \# \#

A2   ratio

Q3   **a.** What is the ratio of 24 years to 9 years? _____

b. What is the ratio of 9 years to 24 years? _____

\# \# \# • \# \# \# • \# \# \# • \# \# \# • \# \# \# • \# \# \# • \# \# \# • \# \# \# • \# \# \# • \# \# \#

A3   **a.** $\frac{8}{3}:$ $\frac{24}{9}=\frac{8}{3}$ **b.** $\frac{3}{8}$

Q4   Find the following ratios as fractions reduced to the lowest terms:

a. 25 to 125   **b.** 25 to 10   **c.** 25 to 5   **d.** 25 to $\frac{1}{5}$

e. $\frac{1}{4}$ to $\frac{1}{2}$ **f.** $\frac{1}{4}$ to 2

\# \# \# • \# \# \# • \# \# \# • \# \# \# • \# \# \# • \# \# \# • \# \# \# • \# \# \# • \# \# \# • \# \# \#

A4   **a.** $\frac{1}{5}$ **b.** $\frac{5}{2}$ **c.** $\frac{5}{1}$ **d.** $\frac{125}{1}$

e. $\frac{1}{2}$ **f.** $\frac{1}{8}$

Q5   The ratio $\frac{1}{2}$ is read "_____."

\# \# \# • \# \# \# • \# \# \# • \# \# \# • \# \# \# • \# \# \# • \# \# \# • \# \# \# • \# \# \# • \# \# \#

A5   one to two

2   Writing the ratio of 2 feet to 15 inches as $\frac{2}{15}$ would be incorrect, because 2 feet is not $\frac{2}{15}$ of 15 inches. Two feet is actually 24 inches, so the ratio is really $\frac{24}{15}$ or $\frac{8}{5}$.

When a comparison between two quantities is desired, the quantities should be expressed in the same unit of measurement. However, the ratio is an abstract number (written without a unit of measurement).

Q6   Determine the ratio of $5 to 40 cents.

\# \# \# • \# \# \# • \# \# \# • \# \# \# • \# \# \# • \# \# \# • \# \# \# • \# \# \# • \# \# \#

A6 $\frac{25}{2}$: $5 = 500 cents, hence, $\frac{500}{40}$

Q7   Express as a ratio:
   a. 15 inches to 2 feet

   b. 10 ounces to 1 pound

   c. 45 minues to 1 hour

   d. a nickel to a dime

\# \# \# • \# \# \# • \# \# \# • \# \# \# • \# \# \# • \# \# \# • \# \# \# • \# \# \# • \# \# \#

A7   **a.** $\frac{5}{8}$:   2 feet = 24 inches   **b.** $\frac{5}{8}$:   1 pound = 16 ounces

   c. $\frac{3}{4}$:   1 hour = 60 minutes   **d.** $\frac{1}{2}$

Q8   Studies indicate that 10 of 12 heroin addicts had histological evidence of alcoholic liver disease on biopsy. Express the ratio of heroin addicts who had histological evidence of alcoholic liver disease, to the total number of heroin addicts which were investigated.

\# \# \# • \# \# \# • \# \# \# • \# \# \# • \# \# \# • \# \# \# • \# \# \# • \# \# \# • \# \# \#

A8 $\frac{5}{6}$

Q9   One of the facts of human reproduction is that almost everywhere in the world, more males are born than females. There are approximately 106 males born for every 100 females. The table below is from Alan S. Parkes, "Sexuality and Reproduction," *Prospectives in Biology and Medicine*, Spring 1974.

   Find the sex ratio for each month:

Sex of Early Human Fetuses

Fetal Month	Male	Female	
2	57	32	**a.** _____
3	253	185	**b.** _____
4	68	58	**c.** _____

\# \# \# • \# \# \# • \# \# \# • \# \# \# • \# \# \# • \# \# \# • \# \# \# • \# \# \# • \# \# \#

A9   **a.** $\dfrac{57}{32}$ **b.** $\dfrac{253}{185}$ **c.** $\dfrac{34}{29}$

Q10   A recent study indicated that 2,600,000 girls aged 15 to 19 have had premarital sexual experience. Of this total about 1,100,000 became pregnant and 830,000 of these had their first pregnancies outside of marriage.

  a. Find the ratio of pregnancies to the total of girls aged 15 to 19 having had premarital sexual experience.

  b. Find the ratio of unwed mothers to pregnancies.

  c. Find the ratio of unwed mothers to the total of girls having had pre-marital sexual experience.

•   # # #   •   # # #   •   # # #   •   # # #   •   # # #   •   # # #   •   # # #   •   # #

A10   **a.** $\dfrac{11}{26}$ **b.** $\dfrac{83}{110}$ **c.** $\dfrac{83}{260}$

---

3   Many ratios are often expressed used the word "per." Such as, miles per gallon, cents per ounce, grams per cm^3, etc. To compute the value of the ratio when the word per is used, it may be helpful to interpret per as "divided by." For example, to find miles per gallon, divide the miles driven by the gallons of gasoline consumed.

Example 1: Determine the miles per gallon if you traveled 140 miles and used 10 gallons of gasoline.

Solution: Miles per gallon means miles divided by gallons

$$\frac{140 \text{ miles}}{10 \text{ gallons}} = 14 \text{ miles per gallon}$$

Example 2: A can of tuna fish costs \$0.45 for 6.5 ounces. Find the cost per ounce.

Solution: Cost per ounce means cost divided by ounces.

$$\frac{\$0.45}{6.5} = \$0.07 \quad \text{(nearest cent)}$$

It is important for all consumers to be able to determine the efficiency of their automobile, by figuring miles per gallon, and to do comparative shopping, by figuring cost per weight.

Q11   Determine the miles per gallon if you travel 220 miles and used 15.8 gallons of gasoline (round off to the nearest tenth).

•   # # #   •   # # #   •   # # #   •   # # #   •   # # #   •   # # #   •   # # #   •   # #

A11   13.9 miles per gallon: 220 miles $\div$ 15.8 gallons

Q12   To determine cost per ounce you would divide _____ by _____.

•   # # #   •   # # #   •   # # #   •   # # #   •   # # #   •   # # #   •   # # #   •   # #

A12   cost by ounces

Q13   A can of corn weighing 12 ounces sells for $0.35. Determine the cost per ounce (round off to the nearest cent).

\# \# \# • \# \# \# • \# \# \# • \# \# \# • \# \# \# • \# \# \# • \# \# \# • \# \# \# • \# \# \#

A13 $0.03: $0.35 ÷ 12 ounces

Q14   Fourteen cubic centimetres of a certain solution weighs 256.2 grams. Find the weight per cm^3.

\# \# \# • \# \# \# • \# \# \# • \# \# \# • \# \# \# • \# \# \# • \# \# \# • \# \# \# • \# \# \#

A14   18.3 g per cm^3

Q15   A local beverage costs $3.19 per 12 pack. If each bottle contains 12 ounces of beer, find the cost of the beverage per ounce.

\# \# \# • \# \# \# • \# \# \# • \# \# \# • \# \# \# • \# \# \# • \# \# \# • \# \# \# • \# \# \#

A15 $0.02: $3.19 ÷ 144 ounces

Q16   A doctor orders 600 ml of glucose to be administered IV to an adult patient in 6 hours. How many millilitres per minute will the patient receive (round off to the nearest tenth)?

\# \# \# • \# \# \# • \# \# \# • \# \# \# • \# \# \# • \# \# \# • \# \# \# • \# \# \# • \# \# \#

A16   1.7 ml per minute: 600 ml ÷ 360 minutes

---

4   A statement of equality between two ratios (or fractions) is called a *proportion*. A proportion is actually a special type of equation. The statement $\frac{1}{3} = \frac{13}{39}$ is a proportion and could be written $1:3 = 13:39$

A proportion consists of four terms labeled as follows:

1st term : 2nd term = 3rd term : 4th term

In the proportion $\frac{1}{3} = \frac{13}{39}$, the first term is 1, the second term is 3, the third term is 13, and the fourth term is 39.

Q17   **a.** A statement of equality between two ratios is called a _____.

b. The four parts of a porportion are called _____.

c. In the proportion $\frac{2}{3} = \frac{10}{15}$, what is the third term? _____

d. In the proportion $1:8 = 2:16$, what is the fourth term? _____

\# \# \# • \# \# \# • \# \# \# • \# \# \# • \# \# \# • \# \# \# • \# \# \# • \# \# \# • \# \# \#

A17   **a.** proportion   **b.** terms   **c.** 10   **d.** 16

Q18   Use colons to write the proportion $\frac{7}{2}=\frac{21}{6}$.

• # # # • # # # • # # # • # # # • # # # • # # # • # # # • # #

A18 $7:2 = 21:6$

Q19   Write the proportion $25:5 = 5:1$ in fraction form.

• # # # • # # # • # # # • # # # • # # # • # # # • # # # • # #

A19 $\dfrac{25}{5}=\dfrac{5}{1}$

---

5   In a proportion, the first and fourth terms are called the *extremes* and the second and third terms are called the *means*. In the proportion

$$\frac{2}{5}=\frac{14}{35}$$

2 and 35 are the extremes and 5 and 14 are the means.

$$2:5 = 14:35$$

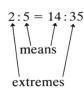

An important property of proportions is that *the product of the means is equal to the product of the extremes.* In the proportion $\frac{2}{5}=\frac{14}{34}$ the product of the means is $5 \cdot 14 = 70$ and the product of the extremes is $2 \cdot 35 = 70$.

Q20   **a.** In a proportion the first and fourth terms are called the _____.

b. In a proportion the product of the _____ is equal to the product of the _____.

c. Name the means of $\frac{7}{21}=\frac{1}{3}$. _____

d. What is the product of the extremes in $\frac{2}{5}=\frac{8}{20}$? _____

• # # # • # # # • # # # • # # # • # # # • # # # • # # # • # #

A20   **a.** extremes   **b.** means, extremes   **c,** 21 and 1   **d.** 40: $2 \cdot 20$

---

6   The truth of a proportion can be determined by using the property that the product of the mean is equal to the product of the extremes. The statement of equality between the ratios will be true only if the above property is satisfied. The proportion $\frac{7}{2}=\frac{14}{4}$ is true because

$$2 \cdot 14 \overset{?}{=} 7 \cdot 4$$

product of means   product of extremes

However, the proportion $\frac{6}{7}=\frac{5}{8}$ is false because

$7 \cdot 5 \neq 6 \cdot 8$

Q21 **a.** In the proportion $\frac{7}{8}=\frac{8}{9}$ the product of the means is _____ and

b. the product of the extremes is _____.

c. Is the proportion true or false? _____.

\# \# \# • \# \# \# • \# \# \# • \# \# \# • \# \# \# • \# \# \# • \# \# \# • \# \# \# • \# \# \#

A21 **a.** $8 \cdot 8 = 64$ **b.** $7 \cdot 9 = 63$ **c.** false

Q22 Express $\frac{7}{3}=\frac{21}{9}$ as a product of its means and extremes.

\# \# \# • \# \# \# • \# \# \# • \# \# \# • \# \# \# • \# \# \# • \# \# \# • \# \# \# • \# \# \#

A22 $3 \cdot 21 = 7 \cdot 9$

7   The property that the product of the means is equal to the product of the extremes, in a proportion, can be developed and generalized using the principles of equality. That is, for the proportion

$$\frac{a}{b}=\frac{c}{d}$$

the means are b and c and the extremes are a and d. The proportion can be written as follows:

$$\frac{a}{b}=\frac{c}{d}$$

$$bd\left(\frac{a}{b}\right)=bd\left(\frac{c}{d}\right)$$ (multiplying both sides by the LCD, bd)

Hence,

$ad = bc$

which states that the products of the extremes is equal to the product of the means. The last equation could also be written

$bc = ad$

Q23 Is $\frac{7}{3}=\frac{21}{9}$ true or false? _____

\# \# \# • \# \# \# • \# \# \# • \# \# \# • \# \# \# • \# \# \# • \# \# \# • \# \# \# • \# \# \#

A23   true: $3 \cdot 21 = 7 \cdot 9$
                          $63 = 63$

Q24   Is each of the following a true proportion?

      a. $\dfrac{7}{14} = \dfrac{21}{42}$ _____   **b.** $\dfrac{4}{6} = \dfrac{20}{24}$ _____

      c. $3:8 = 15:40$ _____   **d.** $6:9 = 48:72$ _____

      e. $\dfrac{15}{20} = \dfrac{5}{4}$ _____   **f.** $\dfrac{9}{15} = \dfrac{72}{120}$ _____

\# \# \#   •   \# \# \#   •   \# \# \#   •   \# \# \#   •   \# \# \#   •   \# \# \#   •   \# \# \#   •   \# \# \#   •   \# \# \#

A24   **a.** yes: $14 \cdot 21 = 7 \cdot 42$ **b.** no: $6 \cdot 20 \neq 4 \cdot 24$
        c. yes: $8 \cdot 15 = 3 \cdot 40$ **d.** yes: $9 \cdot 48 = 6 \cdot 72$
        e. no: $20 \cdot 5 \neq 15 \cdot 4$ **f.** yes: $15 \cdot 72 = 9 \cdot 120$

Q25   Write the proportion $\dfrac{m}{n} = \dfrac{x}{y}$ so that the product of the means is equal to the product of the extremes.

\# \# \#   •   \# \# \#   •   \# \# \#   •   \# \# \#   •   \# \# \#   •   \# \# \#   •   \# \# \#   •   \# \# \#   •   \# \# \#

A25 $nx = my$

This completes the instruction for this section.

8.1   EXERCISE

1. The comparison of one quantity to another by division is called a _____.

2. Find the following ratios in fraction form:

     a. 16 to 8   **b.** $\dfrac{9}{27}$ **c.** 25 to 10   **d.** 6 to 3

     e. $\dfrac{1}{4}$ to $\dfrac{1}{12}$ **f.** 0.2 to 2   **g.** 16 to 64   **h.** 9 to $\dfrac{1}{3}$

     i. 25 to 5   **j.** 6 to 2   **k.** $\dfrac{1}{4}$ to 2   **l.** 0.2 to $\dfrac{1}{10}$

3. Find the following ratios in fraction form:

     a. a quart to a pint   **b.** a quart to a gallon
     c. a yard to two inches   **d.** an inch to a foot
     e. five minutes to an hour   **f.** a day to an hour

4. The American Medical Association (AMA) estimates that more than 22 million Americans alone have high blood pressure, which is a factor in 60,000 deaths a year, and a cause of 1.5 million heart attacks annually.

     a. Find the ratio of deaths caused by high blood pressure to the total Americans that have the disease.

b. Find the ratio of heart attacks caused by high blood pressure to the total of Americans that have high blood pressure.

c. Find the ratio of deaths to heart attacks caused by high blood pressure.

5. The pregnancy of a chronic alcoholic mother is a serious problem. A study of 23 childbirths in women with established diagnoses of chronic alcoholism showed that 4 of the infants died at birth—nearly eight times the rate in a normal control group—and that 6 others suffered from "fetal alcohol syndrome," described to the American Pediatric Society by Kenneth L. Jones, M.D., of the University of Washington School of Medicine, as consisting of stunted growth, smaller head circumference, congenital heart defects, and lowered intelligence.

Find the ratio of childbirths with complications to the number of alcoholic women studied.

6. Diseases of the heart and circulatory system are the leading causes of death in the United States, killing an estimated 1,080,000 of the estimated 2,160,000 people who died in the U.S. in a recent year.

Find the ratio of deaths from heart and circulatory system diseases to the total number of deaths.

7. If you traveled 320 miles and used 22.9 gallons of gasoline, how many miles per gallon is your car getting (nearest tenth)?

8. A can of peas contains 12 ounces and costs $0.44. What is the cost per ounce (round off to the nearest cent)?

9. Five cubic centimetres of mixture weigh 85 grams. Find the weight per cubic centimetre.

10. Which is the better buy? Giant Economy Size $0.98 for 36 oz or Jumbo $1.44 for 48 oz.

11. An adult patient is to receive 1500 ml of 10% glucose IV in 8 hours. How many millilitres will he receive per minute?

12. The statement of equality between two ratios is called a _____.

13. Name the means in the porportion $\dfrac{6}{13} = \dfrac{12}{26}$.

14. Name the extremes in the proportion $1:5 = 7:35$.

15. In a proportion the product of the _____ is equal to the product of the _____ .

16. Which of the following represent true proportions?

    a. $\dfrac{7}{2} = \dfrac{35}{10}$ **b.** $\dfrac{2}{7} = \dfrac{3}{11}$ **c.** $6:2 = 23:8$

    d. $9:11 = 63:77$ **e.** $\dfrac{7}{15} = \dfrac{8}{14}$ **f.** $\dfrac{3}{18} = \dfrac{1}{6}$

8.1 EXERCISE ANSWERS

1. ratio

2. **a.** $\dfrac{2}{1}$ **b.** $\dfrac{1}{3}$ **c.** $\dfrac{5}{2}$ **d.** $\dfrac{2}{1}$

    e. $\dfrac{3}{1}$ **f.** $\dfrac{1}{10}$ **g.** $\dfrac{1}{4}$ **h.** $\dfrac{27}{1}$

    i. $\dfrac{5}{1}$ **j.** $\dfrac{3}{1}$ **k.** $\dfrac{1}{8}$ **l.** $\dfrac{2}{1}$

3. **a.** $\dfrac{2}{1}$ **b.** $\dfrac{1}{4}$ **c.** $\dfrac{18}{1}$

    d. $\dfrac{1}{12}$ **e.** $\dfrac{1}{12}$ **f.** $\dfrac{24}{1}$

4. a. $\dfrac{3}{1100}$ **b.** $\dfrac{3}{44}$ **c.** $\dfrac{1}{25}$

5. $\dfrac{10}{23}$ **6.** $\dfrac{1}{2}$ **7.** 14 miles per gallon

8. \$0.04 per ounce   **9.** 17 g per cm^3 **10.** Giant Economy Size

11. 3.125 ml per minute   **12.** proportion   **13.** 13 and 12

14. 1 and 35   **15.** means, extremes   **16.** a, d, and f

8.2   SOLUTION OF A PROPORTION

1   Since a proportion is a special type of equation, it can be solved using the principles established for solving equations. For example, the proportion

$$\frac{n}{3} = \frac{4}{21}$$

may be solved as follows:

$$\frac{n}{3} = \frac{4}{21}$$

$$3\left(\frac{n}{3}\right) = 3\left(\frac{4}{21}\right) \qquad \text{(multiplying both sides by 3)}$$

$$n = \frac{4}{7}$$

Q1   Solve the proportion $\dfrac{n}{14} = \dfrac{51}{7}$.

• # # # • # # # • # # # • # # # • # # # • # # # • # # # • # #

A1   102: $14\left(\dfrac{n}{14}\right) = 14\left(\dfrac{51}{7}\right)$

$n = 2 \cdot 51$

Q2   Solve the following proportions:

a. $\dfrac{4}{7} = \dfrac{n}{28}$ **b.** $\dfrac{5}{15} = \dfrac{n}{42}$

• # # # • # # # • # # # • # # # • # # # • # # # • # # # • # #

A2   **a.** 16: $28\left(\dfrac{4}{7}\right) = 28\left(\dfrac{n}{28}\right)$ **b.** 14

Q3   Solve the following proportions:

a. $\dfrac{4}{17} = \dfrac{n}{34}$
b. $\dfrac{n}{30} = \dfrac{70}{175}$

•   # # #   •   # # #   •   # # #   •   # # #   •   # # #   •   # # #   •   # # #   •   # #

A3   **a.** 8
b. 12

---

2   The missing term in a proportion can be any of the four terms of the proportion. For example, in the proportion

$$\frac{15}{540} = \frac{2}{n}$$

the missing term is the fourth term. This proportion can be solved using principles of equality; however, the solution is simplified by using the property that the product of the means is equal to the product of the extremes. That is,

$$540 \cdot 2 = 15 \cdot n$$
$$\frac{540 \cdot 2}{15} = n$$
$$72 = n$$

Q4   Solve the proportion $\dfrac{12}{n} = \dfrac{72}{30}$.

•   # # #   •   # # #   •   # # #   •   # # #   •   # # #   •   # # #   •   # # #   •   # #

A4   5: $\quad n \cdot 72 = 12 \cdot 30$
$$n = \frac{12 \cdot 30}{72}$$

Q5   Solve the proportion $\dfrac{2}{n} = \dfrac{6}{15}$.

•   # # #   •   # # #   •   # # #   •   # # #   •   # # #   •   # # #   •   # # #   •   # #

A5   5: $\quad n \cdot 6 = 2 \cdot 15$
$$n = \frac{2 \cdot 15}{6}$$

Q6   Solve the following proportions:

a. $\dfrac{18}{63} = \dfrac{440}{n}$
b. $\dfrac{108}{27} = \dfrac{52}{n}$

•   # # #   •   # # #   •   # # #   •   # # #   •   # # #   •   # # #   •   # # #   •   # #

A6   **a.** 1,540: $63 \cdot 440 = 18 \cdot n$ **b.** 13

$$\frac{63 \cdot 440}{18} = n$$

Q7   Solve the following proportions:

a. $\dfrac{n}{12} = \dfrac{2.5}{5}$ **b.** $\dfrac{0.75}{n} = \dfrac{19}{114}$

\# \# \# • \# \# \# • \# \# \# • \# \# \# • \# \# \# • \# \# \# • \# \# \# • \# \# \# • \# \# \#

A7   **a.** 6   **b.** 4.5

---

3   Various types of problems can be solved by writing the conditions of the problems as a proportion and solving for the missing term. Two general statements will aid in properly placing the conditions of a problem in the proportion.

1. Each ratio should be a comparison of similar things.
2. In every proportion both ratios must be written in the same order of value.

Example: A formula for 1,250 capsules contains 3.25 grams of arsenic trioxide. How much arsenic trioxide should be used in preparing 350 capsules?

Solution: Let *a* represent the amount of arsenic trioxide in 350 capsules and substitute the conditions of the problem in the following proportion:

$$\frac{\text{small number of capsules}}{\text{large number of capsules}} = \frac{\text{small amount of arsenic trioxide}}{\text{large amount of arsenic trioxide}}$$

Each ratio is a comparison of similar things. Each ratio is written in the same order of value. You must decide in your own mind whether the unknown, *a*, is larger or smaller than 3.25 grams. Since *a* is the amount of arsenic trioxide in the smaller number of capsules, *a* must be smaller than 3.25. Therefore, *a* is placed on top in the second fraction. Hence,

$$\frac{350}{1250} = \frac{a}{3.25}$$

$$350 \cdot 3.25 = 1250 \cdot a \qquad \text{and} \qquad \frac{350 \cdot 3.25}{1250} = a$$

$$0.91 = a$$

Therefore, 0.91 grams of arsenic trioxide should be used to prepare 350 capsules. The quantities in the above proportion are *directly* related because an increase in the number of capsules causes a corresponding increase in the amount of arsenic trioxide. Likewise, two quantities are directly related if a decrease in one causes a corresponding decrease in the other.

Q8   If one tablet contains 15 mg of a drug, will it take more or less tablets to fill a prescription of 45 mg?

_____

\# \# \# • \# \# \# • \# \# \# • \# \# \# • \# \# \# • \# \# \# • \# \# \# • \# \# \# • \# \# \#

A8   more

Q9   In a proportion, if an increase in one quantity causes a corresponding increase in another quantity, the quantities are _____ related.

\# \# \# • \# \# \# • \# \# \# • \# \# \# • \# \# \# • \# \# \# • \# \# \# • \# \# \# • \# \# \#

A9   directly

Q10   If one tablet contains 15 mg of a drug, how many tablets are needed to fill a prescription of 45 mg? (Let t equal the amount of tablets needed.)

$$\frac{\text{small no. of tablets}}{\text{large no. of tablets}} = \frac{\text{small amount of drug}}{\text{large amount of drug}}$$

\# \# \#   •   \# \# \#   •   \# \# \#   •   \# \# \#   •   \# \# \#   •   \# \# \#   •   \# \# \#   •   \# \# \#   •   \# \# \#

A10   3 tablets: $\dfrac{1 \text{ tablet}}{t} = \dfrac{15 \text{ mg}}{45 \text{ mg}}$

$1 \cdot 45 = t \cdot 15$

Q11   If 300 cm^3 of a solution contains 2 mg of a drug, how many cubic centimetres will contain 8 mg of the drug?

$$\frac{\text{small no. of cm}^3}{\text{large no. of cm}^3} = \frac{\text{small no. of mg}}{\text{large no. of mg}}$$

\# \# \#   •   \# \# \#   •   \# \# \#   •   \# \# \#   •   \# \# \#   •   \# \# \#   •   \# \# \#   •   \# \# \#   •   \# \# \#

A11   1200 cm^3: $\dfrac{300 \text{ cm}^3}{n} = \dfrac{2 \text{ mg}}{8 \text{ mg}}$

Q12   If 100 capsules contain $\dfrac{3}{8}$ grain of an active ingredient, how much of the ingredient will 48 capsules contain?

$$\frac{\text{large no. of capsules}}{\text{small no. of capsules}} = \frac{\text{large no. of grains}}{\text{small no. of grains}}$$

\# \# \#   •   \# \# \#   •   \# \# \#   •   \# \# \#   •   \# \# \#   •   \# \# \#   •   \# \# \#   •   \# \# \#   •   \# \# \#

A12   0.18 gram: $\dfrac{100 \text{ capsules}}{48 \text{ capsules}} = \dfrac{\frac{3}{8} \text{ gr}}{n}$

Q13   A pharmacist prepared a solution containing 5 million units of penicillin per 10 millilitres. How many units of penicillin will 0.25 millilitre contain?

\# \# \#   •   \# \# \#   •   \# \# \#   •   \# \# \#   •   \# \# \#   •   \# \# \#   •   \# \# \#   •   \# \# \#   •   \# \# \#

A13   125,000 units: $\dfrac{n}{5,000,000} = \dfrac{0.25 \text{ ml}}{10 \text{ ml}}$

---

4   If an increase in one quantity causes a corresponding decrease in another quantity or a decrease in one quantity causes a corresponding increase in the other, the quantities are *indirectly* or inversely related. For example, as the number of workers on a job is increased, the time required to do the work is decreased.

Example: If two workers can paint a hospital wing in 5 days, how long will it take 6 workers, assuming that they all work at the same rate?

Solution: Since the number of days required to paint the wing becomes smaller as the number of workers becomes larger, the quantities vary indirectly. Thus, if N is the number of days it takes 6 workers, N must be smaller than 5. N is therefore placed on top in the second ratio of the proportion.

$$\frac{2(\text{smaller no. workers})}{6(\text{larger no. workers})} = \frac{N(\text{smaller no. days})}{5(\text{larger no. days})}$$

$$6N = 10$$

$$N = 1\frac{2}{3} \text{ days}$$

Hence, it will take 6 workers $1\frac{2}{3}$ days to paint the wing. More specific examples of indirect proportions in health-related areas will be discussed in Sections 8.3 and 8.4.

Q14   Three workers can build a house in 10 days. Will it take 8 workers working at the same rate more or less time to build the house? _____

•   # # #   •   # # #   •   # # #   •   # # #   •   # # #   •   # # #   •   # # #   •   # #

A14   less

Q15   A plane flies from Detroit to Philadelphia in 1 hour and 40 minutes at 440 miles per hour. Will it take more or less time to make the trip flying at 380 miles per hour? _____

•   # # #   •   # # #   •   # # #   •   # # #   •   # # #   •   # # #   •   # # #   •   # #

A15   more

Q16   Eight students sell 3,800 tickets to a football game. Will it take more or fewer students to sell 5,200 tickets selling at the same rate? _____

•   # # #   •   # # #   •   # # #   •   # # #   •   # # #   •   # # #   •   # # #   •   # #

A16   more

Q17   In a proportion, if an increase in one quantity causes a corresponding decrease in another quantity, the proportion is called a/an _____ proportion.

•   # # #   •   # # #   •   # # #   •   # # #   •   # # #   •   # # #   •   # # #   •   # #

A17   indirect

Q18   In a proportion, if a decrease in one quantity causes a corresponding decrease in another quantity, the proportion is called a/an _____ proportion.

•   # # #   •   # # #   •   # # #   •   # # #   •   # # #   •   # # #   •   # # #   •   # #

A18   direct

Q19   If four men can clear the snow near a hospital in 6 hours, how long will it take 12 men working at the same rate to do the job?

$$\frac{4 \text{ men}}{12 \text{ men}} = \frac{\underline{\hspace{2cm}} \text{ (smaller time)}}{\underline{\hspace{2cm}} \text{ (larger time)}}$$

(Let N equal the unknown time and ask yourself, "Is N smaller or larger than 6 hours?" The smaller time must be placed in the numerator and the larger time in the denominator.)

• # # # • # # # • # # # • # # # • # # # • # # # • # # # • # #

A19   2 hours: $\dfrac{4 \text{ men}}{12 \text{ men}} = \dfrac{N \text{ (smaller time)}}{6 \text{ hours (larger time)}}$

Q20   A plane takes 3 hours at a speed of 320 miles per hour to go from Chicago to New York. How fast must the plane fly to make the return trip in 2.5 hours?

• # # # • # # # • # # # • # # # • # # # • # # # • # # # • # #

A20   384 miles per hour: $\dfrac{3 \text{ hours}}{2.5 \text{ hours}} = \dfrac{N \text{ (greater speed)}}{320 \text{ miles per hour}}$

$\left(\text{The problem could have been solved by placing the smaller number on top; that is, } \dfrac{2.5}{3} = \dfrac{320}{N} \right).$

This completes the instruction for this section.

8.2   EXERCISE

1. If an increase in one quantity causes a decrease in another quantity, the quantities are

_____ related.

2. If a decrease in one quantity causes a decrease in another quantity, the quantities are

_____ related.

3. Solve the following proportions:

a. $\dfrac{5}{7} = \dfrac{N}{49}$ b. $\dfrac{49}{98} = \dfrac{7}{N}$ c. $\dfrac{6}{18} = \dfrac{N}{21}$ d. $\dfrac{5}{2} = \dfrac{15}{N}$

e. $\dfrac{4}{3} = \dfrac{N}{21}$ f. $\dfrac{25}{N} = \dfrac{15}{24}$ g. $\dfrac{2}{N} = \dfrac{4}{8}$ h. $\dfrac{3}{N} = \dfrac{18}{27}$

i. $\dfrac{9}{2} = \dfrac{5}{x}$ j. $\dfrac{\frac{2}{3}}{9} = \dfrac{6}{x}$ k. $\dfrac{\frac{1}{2}}{\frac{1}{4}} = \dfrac{x}{\frac{3}{4}}$ l. $\dfrac{0.3}{0.8} = \dfrac{x}{\frac{1}{8}}$

4. If 30 men do a job in 12 days, how long will it take 20 men to do the same work?

5. If the wing area of a model airplane is 3 square feet and it can lift 10 pounds, how much can a wing whose area is 149 square feet lift (nearest pound)?

6. A swimming pool large enough for 6 people must hold 5,000 gallons of water. How much water must a pool large enough for 15 people hold?

7. If a car goes 52 miles on 3 gallons of gas, how far will it go on 11 gallons?

8. If lobster tails are 3 boxes for $3.60, how much will 14 boxes cost?

9. A train takes 24 hours at a rate of 17 miles per hour to travel a certain distance. How fast would a plane have to fly in order to cover the same distance in 3 hours?

10. If electricity costs 10 cents for 4 kilowatt-hours, how many kilowatt-hours could you use for $7.20?

11. If one tablet contains 18 mg of a drug, how many tablets are needed to fill a prescription of 126 mg?

12. If 500 cm^3 of a solution contains 4 mg of a drug, how many mg of the drug are there in 200 cm^3?

13. A solution of digitoxin contains 0.2 milligram per millilitre. How many millilitres will contain 0.03 milligram of digitoxin?

14. The density of a new ointment is 3.2 ounces per cubic inch. What is the weight of the ointment that can fit into a tube that is 2.6 cubic inches in volume?

15. If aspirin contains 15 grains per two tablets, how many grains are contained in a bottle of 100 tablets?

8.2 EXERCISE ANSWERS

1. indirectly   **2.** directly

3. a. 35   **b.** 14   **c.** 7   **d.** 6

    e. 28   **f.** 40   **g.** 4   **h.** $\frac{9}{2}$ or $4\frac{1}{2}$

    i. $\frac{10}{9}$ or $1\frac{1}{9}$ **j.** 81   **k.** $\frac{3}{2}$ or $1\frac{1}{2}$ **l.** $0.046875\left(\frac{3}{64}\right)$

4. 18 days   **5.** 497 pounds   **6.** 12,500 gallons

7. $190\frac{2}{3}$ miles   **8.** $16.80   **9.** 136 miles per hour

10. 288 kilowatt-hours   **11.** 7 tablets   **12.** 1.6 mg

13. 0.15 millilitre   **14.** 8.32 ounces   **15.** 750 grains

8.3 PROPORTIONS USED IN RADIOGRAPHY

1   Radiologists must be able to solve direct and indirect proportions in order to understand and be successful in their work. In working with x-rays, it is important to know the relationships between three quantities each time an x-ray is taken. These three quantities are: the time, t, that the x-ray machine is on, measured in seconds; the current, mA,* flowing through the x-ray machine, measured in milliamperes; and the distance, FFD, from the x-ray machine to the film, usually measured in inches. (With the increased usage of the metric system, centimetres are often used. Both units will be discussed and used in this section.)

    Suppose that the current, mA, the time, t, and the focus–film distance, FFD, have all been determined so that an x-ray is of good quality. If any one of the three quantities is changed the

* In this application mA is a variable and does not mean m times A. In electrical applications, mA is also a symbol used to indicate milliamperes.

others must be adjusted to maintain the same quality of x-ray. If the time is increased the current must be reduced or the focus–film distance increased; if the current is increased the time must be decreased or the focus–film distance increased. If the focus–film distance is increased the current or the time must be increased. These relationships can be shown as ratios and a technician can find the values of each quantity by solving a proportion.

Q1   Identify the following variables:

   a. mA _____

   b. *t* _____

   c. FFD _____

•   # # #   •   # # #   •   # # #   •   # # #   •   # # #   •   # # #   •   # # #   •   # #

A1   **a.** current   **b.** time   **c.** focus–film distance

Q2   Give the standard unit of measure for each:

   a. mA _____

   b. *t* _____

   c. FFD _____

•   # # #   •   # # #   •   # # #   •   # # #   •   # # #   •   # # #   •   # # #   •   # #

A2   **a.** milliamperes   **b.** seconds   **c.** inches or centimetres

2   The first relationship to be considered is that between the current, mA, and the focus–film distance, FFD. If the x-rays emitted at the focal spot, FS, cover an area of 4 square inches when the film is placed 12 inches from the focal spot, then moving the film 24 inches from the focal spot spreads the x-rays over a greater area. As shown on the next page, the new area of the film exposed to the x-rays is 16 square inches. A doubling of the FFD results in the exposed area being 4 times as great. If the time is not increased to keep the intensity of radiation equivalent as before, the current, mA, must be 4 times as great. The current, mA, is directly proportional to the *square* of the focus–film distance. That is

$$\frac{\text{original mA}}{\text{new mA}} = \frac{(\text{original FFD})^2}{(\text{new FFD})^2}$$

   The technician must be careful when the distance is changed to note that the distances themselves are not compared in the ratio, but the squares of each of the distances are compared.

Example: A technician has been taking x-rays at the FFD of 16 inches. The next x-ray must be taken at a distance of 48 inches. What should be the ratio of the original mA to the new mA?

Solution: $\dfrac{\text{original mA}}{\text{new mA}} = \dfrac{(\text{original FFD})^2}{(\text{new FFD})^2}$

   $\dfrac{\text{original mA}}{\text{new mA}} = \dfrac{16^2}{48^2}$

   $\dfrac{\text{original mA}}{\text{new mA}} = \dfrac{256}{2304}$

   $\dfrac{\text{original mA}}{\text{new mA}} = \dfrac{1}{9}$

Which means that if the quality of the x-ray is to remain the same the new current must be 9 times as great as the original current.

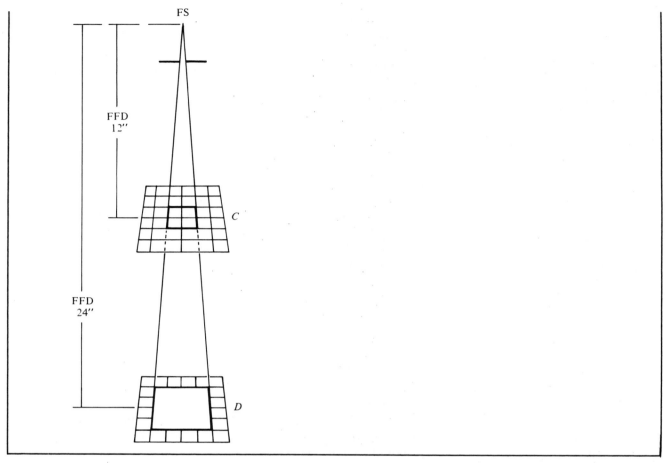

Q3   The film had been 40 inches from the focal spot before a technician moved it to 32 inches. What will be the ratio of the original mA to the new mA in order to keep the intensity the same?

•   # # #   •   # # #   •   # # #   •   # # #   •   # # #   •   # # #   •   # # #   •   # #

A3 $\dfrac{25}{16}$: $\dfrac{\text{original mA}}{\text{new mA}} = \dfrac{(\text{original FFD})^2}{(\text{new FFD})^2}$

$$\frac{\text{original mA}}{\text{new mA}} = \frac{40^2}{32^2}$$

$$\frac{\text{original mA}}{\text{new mA}} = \frac{1600}{1024}$$

Q4   In a given examination the mA employed is 8, and the FFD used is 40 inches. What will be the new mA value at a FFD of 30 inches?

•   # # #   •   # # #   •   # # #   •   # # #   •   # # #   •   # # #   •   # # #   •   # #

A4   4.5 milliamperes: $\dfrac{\text{original mA}}{\text{new mA}} = \dfrac{(\text{original FFD})^2}{(\text{new FFD})^2}$

$$\frac{8}{\text{mA}} = \frac{(40)^2}{(30)^2}$$

$$8 \cdot 900 = \text{mA} \cdot 1600$$

---

3   In actual practice, when the FFD is changed, the current, mA, is usually left the same but the exposure is kept equal, by increasing the time, t. The time is easier to adjust and accomplishes the same result. The ratio of the original time to the new time is still equal to the ratio of the square of the original distance to the square of the new distance. That is,

$$\frac{\text{original } t}{\text{new } t} = \frac{(\text{original FFD})^2}{(\text{new FFD})^2}$$

Q5   The FFD of an x-ray has been 16 inches and the new FFD is to be 48 inches. A technician wishes to keep the same exposure on the film by changing only the time of the exposure. What should the ratio of the original t to the new t be in order to accomplish this?

•   # # #   •   # # #   •   # # #   •   # # #   •   # # #   •   # # #   •   # # #   •   # #

A5 $\dfrac{1}{9}$: $\dfrac{\text{original } t}{\text{new } t} = \dfrac{(\text{original FFD})^2}{(\text{new FFD})^2}$

$$\frac{\text{original } t}{\text{new } t} = \frac{16^2}{48^2}$$

Q6   In Q5 if the original time was $\dfrac{1}{10}$ of a second, what is the new time?

•   # # #   •   # # #   •   # # #   •   # # #   •   # # #   •   # # #   •   # # #   •   # #

A6 $\dfrac{9}{10}$ sec: The ratio of original time to new time is 1 to 9, which means that the new time must be 9 times the original time.

Q7   If the FFD is changed from 25 inches to 35 inches, what is the new time if the original time is 0.2 second (round off to the nearest hundredth)?

•   # # #   •   # # #   •   # # #   •   # # #   •   # # #   •   # # #   •   # # #   •   # #

A7   0.39 sec: $\dfrac{0.2}{t} = \dfrac{(25)^2}{(35)^2}$

$$0.2 \cdot 1225 = 625t$$

$$\frac{0.2 \cdot 1225}{625} = t$$

$$0.392 = t$$

4 The third relationship to be presented is the proportion connecting the current, mA, and the time, t. Assuming that the FFD is kept constant, the current and time vary indirectly. This means that if the current increases, the time must decrease in order for the radiographic exposure to remain the same. That is,

$$\frac{\text{original mA}}{\text{new mA}} = \frac{\text{new } t}{\text{original } t}$$

Example: If the exposure is 2 seconds at 30 milliamperes, what is the exposure time if the current is changed to 200 milliamperes?

Solution: $\dfrac{30 \text{ mA (small value)}}{200 \text{ mA (large value)}} = \dfrac{\text{small } t}{\text{large } t}$

Since the current was increased, the exposure time will decrease, and the new t will be smaller than 2 seconds.

$$\frac{30}{200} = \frac{t}{2}$$
$$60 = 200t$$
$$0.3 = t$$

Hence, the new time is 0.3 second.

Q8 If the exposure time is changed from 2 seconds to 0.5 second, will the current, mA, have to be increased or decreased? _____

\# \# \# • \# \# \# • \# \# \# • \# \# \# • \# \# \# • \# \# \# • \# \# \# • \# \# \# • \# \# \#

A8 increased

Q9 The exposure time is changed from 2 seconds to 0.5 second. What will the new current have to be if the present mA value is 50 milliamperes?

\# \# \# • \# \# \# • \# \# \# • \# \# \# • \# \# \# • \# \# \# • \# \# \# • \# \# \# • \# \# \#

A9 200 milliamperes: $\dfrac{\text{original mA}}{\text{new mA}} = \dfrac{\text{new } t}{\text{original } t}$

$\dfrac{50 \text{ (small mA)}}{\text{mA (large)}} = \dfrac{0.5 \text{ (small } t)}{2 \text{ (large } t)}$

Q10 If the current is changed from 30 milliamperes to 200 milliamperes and the original exposure time is 3 seconds, what will be the new exposure time?

\# \# \# • \# \# \# • \# \# \# • \# \# \# • \# \# \# • \# \# \# • \# \# \# • \# \# \# • \# \# \#

A10   0.45 seconds: $\dfrac{\text{original mA}}{\text{new mA}} = \dfrac{\text{new } t}{\text{original } t}$

$\dfrac{30}{200} = \dfrac{t}{3}$ (exposure time must decrease)

Q11   A certain technique calls for 30 mA and $\dfrac{1}{10}$ sec. If we have an uncooperative patient and wish to

reduce motion by using an exposure time of $\dfrac{1}{60}$ sec, what will be the new mA value?

\# \# \#   •   \# \# \#   •   \# \# \#   •   \# \# \#   •   \# \# \#   •   \# \# \#   •   \# \# \#   •   \# \# \#   •   \# \# \#

A11   180 milliamperes: $\dfrac{\text{original mA}}{\text{new mA}} = \dfrac{\text{new } t}{\text{original } t}$

$\dfrac{30}{\text{mA}} = \dfrac{\dfrac{1}{60}}{\dfrac{1}{10}}$

---

5   Technicians must be acquainted with the techniques of ratio and proportion in order to determine the measurements of objects in a radiograph which may have been magnified in the process of production. One such example is the problem of finding the dimensions of the head of a baby before it is born so that possible problems of delivery, such as insufficient pelvic size, might be ascertained and treatment determined.

Before studying the problem of magnification additional vocabulary is necessary.

FS = focal spot of x-ray tube
FFD = focus–film distance
FOD = focus–object distance
OFD = object–film distance
    J = object
    I = image

Notice that FFD − OFD = FOD

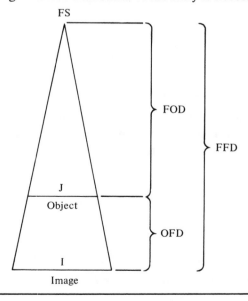

Q12   Identify the following symbols:

a. FS _____   **b.** J _____

c. I _____   **d.** FOD _____

e. OFD _____   **f.** FFD _____

\# \# \#   •   \# \# \#   •   \# \# \#   •   \# \# \#   •   \# \# \#   •   \# \# \#   •   \# \# \#   •   \# \# \#   •   \# \# \#

A12   **a.** focal spot of x-ray tube   **b.** object
       c. image   **d.** focus–object distance
       e. object–film distance   **f.** focus–film distance

---

6   The proportion that is used to relate the above distances is:

$$\frac{\text{image width}}{\text{object width}} = \frac{\text{focus–film distance}}{\text{focus–object distance}}$$

or

$$\frac{I}{J} = \frac{FFD}{FOD}$$

The most common measurement of the fetal head is biparietal diameter. This is, in all but the most exceptional cases, the shortest diameter of the head, and is the easiest to find in a radiograph. The biparietal diameter appears in most views just as the smallest diameter of an egg appears in each shadow of an egg, but the longest diameter does not.

Example: Suppose the focus–film distance of 88 cm was used with the fetal head being 15 cm from the film. If the image of the biparietal diameter is 9.6 cm, what is the actual biparietal diameter of the fetal head?

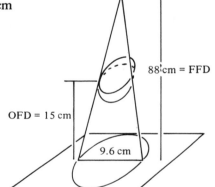

Solution: FFD = 88 cm   OFD = 15 cm   I = 9.6 cm
              FOD = 88 cm − 15 cm = 73 cm

$$\frac{I}{J} = \frac{FFD}{FOD}$$

$$\frac{9.6}{J} = \frac{88}{73}$$

              J = 8.0 cm (rounded off to tenths)

Q13   Using a focus–film distance of 90 cm a technician found that the image of the biparietal diameter was 10.2 cm. If the object–film distance is 18 cm, what is the actual biparietal diameter of the fetal head (rounded off to tenths)?

•   # # #   •   # # #   •   # # #   •   # # #   •   # # #   •   # # #   •   # # #   •   # #

A13   8.2 cm: FOD = 90 cm − 18 cm = 72 cm

$$\frac{I}{J} = \frac{FFD}{FOD}$$

$$\frac{10.2}{J} = \frac{90}{72}$$

Q14   A doctor decides, from pelvic measurements of a pregnant woman, that a Caesarean section would be attempted if the biparietal diameter of the fetus was 9.6 cm or higher. The focus–film distance was 90 cm. The focus–object distance was 70 cm and the image of the biparietal diameter was 12.2 cm. Would a Caesarean section be attempted?

• # # # • # # # • # # # • # # # • # # # • # # # • # # # • # #

A14   no: $\dfrac{I}{J} = \dfrac{FFD}{FOD}$

$$\frac{12.2}{J} = \frac{90}{70}$$

$$J = 9.5 \text{ cm} \qquad \text{(rounded off to tenths)}$$

---

7   The method that has been explained for finding the biparietal diameter has some disadvantages. In order to find the actual dimension of the fetal head, the technician must know numbers not found on the x-ray itself, such as the FFD and the OFD. Therefore, they may become lost. Secondly, the object–film distance is not always accurate or must be taken from another view of the patient.

A second technique that is used to accomplish the same result is to place a measuring rod at the same distance from the film as the object. The measuring rod is then magnified in the x-ray in the same proportion as the object and the actual measurement of the object can be obtained, using the following proportion:

$$\frac{\text{actual measuring rod}}{\text{image of measuring rod}} = \frac{\text{actual diameter}}{\text{image of diameter}}$$

Example: Suppose a calibrated measuring rod which actually is 10 cm appears on an x-ray to be 12.2 cm. What would the actual biparietal diameter of a fetal head be if it measures 9.8 cm on the same x-ray?

Solution: $\dfrac{\text{actual measuring rod}}{\text{image of measuring rod}} = \dfrac{\text{actual diameter}}{\text{image of diameter}}$

$$\frac{10}{12.2} = \frac{n}{9.8}$$

$$n = 8.0 \text{ cm} \qquad \text{(rounded off to tenths)}$$

Q15   The image of the biparietal diameter of the fetal head measures 11.8 cm on the x-ray. A 10 cm measuring rod on the same x-ray measures 12.5 cm. What is the actual biparietal diameter of the fetal head?

• # # # • # # # • # # # • # # # • # # # • # # # • # # # • # #

A15   9.4 cm: $\dfrac{\text{actual measuring rod}}{\text{image of measuring rod}} = \dfrac{\text{actual diameter}}{\text{image of diameter}}$

$$\frac{10}{12.5} = \frac{n}{11.8}$$

Q16 The pelvic measurements of a pregnant woman indicate that if the fetal head has a biparietal diameter of 9.2 cm or higher she might have complications with the delivery. At the full term of her pregnancy, x-rays are taken and the image of the biparietal diameter is 10.5 cm. In the same x-ray the image of a 10 cm measuring rod is 12.8 cm. Should the doctor prepare for complications?

• # # # • # # # • # # # • # # # • # # # • # # # • # # # • # #

A16 no: $\dfrac{\text{actual measuring rod}}{\text{image of measuring rod}} = \dfrac{\text{actual diameter}}{\text{image of diameter}}$

$$\frac{10}{12.8} = \frac{n}{10.5}$$

$$n = 8.2 \text{ cm}$$

This completes the instruction for this section.

8.3   EXERCISE

1. Identify the variables:
   a. mA   **b.** t **c.** FFD   **d.** FS   **e.** J   **f.** I   **g.** FOD   **h.** OFD

2. As the focus–film distance is increased the current must be _____ (assuming time remains constant).

3. The current, mA, is directly proportional to the _____ of the focus–film distance, FFD.

4. If the focus–film distance is increased, and the current is kept constant, then the time must be

   _____ .

5. If the focus–film distance is kept constant and the time is decreased, then the current must be

   _____ .

6. The current and time are directly/indirectly related.

7. Find the ratio of the original time to the new time of exposure if the focus–film distance is changed from 40 inches to a new distance of 25 inches.

8. Find the ratio of the new time of exposure to the old time of exposure if the current is to be changed from 50 milliamperes to 175 milliamperes.

9. In a given examination the mA employed is 10, and the FFD is 6 feet. What will be the new mA value at an FFD of 8 feet (rounded off to the nearest tenth)?

10. If the FFD is changed from 30 cm to 20 cm, what is the time of exposure if the original time was 2 seconds (rounded off to the nearest hundredth)?

11. The exposure time is changed from 2 seconds to 0.5 sec. What will the new mA value have to be if the original mA value is 50 milliamperes (rounded off to the nearest tenth)?

12. If the current is changed from 40 milliamperes to 150 milliamperes and the original exposure time is 3 seconds, what will be the new exposure time?

13. Using a focus–film distance of 80 cm a technician found that the image of the biparietal diameter was 10.2 cm. If the object–film distance is 16 cm, what is the actual biparietal diameter of the fetal head (rounded off to the nearest tenth)?

14. The image of the biparietal diameter of a fetal head measures 10.2 cm on the x-ray. A 10 cm measuring rod on the same x-ray measures 11.8 cm. What is the actual biparietal diameter of the fetal head (rounded off to the nearest tenth)?

15. A doctor determines from pelvic measurements of a pregnant woman that complications could develop in delivery if the fetal biparietal diameter is 8.5 cm or higher. When she is ready to deliver, x-rays indicate the image of the biparietal diameter is 11.2 cm. In the same x-ray the image of a 10 cm rod is 12.8 cm. Should the doctor prepare for complications?

8.3 EXERCISE ANSWERS

1. a. current   **b.** time   **c.** focus–film distance
    d. focal spot   **e.** object   **f.** image
    g. focus–object distance   **h.** object–film distance

2. increased   **3.** square   **4.** increased

5. increased   **6.** indirectly   **7.** $\dfrac{64}{25}$

8. $\dfrac{2}{7}$ **9.** 17.8 milliamperes   **10.** 0.89 sec

11. 200 milliamperes   **12.** 0.8 sec   **13.** 8.2 cm

14. 8.6 cm   **15.** yes: actual diameter = 8.8 cm

8.4 RATIO AND PROPORTION FOR INHALATION THERAPISTS

---

1   Inhalation technicians, as well as certain other medical specialists, must be able to relate *pressure*, *volume*, and *temperature*, which are critical when various gases must be supplied to a patient. To get a feeling for the three variables mentioned, think of a bicycle pump with a handle that goes up and down, building pressure in the bottom of the pump. As the pressure builds air is transferred to the tire through a rubber hose. If the hose is plugged for some reason would you still be able to push the handle down? You would, but two things would happen. The air in the pump would be compressed into a smaller volume and the temperature of the air would rise. You may have noticed how hot the pump gets after extended use. These two results illustrate that as pressure increases, volume decreases, and secondly, as pressure increases, temperature increases.

     The *pressure–volume* relationship is an indirect proportion and can be written as:

$$\frac{\text{original pressure}}{\text{new pressure}} = \frac{\text{new volume}}{\text{original volume}}$$

Q1   **a.** As the pressure increases the volume of a gas _____ .

     b. As the pressure increases the temperature of a gas _____ .

     c. Pressure and volume are directly/indirectly related _____ .

     d. Pressure and temperature are directly/indirectly related _____ .

\# \# \# • \# \# \# • \# \# \# • \# \# \# • \# \# \# • \# \# \# • \# \# \# • \# \# \# • \# \# \#

A1   **a.** decreases   **b.** increases   **c.** indirectly   **d.** directly

---

2   The pressure–volume relationship

$$\frac{\text{original pressure}}{\text{new pressure}} = \frac{\text{new volume}}{\text{original volume}}$$

is usually written

$$\frac{P_1}{P_2}=\frac{V_2}{V_1},$$

where a subscript of 1 represents the original value and a subscript of 2 represents the new value.

Example: If 100 ml of oxygen is under a pressure of 760 mm of mercury, what would be the volume if the pressure is increased to 840 mm of mercury?

Solution: $\frac{P_1}{P_2}=\frac{V_2}{V_1}$

$$\frac{760}{840}=\frac{V_2}{100}$$

$V_2 = 90.5$ ml (rounded off to tenths)

Q2   If the pressure of a gas is decreased, the volume will _____ .

\# \# \#   •   \# \# \#   •   \# \# \#   •   \# \# \#   •   \# \# \#   •   \# \# \#   •   \# \# \#   •   \# \# \#   •   \# \# \#

A2   increase

Q3   If 250 ml of a gas is under a pressure of 820 mm, what would be the volume if the pressure is changed to 500 mm (nearest tenth)?

\# \# \#   •   \# \# \#   •   \# \# \#   •   \# \# \#   •   \# \# \#   •   \# \# \#   •   \# \# \#   •   \# \# \#   •   \# \# \#

A3   410 ml: $\frac{P_1}{P_2}=\frac{V_2}{V_1}$

$$\frac{820}{500}=\frac{V_2}{250}$$

Q4   If 27.3 l of a gas is under a pressure of 7 m, what would be the volume if the pressure is changed to 18 m (nearest tenth)?

\# \# \#   •   \# \# \#   •   \# \# \#   •   \# \# \#   •   \# \# \#   •   \# \# \#   •   \# \# \#   •   \# \# \#   •   \# \# \#

A4   10.6 l: $\frac{P_1}{P_2}=\frac{V_2}{V_1}$

$$\frac{7}{18}=\frac{V_2}{27.3}$$

Q5   If the volume of a gas is decreased is the pressure increased or decreased? _____

\# \# \#   •   \# \# \#   •   \# \# \#   •   \# \# \#   •   \# \# \#   •   \# \# \#   •   \# \# \#   •   \# \# \#   •   \# \# \#

A5   increased

Q6 If 400 ml of oxygen is under a pressure of 2800 mm of mercury, what would be the pressure if the volume is changed to 700 ml?

\# \# \#　•　\# \# \#　•　\# \# \#　•　\# \# \#　•　\# \# \#　•　\# \# \#　•　\# \# \#　•　\# \# \#　•　\# \# \#

A6 1600 mm:
$$\frac{P_1}{P_2} = \frac{V_2}{V_1}$$
$$\frac{2800}{P_2} = \frac{700}{400}$$

3　As previously mentioned, the *pressure–temperature* relationship is a direct proportion. That is, as the pressure is increased the temperature of the gas is also increased. Using a proportion the relationship can be expressed as

$$\frac{\text{original pressure}}{\text{new pressure}} = \frac{\text{original temperature}}{\text{new temperature}}$$

Or, using variables and subscripts, as

$$\frac{P_1}{P_2} = \frac{T_1}{T_2}.$$

The pressure–temperature relationship is valid only if the temperature is expressed using absolute temperature on the *Kelvin* scale. Recall that a Celsius temperature is converted to a Kelvin temperature by adding 273.15° to the Celsius temperature. For use in the section, it will be sufficient to add 273° to the Celsius temperature. That is, $K = °C + 273°$.

Example: A gas is under a pressure of 760 mm of mercury at 37 °C. If the pressure is increased to 800 mm of mercury, what would the new absolute temperature be?

Solution: The Celsius temperature must first be converted to absolute temperature on the Kelvin scale.

$$T_1 = 37\,°C + 273° = 310\,K$$

The new temperature can now be found using

$$\frac{P_1}{P_2} = \frac{T_1}{T_2}$$
$$\frac{760}{800} = \frac{310\,K}{T_2}$$
$$T_2 = 326\,K \quad \text{(rounded off to the nearest degree)}$$

The temperature could be converted to the Celsius scale by subtracting 273°.

$$T_2 = 326\,K - 273° = 53\,°C$$

Q7　**a.** As the pressure of a gas is increased the temperature is _____ .

　　b. Decreasing the temperature of a gas will cause the pressure to _____ .

\# \# \#　•　\# \# \#　•　\# \# \#　•　\# \# \#　•　\# \# \#　•　\# \# \#　•　\# \# \#　•　\# \# \#　•　\# \# \#

A7　**a.** increased　　　　**b.** decrease

Q8   Convert the temperature from Celsius to Kelvin, or conversely:

a. $82\,°C =$ _____   **b.** $273\,K =$ _____   **c.** $0\,K =$ _____

\# \# \# • \# \# \# • \# \# \# • \# \# \# • \# \# \# • \# \# \# • \# \# \# • \# \# \# • \# \# \#

A8   **a.** 355 K   **b.** 0 °C   **c.** ⁻273 °C

Q9   A gas is under a pressure of 760 mm of mercury at 30 °C. If the temperature is decreased to 0 °C, find the new pressure (round off to the nearest tenth).

\# \# \# • \# \# \# • \# \# \# • \# \# \# • \# \# \# • \# \# \# • \# \# \# • \# \# \# • \# \# \#

A9   684.8 mm: $T_1 = 30\,°C + 273° = 303\,K$
$T_2 = 0\,°C + 273° = 273\,K$

$$\frac{P_1}{P_2} = \frac{T_1}{T_2}$$

$$\frac{760}{P_2} = \frac{303\,K}{273\,K}$$

---

4   Under a constant pressure the volume of a gas is directly proportional to the absolute temperature also. As the temperature is increased, the volume increases, or as the volume changes the temperature changes also. The *volume–temperature* relationship can be expressed as

$$\frac{V_1}{V_2} = \frac{T_1}{T_2}$$

Example: Suppose that 100 millilitres of gas is at a temperature of 37 °C. If the temperature is increased to 60 °C, what would be the new volume, if the pressure remains constant?

Solution: The Celsius temperature must first be converted to absolute temperature on the Kelvin scale.

$T_1 = 37\,°C + 273° = 310\,K,$ $T_2 = 60\,°C + 273° = 333\,K$

Then,

$$\frac{V_1}{V_2} = \frac{T_1}{T_2}$$

$$\frac{100}{V_2} = \frac{310\,K}{333\,K}$$

$V_2 = 107.4\,ml$ (rounded off to tenths)

Q10   As the volume of a gas is decreased, the temperature is _____ .

\# \# \# • \# \# \# • \# \# \# • \# \# \# • \# \# \# • \# \# \# • \# \# \# • \# \# \# • \# \# \#

A10   decreased

Q11   One hundred millilitres of gass is at a temperature of ¯10 °C. Find the new volume if the temperature is increased to 40 °C (round off to the nearest tenth).

• # # # • # # # • # # # • # # # • # # # • # # # • # # # • # #

A11   119.0 ml: $T_1 = ¯10\,°C + 273° = 263\ K$
$T_2 = 40\,°C + 273° = 313\ K$

$$\frac{V_1}{V_2} = \frac{T_1}{T_2}$$

$$\frac{100}{V_2} = \frac{263\ K}{313\ K}$$

---

5   It is possible for more than one of the variables that have been discussed to change at the same time. For example, the pressure and temperature could both be changed which would then change the volume. The proportion stating the relationship between the *pressure–temperature–volume* of a gas is

$$\frac{P_1 V_1}{T_1} = \frac{P_2 V_2}{T_2}$$

If you know any five of the six variables you can solve the proportion for the sixth.

Example: Find the new volume if 22 l of oxygen at 15 °C and 730 mm of mercury are converted to 5 °C and 800 mm of mercury.

Solution: $T_1 = 15\,°C + 273° = 288\ K$, $T_2 = 5\,°C + 273° = 278\ K$

$$\frac{P_1 V_1}{T_1} = \frac{P_2 V_2}{T_2}$$
$$\frac{730 \cdot 22}{288} = \frac{800 \cdot V_2}{278}$$
$$730 \cdot 22 \cdot 278 = 288 \cdot 800 \cdot V_2$$

$V_2 = 19.4\ l$ (rounded off to tenths)

Q12   Find the new pressure if 2.5 l of helium at 18 °C and 760 mm of mercury are converted to 37 °C and a volume of 2 l.

$P_1 = 760mm$
$T_1 = 18°C$
$P_2 = x$
$V_1 = 2.5\ L$
$T_2 = 37°C$
$V_2 = 2L$

$$\frac{(2.5)(760)}{18+273} = \frac{(2)(x)}{37+273}$$

$$\frac{1900}{291} = \frac{2x}{310}$$

$$\frac{289000}{1842} = \frac{1842x}{1842}$$

• # # # • # # # • # # # • # # # • # # # • # # # • # # # • # #

A12   1012.0 mm: $T_1 = 18\,°C + 273° = 291\text{ K}$

$$T_2 = 37\,°C + 273° = 310\text{ K}$$

$$\frac{P_1 V_1}{T_1} = \frac{P_2 V_2}{T_2}$$

$$\frac{760 \cdot 2.5}{291} = \frac{P_2 \cdot 2}{310}$$

---

6   Inhalation therapists often work with medications that must be diluted or they must otherwise change the concentration of commercially prepared medications. For this reason, it is necessary to carefully study the material presented in Section 8.5, where this technique is thoroughly discussed.

This completes the instruction for this section.

8.4   EXERCISE

1. As the pressure of a gas increases the volume _____ .

2. As the volume of a gas decreases the pressure _____ .

3. The temperature–pressure relationship, for a certain gas, is an example of a(an) direct/indirect proportion.

4. Using subscripts, express the following relationship as a proportion: **a.** pressure–volume; **b.** pressure–temperature; **c.** temperature volume; **d.** pressure–temperature–volume.

5. If 250 ml of a gas is under a pressure of 800 mm of mercury, what would be the volume if the pressure is changed to 500 mm (nearest tenth)?

6. A gas is under a pressure of 800 mm of mercury at 25 °C. If the temperature is increased to 60 °C, find the new pressure (round off to the nearest tenth).

7. One hundred fifty millilitres of gas is at a room temperature of 20 °C. Find the new volume if the temperature is decreased to 0 °C (round off to the nearest tenth).

8. One hundred twenty millilitres of gas is at a temperature of 30 °C. What would the temperature have to be to increase the volume to 500 ml (round off to the nearest tenth)?

9. Convert 2.0 litres of helium at 20 °C and 760 mm of mercury to 37 °C and a volume of 2.5 litres. What is the new pressure?

10. One hundred fifty millilitres of gas is at a temperature of 10 °C. Find the new volume if the temperature is increased to 60 °C (round off to the nearest tenth).

8.4   EXERCISE ANSWERS

1. decreases   **2.** increases   **3.** direct

4. a. $\dfrac{P_1}{P_2} = \dfrac{V_2}{V_1}$ **b.** $\dfrac{P_1}{P_2} = \dfrac{T_1}{T_2}$

    c. $\dfrac{T_1}{T_2} = \dfrac{V_1}{V_2}$ **d.** $\dfrac{P_1 V_1}{T_1} = \dfrac{P_2 V_2}{T_2}$

5. 400 ml   **6.** 894.0 mm   **7.** 139.8 ml

8. 1262.5 K or 989.5 °C   **9.** 643.3 mm   **10.** 176.5 ml

8.5   SOLUTIONS AND DOSAGES

1   One of the skills which is required of technicians in the health field is the ability to prepare solutions of varying strengths. If the desired solution is not on hand, the solution must be prepared either by diluting a pure drug (usually with sterile water) or diluting a solution which is on hand.

Strengths of solutions are generally expressed with a ratio or a percent.

Example: A $1:10$ (read 1 to 10) solution means that there is 1 part of the drug and 9 parts of water to make a total of 10 parts of solution.

Example 2: A 20% solution means that there are 20 parts of the drug and 80 parts of water to make a total of 100 parts of solution.

Q1   Fill in the blanks:

a. A $1:40$ solution means that there is _____ part of the drug and _____ parts of water to make a

total of _____ parts of the solution.

b. A 25% solution means that there _____ parts of the drug and _____ parts of water to make a

total of _____ parts of the solution.

\# \# \#   •   \# \# \#   •   \# \# \#   •   \# \# \#   •   \# \# \#   •   \# \# \#   •   \# \# \#   •   \# \# \#   •   \# \# \#

A1   **a.** 1, 39, 40   **b.** 25, 75, 100

Q2   Fill in the blanks:

a. A $7:50$ solution means that there are _____ parts of the drug and _____ parts of water to make a total of _____ parts of solution.

b. A 15% solution means that there are _____ parts of the drug and _____ parts of water to make a total of _____ parts of solution.

\# \# \#   •   \# \# \#   •   \# \# \#   •   \# \# \#   •   \# \# \#   •   \# \# \#   •   \# \# \#   •   \# \# \#   •   \# \# \#

A2   **a.** 7, 43, 50   **b.** 15, 85, 100

2   Consider the following order to prepare a solution: Prepare 250 ml of 15% cresol solution from pure liquid cresol. The information which is important for filling the order is:

1. The *desired strength* of the solution. The desired strength of the solution to be prepared is 15%.
2. The *strength* of the drug that is *available* to make the solution. Since the drug is pure, the strength of the available drug is 100%.
3. The amount of the available *drug to use* to prepare the solution. The amount of drug to use to prepare the solution is the "unknown" quantity of the problem. It will be represented by the letter x.
4. The amount of *solution to make*. The order calls for the preparation of 250 ml of solution.

Q3   Answer each question about the following order. Prepare 250 ml of 4% boric acid solution from boric acid crystals.

a. What is the desired strength? _____

b. What is the strength of the available drug? _____

c. What amount of the available drug should be used to prepare the solution? _____

d. How much solution is to be made? _____

\# \# \#   •   \# \# \#   •   \# \# \#   •   \# \# \#   •   \# \# \#   •   \# \# \#   •   \# \# \#   •   \# \# \#   •   \# \# \#

A3   **a.** 4%
      b. 100% (The word crystal implies that the drug is pure.)
      c. x (This is the unknown quantity.)
      d. 250 ml

Q4   Answer each question about the following order. Prepare 500 ml of 2% Lysol solution from pure liquid Lysol.

    a. What is the desired strength? _____

    b. What is the strength of the available drug? _____

    c. What amount of drug should be used to prepare the solution? _____

    d. How much solution is to be made? _____

• # # # • # # # • # # # • # # # • # # # • # # # • # # # • # #

A4   **a.** 2%   **b.** 100%   **c.** x **d.** 500 ml

---

3   The following proportion may be used in preparing solutions of varying strengths:

$$\frac{\text{desired strength}}{\text{available strength}} = \frac{\text{drug to use}}{\text{solution to make}}$$

Example: Prepare 100 ml of 5% cresol solution from pure liquid cresol.

Solution: It is first necessary to identify the information which is to be substituted into the proportion.

The desired strength is __5%__ .
The available strength is __100%__ .
The amount of available drug to use is __x__ .
The amount of solution to make is __100 ml__ .

Substituting this information into the proportion we obtain:

$$\frac{5\%}{100\%} = \frac{x}{100\ ml}$$

Since both numerator and denominator of the left side of the equation have a % sign, it may be eliminated. The proportion can then be solved using the procedure of Section 8.2.

$$\frac{5\%}{100\%} = \frac{x}{100\ ml}$$

$$\frac{5}{100} = \frac{x}{100}$$

$$100x = 500$$

$$\frac{100x}{100} = \frac{500}{100}$$

$$x = 5$$

Thus, the amount of the available drug which should be used to prepare the solution is 5 ml.

Q5   Prepare 1000 ml of 10% Lysol solution from pure liquid Lysol.

• # # # • # # # • # # # • # # # • # # # • # # # • # # # • # #

A5   100 ml: The desired strength is 10%.
The available strength is 100%.
The amount of drug to use is x.
The amount of solution to make is 1000 ml.

$$\frac{10\%}{100\%} = \frac{x}{1000 \text{ ml}}$$
$$100x = 10\,000$$
$$x = 100$$

---

4   Consider the following:

Example: Prepare 400 ml of 10% sodium bicarbonate solution from sodium bicarbonate powder.

Solution: The desired strength is 10%.
The available strength is 100%. (The word powder implies that the drug is pure.)
The amount of drug to use is x.
The amount of solution to make is 400 ml.

Substituting this information into the proportion we obtain:

$$\frac{10\%}{100\%} = \frac{x}{400 \text{ ml}}$$
$$100x = 4000$$
$$x = 40$$

Since the solution is to be prepared from powder, the amount of available drug to use must be given with a unit of measure for solids. 1 g is the mass (weight) equivalent of 1 ml. Since the amount of solution to make is measured in millilitres, the amount of solid substance to use is measured in grams. Thus, the amount of the available drug which should be used to prepare the solution is 40 g.
   Whenever the available drug is in solid form, and the amount of solution to make is measured in millilitres, the available drug to use should always be measured in grams.

Q6   Determine the amount of drug needed to prepare the following solution. Prepare 250 ml of 5% glucose solution from crystalline glucose.

\# \# \# • \# \# \# • \# \# \# • \# \# \# • \# \# \# • \# \# \# • \# \# \# • \# \# \# • \# \# \#

A6   12.5 g: The desired strength is 5%.
The available strength is 100%.
The amount of drug to use is x.
The amount of solution to make is 250 ml.

$$\frac{5\%}{100\%} = \frac{x}{250 \text{ ml}}$$
$$100x = 1250$$
$$x = 12.5$$

---

5   When the strength of the desired solution is expressed as a ratio, the approach is very similar to that already presented.

Example: Prepare 1500 ml of 1:1000 epinephrine solution from solid epinephrine.

Solution: The desired strength is 1:1000.
The available strength is 100%.
The amount of drug to use is x.
The amount of solution to make is 1500 ml.

$$\frac{\frac{1}{1000}}{100\%} = \frac{x}{1500 \text{ ml}}$$

Before the proportion can be solved, the numerator and denominator of the left side of the equation must be expressed in similar units. That is, either $\frac{1}{1000}$ must be written as a percent or 100% must be written as a number. Since $100\% = \frac{100}{100} = 1$, it is convenient to replace 100% by 1. The proportion can now be solved.

$$\frac{\frac{1}{1000}}{1} = \frac{x}{1500 \text{ ml}}$$

$$1x = \frac{1}{\cancel{1000}_{2}} \cdot \cancel{1500}^{3}$$

$$x = 1.5$$

Thus, 1.5 g of drug are needed to prepare the solution. The preceding problem demonstrates the use of the following procedure. *Whenever the desired strength is expressed as a ratio, the available strength of a pure drug is expressed as 1.*

Q7   Determine the amount of Lysol to use in preparing the following solution. Prepare 750 ml of 1:5 Lysol solution from pure liquid Lysol.

\# \# \#   •   \# \# \#   •   \# \# \#   •   \# \# \#   •   \# \# \#   •   \# \# \#   •   \# \# \#   •   \# \# \#   •   \# \# \#

A7   150 ml: $\dfrac{\frac{1}{5}}{1} = \dfrac{x}{750 \text{ ml}}$

$1x = \dfrac{1}{5} \cdot 750$

$x = 150$

Q8   Determine the amount of drug needed to fill the following order. Prepare 50 ml of 7:100 potassium citrate solution from potassium citrate crystals.

\# \# \#   •   \# \# \#   •   \# \# \#   •   \# \# \#   •   \# \# \#   •   \# \# \#   •   \# \# \#   •   \# \# \#   •   \# \# \#

A8   3.5 g: $\dfrac{\dfrac{7}{100}}{1}=\dfrac{x}{50\ \text{ml}}$

$1x=\dfrac{7}{100}\cdot 50$

$x=3.5$

---

6   The response to a solution order is usually written in the form of a statement. The statement for the order in Q8 is given as follows:

> To prepare 50 ml of 7:100 potassium citrate solution from potassium citrate crystals, take 3.5 g of potassium citrate crystals, dissolve in water, and dilute to 50 ml.

Notice that the statement begins with the word "To" and then repeats the order as originally given. The drug available for the solution is solid, and therefore must be dissolved in a small amount of water before being diluted to the desired 50 ml.

If the available drug is already in liquid form, it need not be dissolved.

Example: Write the statement of the order from Q7.

Solution: To prepare 750 ml of 1:5 Lysol solution from pure liquid Lysol, take 150 ml pure liquid Lysol and dilute to 750 ml.

Q9   Write the statement for the order in Q6.

\# \# \#   •   \# \# \#   •   \# \# \#   •   \# \# \#   •   \# \# \#   •   \# \# \#   •   \# \# \#   •   \# \# \#   •   \# \# \#

A9   To prepare 250 ml of 5% glucose solution from crystalline glucose, take 12.5 g of crystalline glucose, dissolve in water, and dilute to 250 ml.

Q10   Write the statement for the order in Q5.

\# \# \#   •   \# \# \#   •   \# \# \#   •   \# \# \#   •   \# \# \#   •   \# \# \#   •   \# \# \#   •   \# \# \#   •   \# \# \#

A10   To prepare 1000 ml of 10% Lysol solution from pure liquid Lysol, take 100 ml of pure liquid Lysol and dilute to 1000 ml.

Q11   Prepare 500 ml of 3% cresol solution from pure liquid cresol.
   a. Determine the amount of drug to use in preparing the solution.

   b. Write the statement of the answer.

\# \# \#   •   \# \# \#   •   \# \# \#   •   \# \# \#   •   \# \# \#   •   \# \# \#   •   \# \# \#   •   \# \# \#   •   \# \# \#

A11   **a.** 15 ml: $\dfrac{3\%}{100\%} = \dfrac{x}{500\ \text{ml}}$

b. To prepare 500 ml of 3% cresol solution from pure liquid cresol, take 15 ml of pure liquid cresol and dilute to 500 ml.

Q12   Prepare 20 ml of 1:200 silver nitrate solution from silver nitrate crystals.
a. Determine the amount of drug to use in preparing the answer.

b. Write the statement of the answer.

\# \# \#   •   \# \# \#   •   \# \# \#   •   \# \# \#   •   \# \# \#   •   \# \# \#   •   \# \# \#   •   \# \# \#   •   \# \# \#

A12   0.1 g: $\dfrac{\frac{1}{200}}{1} = \dfrac{x}{20\ \text{ml}}$

b. To prepare 20 ml of 1:200 silver nitrate solution from silver nitrate crystals, take 0.1 g of silver nitrate crystals, dissolve in water, and dilute to 20 ml.

---

7   To this point we have used the following proportion to find the amount of an available drug to use to prepare a given strength of solution.

$$\frac{\text{desired strength}}{\text{available strength}} = \frac{\text{drug to use}}{\text{solution to make}}$$

This proportion can also be used to determine how much of a given strength solution *can be made* from the drug that is available.

Example: How much 50% magnesium sulfate solution can be made from 20 g of magnesium sulfate crystals?

Solution: The desired strength is 50%.
The available strength is 100%.
The amount of available drug to use to prepare the solution is 20 g.
The amount of solution that can be made is the unknown quantity, x.

$$\frac{50\%}{100\%} = \frac{20\ \text{g}}{x}$$
$$50x = 2000$$
$$x = 40$$

Thus, the amount of solution that can be made is 40 ml. The formal statement of the answer is: 40 ml of 50% magnesium sulfate solution can be made from 20 g of magnesium sulfate crystals.

Q13   How much 5% boric acid solution can be made from 10 g of boric acid crystals?

\# \# \#   •   \# \# \#   •   \# \# \#   •   \# \# \#   •   \# \# \#   •   \# \# \#   •   \# \# \#   •   \# \# \#   •   \# \# \#

A13   200 ml: $\dfrac{5\%}{100\%} = \dfrac{10\,g}{x}$

$$5x = 1000$$
$$x = 200$$

Q14   Write a statement for the answer to Q13.

\# \# \#   •   \# \# \#   •   \# \# \#   •   \# \# \#   •   \# \# \#   •   \# \# \#   •   \# \# \#   •   \# \# \#   •   \# \# \#

A14   200 ml of 5% boric acid solution can be made from 10 g of boric acid crystals.

Q15   How many millilitres of 1 : 5000 potassium permanganate solution can be made from 1 g of potassium permanganate crystals?

\# \# \#   •   \# \# \#   •   \# \# \#   •   \# \# \#   •   \# \# \#   •   \# \# \#   •   \# \# \#   •   \# \# \#   •   \# \# \#

A15   5000 ml: $\dfrac{\frac{1}{5000}}{1} = \dfrac{1\,g}{x}$

$$\frac{1}{5000}x = 1$$
$$5000\left(\frac{1}{5000}x\right) = 5000(1)$$
$$x = 5000$$

Q16   Write a statement for the answer to Q15.

\# \# \#   •   \# \# \#   •   \# \# \#   •   \# \# \#   •   \# \# \#   •   \# \# \#   •   \# \# \#   •   \# \# \#   •   \# \# \#

A16   5000 ml of 1 : 5000 potassium permanganate solution can be made from 1 g of potassium permanganate crystals.

Q17   How much 0.9% saline solution can be made from 4.5 g of sodium chloride crystals?

\# \# \#   •   \# \# \#   •   \# \# \#   •   \# \# \#   •   \# \# \#   •   \# \# \#   •   \# \# \#   •   \# \# \#   •   \# \# \#

A17   500 ml: $\dfrac{0.9\%}{100\%} = \dfrac{4.5\,g}{x}$

$$0.9x = 450$$

$$\dfrac{0.9x}{0.9} = \dfrac{450}{0.9}$$

$$x = 500$$

Q18   Write a statement for the answer to Q17.

•   # # #   •   # # #   •   # # #   •   # # #   •   # # #   •   # # #   •   # # #   •   # #

A18   500 ml of 0.9% saline solution can be made from 4.5 g of sodium chloride crystals.

---

8   At times you will be required to prepare solutions from other solutions rather than from pure drugs. Regardless, the same proportion is used to determine the amount of solution needed.

Example: Prepare 50 ml of 1% boric acid solution from 5% boric acid solution.

Solution: The desired strength is 1%.
The available strength is 5%.
The amount of drug to use is x.
The amount of solution to make is 50 ml.

$$\dfrac{\text{desired strength}}{\text{available strength}} = \dfrac{\text{drug to use}}{\text{solution to make}}$$

$$\dfrac{1\%}{5\%} = \dfrac{x}{50\,ml}$$

$$5x = 50$$

$$x = 10$$

Thus the amount of 5% solution to use to prepare the desired solution is 10 ml. The formal statement of the answer is:

To prepare 50 ml of 1% boric acid solution from 5% boric acid solution, take 10 ml of 5% boric acid solution and dilute to 50 ml.

Q19   Consider the following order. Prepare 200 ml of 20% sodium bromide solution from 25% sodium bromide solution.
   a. Determine the amount of solution to use to prepare the desired solution.

   b. Write a statement of the answer.

•   # # #   •   # # #   •   # # #   •   # # #   •   # # #   •   # # #   •   # # #   •   # #

A19 **a.** 160 ml: $\dfrac{20\%}{25\%} = \dfrac{x}{200\ \text{ml}}$

$$25x = 4000$$
$$x = 160$$

b. To prepare 200 ml of 20% sodium bromide solution from 25% sodium bromide solution, take 160 ml of 25% sodium bromide solution and dilute to 200 ml.

---

9 Consider the following example.

Example: Prepare 1000 ml of $1:200$ solution from 2% solution.

Solution: $\dfrac{\text{desired strength}}{\text{available strength}} = \dfrac{\text{drug to use}}{\text{solution to make}}$

$$\dfrac{\dfrac{1}{200}}{2\%} = \dfrac{x}{1000\ \text{ml}}$$

Notice that the left side numerator and denominator do not have the same form. That is, one is a percent while the other is a number. Thus, before proceeding either the number $\dfrac{1}{200}$ must be changed to a percent or the 2% must be changed to a number. In this case 2% is easily changed to a number since $2\% = \dfrac{2}{100} = \dfrac{1}{50}$. Thus, the proportion becomes:

$$\dfrac{\dfrac{1}{200}}{\dfrac{1}{50}} = \dfrac{x}{1000\ \text{ml}}$$

$$\dfrac{1}{50}x = \dfrac{1}{200} \cdot 1000$$

$$\dfrac{1}{50}x = 5$$

$$50\left(\dfrac{1}{50}x\right) = 50(5)$$

$$x = 250$$

The formal statement of the answer is given as follows:

To prepare 1000 ml of 1:200 solution from 2% solution, take 250 ml of 2% solution, and dilute to 1000 ml.

Q20 Consider the following order. Prepare 2000 ml of 4% solution from $2:5$ solution.
a. Determine the amount of solution to use to prepare the desired solution.

b. Write a statement for the answer.

• # # # • # # # • # # # • # # # • # # # • # # # • # # # • # #

A20   **a.** 200 ml:

$$\frac{4\%}{\frac{2}{5}}=\frac{x}{2000\text{ ml}}$$

$$\frac{\frac{1}{25}}{\frac{2}{5}}=\frac{x}{2000}$$

$$\frac{2}{5}x=\frac{1}{25}\cdot 2000$$

$$\frac{2}{5}x=80$$

$$\frac{5}{2}\left(\frac{2}{5}x\right)=\frac{5}{2}(80)$$

$$x=200$$

b. To prepare 2000 ml of 4% solution from 2:5 solution, take 200 ml of 2:5 solution and dilute to 2000 ml.

Q21   Consider the following order. Prepare 2500 ml of 1:400 solution from 1% solution.
a. Determine the amount of solution to use to prepare the desired solution.

b. Write a statement for the answer.

\# \# \#   •   \# \# \#   •   \# \# \#   •   \# \# \#   •   \# \# \#   •   \# \# \#   •   \# \# \#   •   \# \# \#   •   \# \# \#

A21   **a.** 625 ml:

$$\frac{\frac{1}{400}}{1\%}=\frac{x}{2500\text{ ml}}$$

$$\frac{\frac{1}{400}}{\frac{1}{100}}=\frac{x}{2500}\qquad\left(1\%=\frac{1}{100}\right)$$

$$\frac{1}{100}x=\frac{1}{400}\cdot 2500$$

$$\frac{1}{100}x=\frac{25}{4}$$

$$100\left(\frac{1}{100}x\right)=100\left(\frac{25}{4}\right)$$

$$x=625$$

b. To prepare 2500 ml of 1:400 solution from 1% solution, take 625 ml 1% solution and dilute to 2500 ml.

10   **Example:** How much 2% Lysol solution can be made from 20 ml of 1 : 10 solution?

$$\frac{\text{desired strength}}{\text{available strength}} = \frac{\text{drug to use}}{\text{solution to make}}$$

Solution: $\dfrac{2\%}{\dfrac{1}{10}} = \dfrac{20 \text{ ml}}{x}$

Notice that the unknown is the amount of solution that can be made. Notice also that the numerator and denominator on the left must be expressed in the same form before the proportion can be solved. Thus, since $2\% = \dfrac{2}{100} = \dfrac{1}{50}$, the proportion is solved as follows:

$$\frac{\dfrac{1}{50}}{\dfrac{1}{10}} = \frac{20 \text{ ml}}{x}$$

$$\frac{1}{50}x = \frac{1}{10} \cdot 20$$

$$\frac{1}{50}x = 2$$

$$50\left(\frac{1}{50}x\right) = 50(2)$$

$$x = 100$$

The statement of the answer can now be given:

100 ml of 2% Lysol solution can be made from 20 ml of 1 : 10 solution.

Q22   How much 5% phenol solution can be made from 10 ml of 1 : 10 phenol?

• # # # • # # # • # # # • # # # • # # # • # # # • # # # • # #

A22   20 ml: $\dfrac{5\%}{\dfrac{1}{10}} = \dfrac{10 \text{ ml}}{x}$

$$\frac{\dfrac{1}{20}}{\dfrac{1}{10}} = \frac{10}{x} \qquad \left(5\% = \frac{5}{100} = \frac{1}{20}\right)$$

$$\frac{1}{20}x = 1$$

$$20\left(\frac{1}{20}x\right) = 20(1)$$

$$x = 20$$

Q23   Write a statement for the answer to Q22.

•   # # #   •   # # #   •   # # #   •   # # #   •   # # #   •   # # #   •   # # #   •   # #

A23   20 ml of 5% phenol solution can be made from 10 ml of 1 : 10 phenol.

Q24   How much 1 : 50 formaldehyde solution can be made from 500 ml of 40% solution?

•   # # #   •   # # #   •   # # #   •   # # #   •   # # #   •   # # #   •   # # #   •   # #

A24   10 000 ml:

$$\frac{\frac{1}{50}}{\frac{2}{5}} = \frac{500 \text{ ml}}{x}$$

$$\frac{1}{50}x = \frac{2}{5} \cdot 500$$

$$\frac{1}{50}x = 200$$

$$50\left(\frac{1}{50}x\right) = 50(200)$$

$$x = 10\,000$$

Q25   Write a statement for the answer to Q24.

•   # # #   •   # # #   •   # # #   •   # # #   •   # # #   •   # # #   •   # # #   •   # #

A25   10 000 ml of 1 : 50 formaldehyde solution can be made from 500 ml of 40% solution.

---

11   Often times patients are administered medications orally, intramuscularly (IM), intravenously (IV), or subcutaneously (SC) from a prepared solution. When medication is supplied in liquid form, it is necessary to calculate the volume of liquid that contains the proper amount of the drug.

Example: The physician orders 500 mg IM of a drug. How many minims should be administered if the ampul* reads 5000 mg = 150 minims?

Solution: The correct amount can be calculated using a slight variation of the previously used proportion.

$$\frac{\text{desired amount}}{\text{available amount}} = \frac{\text{solution to use}}{\text{solution on hand}}$$

The desired amount is 500 mg.
The available amount is 5000 mg.
The amount of solution to use is x.
The amount of solution on hand is 150 minims.

*An ampul is a small sealed glass vessel used to hold sufficient solution for a single parenteral (intravenous or intramuscular) injection.

$$\frac{500 \text{ mg}}{5000 \text{ mg}} = \frac{x}{150 \text{ minims}}$$

$$5000\, x = 500(150)$$
$$5000x = 75\,000$$
$$x = 15$$

Thus, 15 minims should be injected IM. Notice that if the proportion is set up correctly, the denominators repeat the equation on the ampul. That is, the equation on the ampul reads 5000 mg = 150 minims and this was repeated in the left and right denominators of the proportion.

Q26   Consider the following order:
Give thiamine 75 mg IM from a vial* labeled 100 mg = 1 ml.

  a. What is the desired amount? _____

  b. What is the available amount? _____

  c. What is the amount of solution to use? _____

  d. What is the amount of solution on hand? _____
  e. Determine the amount of solution to use.

*A vial is similar to an ampul in that it is a stoppered glass vessel containing sufficient solution for multiple parenteral injections.

\# \# \#   •   \# \# \#   •   \# \# \#   •   \# \# \#   •   \# \# \#   •   \# \# \#   •   \# \# \#   •   \# \# \#   •   \# \# \#

  A26   **a.** 75 mg   **b.** 100 mg   **c.** x **d.** 1 ml

  e. 0.75 m: $\dfrac{75 \text{ mg}}{100 \text{ mg}} = \dfrac{x}{1 \text{ ml}}$

  $$100x = 75$$
  $$x = 0.75$$

Q27   Solve the following order for the amount of solution to use: The doctor orders penicillin G procaine 300,000 units IM. The available strength is 400,000 units per ml.

\# \# \#   •   \# \# \#   •   \# \# \#   •   \# \# \#   •   \# \# \#   •   \# \# \#   •   \# \# \#   •   \# \# \#   •   \# \# \#

  A27   0.75 ml: $\dfrac{300,000 \text{ units}}{400,000 \text{ units}} = \dfrac{x}{1 \text{ ml}}$

  $$400,000x = 300,000$$
  $$x = 0.75$$

---

12   Consider the statement of the answer to Q26.

To give 75 mg IM from a vial labeled 100 mg = 1 ml, withdraw 0.75 ml and administer IM.

Notice that since the medication is given IM (intramuscularly), it must first be withdrawn from the vial before it is administered. If no indication is given in the order about how the medication is to be administered, the physician in charge should be consulted.

Q28   Write the statement for the answer to Q27.

•   # # #   •   # # #   •   # # #   •   # # #   •   # # #   •   # # #   •   # # #   •   # #

A28   To give penicillin G procaine 300,000 units IM from an available strength of 400,000 units per ml, withdraw 0.75 ml and administer IM.

Q29   Solve the following order for the amount of solution to use. Give 4 g (4000 mg) of a drug orally from a solution labeled 250 mg per ml.

•   # # #   •   # # #   •   # # #   •   # # #   •   # # #   •   # # #   •   # # #   •   # #

A29   16 ml: $\dfrac{4000 \text{ mg}}{250 \text{ mg}} = \dfrac{x}{1 \text{ ml}}$

$$250x = 4000$$
$$x = 16$$

Q30   Write the statement for the answer to Q29.

•   # # #   •   # # #   •   # # #   •   # # #   •   # # #   •   # # #   •   # # #   •   # #

A30   To give 4 g of a drug from a solution labeled 250 mg per ml, pour out 16 ml and administer orally.

---

13   Sometimes it is necessary to convert portions of the order from one system of measure to another to ensure that the left side numerator and denominator are the same unit.

Example: Give codeine 30 mg SC (subcutaneously) from a vial of codeine labeled gr i = 1 ml.

Solution: $\dfrac{30 \text{ mg}}{1 \text{ grain}} = \dfrac{x}{1 \text{ ml}}$

Since the left-side units are not the same, either 30 mg must be converted to grains or 1 grain must be converted to milligrams. 1 grain is easily converted to milligrams using the fact that 60 mg = 1 grain.

$$\dfrac{30 \text{ mg}}{60 \text{ mg}} = \dfrac{x}{1 \text{ ml}}$$
$$60x = 30$$
$$x = 0.5$$

The statement of the answer can now be written:

To give codeine 30 mg SC from a vial of codeine labeled gr i = 1 ml, withdraw 0.5 ml and administer SC.

Q31   Determine the amount of medication to administer in the following order. Give 10 mg of morphine sulfate IM from a morphine sulfate solution labeled gr $\frac{1}{4}$ = 1 ml.

• # # # • # # # • # # # • # # # • # # # • # # # • # # # • # #

A31 $\frac{2}{3}$ or 0.67 ml: $\dfrac{10\ \text{mg}}{\frac{1}{4}\ \text{grain}} = \dfrac{x}{1\ \text{ml}}$

$\dfrac{10\ \text{mg}}{15\ \text{mg}} = \dfrac{x}{1\ \text{ml}}$ $\left[\dfrac{1}{4}\,\text{gr} = \dfrac{1}{4}(60\ \text{mg})\right]$

$15x = 10$

$x = \dfrac{2}{3}$ or 0.67

Q32   Write the statement for the answer to Q31.

• # # # • # # # • # # # • # # # • # # # • # # # • # # # • # #

A32   To give 10 mg of morphine sulfate IM from a morphine sulfate solution labeled gr $\frac{1}{4}$ = 1 ml, withdraw 0.67 ml and administer IM.

Q33   Determine the amount of medication to administer in the following order. Give thiamine gr ss IM from a vial of thiamine labeled 100 mg = 1 ml.

• # # # • # # # • # # # • # # # • # # # • # # # • # # # • # #

A33   0.3 ml: $\dfrac{\frac{1}{2}\ \text{grain}}{100\ \text{mg}} = \dfrac{x}{1\ \text{ml}}$

$\dfrac{30\ \text{mg}}{100\ \text{mg}} = \dfrac{x}{1}$ $\left[\dfrac{1}{2}\,\text{gr} = \dfrac{1}{2}(60\ \text{mg})\right]$

$100x = 30$

$x = 0.3$

Q34   Write the statement for the answer to Q33.

• # # # • # # # • # # # • # # # • # # # • # # # • # # # • # #

A34   To give thiamine gr ss from a vial of thiamine labeled 100 mg in 1 ml, withdraw 0.3 ml and administer IM.

This completes the instruction for this section.

8.5   EXERCISE

1. Fill in the blanks:

   a. A 5% solution means that there is/are _____ part(s) of the drug and _____ parts of water to make a total of _____ parts of the solution.

   b. A 1 : 20 solution means that there is/are _____ part(s) of the drug and _____ parts of water to make a total of _____ parts of solution.

2. Answer each question about the following order. Prepare 500 ml of 4% boric acid solution from boric acid crystals.

   a. What is the desired strength?

   b. What is the available strength?

   c. What amount of the available drug should be used to prepare the solution?

   d. How much solution is to be made?

3. Answer each question about the following order. Prepare 200 ml of 1:20 boric acid solution from boric acid powder.

   a. What is the desired strength?

   b. What is the available strength?

   c. What amount of the available drug should be used to prepare the solution?

   d. How much solution is to be made?

4. Determine the amount of the available drug that should be used to prepare the solution ordered in problem 2.

5. Write the statement for the answer to problem 4.

6. Determine the amount of the available drug that should be used to prepare the solution ordered in problem 3.

7. Write the statement for the answer to problem 6.

8. Determine the amount of the available solution that should be used to prepare the solution in the following order. Prepare 20 ml of 1:100 cocaine solution from 10% cocaine solution.

9. Write a statement for the answer to problem 8.

10. How much 1% silver nitrate solution can be made from 50 ml of 10% silver nitrate solution?

11. How much 2% phenol solution can be made from 10 ml of 1:10 phenol?

12. Solve the following orders for the amount of solution to use:

    a. Give 75 mg of promazine IM from a vial of promazine labeled 50 mg = 1 ml.

    b. Give 2 g of sodium bromide orally from a sodium bromide solution labeled gr xv = 3i.

13. Write the statement for the answer to problem 12a.

14. Write the statement for the answer to problem 12b.

8.5   EXERCISE ANSWERS

1. a. 5, 95, 100   b. 1, 19, 20
2. a. 4%   b. 100%   c. x d. 500 ml

3. a. 1:20   **b.** 1   **c.** *x*   **d.** 200 ml

4. 20 g

5. To prepare 500 ml of 4% boric acid solution from boric acid crystals, take 20 g of boric acid crystals, dissolve in water, and dilute to 500 ml.

6. 10 g

7. To prepare 200 ml of 1:20 boric acid solution from boric acid powder, take 10 g boric acid powder, dissolve in water, and dilute to 200 ml.

8. 2 ml

9. To prepare 20 ml of 1:100 cocaine solution from 10% cocaine solution, take 2 ml cocaine solution and dilute to 20 ml.

10. 500 ml   **11.** 50 ml   **12. a.** 1.5 ml   **b.** 2 drams

13. To give 75 mg of promazine IM from a vial of promazine labeled 50 mg = 1 ml, withdraw 1.5 ml of promazine and administer IM.

14. To give 2 g of sodium bromide from a sodium bromide solution labeled gr xv = ℨi take 2 drams of sodium bromide solution and administer orally.

CHAPTER 8 SAMPLE TEST

At the completion of Chapter 8 you should be able to work the following problems.

8.1   INTRODUCTION TO RATIO AND PROPORTION

1. Determine the ratio of (write in fraction form):
   a. 15 years to 10 years   **b.** $5.00 to 60 cents
   c. 1 foot to 4 yards   **d.** $2\frac{1}{2}$ to $3\frac{1}{4}$

2. Determine the miles per gallon if you travel 364.8 miles and use 16 gallons of gasoline.

3. Eighteen cubic centimetres of a solution weighs 242 grams. Find the weight per cm^3 (nearest tenth).

4. A patient receives 500 ml glucose in 4 hours. How many millilitres per minute will the patient receive (nearest hundredth)?

5. a. Name the means in the proportion $\frac{3}{8}=\frac{12}{32}$.
   b. What is the product of the extremes in the proportion $7:12 = 14:24$?
   c. Is $\frac{2}{3}=\frac{4}{5}$ a true proportion?
   d. Why?

8.2   SOLUTION OF A PROPORTION

6. Solve the following proportions:
   a. $\frac{16}{52}=\frac{M}{36}$ **b.** $\frac{5}{12}=\frac{M}{36}$ **c.** $\frac{M}{12}=\frac{2.5}{5}$ **d.** $\frac{4}{5}=\frac{7}{M}$

7. Solve the following problems:
   a. Four bricklayers can brick a building in 15 hours. Working at the same rate, how long would it take with six men?

b. If rain is falling at the rate of 0.5 inch per hour, how many inches will fall in 15 minutes?

c. A well produces 4,800 gallons of water in 120 minutes. How long will it take to produce 5,700 gallons of water?

d. An airplane travels from one city to another in 160 minutes at the rate of 270 miles per hour. How long will it take to make the return trip, traveling at 240 miles per hour?

8. If one tablet contains 16 mg of a drug, how many tablets are needed to fill a prescription of 208 mg?

9. If 50 capsules contain 0.375 grain of an active ingredient, how much of the ingredient will 18 capsules contain?

10. If aspirin contains 10 grains per two tablets, how many grains are contained in a bottle of 75 tablets?

8.3 PROPORTIONS USED IN RADIOGRAPHY

11. Identify the variables:
    a. FFD   **b.** mA   **c.** FOD   **d.** J

12. The time is **(a)** directly/indirectly proportional to the **(b)** _____ of the focus–film distance.

13. If the FFD is changed from 15 inches to 20 inches, what is the new time if the original time is 0.2 second (nearest hundredth)?

14. A certain technique calls for 40 milliamperes for 1.5 seconds. If we reduce exposure time to 0.5 second, what will the current have to be?

15. The image of the biparietal diameter of a fetal head measure 9.9 cm on the x-ray. A 10 cm measuring rod on the same x-ray measures 11.2 cm. What is the actual biparietal diameter of the fetal head (nearest tenth)?

8.4 RATIO AND PROPORTION FOR INHALATION THERAPISTS

16. a. The pressure–volume relationship is usually written (using variables):
    b. The pressure–temperature relationship is usually written:
    c. The pressure–temperature–volume relationship is usually written:

17. If 150 ml of oxygen is under a pressure of 700 mm of mercury, what would be the volume if the pressure is increased to 850 mm of mercury (round off to the nearest tenth)?

18. Suppose that 150 ml of gas is at a temperature of 32 °C. If the temperature is increased to 65 °C, what would be the new volume, if the pressure remains constant (round off to the nearest tenth)?

19. Find the new pressure if 2.5 l of helium at 30 °C and 800 mm of mercury are converted to 10 °C and a volume of 4.2 l.

20. Convert 2.8 litres of helium at 30 °C and 750 mm of mercury to 42 °C and a volume of 4.3 litres. What is the new pressure (round off to the nearest tenth)?

8.5 SOLUTIONS AND DOSAGES

21. Determine the amount of the available solution that should be used to prepare the solution in the following orders:
    a. Prepare 1000 ml of a 10% glucose solution from a 50% stock solution of glucose.

    b. Prepare 2000 ml of a 5% solution of potassium permanganate from potassium permanganate crystals.

    c. Prepare 1000 ml of a 10% solution of magnesium sulfate from a 1:5 stock solution.

    d. Prepare 1500 ml of a $\frac{1}{4}$% solution of bichloride of mercury using pure bichloride of mercury liquid.

22. Write a statement for each of the answers in problem 21.

23. Complete each of the following:

    a. How much 5% glucose solution can be made from 120 ml of 1:4 glucose solution?

    b. How much 2% boric acid solution can be made from 8 g of boric acid crystals?

    c. How much 1:100 solution can be made from 50 ml of 25% solution?

    d. How much 5% glucose solution can be made from 15 g of glucose?

24. Solve the following orders for the amount of solution to use:

    a. Give caffeine and sodium benzoate gr viiss IM from an ampul labeled 0.5 g = 2 ml.

    b. Give thiamine 0.05 g IM from an ampul labeled 100 mg = 1 ml.

    c. Give 2.5 g of sodium bicarbonate orally from a bottle of sodium bicarbonate labeled gr v = 4 ml.

    d. Give 4 g of a medication from a vial labeled gr v = 3 ml.

25. Write a statement for each of the answers in problem 24.

CHAPTER 8 SAMPLE TEST ANSWERS

1. a. $\frac{3}{2}$ **b.** $\frac{25}{3}$ **c.** $\frac{1}{12}$ **d.** $\frac{10}{13}$

2. 22.8 mi per gal   **3.** 13.4 g per cm^3 **4.** 2.08 ml per min

5. a. 8 and 12   **b.** 168   **c.** no   **d.** $3 \times 4 \neq 2 \times 5$

6. a. $11\frac{1}{13}$ **b.** 15   **c.** 6   **d.** $8\frac{3}{4}$

7. a. 10 hours   **b.** $\frac{1}{8}$ inch (0.125)   **c.** 142 min 30 sec   **d.** 180 min

8. 13 tablets   **9.** 0.135 gr   **10.** 375 gr

11. a. focus–film distance   **b.** current in milliamperes

    c. focus–object distance   **d.** object

12. a. directly   **b.** square

13. 0.36 sec   **14.** 120 milliamperes   **15.** 8.8 cm

16. a. $\dfrac{P_1}{P_2} = \dfrac{V_2}{V_1}$ **b.** $\dfrac{P_1}{P_2} = \dfrac{T_1}{T_2}$ **c.** $\dfrac{P_1 V_1}{T_1} = \dfrac{P_2 V_2}{T_2}$

17. 123.5 ml   **18.** 166.22 ml   **19.** 444.8 mm   **20.** 507.7 mm

21. a. 200 ml   **b.** 100 g   **c.** 500 ml   **d.** 3.75 ml

22. a. To prepare 1000 ml of a 10% glucose solution from a 50% stock solution of glucose, take 200 ml and dilute to 1000 ml.

    b. To prepare 2000 ml of a 5% solution of potassium permanganate from potassium permanganate crystals, take 100 g of potassium permanganate crystals, dissolve in water, and dilute to 2000 ml.

    c. To prepare 1000 ml of a 10% solution of magnesium sulfate from a 1:5 stock solution, take 500 ml of 1:5 stock solution and dilute to 1000 ml.

    d. To prepare 1500 ml of a $\frac{1}{4}$% solution of bichloride of mercury using pure drug, take 3.75 ml of pure bichloride of mercury liquid and dilute to 1500 ml.

23. a. 600 ml   **b.** 400 ml   **c.** 1250 ml   **d.** 300 ml
24. a. 2 ml   **b.** 0.5 ml   **c.** 30 ml   **d.** 36 ml
25. a. To give caffeine and sodium benzoate gr viiss IM from an ampul labeled 0.5 g = 2 ml, withdraw 2 ml and administer IM.
   b. To give thiamine 0.05 g IM from an ampul labeled 100 mg = 1 ml, withdraw 0.5 ml and administer IM.
   c. To give 2.5 g of sodium bicarbonate from a bottle of sodium bicarbonate labeled gr v = 4 ml, pour out 30 ml and administer orally.
   d. To give 4 g of a medication from a bottle labeled gr v = 3 ml, pour out 36 ml and administer orally.

CHAPTER 9

INSTRUMENTATION

The students studying in an allied health field will be exposed to hundreds of measuring devices. Accuracy in reading the measurement is extremely important. This chapter will present numerous dials, gauges, and scales which may be encountered.

9.1   UNIFORM AND NONUNIFORM SCALES

1   There are two types of scales common to most measuring devices: uniform and nonuniform.

In a *uniform scale*, each graduation (space) is of the same length and represents the same value as all other graduations on the scale.

Example:

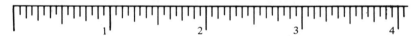

The portion of the ruler above is an example of a uniform scale in which each graduation represents $\frac{1}{16}$ of an inch.

A *nonuniform scale* is one in which the graduations vary in length and/or value.

Examples:

1.

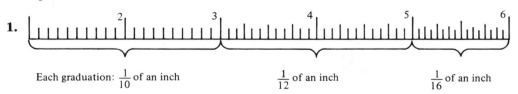

Each graduation: $\frac{1}{10}$ of an inch $\frac{1}{12}$ of an inch $\frac{1}{16}$ of an inch

2.

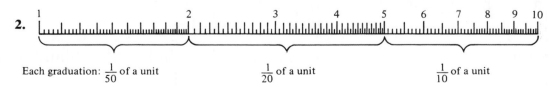

Each graduation: $\frac{1}{50}$ of a unit $\frac{1}{20}$ of a unit $\frac{1}{10}$ of a unit

In addition to the difference in value of graduations, in this example the length of each graduation varies as well. Notice that the space between graduation marks gets smaller as you go from left to right.

Q1   Indicate whether each scale represents a uniform or nonuniform scale:

a.

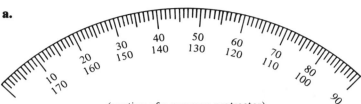

(portion of a common protractor)

_____

b.

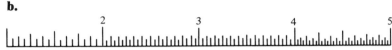

_____

•   # # #   •   # # #   •   # # #   •   # # #   •   # # #   •   # # #   •   # # #   •   # #

A1   **a.** uniform   **b.** nonuniform

---

2   When using uniform or nonuniform scales to determine a measurement, it is necessary to determine the value of the graduations of the scale being used.

Example: What is the length of the nail below?

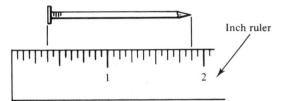

Solution:

Step 1: Count the number of graduations per inch. There are 16; hence, each graduation represents $\frac{1}{16}$ of an inch.

Step 2: Count the total number of graduations in the length of the nail. There are 24; hence, the length of the nail is $\frac{24}{16}$ or $1\frac{1}{2}$ inches long.

Q2   Determine the lengths of the items below:

a. _____ unit   **b.** _____ unit   **c.** _____ unit

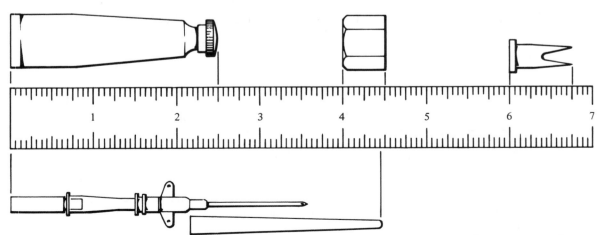

d. _____ unit

A2   **a.** $2\frac{1}{2}$ **b.** $\frac{1}{2}$ **c.** $\frac{3}{4}$ **d.** $4\frac{7}{16}$

---

3   A convenient method to determine the value of each graduation is to divide the value between two known graduation marks by the number of graduations (spaces).

Example 1: What is the value of each graduation?

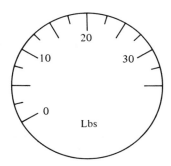

Solution: Between 0 and 10 there are 4 graduations. Count the spaces between 0 and 10, *not* the marks. Therefore, each graduation represents $\frac{10}{4}$ or 2.5 lbs.

Example 2: What is the value of each graduation?

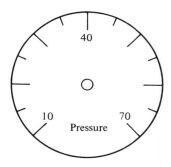

Solution: Between 10 and 40 there are 6 graduations (spaces). Therefore, each graduation represents a pressure of $\frac{40-10}{6}$ or 5 lbs.

Q3   Determine the value of each graduation:

a. _____ gallons

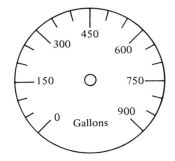

b. _____ unit

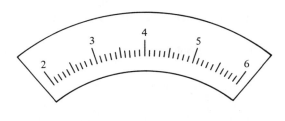

c. _____°

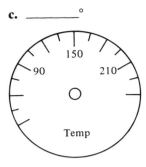

Temp

d. _____ unit

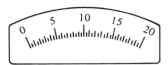

•   # # #   •   # # #   •   # # #   •   # # #   •   # # #   •   # # #   •   # # #   •   # #

A3   **a.** 50: $\dfrac{150}{3}$

b. 0.1: $\dfrac{1}{10}$

c. 15: $\dfrac{150-90}{4}$

d. 0.5: $\dfrac{5}{10}$ or $\dfrac{1}{2}$

---

4   When obtaining a reading from a dial, gauge, or scale, be sure to first determine the value of each graduation.

Example: What is the reading on the gauge below?

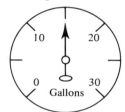

Solution: Each graduation represents 5 gallons. Hence, the reading is 15 gallons.

Q4   Determine the readings:

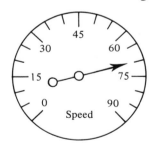

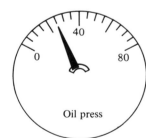

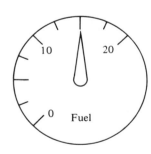

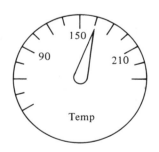

a. _____ rpm   **b.** _____ lbs   **c.** _____ gallons   **d.** _____°

•   # # #   •   # # #   •   # # #   •   # # #   •   # # #   •   # # #   •   # # #   •   # #

A4   **a.** 70:   Each graduation represents $\dfrac{15}{3} = 5$ rpm.

b. 25:   Each graduation represents $\dfrac{40}{8} = 5$ lbs.

c. 15:   Each graduation represents $\dfrac{10}{4} = 2.5$ gallons.

d. 165:   Each graduation represents $\dfrac{60}{4} = 15°$.

Q5   Determine the readings:

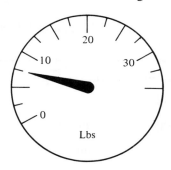

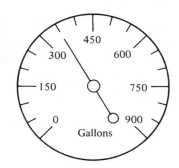

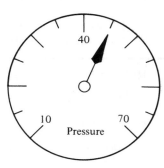

a. _____ lbs   **b.** _____ gallons   **c.** _____ lbs

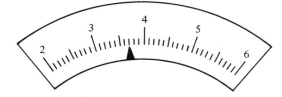

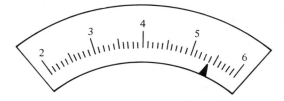

d. _____ ft   **e.** _____ ft

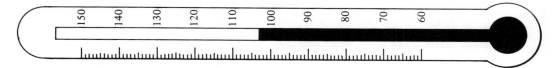

f. _____ °

\# \# \#   •   \# \# \#   •   \# \# \#   •   \# \# \#   •   \# \# \#   •   \# \# \#   •   \# \# \#   •   \# \# \#   •   \# \# \#

A5   **a.** 7.5   **b.** 350   **c.** 45   **d.** 3.7   **e.** 5.4   **f.** 103

---

5   Reading nonuniform scales requires special care since graduations have different values depending on their location on the scale. On the ohmmeter (a device for measuring electrical resistance) observe the following:

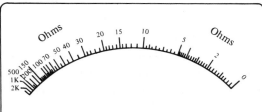

1. Between 0 and 5 each graduation represents $\frac{1}{5}$ or 0.2 ohms.

2. Between 5 and 10 each graduation represents $\frac{10-5}{10} = \frac{1}{2}$ or 0.5 ohms.

3. Between 10 and 20 each graduation represents $\frac{20-10}{10} = 1$ ohm. The same result can be obtained

by $\frac{15-10}{5} = 1$ ohm.

4. Between 20 and 30 each graduation represents $\dfrac{30-20}{5} = 2$ ohms.

5. The values of graduations between 30 and 100, 100 and 150, 150 and 200, 200 and 300, 300 and 500, 500 and 1 K (thousand), and 1 K and 2 K are all different.

Q6   Refer to the scale in Frame 5. What is the value of each graduation between:

a. 30 and 100? _____ ohms   **b.** 100 and 150? _____ ohms

c. 150 and 200? _____ ohms   **d.** 200 and 500? _____ ohms

e. 500 and 1 K? _____ ohms   **f.** 1 K and 2 K _____ ohms

\# \# \# • \# \# \# • \# \# \# • \# \# \# • \# \# \# • \# \# \# • \# \# \# • \# \# \# • \# \# \#

A6   **a.** 5   **b.** 10   **c.** 50   **d.** 100   **e.** 500   **f.** 1000

Q7   Determine the readings:

a. _____ ohms   **b.** _____ ohms

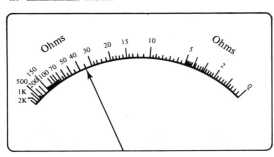
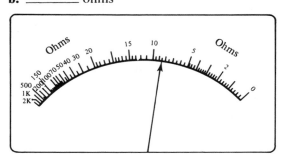

c. _____ ohms   **d.** _____ ohms

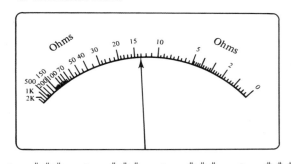
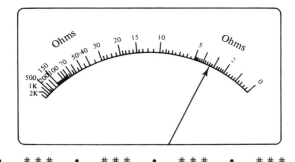

\# \# \# • \# \# \# • \# \# \# • \# \# \# • \# \# \# • \# \# \# • \# \# \# • \# \# \# • \# \# \#

A7   **a.** 35   **b.** 8.5   **c.** 13   **d.** 3.4

6   The diagram below shows the AC (alternating current) scale which is typical of the one found on a volt-ohm milliameter (VOM). It is used to measure AC voltage in electrical circuits. Each graduation represents $\dfrac{1}{5}$ or 0.2 volts.

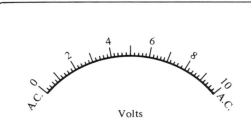

Q8   Indicate the reading of the scales:

a. _____ volts   **b.** _____ volts

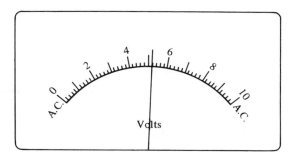   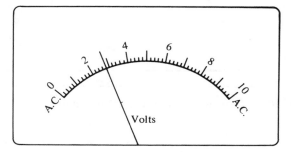

• # # # • # # # • # # # • # # # • # # # • # # # • # # # • # #

A8   **a.** 5.2   **b.** 2.8

---

7   The diagram below shows an 2.5 AC volt scale (VAC) which is typical of the one found on a VOM. Each graduation represents 0.1 of a volt.

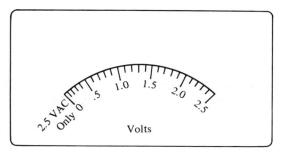

Q9   Indicate the reading of the scale:

a. _____ volts   **b.** _____ volts

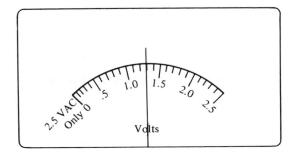   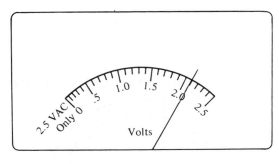

• # # # • # # # • # # # • # # # • # # # • # # # • # # # • # #

A9   **a.** 1.3   **b.** 2.1

---

8   The diagram below shows a DC (direct current) scale which is typical of the one found on a VOM. Each graduation represents 5 volts.

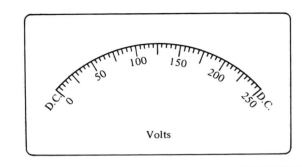

Volts

Q10   Indicate the reading of the scale:

a. _____ volts   **b.** _____ volts

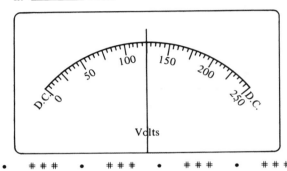

Volts

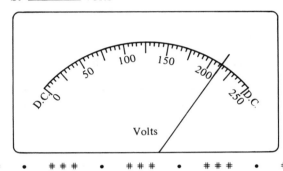

Volts

•   # # #   •   # # #   •   # # #   •   # # #   •   # # #   •   # # #   •   # # #   •   # #

A10   **a.** 125   **b.** 212

9   A *tachometer* is used to measure the number of revolutions the shaft of a motor makes with respect to a unit of time, usually minutes. Thus, a reading from a tachometer is generally in revolutions per minute (rpm).

The reading from the tachometer in Figure 1 would be 55 hundred or 5500 rpm.

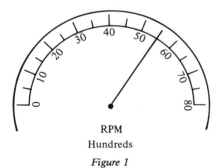

RPM
Hundreds

Figure 1

Tachometers are available in a variety of calibrations. The one in Figure 2 permits readings to

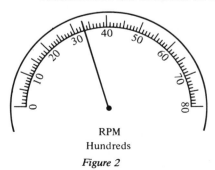

RPM
Hundreds

Figure 2

the nearest hundred rpm. It reads 3300 (33 hundred) rpm. Tachometers also are available for higher speed motors. The tachometer in Figure 3 registers 105 thousand or 105,000 rpm.

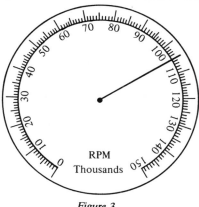

Figure 3

Q11   What is the indicated rpm?

a. _____ rpm   **b.** _____ rpm

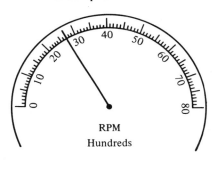   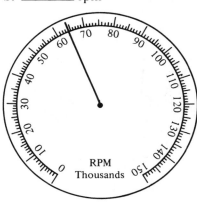

• # # # • # # # • # # # • # # # • # # # • # # # • # # # • # #

A11   **a.** 2700   **b.** 64,000

---

10   A *radiation survey meter* is an instrument designed for making general surveys of x-ray and gamma activity. It determines any increase in radiation intensities coming from radioactive sources, radiation areas, and x-ray machines. A gauge from such an instrument is pictured. You should observe that the gauge has two ranges:

1. top: 0–50 mR/hr (milli-Roentgens per hour)
2. bottom: 0–5 R/hr (Roentgens per hour)

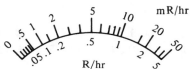

(*Note*: Both scales are nonuniform. In fact, they are logarithmic scales. Chapter 12 will discuss logarithms.)

Q12   Use the illustration from Frame 10 to answer these questions.
On the mR/hr scale (top):

a. From 0–0.5, each graduation represents _____mR/hr.

b. From 0.5–2, each graduation represents _____mR/hr.

c. From 2–10, each graduation represents _____mR/hr.

d. From 10–20, each graduation represents _____mR/hr.

e. From 20–50, each graduation represents _____mR/hr.

On the R/hr scale (bottom):

f. From 0–0.05, each graduation represents _____R/hr.

g. From 0.05–0.2, each graduation represents _____R/hr.

h. From 0.2–1, each graduation represents _____R/hr.

i. From 1–2, each graduation represents _____R/hr.

j. From 2–5, each graduation represents _____R/hr.

#　•　# # #　•　# # #　•　# # #　•　# # #　•　# # #　•　# # #　•　# # #　•　# #

A12　　a. 0.1　　b. 0.5　　c. 1　　d. 5　　e. 10
　　　　f. 0.01　　g. 0.05　　h. 0.1　　i. 0.5　　j. 1

Q13　　Read the following:

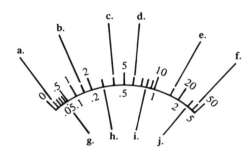

a. _____mR/hr　　f. _____mR/hr

b. _____mR/hr　　g. _____R/hr

c. _____mR/hr　　h. _____R/hr

d. _____mR/hr　　i. _____R/hr

e. _____mR/hr　　j. _____R/hr

#　•　# # #　•　# # #　•　# # #　•　# # #　•　# # #　•　# # #　•　# # #　•　# #

A13　　a. 0.1　　b. 1.5　　c. 4　　d. 6　　e. 15
　　　　f. 40　　g. 0.04　　h. 0.3　　i. 0.8　　j. 3

11　　It would be impractical to attempt to illustrate all of the possible dials, gauges, meters, etc. which might be unique to each specific health area. However, in each case the techniques discussed here should enable you to analyze the value of each graduation on the scale of the instrument in order to give an accurate reading. The exercise which accompanies this section and the sample test at the end of this chapter will contain scales which might not have been used here. Nevertheless, you should be able to read the scales correctly.

This completes the instruction for this section.

9.1   EXERCISE

1. Determine the following measurements with the inch ruler provided:

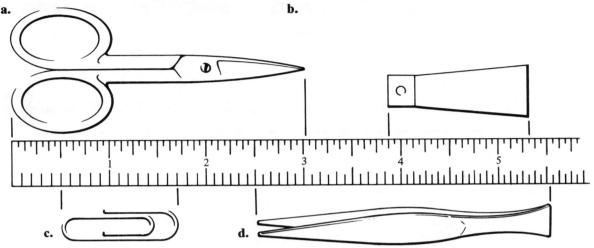

a.

b.

c.

d.

2. Determine the following measurements with the metric ruler provided (the numbers indicate centimeters):

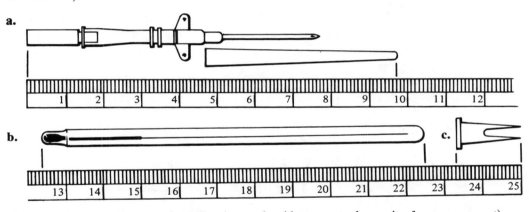

a.

b.

c.

3. Determine the readings on the following scales (do not attach a unit of measurement):

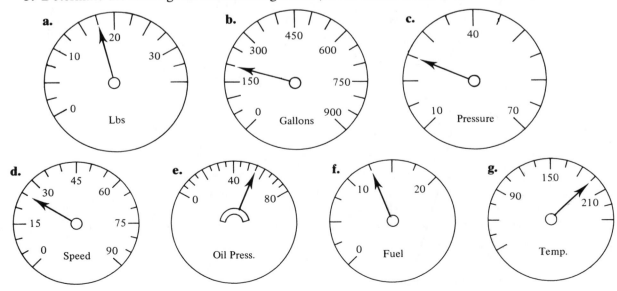

a.

b.

c.

d.

e.

f.

g.

h.

i.

j.

k.

l.

m.

n.

o.

p.

q.

r.

s.

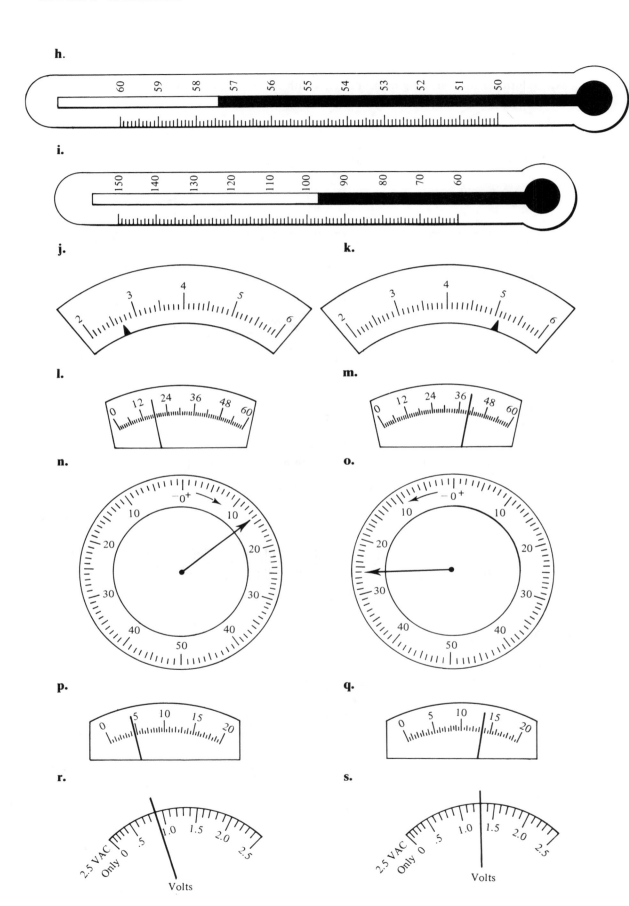

t.

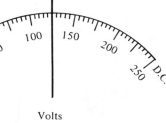

Volts

u.

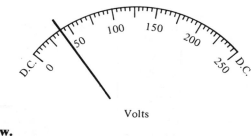

Volts

v.

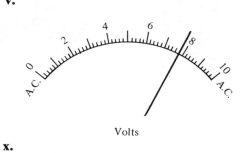

Volts

w.

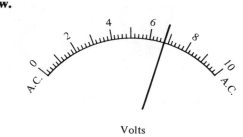

Volts

x.

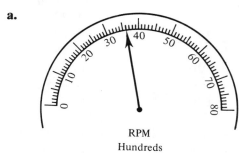

y.

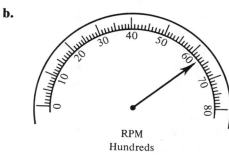

4. Determine the rpm:

a.

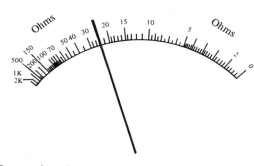

RPM
Hundreds

b.

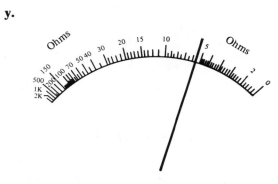

RPM
Hundreds

c.

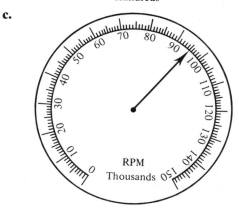

RPM
Thousands

d.

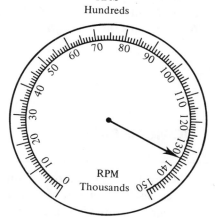

RPM
Thousands

5. Determine the measurement:

a.   **b.**   **c.**   **d.**

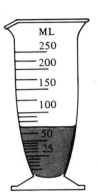
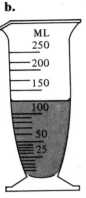
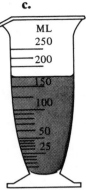
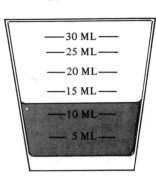

6. Read the given scale:

9.1   EXERCISE ANSWERS

1. a. $3\frac{1}{16}$ in.   **b.** $1\frac{7}{16}$ in.   **c.** 1.2 in.   **d.** $3\frac{1}{16}$ in.

2. a. 9.7 cm or 97 mm   **b.** 10.1 cm or 101 mm   **c.** 1.7 cm or 17 mm

3. a. 17.5   **b.** 200   **c.** 25   **d.** 25
   e. 55   **f.** 12.5   **g.** 195   **h.** 57.4
   i. 97   **j.** 2.7   **k.** 5.1   **l.** 18
   m. 40   **n.** $^{+}14$ **o.** $^{-}26$ **p.** 4.6
   q. 13.5   **r.** 0.9   **s.** 1.3   **t.** 125
   u. 40   **v.** 7.8   **w.** 6.8   **x.** 24
   y. 5.5
4. a. 3600 rpm   **b.** 6300 rpm   **c.** 95,000 rpm   **d.** 134,000 rpm
5. a. 70 ml   **b.** 125 ml   **c.** 175 ml   **d.** 12.5 ml
6. a. 2.5 mR/hr   **b.** 0.25 R/hr   **c.** 1.5 mR/hr   **d.** 0.15 R/hr

9.2   NOMOGRAMS

1   Whenever three or more variables are related in a specific manner the relationship between these values can be shown by means of a *nomogram* (sometimes referred to as a *nomograph*). Basically, a nomogram consists of three or more parallel and equally spaced scales constructed in a particular way.* If at least two of the variables are known, the remaining value(s) may be found by passing a straight line through the known values. The intersection of this line with the other scale(s) determines the remaining value(s).

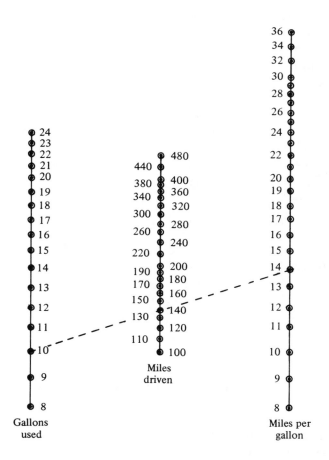

Gallons used

Miles driven

Miles per gallon

A simple nomogram relating miles per gallon, gallons (fuel) used, and miles driven is shown. The dashed line indicates that if 140 miles were driven on 10 gallons of fuel, the driver would have obtained 14 miles per gallon (mpg).

*Information on the construction of nomograms can be found in *A First Course in Nomography* by S. Brodetsky, G. Bell and Sons, Ltd.

Q1   Use the nomogram of Frame 1 and a straightedge to answer the following:

On a recent trip Ms. Rose Creed drove 380 miles on 17 gallons of gasoline. How many miles per gallon did she get on the trip? _____

\# \# \# • \# \# \# • \# \# \# • \# \# \# • \# \# \# • \# \# \# • \# \# \# • \# \# \# • \# \# \#

A1   22.4 mpg (just over 22 mpg)

2   A very useful nomogram appears on the next page. Scale B indicates the factor relating a metric unit from Scale A to another metric unit found on Scale C.

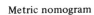

Metric nomogram

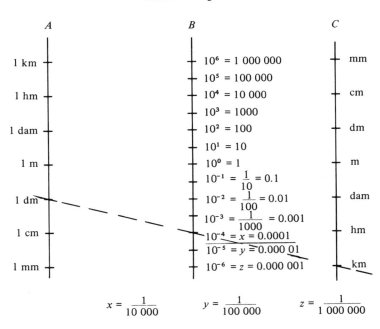

$$x = \frac{1}{10\ 000} \qquad y = \frac{1}{100\ 000} \qquad z = \frac{1}{1\ 000\ 000}$$

The dashed line indicates that

1 decimetre (dm) $= 10^{-4}$ kilometre (km)

or

1 dm $= 0.0001$ km

Note: The exponent on the power of 10 indicates the movement of the decimal point.

Examples:

1. 10^4 indicates a shift of the decimal point four places to the right.
2. 10^{-3} indicates a shift of the decimal point three places to the left.

Integer exponents will be discussed in detail in Section 1 of Chapter 12.

Q2   Use the nomogram of Frame 2 to complete the following:

a. 1 km = _____cm   **b.** 1 dam = _____mm   **c.** 1 dm = _____mm

d. 1 mm = _____hm   **e.** 1 cm = _____dm   **f.** 1 hm = _____dam

g. 1 m = _____hm   **h.** 1 m = _____mm   **i.** 1 cm = _____dam

j. 1 dam = _____dm

\# \# \#   •   \# \# \#   •   \# \# \#   •   \# \# \#   •   \# \# \#   •   \# \# \#   •   \# \# \#   •   \# \# \#   •   \# \# \#

A2   **a.** 10^5 (100 000)   **b.** 10^4 (10 000)   **c.** 10^2 (100)
     d. 10^{-5} (0.000 01)   **e.** 10^{-1} (0.1)   **f.** 10^1 (10)
     g. 10^{-2} (0.01)   **h.** 10^3 (1000)   **i.** 10^{-3} (0.001)
     j. 10^2 (100)

---

3   The nomogram illustrated in this frame relates the blood–alcohol concentration percent by weight to a person's body weight to the ounces of 80 proof liquor consumed in one hour. The dashed lines indicate the amount of 80 proof liquor a 150 pound person would have to consume in a one-hour period to reach the 0.07% and 0.10% blood–alcohol levels.

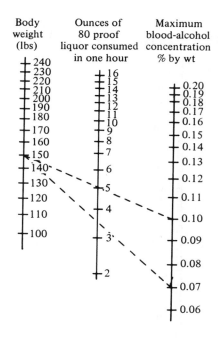

According to many state laws, at a 0.10% (and over) blood–alcohol level a driver is considered to be "under the influence." Above 0.07% a person's driving is considered to be "impaired." At 0.15% blood–alcohol level and above the same driver would be "seriously drunk."

Q3   Use the nomogram in Frame 3 to complete the following. To determine the amount of liquor (or beer) needed in a one-hour period to reach 0.10% blood–alcohol level, draw a line from *your* body weight to 0.10%. Also draw a line from *your* weight to 0.07%. According to the state laws mentioned in Frame 3, approximately what is the maximum number of ounces of 80 proof liquor you should consume in one-hour before:

a. your driving would become "impaired"? _____

b. you would be driving "under the influence"? _____

c. you would be "seriously drunk"? _____

•   # # #   •   # # #   •   # # #   •   # # #   •   # # #   •   # # #   •   # # #   •   # #

A3   Answers will vary! (*Note*: Alcohol is eliminated from the blood at the rate of only one drink per hour. Also, the amount of food in the stomach slows down the absorption of alcohol into the blood.)

---

4   Many nomograms are useful in health-related technologies. The accompanying nomogram is used to estimate body surface area when a patient's height and weight are known. To find body surface, locate the patient's height and weight on Scales I and II. Place a straightedge between these two points. The point where the straightedge intersects Scale III is the patient's estimated body surface area.

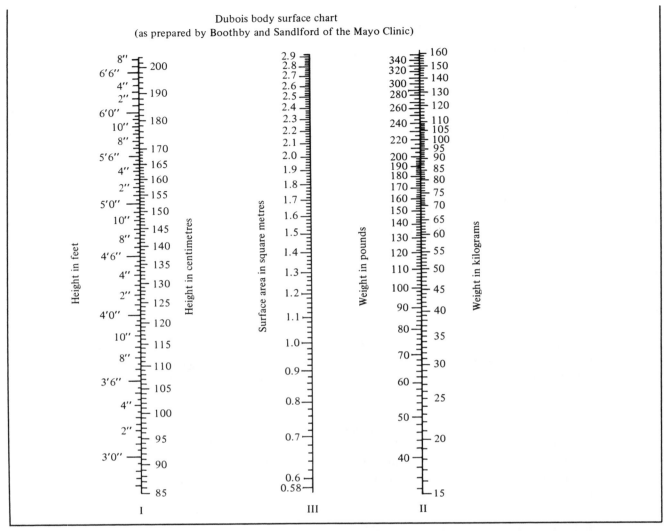

Dubois body surface chart
(as prepared by Boothby and Sandlford of the Mayo Clinic)

Q4   **a.** Find the estimated body surface area of a person 165 centimetres tall who weighs 60 kilograms.

_____

b. Charlotte Stieve, a nurse, measured a patient's height to be 147 centimetres. The patient weighs 55 kilograms. According to the Dubois Body Surface Chart, what is the patient's estimated body surface? _____

c. Determine your own estimated body surface area.

•   # # #   •   # # #   •   # # #   •   # # #   •   # # #   •   # # #   •   # # #   •   # #

A4   **a.** 1.66 m^2 (1.66 square metres)   **b.** 1.46 m^2
      c. Answers will vary! (We hope you are not alarmed.)

---

5   It would be impractical to illustrate all the nomograms used in the various allied health programs. In many cases, a great deal of medical background might be required in order to understand the data and implications received from a particular nomogram. At any rate, your ability to read uniform and nonuniform scales is essential to the correct application and use of the nomogram. The experience gained in this chapter should aid you in the future when you are confronted with a nomogram specific to your area of interest.

This completes the instruction for this section.

9.2   EXERCISE

1. Use the nomogram in Frame 1 of Section 9.2 to answer these questions:

   a. A trip of 280 miles required 16.5 gallons of gasoline. What was the miles per gallons on the trip?

   b. Alan Creed figured his weekly mileage based on 350 miles for 21.5 gallons of gasoline. How many miles per gallon did he get from his automobile?

2. Use the metric nomogram in Frame 2 of Section 9.2 to make these conversions:

   a. 1 mm = _____dm   **b.** 1 km = _____cm

   c. 1 dm = _____cm   **d.** 1 hm = _____km

3. Use the nomogram in Frame 3 of Section 9.2 to answer the following questions:

   a. Harold Lindbery weighs 185 pounds. He drank 8 ounces of 80 proof liquor in a one-hour period. What was his blood–alcohol level?

   b. Harold's wife, who weighs 100 pounds, consumed 4 ounces of 80 proof liquor during the same period. What was her blood–alcohol level?

4. Use the Dubois Body Surface Chart in Frame 4 of Section 9.2 to answer the following question:

   a. Terri Lynn is 5 feet 2 inches tall. She weighs 104 pounds. What is her estimated body surface in square metres?

   b. Robert Nelson measured his height to be 177 centimetres. He estimated his weight to be 75 kilograms. What was his estimated body surface in square metres?

9.2   EXERCISE ANSWERS

1. a. 17 mpg   **b.** 16.5 mpg
2. a. 10^{-2} (0.01)   **b.** 10^5 (100 000)
   c. 10^1 (10)   **d.** 10^{-1} (0.1)

3. a. Just under $0.12\frac{1}{2}\%$, approximately 0.124%.

   b. Just over $0.11\frac{1}{2}\%$, approximately 0.117%.

4. a. Just slightly over 1.44 m^2.
   b. 1.92 m^2

CHAPTER 9 SAMPLE TEST

At the completion of Chapter 9 you should be able to work the following problems.

9.1   UNIFORM AND NONUNIFORM SCALES

1. Determine the following measurements with the inch ruler provided:

a.   **b.**

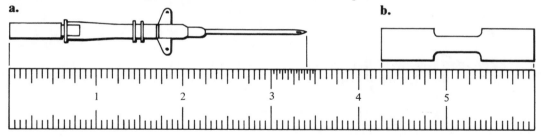

2. Determine the following measurements with the metric ruler provided (the numbers indicate centimetres):

a.

b.

| 1 | 2 | 3 | 4 | 5 | 6 | 7 | 8 | 9 | 10 | 11 | 12 | 13 | 14 | 15 |

3. Determine the readings on the following scales (do not attach a unit of measurement):

a.

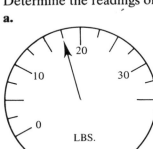

LBS.

b.

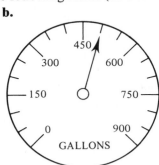

GALLONS

c.

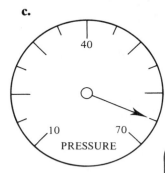

PRESSURE

d.

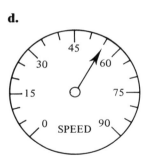

SPEED

e.

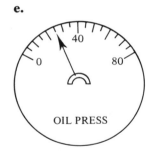

OIL PRESS

f.

g.

h.

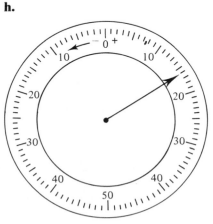

i.

j.

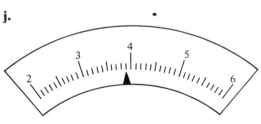

k.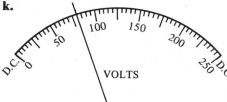

l.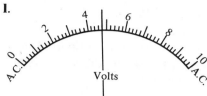

m.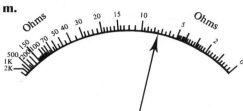

n.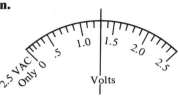

4. Determine the rpm:

a.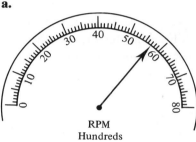

b.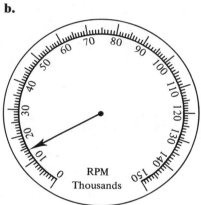

5. Determine the following readings:

a. 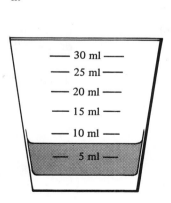   **b.**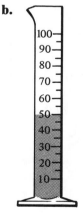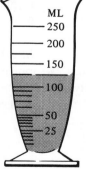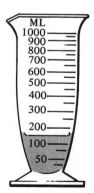

6. Read the following scales.

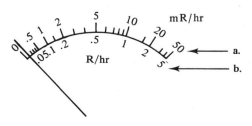   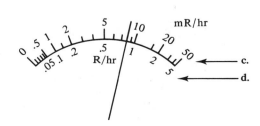

9.2   NOMOGRAMS

7. Use the nomogram in Frame 1 of Section 9.2 to answer the following:
   a. Carl Hammond drove 240 miles on 13 gallons of gasoline. What mileage (miles per gallon) did he get?
   b. Jerry Baker claimed he got 34 miles to the gallon on 14 gallons of gasoline. How many miles did he travel?

8. Use the nomogram in Frame 3 of Section 9.2 to answer the following:

   a. 1 m = _____mm   b. 1 mm = _____hm

   c. 1 hm = _____m   d. 1 cm = _____mm

9. Use the nomogram in 9.2 Exercise, problem 3, to answer the following:
   a. Steve Wallace weighs 200 pounds. He drank 5 ounces of 80 proof liquor during a one-hour period. What was his blood–alcohol level?
   b. Sue Wallace, Steve's mother, drank the same amount at the same time. She weighs 110 pounds. What was her blood–alcohol level?

10. Use the Dubois Body Surface Chart in Frame 4 of Section 9.2 to answer the following:
   a. Steve Wallace (9a) is 6 feet 4 inches tall. What is his estimated body surface.
   b. Mrs. Wallace (9b) is 167 centimetres tall. What is her estimated body surface.

CHAPTER 9 SAMPLE TEST ANSWERS

1. a. $3\frac{13}{32}$ in.   b. $1\frac{3}{4}$ in.   2. a. 7.8 cm (78 mm)   b. 4.5 cm (45 mm)

3. a. 17.5   b. 500   c. 65   d. 55
   e. 25   f. 57.8   g. 7   h. $^-$84
   i. 7.5   j. 3.9   k. 80   l. 4.8
   m. 7.5   n. 1.3

4. a. 5700 rpm   b. 14,000 rpm

5. a. 7–8 ml   b. 50 ml   c. 125 ml   d. 150 ml

6. a. 0.1 mR/hr   b. 0.01 R/hr   c. 8 mR/hr   d. 0.8 R/hr

7. a. 18.5 mpg   b. Just under 480 miles.

8. a. 10^3 (1000)   b. 10^{-5} (0.000 01)   c. 10^2 (100)   d. 10^1 (10)

9. a. Just over 0.07%, approximately 0.072%.
   b. Just slightly over 0.13%.

10. a. 2.22 m^2 b. 1.54–1.56 m^2

CHAPTER 10

INTERPRETATION AND CONSTRUCTION OF CIRCLE, BAR, AND LINE GRAPHS

One of the most common methods of communicating in the health sciences is with graphs. Some machines used in patient care are designed to provide information on a patient in graph form. It is therefore extremely important to understand the principles on which graphs are constructed and interpreted.

10.1 CHOOSING THE TYPE OF GRAPH

<table>
<tr><td>1</td><td>

Frequently people are asked to read and understand material that contains many numbers. The method of presentation of those numbers determines the ease with which the number relationships are understood. Written paragraphs containing numbers are difficult to understand unless there are very few numbers. Tables in which numbers are located in a uniform pattern are more easily read, and graphs will often show relationships much more forcefully and possibly help the reader recognize and remember relationships.

A graph is used to present information artistically and accurately. A few mathematical principles are used which help to ensure that the graphs convey the truth. If these principles are ignored, the relationships between the numbers are distorted and the reader is left with an inaccurate impression of the facts. A person should be able to recognize distortions of graphs that he reads and avoid introducing distortions in graphs that he constructs.

Three types of graphs are used so frequently that everyone should be able to interpret and construct them. They are the *circle graph*, the *bar graph*, and the *line graph*. The name of the type of graph describes its character. Numbers are represented by sectors* of a circle on a circle graph, by bars in a bar graph, and by a broken line on a line graph.

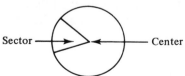

* A sector is a section of a circle shaped like a piece of pie.
</td></tr>
</table>

Q1 Examine the differences in the following graphs and identify each type of graph by writing its name on the line under the graph.

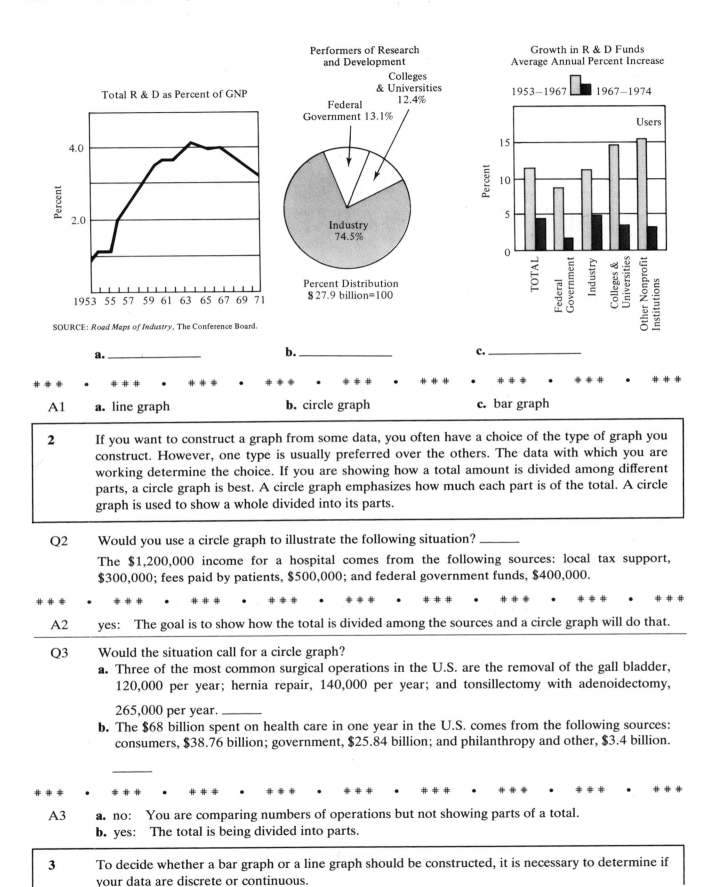

Total R & D as Percent of GNP

Performers of Research
and Development

Growth in R & D Funds
Average Annual Percent Increase

SOURCE: *Road Maps of Industry*, The Conference Board.

a. _____   b. _____   c. _____

\# \# \# • \# \# \# • \# \# \# • \# \# \# • \# \# \# • \# \# \# • \# \# \# • \# \# \# • \# \# \#

A1   **a.** line graph   **b.** circle graph   **c.** bar graph

---

2   If you want to construct a graph from some data, you often have a choice of the type of graph you construct. However, one type is usually preferred over the others. The data with which you are working determine the choice. If you are showing how a total amount is divided among different parts, a circle graph is best. A circle graph emphasizes how much each part is of the total. A circle graph is used to show a whole divided into its parts.

Q2   Would you use a circle graph to illustrate the following situation? _____

The $1,200,000 income for a hospital comes from the following sources: local tax support, $300,000; fees paid by patients, $500,000; and federal government funds, $400,000.

\# \# \# • \# \# \# • \# \# \# • \# \# \# • \# \# \# • \# \# \# • \# \# \# • \# \# \# • \# \# \#

A2   yes: The goal is to show how the total is divided among the sources and a circle graph will do that.

Q3   Would the situation call for a circle graph?
   a. Three of the most common surgical operations in the U.S. are the removal of the gall bladder, 120,000 per year; hernia repair, 140,000 per year; and tonsillectomy with adenoidectomy, 265,000 per year. _____
   b. The $68 billion spent on health care in one year in the U.S. comes from the following sources: consumers, $38.76 billion; government, $25.84 billion; and philanthropy and other, $3.4 billion.

   _____

\# \# \# • \# \# \# • \# \# \# • \# \# \# • \# \# \# • \# \# \# • \# \# \# • \# \# \# • \# \# \#

A3   **a.** no: You are comparing numbers of operations but not showing parts of a total.
      b. yes: The total is being divided into parts.

---

3   To decide whether a bar graph or a line graph should be constructed, it is necessary to determine if your data are discrete or continuous.

Continuous data consist of measurements that can be made more precise if a person chooses. For example, if the data are the amount of time spent on a project, it might be measured in days. If this is not satisfactory for some reason, time could be measured in hours or, more precisely, in minutes or seconds. Therefore, time is a continuous variable.

Discrete data allow no interpretation between the values of the data. For example, in a football game there may be 2 field goals scored or 3, but it is impossible to score $2\frac{1}{2}$ field goals. The number of field goals is a discrete variable.

Examples of continuous data:

1. Height: 60 in., 60.25 in., 6.2546 in. (the number of decimal places is dependent on the precision of the measurement)

2. Time measured in hours: 4 hours, $4\frac{1}{2}$ hours, 4.2576 hours

Examples of discrete data:

1. Makes of automobiles: Ford, Chevrolet, VW (there is no interpretation of halfway between a Chevrolet and a Ford)

2. Number of people in a classroom: 42, 16, 4 (you would not count people in fractional parts)

Sometimes there is no natural order for discrete data. For example, it makes no difference which make of automobile is listed first. When there is an order to discrete data, the numbers change in incremental steps, usually increasing by one each time.

Q4   Indicate whether the variable is continuous or discrete:

   a. number of suicides in a year _____

   b. dosage of insulin in an injection _____

   c. weight of a person _____

   d. number of teeth in your mouth _____

   e. time since an injection was made _____

   f. distance from an x-ray tube to the film _____

   g. measurement of a person's blood pressure _____

•   # # #   •   # # #   •   # # #   •   # # #   •   # # #   •   # # #   •   # # #   •   # #

A4   **a.** discrete   **b.** continuous   **c.** continuous   **d.** discrete
      e. continuous   **f.** continuous   **g.** continuous

4   Both bar graphs and line graphs have a vertical axis and a horizontal axis. Both bar and line graphs are used to show a numerical value measured on the scale on the vertical axis for various values located on the horizontal axis. Bar graphs are used when the horizontal axis of the graph represents discrete values. Line graphs are used when the horizontal axis of the graph represents continuous values.

   The horizontal axis on the accompanying figure represents new prescriptions (Rx's), refill prescriptions, and total prescriptions. These are discrete values, so a bar graph is used.

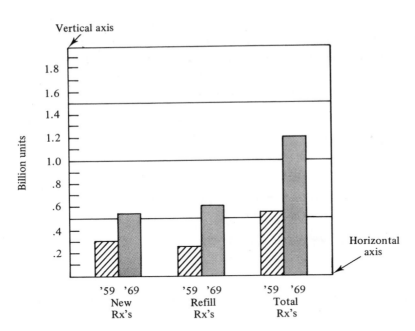

The horizontal axis on the next figure represents time measured in hours. Since time is a continuous variable, the graph should be readable between numbers on the horizontal axis. Therefore, a line graph is constructed.

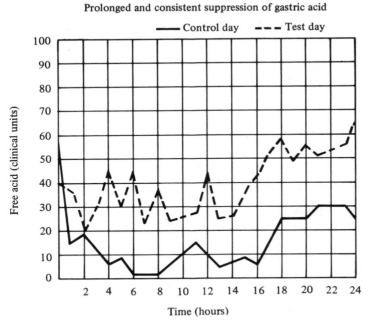

Thus, in order to tell what type of graph to construct, first determine the type (continuous or discrete) of data on the horizontal axis.

Q5   Suppose that the amount of food consumed per day were being compared for college freshmen of various weights. Are the data on the horizontal axis continuous or discrete (see figure at top of next page)? _____

Food consumed (vertical axis) — Weight of freshmen (horizontal axis)

\# \# \# • \# \# \# • \# \# \# • \# \# \# • \# \# \# • \# \# \# • \# \# \# • \# \# \# • \# \# \#

A5 continuous: You can interpret the data no matter how precisely it is reported. 100 lb, 112.5 lb, 149.275 lb.

Q6 What type of graph would you use in Q5? _____

\# \# \# • \# \# \# • \# \# \# • \# \# \# • \# \# \# • \# \# \# • \# \# \# • \# \# \# • \# \# \#

A6 line graph

Q7 Suppose that a graph were to be made that shows the average weekly food budget for families with various numbers of children.

a. Is the number of children continuous or discrete? _____

b. What type of graph should be drawn? _____

Budget (vertical axis) — Number of children (horizontal axis)

\# \# \# • \# \# \# • \# \# \# • \# \# \# • \# \# \# • \# \# \# • \# \# \# • \# \# \# • \# \# \#

A7 **a.** discrete: A family could not have $\frac{1}{2}$ a child. **b.** bar graph

---

Q8 Assume that the variable listed is on the horizontal axis of a graph. Indicate whether the data are continuous or discrete and what type of graph would be drawn.

Data	Type data	Type graph
a. countries: USA, France, USSR	_____	_____
b. months: 3 mo, $3\frac{1}{2}$ mo, $4\frac{2}{3}$ mo	_____	_____
c. number of births	_____	_____
d. temperature	_____	_____
e. age	_____	_____

\# \# \# • \# \# \# • \# \# \# • \# \# \# • \# \# \# • \# \# \# • \# \# \# • \# \# \# • \# \# \#

A8 **a.** discrete, bar graph   **b.** continuous, line graph
c. discrete, bar graph   **d.** continuous, line graph
e. continuous, line graph

(*Note*: Age is continuous, since the time since birth is continually changing; however, the general practice of not changing your age until your birthday causes it to be used like a discrete variable.)

This completes the instruction for this section.

10.1 EXERCISE

1. Indicate whether each of the following variables is continuous or discrete:
   a. number of creditors of a medical office
   b. cubic centimetres of blood in the body
   c. number of deaths in a city in one day
   d. amount of oxygen in a tank
   e. votes cast in an election
   f. number of coins in your pocket
   g. amount of radiation that a technician is exposed to in a day
2. Indicate what type of graph should be used:
   a. You want to show the survival rate of children for the immediate 5 years after a kidney transplant.
   b. A drug is made of a mixture of several ingredients. You want to show the percent of each ingredient as a part of the total.
   c. You want to show how the 4.4 million health care personnel are divided into service workers, managerial workers, and professional and technical workers.
   d. The dosage of medicine changes according to the amount of fever a patient has. You want to illustrate the dosage for body temperatures between 98.6 °F and 105 °F.
   e. You want to compare the number of new cavities in children at a six-month checkup for 12 toothpastes.

10.1 EXERCISE ANSWERS

1. a. discrete   b. continuous   c. discrete   d. continuous
   e. discrete   f. discrete   g. continuous
2. a. line graph: Time is a continuous variable.
   b. circle graph: You are showing parts of a total.
   c. circle graph: You are showing parts of a total.
   d. line graph: Temperature is a continuous variable.
   e. bar graph: The different toothpastes are discrete variables.

10.2 CIRCLE GRAPHS

1   A circle graph has the general appearance of a pie cut into uneven wedges. The geometric name of each wedge is a *sector*. The angle whose vertex is located at the center of the circle in each sector is called the *central angle* of the sector. Three sectors are shown. Each has a central angle.

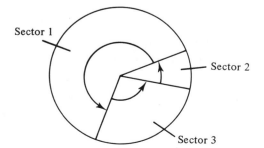

To interpret a circle graph you must know that the complete circle represents the total amount and that each sector represents a part of the total amount in the same ratio as the measure of its central angle is to 360°.

Example: If the circle above represented 8,000 people and the central angle for sector 3 measured 100°, how many people are represented by sector 3?

Solution: 2,222 people: $\dfrac{100°}{360°} = \dfrac{x}{8,000}$

$$x = \dfrac{100°}{360°}(8,000)$$

Q1   **a.** In the circle graph of Frame 1, if the measure of the central angle for sector 2 measured 30°, how many people does sector 2 represent?

b. How many people out of the 8,000 are left for sector 1?

\# \# \# • \# \# \# • \# \# \# • \# \# \# • \# \# \# • \# \# \# • \# \# \# • \# \# \# • \# \# \#

A1   **a.** 667 people: $\dfrac{30°}{360°} = \dfrac{x}{8,000}$ **b.** 5,111: $8,000 - (2,222 + 667)$

Q2   If a circle graph has a sector with a central angle of 90°, what percent of the total does that sector represent?

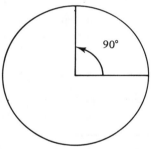

\# \# \# • \# \# \# • \# \# \# • \# \# \# • \# \# \# • \# \# \# • \# \# \# • \# \# \# • \# \# \#

A2   25%: $\dfrac{90°}{360°} = \dfrac{x}{100\%}$

2   Just as the sum of the parts must equal the total amount represented, the sum of the percent of all sectors must be 100 percent and the sum of the central angles must be 360°.

Q3   Consider the circle graph and find the percent for the category "miscellaneous."

Distribution of
Expenses for an
Average Family

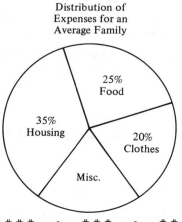

\# \# \# • \# \# \# • \# \# \# • \# \# \# • \# \# \# • \# \# \# • \# \# \# • \# \# \# • \# \# \#

A3   20%: $35\% + 25\% + 20\% = 80\%$
$100\% - 80\% = 20\%$ for miscellaneous

---

3   Usually the total amount that the whole circle represents is given in the title of the circle graph. To find the amount that each sector represents, multiply the total amount represented times the percent of the total included in the sector. For example, in the circle graph shown, to find the number of dollars used for housing in a family with income $8,500, we would find 35% of $8,500 = $0.35 \times \$8,500 = \$2,975$.

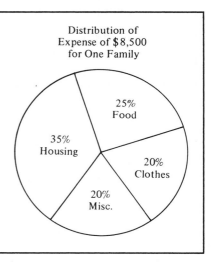

Distribution of
Expense of $8,500
for One Family

25% Food

35% Housing

20% Clothes

20% Misc.

Q4   **a.** Find the amount spent on food for the family whose expenses are shown in the preceding circle graph (Frame 3).

b. Find the amount spent on clothes for the same family.

\# \# \#   •   \# \# \#   •   \# \# \#   •   \# \# \#   •   \# \# \#   •   \# \# \#   •   \# \# \#   •   \# \# \#   •   \# \# \#

A4   **a.** $2,125:   25% of $8,500 = $0.25 \times \$8,500 = \$2,125$
b. $1,700:   20% of $8,500 = $0.20 \times \$8,500 = \$1,700$

---

4   To construct a circle graph you must find the number of degrees to use for the central angle for each sector.

If you are representing percents on a circle graph, the degrees of each sector can be found by multiplying the percent of each sector times 360°.

Example: 10% of all poisoning cases are adults. 12.6% are children 5 years or older, and 77.4% are children under 5. Find the number of degrees in the sector of a circle graph representing children 5 or older. Round off to the nearest degree.

Solution: 12.6% of $360 = 0.126(360°) = 45.36° = 45°$

Q5   In the example dealing with poisonings given in Frame 4 find:
a. The degrees in the sector of a circle graph representing poisoning of adults.

b. The degrees in the sector representing children under 5. Round off to the nearest degree.

\# \# \#   •   \# \# \#   •   \# \# \#   •   \# \# \#   •   \# \# \#   •   \# \# \#   •   \# \# \#   •   \# \# \#   •   \# \# \#

A5   **a.** 36°: $0.10(360°) = 36°$ **b.** 279°: $0.774(360°) = 278.64°$

5   If the data is not given by percents, the degrees of the central angle of each sector of a circle graph can be found by using proportions.

$$\frac{x}{360°} = \frac{\text{amount of part}}{\text{amount of total}}$$ where x = number of degrees in the sector

Solving the proportion for x will give the measure of the central angle of the sector. To draw the angle you will need a protractor.

Example: Find the number of degrees in the central angle of the sector of a circle graph which represents bedroom accidents. Round off to the nearest degree.

Where Poisoning Accidents Occur (900 cases)

Kitchen	369 cases
Bathroom	189 cases
Bedroom	108 cases
All other Places	234 cases

Solution: $\dfrac{x}{360°} = \dfrac{108}{900}$

$x = \dfrac{108}{900}(360°)$

$x = 43.2°$

Hence, the number of degrees in the central angle is 43°.

Q6   **a.** Determine the central angle for kitchen accidents, bathroom accidents, and accidents in all other places for the information in Frame 5. Round off to the nearest degree.

b. Construct a circle graph by using the results of part **a** and the example in Frame 5. Write a title and label each sector.

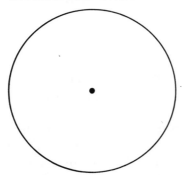

•   # # #   •   # # #   •   # # #   •   # # #   •   # # #   •   # # #   •   # # #   •   # #

A6   **a.**   148°: $\dfrac{x}{360°} = \dfrac{369}{900}$ 76°: $\dfrac{x}{360°} = \dfrac{189}{900}$ 94°: $\dfrac{x}{360°} = \dfrac{234}{900}$

$x = \dfrac{369}{900}(360°)$ $x = \dfrac{189}{900}(360°)$ $x = \dfrac{234}{900}(360°)$

$x = 147.6°$ $x = 75.6°$ $x = 93.6°$

b.   Where poisoning cases occur (900 cases)

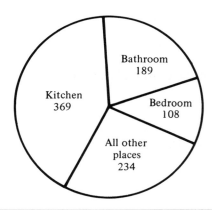

This completes the instruction for this section.

10.2   EXERCISE

Use the circle graph below to answer problems 1–5.

Health care costs
Total costs: 68 Billion

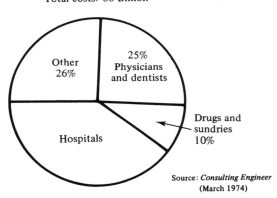

Source: *Consulting Engineer*
(March 1974)

1. Determine the percent of health care costs for hospitals.
2. Find the cost in dollars for physicians and dentists.
3. Use your answer to problem 1 to determine the cost in dollars for hospitals.
4. Find the number of degrees in the central angle of the sector that represents other health care costs.
5. Determine the number of degrees in the central angle of the sector representing hospitals.
6. Suppose you are constructing a circle graph to represent the sources of funds for health care. Your data indicates that philanthropy contributes 3.4 billion dollars, consumers contribute 38.76 billion dollars, and government contributes 25.84 billion dollars. Find the number of degrees in the central angle of each sector.

10.2   EXERCISE ANSWERS

1. 39%   **2.** $17 billion   **3.** $26.52 billion
4. 93.6°   **5.** 140.4°
6. philanthropy 18°, consumers 205.2°, government 136.8°

10.3 BAR GRAPHS

1   A bar graph is useful when a quick visual impression of the relative sizes of various quantities is to be communicated. If the actual numbers desired correspond to the heights of the bars, they should certainly be obtainable on a scale given as a part of the graph. The values will, by necessity, be approximate. However, the goal of a bar graph is not to communicate numbers associated with each bar as much as it is to show an accurate comparison of sizes of these numbers.

     A bar graph is used to compare items of discrete data. A bar graph is appropriate for this example because the set of organs represented on the horizontal axis is a set of discrete data.

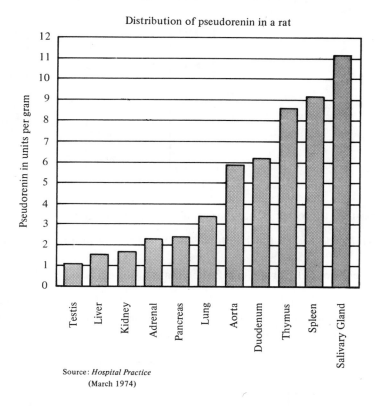

Distribution of pseudorenin in a rat

Source: *Hospital Practice*
(March 1974)

     If a short bar is placed next to a tall bar, it accents the shortness of the bar. To avoid the criticism that the maker of the graph is deliberately trying to distort the relationships among the numbers, two procedures have been developed for arranging discrete data that have no natural order. The first procedure is to arrange the data alphabetically. The second procedure is to arrange the bars in order of height. Notice that the second procedure was used in the bar graph in this frame.

Q1   Use the graph in Frame 1 to answer the following questions:

     a. What organ has the highest concentration of pseudorenin? _____

     b. What organ is third highest in concentration? _____

     c. How many organs have a concentration of over 5 units per gram? _____

     d. What is the concentration of pseudorenin in the lung? _____

     e. What is the concentration in the spleen? _____

     f. What is the concentration in the aorta? _____

•   # # #   •   # # #   •   # # #   •   # # #   •   # # #   •   # # #   •   # # #   •   # #

A1   **a.** salivary gland   **b.** thymus   **c.** 5
          d. 3.4 units per gram   **e.** 9.1 units per gram   **f.** 5.9 units per gram

---

2   A bar graph consists of a series of vertical or horizontal bars drawn according to scale. When constructing a bar graph one must be careful not to introduce a distortion in the impression left with the reader. The visual impression should match the actual relationships between the numbers being represented. An example will show how a bar graph can leave the wrong impression when not constructed correctly. Study the data in the table and the bar graph and see if you can locate the distortion.

Average Weekly Earnings	
Ardis	$300
Baker	$400
Chambers	$600

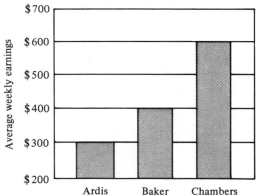

The relationships that exist in the chart (Chambers making twice as much as Ardis, Baker making $\frac{2}{3}$ of Chambers) are not reflected in the height of the bars. In the graph it appears that Chambers makes 4 times the earnings of Ardis and Baker makes $\frac{1}{2}$ the earnings of Chambers.

Although the top of the bar corresponds to the correct dollar amounts, the visual impression (some say this is what people usually remember) is inaccurate. The graph shown is actually only the top portion of a graph as it should be drawn. Compare the two graphs.

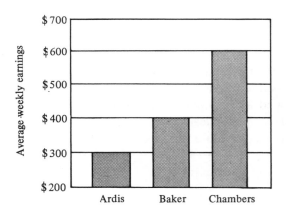

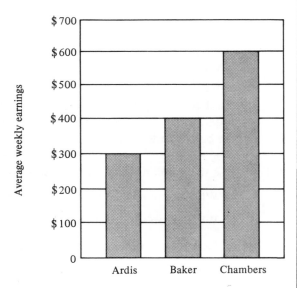

Notice that starting the vertical scale at zero instead of a larger number causes the heights of the bars to be in the same proportion as the numbers they represent. Using any other number as the smallest value on the vertical scale will distort the impression. Therefore, remember—*always start*

the vertical scale on a bar graph at the number zero. Removing a section of a bar or removing a section of the vertical scale also distorts the ratios of the bars of a bar graph. The omissions are usually indicated with a jagged line. If you see such a jagged line, be on the lookout for a distorted graph.

Q2   Use the accompanying graph to answer the following questions:

Deaths in city hospitals

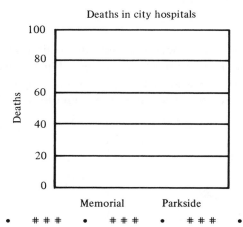

Memorial   Parkside

a. What are the number of deaths in the hospitals? _____

b. What is the ratio of Memorial deaths to Parkside deaths? _____

c. What is the ratio of the height of the Memorial bar to the height of the Parkside bar? _____

d. If an unethical reporter were to use this graph in an article stressing the high number of deaths in the local hospitals, which hospital would look much worse than the numerical value of the deaths

   indicate? _____

e. What other information would help you determine the significance of the graphs? _____

f. Draw the graph with the vertical scale starting at zero.

Deaths in city hospitals

Memorial   Parkside

•   # # #   •   # # #   •   # # #   •   # # #   •   # # #   •   # # #   •   # # #   •   # #

A2   a. Memorial 80, Parkside 60

b. $\frac{4}{3}$ c. $\frac{3}{1}$

d. Memorial: It looks as though it has 3 times as many deaths when it actually has $\frac{4}{3}$ as many.

e. Number of beds in each hospital. Time over which the data was collected.

f.

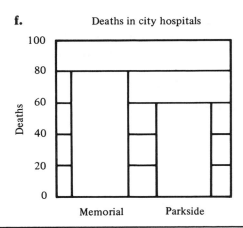

Deaths in city hospitals

3   Another way of introducing a distortion in a graph is to remove a section of the vertical scale. These omissions are usually indicated with a jagged line. If you see a jagged line on a bar graph look out for a distorted graph.

The accompanying graph shows how a drug is useful in keeping a patient asleep. The first bar was without medication, although placebos (tablets without active medication) were administered. It is shown in order to compare the other bars to it. The second bar is the length of a person's sleep as a percent of the first bar on the first three nights under medication. The third bar is on the 12th–14th nights of medication.

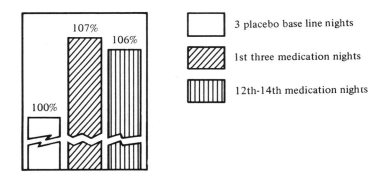

The next graph represents the same data as the previous one, but without the sections removed. Notice that the real differences in the bars are slight. This graph actually appeared in an advertisement in a nationwide magazine drawn as the first graph is drawn. The name of the drug company will remain anonymous to protect the guilty. If they drew it accurately the "superiority" of their product would not have been apparent.

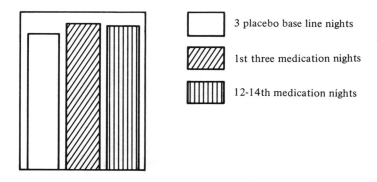

Q3   **a.** In favor of which toothpaste is the graph biased? _____
      b. Draw an unbiased graph in the space provided.

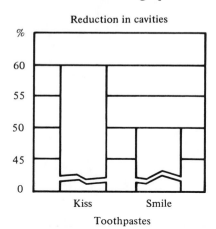
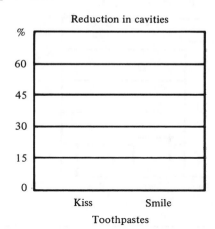

\# \# \#   •   \# \# \#   •   \# \# \#   •   \# \# \#   •   \# \# \#   •   \# \# \#   •   \# \# \#   •   \# \# \#   •   \# \# \#

A3   **a.** Kiss: It appears that Kiss toothpaste is associated with a reduction in cavities twice as large as Smile.

      b.
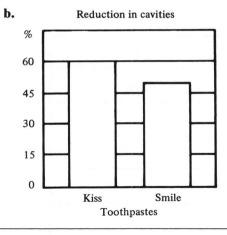

Q4   **a.** Which physician is the graph biased against? _____
      b. Draw an unbiased graph.

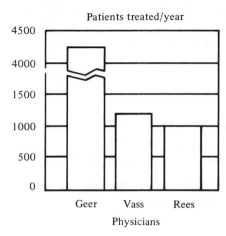
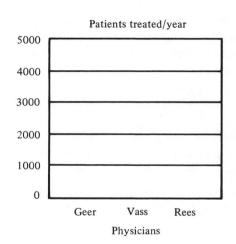

\# \# \#   •   \# \# \#   •   \# \# \#   •   \# \# \#   •   \# \# \#   •   \# \# \#   •   \# \# \#   •   \# \# \#   •   \# \# \#

A4   **a.** Geer

b.

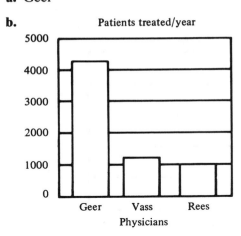

Patients treated/year

4.   The most important part of drawing a bar graph is determining the scale. You must be able to represent the largest number by a bar that fits into the available space. Suppose that you were to graph the data from the chart below on the space provided.

Population of the Five Largest Metropolitan
Areas (in millions of persons)

New York	11.5
Los Angeles	6.7
Chicago	6.5
Philadelphia	4.7
Detroit	4.0

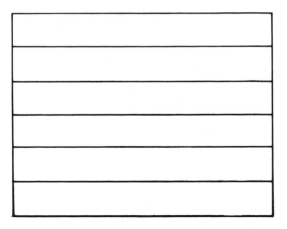

The population of the New York metropolitan area would have to be represented by a bar no longer than 6 units because there are six spaces available. *To find the scale, divide the amount to be represented by the longest bar by the number of available spaces.* (If your paper is unlined, divide by the number of inches available.) Round the resulting value up to a convenient *larger* value. In the example given:

$$11.5 \div 6 = 1.9\frac{1}{6} = 2.0 \text{ million rounded up}$$

Before you are given an opportunity to complete the bar graph of this example, you will be given a chance to practice determining the scale for various graphs.

Q5   Suppose that the largest number to be represented was 426 and you wanted to draw your graph on a location that had 10 vertical spaces. What would you use for a scale?

• # # # • # # # • # # # • # # # • # # # • # # # • # # # • # #

A5   Use 50 units per space: $426 \div 10 = 42.6$ rounded upward would be 50. (45 would not be incorrect.)

Q6   If the longest bar on a bar graph was to represent 45,050 and you had 7 inches in the vertical direction available, what would you use for a scale?

•   # # #   •   # # #   •   # # #   •   # # #   •   # # #   •   # # #   •   # # #   •   # #

A6   7,000 per inch: $45,050 \div 7 = 6,436$ rounded up to 7,000. Therefore, use 7,000 per inch. In this case 8,000, or even 10,000, would not be incorrect. Use of 10,000 would cause your bars to be much shorter, and you would not be using as much of your available space.

Q7   The longest bar should represent $44, and there are 6 vertical spaces available. What should be used for the vertical scale?

•   # # #   •   # # #   •   # # #   •   # # #   •   # # #   •   # # #   •   # # #   •   # #

A7 $8 per space: $\$44 \div 6 = \$7.33$ rounded upward would be 8. It would also be correct to use $10 per space.

Q8   Use the scale of 2.0 million people per vertical space and complete the bar graph in Frame 4. Be sure that both scales are labeled and that a title is included.

•   # # #   •   # # #   •   # # #   •   # # #   •   # # #   •   # # #   •   # # #   •   # #

A8

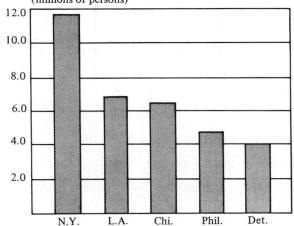

Population of the Five Largest Metropolitan Areas (millions of persons)

(*Note*: The lengths of each bar must be approximated as nearly as possible.)

5 In some cases the horizontal axis represents a continuous variable such as time, but it is grouped into intervals. A bar graph can then be constructed representing the frequency with which numbers in each interval occur. In this case no space is left between the bars. The resulting graph is called a *histogram*.

The data gives the highest temperature observed in 200 patients with infectious mononucleosis. Since the highest bar must represent 58 and must fit on 5 spaces, each space should represent 15 ($58 \div 5 = 11.6$ would be rounded off to 15).

Highest Degree of Fever

°F	Number
no fever	5
99–99.5	16
100–100.9	58
101–101.9	44
102–102.9	44
103–103.9	28
104–104.9	5

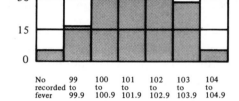

From the graph it can be seen that the most common fever for infectious mononucleosis is between 100 and 100.9, but that the fever could go as high as 104 °F. It is possible to have a higher fever but it would be very uncommon.

Q9 **a.** Use the data below to construct a histogram showing the duration of the fever from infectious mononucleosis. You must determine the vertical scale.

Days	Frequency
1–7	24
8–14	93
15–20	52
21–28	28
28–34	3
total	200

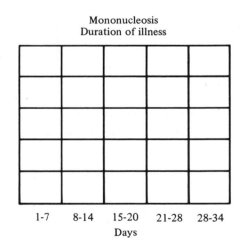

Mononucleosis
Duration of illness

b. What is the most common length of time for fever from mononucleosis to last? _____

c. Is it common for the fever from mononucleosis to last over one month? _____

d. Which is more likely to happen: The fever from mononucleosis will subside in the first week or the fever will subside in the fourth week? _____

\# \# \# • \# \# \# • \# \# \# • \# \# \# • \# \# \# • \# \# \# • \# \# \# • \# \# \# • \# \# \#

A9   **a.**

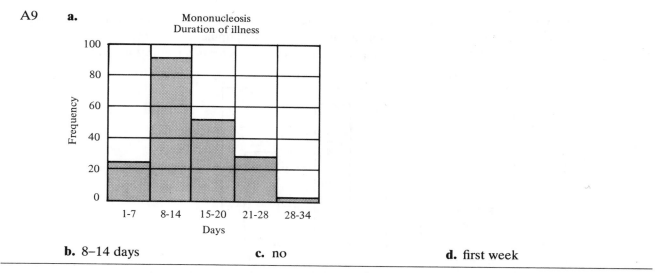

b. 8–14 days   **c.** no   **d.** first week

This completes the instruction for this section.

10.3   EXERCISE

1. The accompanying bar graph shows the excess mortality of overweight women. (Mortality rate is the number of people in a group who are expected to die in a year compared to the number of people in the group.)

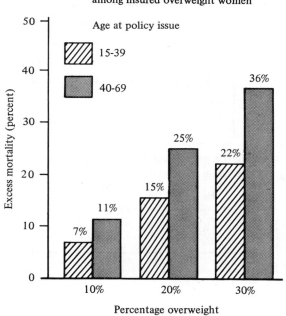

a. What is the percent of excess mortality for women 40–69 years old at policy issue and 20% overweight?

b. What is the percent of excess mortality for women 15–39 years old at policy issue who are 10% overweight?

c. The trend is for the excess mortality to _____ as the percentage overweight
increase/decrease
increases.

d. Would the following conclusion be supported by the graph? Women who are more overweight are more likely to die at a given age than those in the population at large.

2. The following graph appeared in an article discussing diabetes in a medical journal.

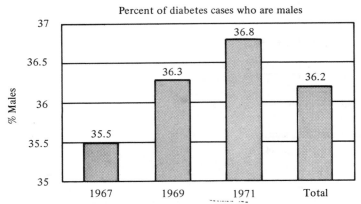

Percent of diabetes cases who are males

a. What flaw in the construction of the graph distorts the image the reader obtains?

b. After considering the effect of the distortion, guess what the point was of the article which accompanied the graph:

1. The percentage of males out of the total diabetes patients is about the same for 4 years.

2. The percentage of males out of the total diabetes patients is increasing dramatically.

3. The percentage of males out of the total diabetes patients is decreasing.

c. If the longest bar of length 36.8 is to be represented on a scale with 8 divisions, then each division should represent how much?

d. Graph the same information with a vertical scale that starts at zero.

3. Construct a graph for the data below showing the trend in the percentage of people who say they would prefer living in a city to living in other areas of the country.

Those preferring city life

Those preferring city life

1968	22%
1970	18%
1972	17%
1974	13%
1976	12%

1968   1970   1972   1974   1976

4. Consider the graph below.

Ages of patients
with infectious mononucleosis
during a fifteen-year period

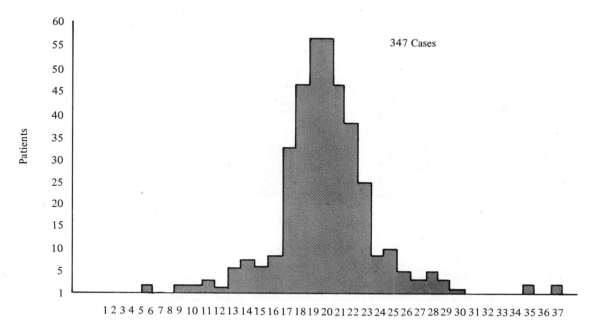

Source: *Hospital Medicine* (March 1973)

a. A graph where the bars are not separated is called a _____.

b. At what age do the most cases of infectious mononucleosis occur according to the graph?

c. Which of the age groups would complete the following statement most accurately? Mononucleosis is a disease which occurs in people predominantly between the ages of

_____. 1. 12–17 yr   2. 17–23 yr   3. 21–26 yr   4. 25–30 yr.

d. Which of the age groups would complete the following statement most accurately: Mononucleosis rarely strikes a person _____. 1. under 6   2. under 20   3. over 25   4. over 31.

10.3   EXERCISE ANSWERS

1. a. 25%   **b.** 7%   **c.** increase   **d.** yes

2. a. The vertical scale does not start at zero.

b. 2   **c.** 5

d.

Percent of diabetes cases who are males

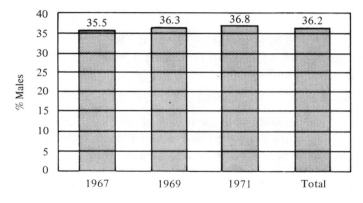

3.

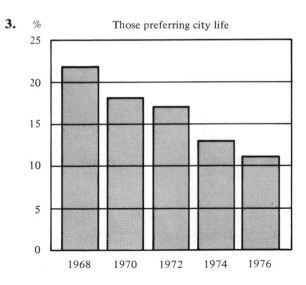

Those preferring city life

4. a. histogram   **b.** 19 and 20
   c. 2 (17–23 yrs)   **d.** 1 and 4

10.4 LINE GRAPHS

1   Line graphs are used when the horizontal scale indicates continuous data. The line graph is particularly useful for showing a continuous trend over a period of time. Time is located on the horizontal axis. You can read a line graph for values in between the numbers shown on the horizontal scale. The accompanying line graph shows the course of fever in measles for the first four days of a patient's illness.

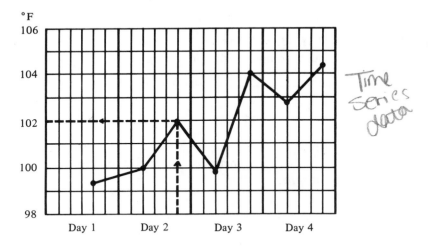

The fever at a given time is found by locating the time on the horizontal axis. Each 24-hour day is divided into 6 subdivisions so each subdivision represents 4 hours. The first temperature was recorded at 4:00 P.M. of the first day and was about 99.4 °F.

Example: What was the temperature of the patient at 8:00 P.M. of the second day?

Solution: 102 °F: 8:00 P.M. of the second day is located 5 subdivisions into the second day. The temperature is found by moving vertically to the graph and then horizontally to find the temperature. A dotted arrow shows the path used to read the temperature at 8:00 P.M. of the second day.

Q1   Use the line graph in Frame 1 to find the temperature at:

   a. 8:00 A.M. of 3rd Day _____   **b.** 8:00 P.M. of 3rd day _____

   c. 8:00 A.M. of 4th Day _____   **d.** 8:00 P.M. of 4th Day _____

•   # # #   •   # # #   •   # # #   •   # # #   •   # # #   •   # # #   •   # # #   •   # #

A1   **a.** 99.8 °F   **b.** 104 °F   **c.** 102.8 °F   **d.** 104.4 °F:

   These temperatures are obtained by following the arrows shown on the graph below.

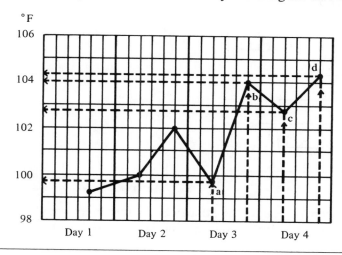

Q2   By comparing the temperature at 8:00 A.M. to that at 8:00 P.M. each day, would you say that it is

   more common to have a higher temperature in the morning or in the evening? _____

•   # # #   •   # # #   •   # # #   •   # # #   •   # # #   •   # # #   •   # # #   •   # #

A2   evening

Q3   Although there are up-and-down fluctuations of temperature, what is the general trend for the

   temperature of a measles patient for the first four days? _____

•   # # #   •   # # #   •   # # #   •   # # #   •   # # #   •   # # #   •   # # #   •   # #

A3   The temperature rises.

2   In a situation where there are many fluctuations in a line graph the general trend of the graph is
     important. The graph shows the temperature of a patient with osteomyelitis of the hip for 48 days.
     The temperature is measured in Celsius units where 37 °C is normal.

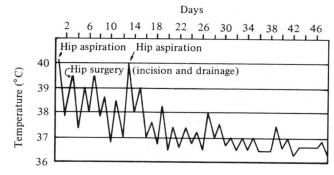

Example: How many days did it take before the patient's temperature was brought down to normal to remain approximately normal?

Solution: The temperature became normal on the 16th day and remained approximately normal thereafter.

Q4   On what day was the temperature brought down to normal to remain approximately so? _____

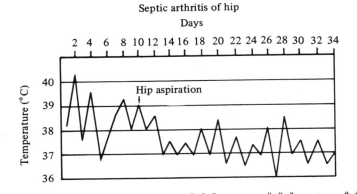

•   # # #   •   # # #   •   # # #   •   # # #   •   # # #   •   # # #   •   # # #   •   # #

A4   13th day: The temperature was below normal on the 5th day but immediately went back up and did not return to normal until the 13th day. It then stayed approximately normal but with rather wide fluctuations.

Q5   Describe the general trend of the temperature graph below.

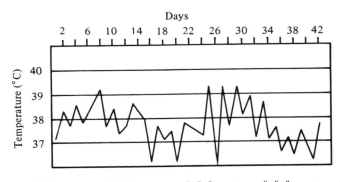

•   # # #   •   # # #   •   # # #   •   # # #   •   # # #   •   # # #   •   # # #   •   # #

A5   The patient has a fever for about 14 days, then becomes normal for about 7 days, before the temperature goes up again until the 32nd day at which time it returns to normal.

3   Line graphs are sometimes used for showing relationships between quantities over the same time span by putting more than one line graph on the same set of axes. The graph below compares survival rates for patients treated with penicillin and a type-specific antiserum with untreated patients. All had pneumococcal pneumonia.

Example: What percent survived under each treatment at the 10th day of illness?

Solution: penicillin 86%, serum 63%, and untreated 42%

Example 2: Which treatment was superior at the end of the 10th day?

Solution: penicillin: 86% of the patients treated with penicillin were still alive which was the highest of the three treatments.

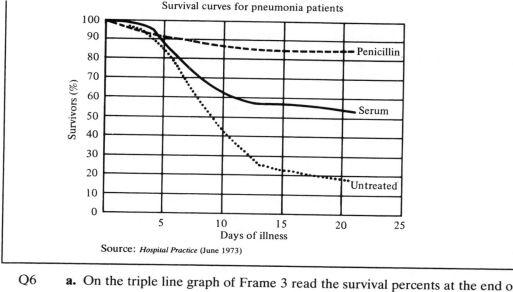

Survival curves for pneumonia patients

Source: *Hospital Practice* (June 1973)

Q6   **a.** On the triple line graph of Frame 3 read the survival percents at the end of the 20th day.

penicillin _____ serum _____ untreated _____

b. What treatment was superior for the first few days of treatment? _____

c. On which day did the penicillin start to show its superiority? _____

\# \# \# • \# \# \# • \# \# \# • \# \# \# • \# \# \# • \# \# \# • \# \# \# • \# \# \# • \# \# \#

A6   **a.** 84%, 54%, 18%   **b.** serum   **c.** 4th

Q7   The following line graph shows the distribution of leukemia cases. The vertical scale represents number of cases but has no numerical values since the purpose of the graph is to show comparisons of the different kinds of leukemia.

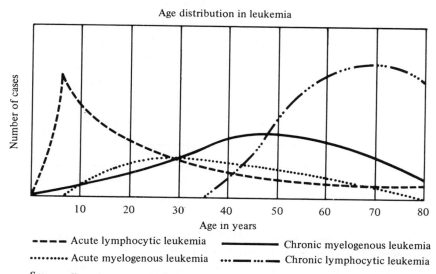

Age distribution in leukemia

- - - - Acute lymphocytic leukemia   ———— Chronic myelogenous leukemia

·········· Acute myelogenous leukemia   ···———···— Chronic lymphocytic leukemia

Source: *Hospital Medicine* (December 1970)

a. Match the name of the leukemia with its description:

1. Acute lymphocytic   i. dominant in the elderly
2. Acute myelogenous   ii. crests at age 30
3. Chronic myelogenous   iii. dominant in children
4. Chronic lymphocytic   iv. crests at age between 40 and 50

b. At what age does acute lymphocytic leukemia occur with greatest frequency? _____

c. At what age does acute myelogenous leukemia surpass acute lymphocytic leukemia? _____

d. Between what ages is chronic myelogenous leukemia the dominant form of leukemia in number of cases? _____

e. There are virtually no cases of chronic lymphocytic leukemia below what age? _____

• # # # • # # # • # # # • # # # • # # # • # # # • # # # • # #

A7   **a.** 1-iii, 2-ii, 3-iv, 4-i   **b.** 7 years   **c.** 29 or 30 years

      d. 30-48 years   **e.** 35 years

---

4   Since line graphs are used with continuous data on the horizontal axis, they represent a continuous change in the variable being represented. Although the graph may be constructed by locating only a few points on the graph, the line graph allows you to read the graph for values in between the points plotted. Approximating values in between known values on the graph is called *interpolation*.

This graph shows systolic and diastolic blood pressure for a patient at various times in a 14-minute period. The two blood pressures could be read at 1 minute on the graph even though 1

Time (min)	Diastolic (mm Hg)	Systolic (mm Hg)
0	60	120
2	95	215
4	80	175
6	75	120
8	65	95
14	95	120

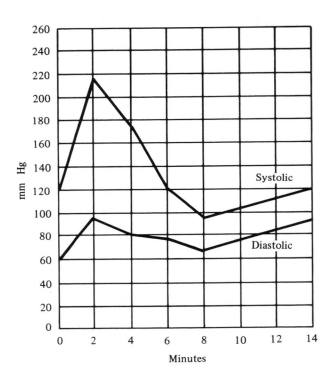

minute was not in the table. The interpolated values for 1 minute are 170 systolic and 79 diastolic. The interpolated values for 3 minutes are 195 systolic and 87 diastolic.

Interpolation sometimes does not predict the actual readings. If the graph fluctuates widely there may actually be a fluctuation where you assume it is straight. The graph at the top of the next page is of the same person's blood pressure over the same time which includes the previously graphed points. It also has some additional values. Notice that the interpolated values for one minute and three minutes were inaccurate because these were locations where fluctuations occurred. On the other hand, an interpolated value for nine minutes on the diastolic graph would have been quite accurate.

Time (min)	Diastolic (mm Hg)	Systolic (mm Hg)
1	50	85
3	135	250
5	70	135
7	75	100
9	75	120
11	90	140

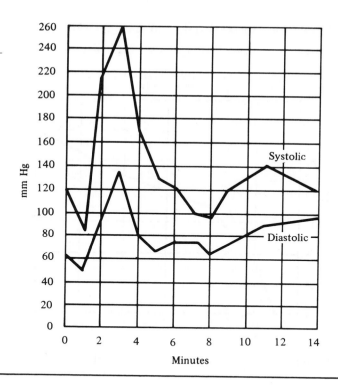

Q8   What is the process of approximating between two known values on a graph called? _____

\# \# \# • \# \# \# • \# \# \# • \# \# \# • \# \# \# • \# \# \# • \# \# \# • \# \# \# • \# \# \#

A8   interpolation

Q9   **a.** Plot the number of decayed, filled, or missing teeth at each age. Connect the points to make a line graph.

Age	Number of decayed, filled, or missing teeth
5	0
10	7
20	14
40	18
60	24

Source: *Dental Economics*, July 1973

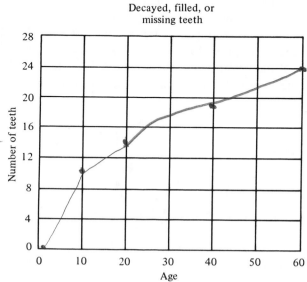

Decayed, filled, or missing teeth

- Interpolation: predicting
what will happen between 2 data
points.

- Extrapolation: predicting what
will happen outside the range
of data. (RISKY!)

b. Use your line graph from part **a** to interpolate the number of teeth decayed, filled, or missing at age 15. _____

c. Interpolate to find how many teeth are decayed, filled, or missing at age 30. _____

d. Would you expect this graph to fluctuate widely or be a smoothly rising graph? _____

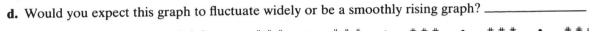

A9 **a.**

Decayed, filled, or
missing teeth

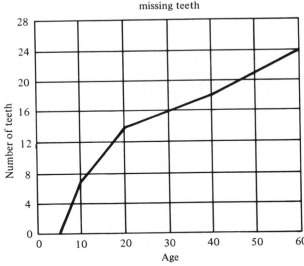

b. 10 teeth   **c.** 16 teeth   **d.** smoothly rising

---

5 If the graph is extended beyond the last point that was graphed and values are read in the extended portion of the graph, these are *extrapolated* values. Extrapolation is usually a risky thing to do with a fluctuating graph, but with a smoothly changing graph a fairly accurate reading is obtained over a small interval.

In the following example approximate information is obtained in a region in which it would be virtually impossible to obtain experimental readings. X-ray dose rates may be measured by means of a probe which is placed into the x-ray beams. The x-rays emerge from a cone which ensures that the patient's skin is the proper distance from the x-ray source. The end of the cone through which the x-rays emerge is usually closed by a thin sheet of plastic. It is the dose rate at the surface of the cone end which is required for treatment purposes. However, because of the thickness of the probe, the center of the probe where the dose rate reading is made cannot be placed nearer to the surface of the cone than a distance equal to the radius of the probe. To solve this problem extrapolation is

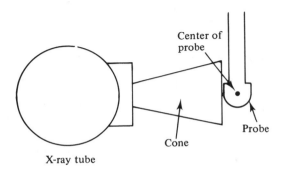

used. The distance from the cone end to the probe is put on the horizontal axis, and the dose rate is located on the vertical scale. Dose rates are observed to be a series of points approaching more and more closely to the cone surface until the probe touches the surface. The curve is then extended back (extrapolated) to find the dose rate at zero centimetres from the cone end.

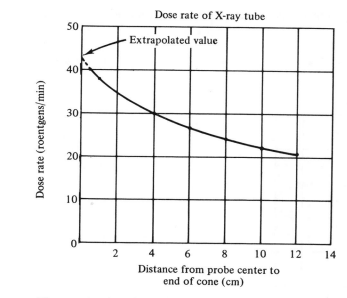

The extrapolated value of the dose rate appears to be 43 roentgens/min at the end of the cone.

Q10 **a.** Plot the double line graph showing suicide and homicide rates in the United States from 1930 to 1970.

Year	Suicides	Homicides
1930	21.5	12.2
1935	20.0	11.6
1940	19.5	8.6
1945	14.2	7.0
1950	15.5	7.0
1955	14.5	6.5
1960	15.5	7.0
1965	16.2	8.0
1970	15.8	10.8

Source: Bureau of the Census

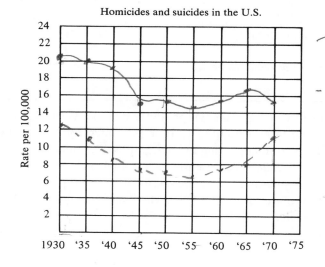

~ = suicides

---- = homicides

b. What is the trend for suicides from 1930 to 1945? _decrease_

c. What is the trend for suicides from 1945 to 1970? _pretty level_

d. What is the trend for homicides from 1930 to 1955? _decrease_

e. What is the trend for homicides from 1955 to 1970? _increasing_

f. Are Americans more inclined to kill themselves or to kill someone else? _themselves_

g. Interpolate to determine the suicide rate in 1948. _____

h. Extrapolate to determine the suicide rate in 1975. _____

i. Extrapolate to determine the homicide rate in 1975. _____

j. On the basis of the data above will the homicide rate overtake the suicide rate in the future?

_____

\# \# \#   •   \# \# \#   •   \# \# \#   •   \# \# \#   •   \# \# \#   •   \# \# \#   •   \# \# \#   •   \# \# \#   •   \# \# \#

A10   **a.**

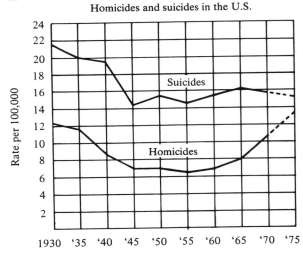

Homicides and suicides in the U.S.

b. the suicide rate declined

c. stable to slowly rising

d. declined

e. increasing more rapidly

f. kill themselves

g. 15

h. 15

i. 13.5

j. yes: It appears to be so.

---

6   When constructing a line graph, determine the vertical scale in the same manner as the bar graph. Divide the largest number to be represented by the number of spaces available. This will keep distortions from appearing in your graphs. The only exception to this rule would be in a case where the vertical scale is representing a variable such as temperature where the zero point is arbitrary. The zero point on a temperature scale does not represent the absence of all temperature but is only used as a reference point. (This is the reason the graphs in Frame 1 and 2 do not start at zero on the vertical scale.)

Q11   **a.** Determine the scale markings for the data below if the line graph is to be placed on a graph with 8 vertical spaces.

Average Annual Death Rate among Tuberculosis Patients and among the General Population in Age Groups

Age	Tuberculosis Patients	General Population
20	0.5	0.1
30	0.7	0.2
40	1.2	0.3
50	2.2	0.8
60	6.0	2.1
70	12.8	5.8
greater than 75	14.6	12.8

b. Mark the vertical and horizontal scales and graph the data.

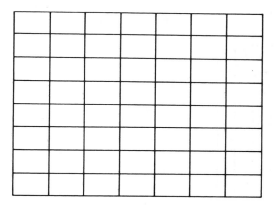

\# \# \#   •   \# \# \#   •   \# \# \#   •   \# \# \#   •   \# \# \#   •   \# \# \#   •   \# \# \#   •   \# \# \#   •   \# \# \#

A11   **a.** 2: $14.6 \div 8 = 1.825$ which would be rounded to 2

b.

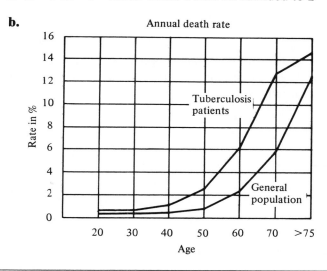

Annual death rate

This completes the instruction for this section.

10.4   EXERCISE

1. Use the graph of the incidence of venereal diseases (top of next page) to answer the following questions.

   a. What is the trend for the incidence of syphilis?

   b. What is the trend for the incidence of gonorrhea?

   c. Read the incidence of gonorrhea for 1967.

   d. Is the answer to part **c** the result of interpolation or extrapolation?

   e. Predict the incidence of gonorrhea in 1976.

   f. Is the answer to part **e** the result of interpolation or extrapolation?

   g. The incidence of gonorrhea was 200,000 cases in 1958. How many years did it take to double in frequency?

   h. How many years did it take for the gonorrhea incidence to double from 400,000 to 800,000 cases?

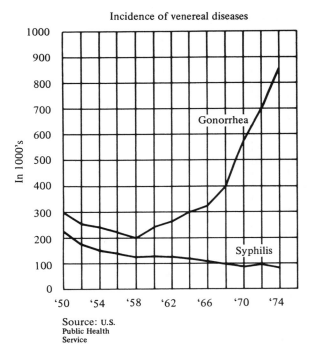

Incidence of venereal diseases

Source: U.S.
Public Health
Service

2. The following data was obtained by placing different thicknesses of copper before an x-ray beam and recording the intensity of the beam on the other side. The intensities are expressed as percentages of the beam with no obstructions.

Thickness of copper (mm)	Intensity
0.0	100
0.2	70
0.4	55
0.7	40
1.0	35
1.5	25
2.0	23

a. Determine the scale on the vertical axis and graph the data.

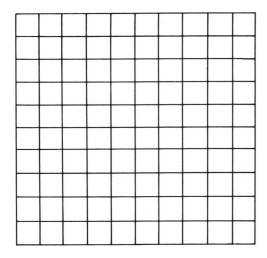

b. Read the intensity of the beam for a thickness of 1.2 mm of copper.
c. What is the name of the process employed in part b?

d. The thickness of copper required to reduce the intensity to $\frac{1}{2}$ the original is called the half-value layer of the beam in copper. What is the half-value layer of the beam?

10.4   EXERCISE ANSWERS

1. a. It is decreasing slowly.
   c. 370,000 cases
   e. 1,000,000 cases
   g. 10 years

   b. It is increasing rapidly.
   d. interpolation
   f. extrapolation
   h. 5 years

2. a.

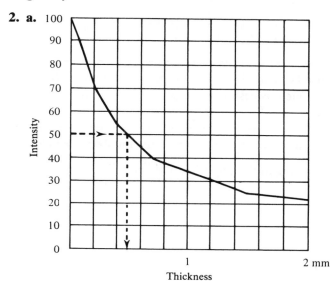

   b. 32
   c. interpolation
   d. 0.5 mm (see graph)

10.5   THE RECTANGULAR COORDINATE SYSTEM

1   Some graphs illustrate the physical world more clearly by using negative numbers. These graphs will be discussed in this section. We begin by reviewing the number line.

A *number line* is a line with points corresponding to each integer. Fractions can also be located on a number line. The following section of a number line has a few integers shown. Of course, the line extends forever in each direction just as the integers continue in both the positive and negative directions.

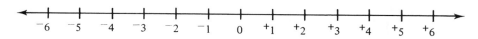

Q1   What numbers correspond to the points indicated by the arrows?

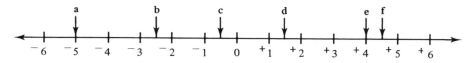

  a. _____ **b.** _____ **c.** _____ **d.** _____ **e.** _____ **f.** _____

• # # # • # # # • # # # • # # # • # # # • # # # • # # # • # #

A1   **a.** $^-5$ **b.** $^-2\frac{1}{2}$ **c.** $\frac{^-1}{2}$ **d.** $1\frac{1}{2}$ **e.** 4   **f.** $4\frac{1}{2}$

Q2   Place arrows at the points that correspond to the numbers below:

a. 3   **b.** $^-4$ **c.** $\frac{1}{2}$ **d.** $^-1\frac{1}{2}$ **e.** 4   **f.** $^-3$

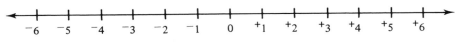

A2

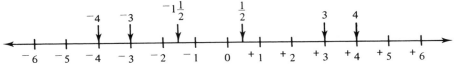

| 2 | Mathematicians use the right side of a horizontal line for the positive numbers. Number lines can also be drawn vertically. On a vertical line it is customary to place the positive numbers above zero and the negative numbers below zero. |

Q3   **a.** Select a point to correspond to zero and label the integers on the number line below.

b. Place arrows at the points corresponding to the following numbers: $^-3, \frac{^-1}{2}, \frac{3}{4}, 2\frac{1}{2}$

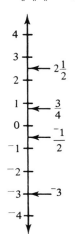

A3

3   A *rectangular coordinate system* is formed by crossing one number line in a vertical position over another number line in a horizontal position. The horizontal line is called the *x axis* and the vertical line is the *y axis*. Together they are called the *coordinate axes*. The two lines intersect at the zero point on each axis. This point is called the *origin*. A rectangular coordinate system looks as follows:

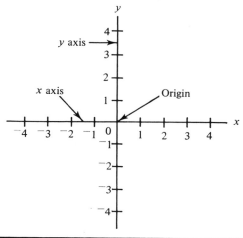

Q4   **a.** The horizontal number line of a coordinate system is called the _____.

b. The vertical number line of a coordinate system is called the _____.

c. The point where the number lines cross in a coordinate system is called the _____.

d. The vertical and horizontal number lines together in a rectangular coordinate system are called

_____ _____.

•   # # #   •   # # #   •   # # #   •   # # #   •   # # #   •   # # #   •   # # #   •   # #

A4   **a.** *x* axis   **b.** *y* axis   **c.** origin   **d.** coordinate axes
       (*Note*: "axes" is plural, "axis" is singular.)

4   Each point in the plane has a name determined by its relationship to the origin. To determine this name, distances are measured on horizontal or vertical lines. A point is named with two numbers called *coordinates* placed in a set of parentheses such as (3, 2). The expression (x, y) is called an *ordered pair*. To locate the ordered pair (x, y), move *x* units horizontally from the origin, and from that location move *y* units vertically. Below is the location of the ordered pair (3, 2) with *x* coordinate, 3, and *y* coordinate, 2.

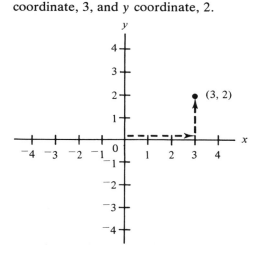

> Although the y value is determined by the scale on the y axis, the path taken in the vertical direction is not on the y axis but is on a line parallel to it.

Q5   Use the paths shown to name the points on the coordinate system:

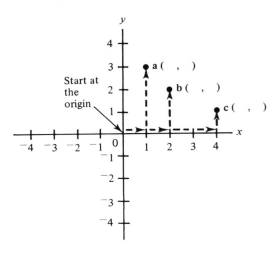

•   # # #   •   # # #   •   # # #   •   # # #   •   # # #   •   # # #   •   # # #   •   # #

A5   **a.** (1, 3)   **b.** (2, 2)   **c.** (4, 1)

Q6   Is the point that corresponds with (3, 1) the same point as the point that corresponds with (1, 3)?

_____

•   # # #   •   # # #   •   # # #   •   # # #   •   # # #   •   # # #   •   # # #   •   # #

A6   no

---

5   If a point is to the left of the y axis, its x coordinate is negative. A point below the x axis has a negative y coordinate. Study the coordinates of the following points:

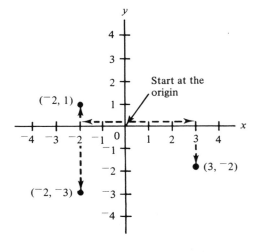

Q7   Name the points on the coordinate system:

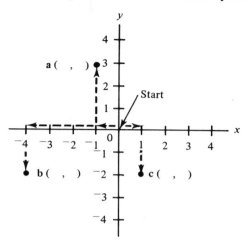

• # # # • # # # • # # # • # # # • # # # • # # # • # # # • # #

A7   **a.** ($^-$1, 3)   **b.** ($^-$4, $^-$2)   **c.** (1, $^-$2)

Q8   Name the coordinates of each of the following points:

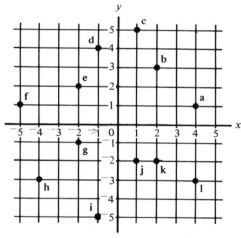

a. 4,1   **b.** 2,3   **c.** 1,5   **d.** -1,4

e. -2,2   **f.** -5,1   **g.** -3,-1   **h.** -4,-3

i. -1,-5   **j.** 1,-2   **k.** 2,-2   **l.** 4,-3

• # # # • # # # • # # # • # # # • # # # • # # # • # # # • # #

A8   **a.** (4, 1)   **b.** (2, 3)   **c.** (1, 5)   **d.** ($^-$1, 4)
      e. ($^-$2, 2)   **f.** ($^-$5, 1)   **g.** ($^-$2, $^-$1)   **h.** ($^-$4, $^-$3)
      i. ($^-$1, $^-$5)   **j.** (1, $^-$2)   **k.** (2, $^-$2)   **l.** (4, $^-$3)

6   A point is always named with an ordered pair of numbers. If a point is on the axes, one of its coordinates will be zero. For example, point a on the following coordinate system is 3 units from the origin in the horizontal direction but it is zero units from the x axis. It is named (3, 0). Point b is zero units from the y axis but 2 units up. It is named (0, 2). Study the names of each of the points.

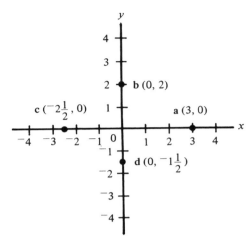

When graphing, numbers are more easily located if written in mixed-number form.

Q9   Name each point on the coordinate axes:

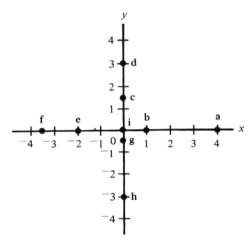

a. _____   b. _____   c. _____   d. _____

e. _____   f. _____   g. _____   h. _____

i. _____

\# \# \#   •   \# \# \#   •   \# \# \#   •   \# \# \#   •   \# \# \#   •   \# \# \#   •   \# \# \#   •   \# \# \#   •   \# \# \#

A9   **a.** $(4, 0)$ **b.** $(1, 0)$ **c.** $\left(0, 1\frac{1}{2}\right)$ **d.** $(0, 3)$

     e. $(^-2, 0)$ **f.** $\left(^-3\frac{1}{2}, 0\right)$ **g.** $\left(0, \frac{^-1}{2}\right)$ **h.** $(0, ^-3)$

     i. $(0, 0)$

[*Note*: If your point has the coordinates in the opposite order from the answers given, it is incorrect. For example, $(4, 0) \neq (0, 4)$.]

Q10   Name the points on the coordinate system (see top of page 415):

a. _____   b. _____   c. _____   d. _____

e. _____   f. _____   g. _____   h. _____

i. _____   **j.** _____   **k.** _____   **l.** _____

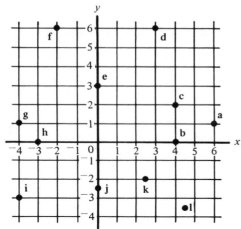

• # # # • # # # • # # # • # # # • # # # • # # # • # # # • # #

A10   **a.** (6, 1)   **b.** (4, 0)   **c.** (4, 2)   **d.** (3, 6)
      e. (0, 3)   **f.** ($^-$2, 6)   **g.** ($^-$4, 1)   **h.** ($^-$3, 0)

i. ($^-$4, $^-$3)   **j.** $\left(0, ^-2\frac{1}{2}\right)$ **k.** $\left(2\frac{1}{2}, ^-2\right)$ **l.** $\left(4\frac{1}{2}, ^-3\frac{1}{2}\right)$

---

8   The coordinate plane extends forever in each direction. The portion shown is only a finite portion of it. The coordinate axes do not have to be centered on the portion of the planes on which you graph. For instance, if you were only interested in graphing points with positive coordinates, the axes may be drawn as shown.

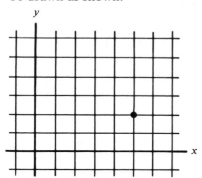

   If numbers are not written along the axes, each space is assumed to represent 1 unit. Therefore, the point shown above is (5, 2).

   The plane is separated (by the coordinate axes) into four parts called *quadrants*. The quadrants are numbered counterclockwise. A point on an axis is not in any quadrant.

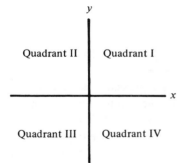

Q11   Draw the x and y axes on the plane and graph the points. Write the points that are in each of the four quadrants.

(5, 2), (3, ⁻3), (3, 1), (⁻2, 1), (⁻1, 4), (1, 5), (⁻2, ⁻1), (3, ⁻4), (⁻4, 1), (⁻4, ⁻1), (⁻1, ⁻4), (1, ⁻4)

a. quadrant I   _____

b. quadrant II   _____

c. quadrant III   _____

d. quadrant IV   _____

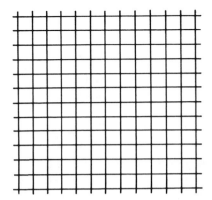

•   # # #   •   # # #   •   # # #   •   # # #   •   # # #   •   # # #   •   # # #   •   # #

A11   **a.** (5, 2), (3, 1), (1, 5)   **b.** (⁻2, 1), (⁻1, 4), (⁻4, 1)
       c. (⁻2, ⁻1), (⁻4, ⁻1), (⁻1, ⁻4)   **d.** (3, ⁻3), (3, ⁻4), (1, ⁻4)

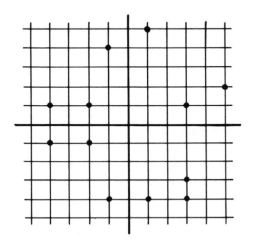

9   A medical doctor did a study on the effects of a certain appetite suppressant by selecting two groups who wanted to lose weight. She recorded the average weight of the groups for 2 weeks, then gave each group tablets which she told each group were appetite suppressants. This was true for Group I, but Group II was given placebos. The groups were asked to follow the same dosages of the tablets and the same procedures for diet and exercise. The results are illustrated with a line graph as well as a chart.

Time (weeks)	Weight Change (lb) Group I	Group II
¯2	0.2	¯0.1
¯1	0.1	¯0.1
0	0.0	0.0
1	¯1.0	¯1.0
2	¯2.2	¯2.0
3	¯3.8	¯2.2
4	¯4.5	¯2.5
6	¯7.0	¯3.0
8	¯8.0	¯3.0
10	¯9.5	¯3.5
12	¯10.0	¯4.2

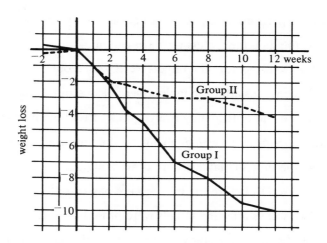

The x axis is the time measured in weeks. The zero point represents the time when the tablets were given to the groups. The two weeks before that time are recorded as negative values of time.

The y axis represents the weight measured in pounds. The zero point is the average weight of the groups when the tablets were administered. Positive numbers on the weight axis represent a gain in weight while negative numbers represent a weight loss.

Q12 Use the graph in Frame 9 to answer the following questions:

a. Which quadrant contains most of the line graph? _____

b. What other quadrants also contain a portion of the graph? _____

c. What was the weight change for Group I at 7 weeks? _____

d. What was the weight change for Group II at 7 weeks? _____

e. Did the group with the actual appetite supressant lose the most weight? _____

• # # # • # # # • # # # • # # # • # # # • # # # • # # # • # #

A12 **a.** IV **b.** II and III **c.** ¯7.5 lb **d.** ¯3 lb **e.** yes

Q13 Two participants in the study of Frame 9 kept records of their weight changes for the same 14-week period as the study. Use the graph of their weight changes to answer the questions.

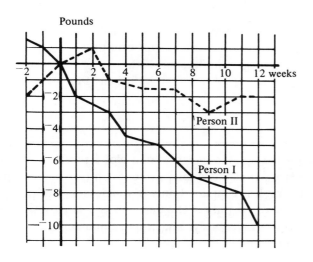

a. Indicate person I's weight change at the following times:

1. At the time the tablets were passed out. _____

2. Two weeks before the tablets were passed out. _____

3. Three weeks after the tablets were passed out. _____

4. At the end of the study twelve weeks after the tablets were passed out. _____

b. Indicate person II's weight change at the following times:

1. At the time the tablets were passed out. _____

2. Two weeks before the tablets were passed out. _____

3. Two weeks after the tablets were passed out. _____

4. At the end of the study 12 weeks after the tablets were passed out. _____

c. For the two weeks before the tablets were made available was person II gaining weight or losing weight? _____

d. For the two weeks before the tablets were made available was person I gaining weight or losing weight? _____

e. What happened to person II's weight during the first week after the tablets were given?

_____

f. What other weeks after the tablets were given did person II gain weight? _____

g. What weeks did person II's weight make no change? _____

h. Did person I ever make a weight gain over a weeks time? _____

i. Did person I's weight ever make no change for a week? _____

j. In what weeks did person II lose more weight than person I? _____

k. How much weight did person I lose over the 14 weeks? _____

l. How much weight did person II lose over the 14 weeks? _____

\# \# \#   •   \# \# \#   •   \# \# \#   •   \# \# \#   •   \# \# \#   •   \# \# \#   •   \# \# \#   •   \# \# \#   •   \# \# \#

A13   **a.** 1. 0 lb   2. $1\frac{1}{2}$ lb   3. ⁻3 lb   4. ⁻10 lb

b. 1. 0 lb   2. ⁻2 lb   3. 1 lb   4. ⁻2 lb

c. gaining   **d.** losing   **e.** went up

f. 2nd, 10th, and 11th weeks   **g.** 6th, 7th, and 12th

h. no   **i.** no   **j.** 3rd and 9th

k. $11\frac{1}{2}$ lb   **l.** 0 lb

---

10   The following example of a graph shows the systolic and diastolic blood pressure of a patient measured in mm Hg (millimetres of mercury). It also contains a line graph for the same person's pulse measured in beats per minute. The graph is contained only in quadrants I and II since it is impossible to have a negative blood pressure or pulse. The zero on the horizontal time axis corresponds to the time of injection of a drug intravenously. The negative numbers on the time axis refer to the number of minutes before the injection of the drug.

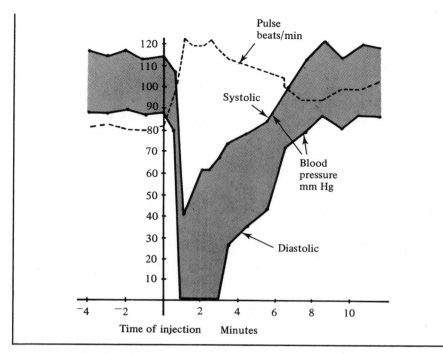

Q14 Use the graph of Frame 10 to answer the following questions:

a. What was the pulse three minutes before the injection?_____ At the time of the injection? _____ Two minutes after the injection? _____ Eight minutes after the injection? _____

b. What was the systolic blood pressure in mm Hg one minute before the injection? _____ At the time of the injection? _____ One-half minute after the injection? _____ One minute after the injection? _____ Seven minutes after the injection? _____

c. What was the diastolic blood pressure in mm Hg two minutes before the injection? _____ At the time of the injection? _____ One-half minute after the injection? _____ One minute after the injection? _____ Three minutes after the injection? _____ Four and one-half minutes after the injection? _____ Ten and one-half minutes after the injection? _____

• # # # • # # # • # # # • # # # • # # # • # # # • # # # • # #

A14 **a.** 83, 82, 119, 95 **b.** 113, 114, 108, 40, 105
c. 90, 88, 80, 0, 0, 35, 88

Q15 A graph can be used to show the relationship between Celsius temperature units and Fahrenheit temperature units represented by the equation $F = 1.8C + 32$. A table is partially filled in showing some commonly used temperatures.
a. Use the equation to determine the value for F corresponding to each value of C in the table.

	Celsius (°C)	Fahrenheit (°F)
water freezes	0	32
water boils	100	212
normal oral body temperature	37	_____
	20	_____
	⁻40	_____

b. Graph the resulting points and draw a line through them. This produces a line graph relating Celsius and Fahrenheit temperatures.

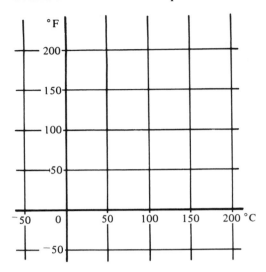

c. Use the graph to locate the Fahrenheit temperatures for:

75 °C _____   ⁻30 °C _____   ⁻10 °C _____   60 °C _____

\# \# \# • \# \# \# • \# \# \# • \# \# \# • \# \# \# • \# \# \# • \# \# \# • \# \# \# • \# \# \#

A15   **a.** (37, 98.6), (20, 68)
and (⁻40, ⁻40):
$$F = 1.8C + 32$$
$$= 1.8(37) + 32$$
$$= 66.6 + 32$$
$$= 98.6$$
$$F = 1.8(20) + 32$$
$$= 36 + 32$$
$$= 68$$
$$F = 1.8(⁻40) + 32$$
$$= ⁻72 + 32$$
$$= ⁻40$$
c. (75, 165), (⁻30, ⁻22)
(⁻10, 14), (60, 140)

b.

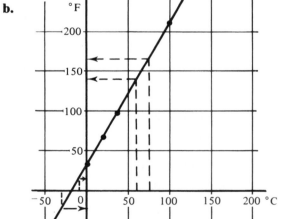

11   There are many examples in such allied health fields where two quantities are related in such a fashion that a graph continues to repeat the same pattern over and over again. These graphs are called *periodic* graphs. A few of these periodic line graphs will be examined.

A very fundamental graph that often arises is the sine curve (sine rhymes with mine). One example of where a sine curve is produced is on the simple alternating current generator. A coil rotates counterclockwise between the north and south poles of a magnet. Magnetic field lines flow between these poles. When a coil cuts across these lines a current is produced. As the coil rotates through the magnetic field the current in the coil will be maintained in one direction for one half a turn and reversed in the next half turn.

The graph is constructed by placing time on the horizontal axis. (You could also put the angle turned by the coil on the horizontal axis.) Current is placed on the vertical axis. A positive number represents current flow in one direction in the wire, and a negative number represents current flow in the opposite direction.

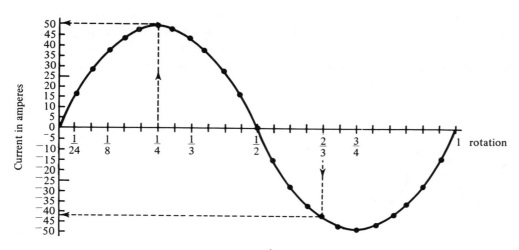

Example 1: What is the current in the line $\frac{1}{4}$ of the way through one rotation?

Solution: 50 amperes: The reading is made as the arrow on the graph indicates.

Example 2: What is the current in the line at $\frac{2}{3}$ rotation?

Solution: $^-43$ amperes

Q16   Use the graph in Frame 11 to answer the following:

a. What is the current at $\frac{1}{8}$ of a rotation? _____

b. What is the current at $\frac{1}{24}$ of a rotation? _____

c. What is the current at $\frac{3}{4}$ of one rotation? _____

d. What is the current at the beginning of the rotation? _____

e. What is the current $\frac{1}{2}$ way through the rotation? _____

f. What is the current at the end of the rotation? _____

#　•　# # #　•　# # #　•　# # #　•　# # #　•　# # #　•　# # #　•　# # #　•　# #

A16   **a.** 36 amperes   **b.** 17 amperes   **c.** −50 amperes
       d. 0 ampere   **e.** 0 ampere   **f.** 0 ampere

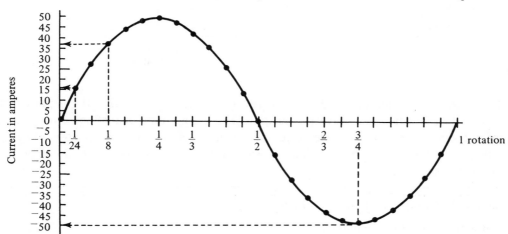

12   The sine curve shown in Frame 11 is one cycle of a graph of an alternating current. In North America power is generated at 60 Hertz which means that there are 60 cycles in one second. The graph below shows several cycles each one repeating the former. One cycle extends from point O on the *x* axis to point A on the *x* axis.

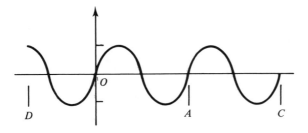

Q17   Use the graph in Frame 12 to answer the questions:

a. How many cycles are contained in the curve from O to C? _____

b. How many cycles are contained in the curve from D to C? _____

c. If there are 60 cycles in 1 second on the *x* axis, what fraction of a second does it take to complete

one cycle? _____

•   # # #   •   # # #   •   # # #   •   # # #   •   # # #   •   # # #   •   # # #   •   # #

A17   **a.** 2 cycles   **b.** $2\frac{3}{4}$ cycles   **c.** $\frac{1}{60}$ or 0.0167 second
                                                                            (rounded to ten thousandths)

13   For maximum efficiency modern x-ray equipment uses direct current rather than alternating current. Alternating current can be converted to direct current by special electrical devices. The process of changing an alternating current to direct current is called *rectification*.

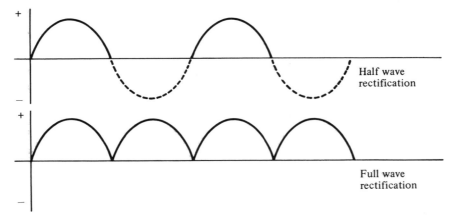

There are two commonly used types of rectified circuits. In the first the negative current is suppressed. This is called half-wave rectification. The second type of rectified circuit reverses the current in the negative section of the graph thereby inverting the negative portion of the graph so that it lies above the *x* axis. This is called full-wave rectification. Notice that both methods produce uneven, pulsating, direct current.

Q18   Use the graph in Frame 13 to answer the following:

a. What is the process of changing alternating current to direct current called? _____

b. Is the curve that results from full-wave rectification a periodic curve? _____

c. If the cycle for the half-wave rectification is $\frac{1}{60}$ of a second, how long is the cycle for full wave rectification of the same current? _____

•   # # #   •   # # #   •   # # #   •   # # #   •   # # #   •   # # #   •   # # #   •   # #

A18   **a.** rectification   **b.** yes   **c.** $\frac{1}{120}$ second

---

14   When the intra-alveolar pressure of the lung is plotted with time on the x axis, a periodic graph results. It looks a little like the sine curve, but each peak does not have the symmetry of the sine curve.

  The vertical axis is marked to show pressure. A positive pressure will force air from the lungs, while a negative pressure will cause air to flow into the lungs. The unit for measuring air pressure in this case is cm H_2O (centimeters of water).

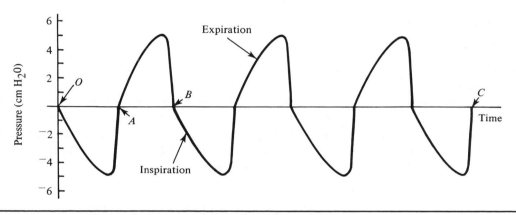

Q19   Use the graph in Frame 14 to answer the following:

  a. The cycle that starts at O ends at _____?

  b. How many cycles are shown on the graph from O to C? _____

  c. If a person takes 15 breaths per minute, how many seconds does it take for one cycle? _____

  d. How many seconds are shown on the horizontal time axis from O to C under the assumption of part **c**? _____

•   # # #   •   # # #   •   # # #   •   # # #   •   # # #   •   # # #   •   # # #   •   # #

A19   **a.** B   **b.** $3\frac{1}{2}$ cycles   **c.** 4 seconds: $60 \div 15$

  d. 14 seconds: $\left(3\frac{1}{2}\right)(4)$

---

15   Equipment has been developed which automatically records information on patients which many times is periodic. One of these is the electrocardiogram (EKG). Invented by Wilhelm Einthoven, it won him the Nobel Prize in 1906. The EKG is a line graph (see next page) with time on the horizontal axis and voltage on the vertical. An example of an EKG is shown here. The muscles of the heart are stimulated by electrochemical impulses. These electrical currents spread through the heart passing through surrounding tissue with some spreading to the surface of the body. Electrodes placed on opposite sides of the body record the impulses on a line graph.

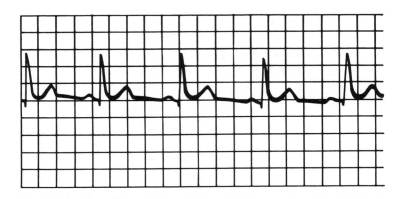

Q20   **a.** What is the abbreviation for electrocardiogram? _____

　　　　b. What is represented on the horizontal axis of the graph? _____

　　　　c. What is represented on the vertical axis of the graph? _____

　　　　d. What does the EKG measure? _____

\# \# \# • \# \# \# • \# \# \# • \# \# \# • \# \# \# • \# \# \# • \# \# \# • \# \# \# • \# \# \#

A20   **a.** EKG   **b.** time   **c.** voltage
　　　　d. electrical impulses originating in the heart

---

16   The normal EKG has 5 or 6 parts: the P, Q, R, S, T, and U waves. It is not abnormal if the U wave does not appear. These waves are labeled on the first cycle of a magnified graph. The second cycle is shown with the graph background that appears on the EKG strip. Each horizontal interval represents 0.04 second. Each vertical interval represents 0.1 millivolt (mV).

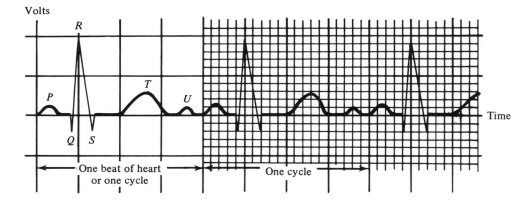

Example 1: If one cycle lasts for 22 subdivisions, how many seconds does it last?

Solution: 0.88 second: $(22)(0.04) = 0.88$

Example 2: If a P wave is $2\frac{1}{2}$ intervals high, how many millivolts does that represent?

Solution: 0.25 millivolt: $\left(2\frac{1}{2}\right)(0.1) = 0.25$

Q21   Use the graph in Frame 16 to answer the following:
　　　　a. Label the waves in the second and third cycles.

b. Count the intervals between the R wave of the 2nd cycle and the R wave of the third cycle.

_____

c. How many seconds does this represent? _____

d. Count the intervals from the top of the P wave in the second cycle to the top of the P wave in the third cycle. _____

e. How many seconds does this represent? _____

#　•　# # #　•　# # #　•　# # #　•　# # #　•　# # #　•　# # #　•　# # #　•　# #

A21　**a.**

b. 20　　　　　　　**c.** 0.8 second　　　　　**d.** 20　　　　　**e.** 0.8 second

Q22　Divide 60 seconds by 0.04 second to find the number of horizontal subdivisions in a minute.

#　•　# # #　•　# # #　•　# # #　•　# # #　•　# # #　•　# # #　•　# # #　•　# #

A22　1500

Q23　If a cycle lasts for 25 subdivisions divide 1500 by 25 to find the number of cycles per minute (this is the pulse).

#　•　# # #　•　# # #　•　# # #　•　# # #　•　# # #　•　# # #　•　# # #　•　# #

A23　60 cycles per minute:　This also means the heart is beating at 60 beats per minute.

Q24　Determine the cycles per minute (pulse) for the EKG in Frame 16.

#　•　# # #　•　# # #　•　# # #　•　# # #　•　# # #　•　# # #　•　# # #　•　# #

A24　75 cycles per minute:　$1500 \div 20 = 75$

Q25　**a.** A P wave should not exceed 0.25 millivolt. Is the P wave in Frame 16 normal? _____
　　　b. A P wave should not last longer than 0.11 second. Is the P wave in Frame 16 normal in this regard? _____
　　　c. The QRS complex is the portion or the curve which starts at the beginning of the Q wave and ends at the end of the S wave. The QRS complex should not be longer than 0.1 second. Is the QRS complex of the 2nd cycle in the EKG of Frame 16 normal in this regard? _____

d. The R wave should not exceed 2.7 millivolts. Is the R wave of Frame 16 normal in this regard? _____

\# \# \#   •   \# \# \#   •   \# \# \#   •   \# \# \#   •   \# \# \#   •   \# \# \#   •   \# \# \#   •   \# \# \#   •   \# \# \#

A25   **a.** yes: It is 0.15 mV.   **b.** yes: It is borderline however.
      c. no: It lasts 0.12 second.   **d.** yes: It is 1.0 mV.

---

17   Variations in the shape and length of segments of the curve in an EKG allow a physician to diagnose heart conditions. The EKG shown here differs in the second cycle from the first. Remember from Q23 that the number of beats per minute can be obtained by dividing 1500 by the number of intervals in the cycle.

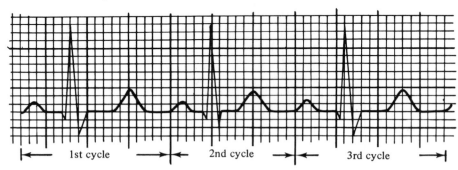

|← 1st cycle →|← 2nd cycle →|← 3rd cycle →|

Q26   **a.** By comparing the EKG of Frame 17 to the EKG of Frame 16 determine which wave is missing in each cycle. _____

b. Label the waves in the EKG of Frame 17.

c. The P wave is indicative of atrial activity. Determine the atrial rate in cycles per minute by using the number of intervals between the P wave of the 1st cycle and the P wave of the second cycle. _____

d. Determine the atrial rate in cycles per minute by using the second cycle. _____

e. Determine the length of the QRS complex in the first cycle (from the start of the Q wave to the end of the S wave). _____

f. Determine the length of the QRS complex in the second cycle. _____

g. The R wave is indicative of ventrical activity. Count the intervals between R waves to determine if the ventrical rate is regular or irregular. _____

\# \# \#   •   \# \# \#   •   \# \# \#   •   \# \# \#   •   \# \# \#   •   \# \# \#   •   \# \# \#   •   \# \# \#   •   \# \# \#

A26   **a.** U waves: This is not uncommon.   **b.** As Frame 16 indicates.
      c. 83 cycles per min: $1500 \div 18$
      d. 100 cycles per min: $1500 \div 15$. This rate compared with answer c shows that the atrial rate is irregular.
      e. 0.12 second   **f.** 0.08 second
      g. irregular: There are 16.8 intervals between R waves of the 1st and 2nd cycles compared to 16.2 intervals between the R waves of the 2nd and 3rd cycles. This is not much difference, however.

---

18   These questions give a short introduction to EKG's. For further elementary reading on EKG's, see "What Every Nurse Should Know about EKG's" by Margaret Van Meter and Peter G. Lavine in *Nursing* 75 April, May, June, and July 1975.

This completes the instruction for this section.

10.5   EXERCISE

1. Write the coordinates of the points shown on the coordinate system:

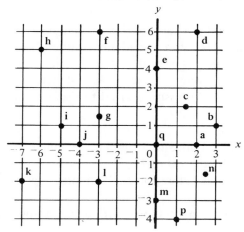

2. Name the letters of the points on the coordinate system in problem 1 in each of the following:
  a. quadrant I   **b.** quadrant II   **c.** quadrant III   **d.** quadrant IV

3. Graph the ordered pairs: $(^-5, 2), (^-2, 2), (2, ^-4), (^-2, ^-3), (^-4, 0), (0, 3), (3, 2), (^-5, ^-5), (0, ^-2), (1, 2), (1, 0), (4, 0), (4, ^-2)$.

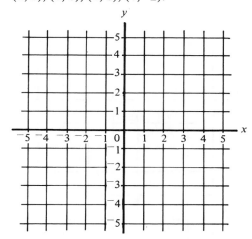

4. The graph below indicates the change in blood pressure for a patient 2 minutes before and 8 minutes after a drug was administered. The drug was administered at 0 on the x axis.

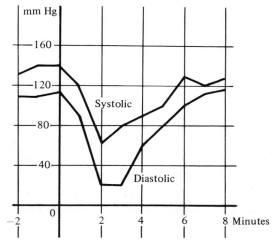

    a. What was the systolic blood pressure 2 minutes before the drug was administered? At the time the drug was administered? Eight minutes after the drug was administered?

    b. For how long was the graph of the systolic blood pressure falling?

    c. How low did the systolic blood pressure drop?

    d. What was the amount of drop in systolic blood pressure from 0 to 2 minutes?

    e. What was the diastolic blood pressure 2 minutes before the administration of the drug? At the time of the administration of the drug? Six minutes after the administration of the drug?

    f. How long did it take for the diastolic blood pressure to reach its lowest value?

    g. How long did it take before the diastolic blood pressure started to rise measuring from the administration of the drug?

    h. What was the lowest diastolic blood pressure?

    i. What was the amount of drop in diastolic blood pressure from 0 to 2 minutes?

    j. Which dropped more, systolic or diastolic blood pressure?

    k. From the time the systolic blood pressure was at its low point at 2 minutes how long did it take to return above 120 mm Hg?

5. The relationship between pressure and volume can be shown with a line graph. As pressure increases the volume decreases according to the equation $V = \dfrac{30}{P}$ (one mole of an ideal gas at 92 °F) if V is measured in liters and P in atmospheres (atm). Some values have been calculated in the chart below by using the formula.

    a. Calculate the remaining values of V.

    b. Plot the points (P, V) and draw a line graph.

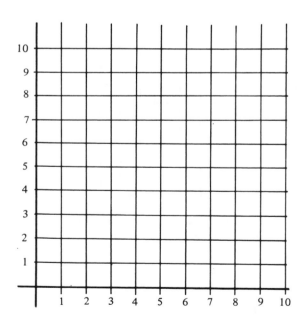

P(atms)	V(litres)
3	$V = \dfrac{30}{3} = 10$
4	$V = \dfrac{30}{4} = 7.5$
5	
6	
7	
8	
9	
10	

    c. Use the graph to find V when $P = 4.5$.

    d. What is the process of part **c** called?

    e. Use the graph to find V when $P = 8.5$.

6. Some mechanical ventilating machines assist patients in breathing by filling the lungs under a positive pressure and then releasing that pressure to allow the patient to exhale. The positive pressure in the lungs has the side effect of decreasing circulation of the blood in the veins. Therefore, other ventilating machines follow each period of positive pressure with a period of negative pressure to allow increased return of blood through the veins during exhalation. Such a machine has the accompanying graph of pressure compared to time.

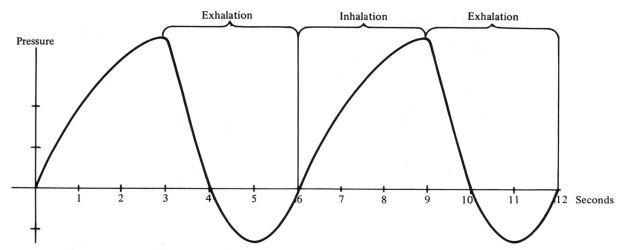

a. What is a graph called that repeats the same pattern again and again?

b. How long is each cycle?

c. How many cycles of respiration are shown?

d. If the ventilating machine is set as the graph shows, how many breaths per minute will the patient receive?

e. Inhalation takes place while positive pressure builds up. How many seconds of inhalation are there in each cycle?

f. Exhalation takes place during the rest of the cycle. How many seconds of exhalation are there in each cycle?

g. How many seconds of negative pressure in the lung are there during each cycle?

h. Under normal unassisted breathing there is negative pressure in the lungs during 0.5 of the cycle. What fraction of the cycle is there negative pressure in the lungs under the type of assisted breathing shown in the graph?

10.5   EXERCISE ANSWERS

1. a. $(2, 0)$ **b.** $(3, 1)$ **c.** $\left(1\frac{1}{2}, 2\right)$ **d.** $(2, 6)$

e. $(0, 4)$ **f.** $(^-3, 6)$ **g.** $\left(^-3, 1\frac{1}{2}\right)$ **h.** $(^-6, 5)$

i. $(^-5, 1)$ **j.** $(^-4, 0)$ **k.** $(^-7, ^-2)$ **l.** $(^-3, ^-2)$

m. $(0, ^-3)$ **n.** $\left(2\frac{1}{2}, ^-1\frac{1}{2}\right)$ **p.** $(1, ^-4)$ **q.** $(0, 0)$

2. a. b, c, and d   **b.** f, g, h, and i   **c.** k and l   **d.** n and p

3.

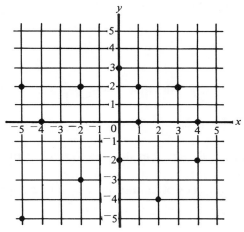

4. a. 130 mm Hg, 140 mm Hg, 130 mm Hg
   b. 2 min   **c.** 65 mm Hg   **d.** 75 mm Hg
   e. 110 mm Hg, 115 mm Hg, 100 mm Hg
   f. 2 min   **g.** 3 min   **h.** 20 mm Hg
   i. 95 mm Hg   **j.** diastolic   **k.** 3.5 min

5. a.

P(atms)	V(liters)
3	10
4	7.5
5	6
6	5
7	4.3
8	3.8
9	3.3
10	3

b.

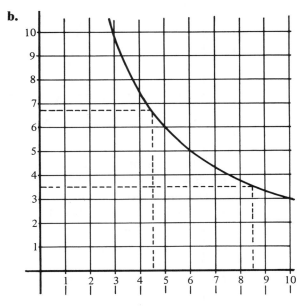

   c. (4.5, 6.7)   **d.** interpolation   **e.** (8.5, 3.5)
6. a. periodic   **b.** 6 sec   **c.** 2 cycles   **d.** 10 breaths/min
   e. 3 sec   **f.** 3 sec   **g.** 2 sec   **h.** 0.3

CHAPTER 10 SAMPLE TEST

At the completion of Chapter 10 you should be able to work the following problems.

10.1   CHOOSING THE TYPE OF GRAPH

1. Identify each of the following variables as continuous or discrete:
   a. measurement in inches of a person's waist
   b. number of players on a hockey team
   c. miles per hour that a motorcycle travels
   d. hourly temperatures throughout a day
2. Choose the type of graph (bar graph or circle graph) that would be used to illustrate the following data:
   a. You want to compare the inventories of a drugstore at the end of each of the last five years.
   b. You want to examine the total inventory of a department store by comparing the inventories of all five departments.
   c. You want to examine the total income from sales of an insurance agency by comparing the total sales of all of its four salesmen.

3. Choose the type of graph (line graph or bar graph) that would be used to illustrate the following data:

a. You want to show the total sales for Chrysler, Ford, and General Motors last year.

b. You want to show the changes in the price of a stock over the course of a year.

c. You want to compare the dollars per capita that each of the fifty states in the United States spent on education last year.

10.2   CIRCLE GRAPHS

**Distribution of Foreign Direct
Investments in the U.S. by Country
of Ownership, 1971 ($15 billion)**

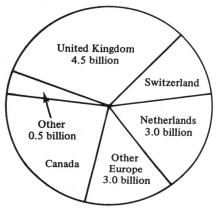

4. If Switzerland controls 10% of the foreign investments in the United States, what is its investment in the United States?

5. Find the dollars invested by Canada in the United States.

6. What is the sum of all the central angles of the sectors of a circle?

7. Find the number of degrees in the central angle of the sector representing Switzerland.

8. Find the number of degrees in the central angle of the sector representing Netherlands.

10.3   BAR GRAPHS

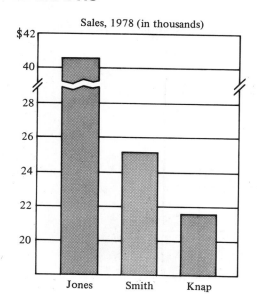

Use the graph to answer questions 9–11.

9. Give two reasons why the bar graph is a distortion of the data on which it is based.
10. What were the total sales of Smith in the graph?
11. What were the total sales of Knap in the graph?
12. If you were constructing a bar graph and had to draw the longest bar representing 108 million on a graph with six vertical spaces, what scale would you use?
13. Graph the following data.

Retirement Income/Month

Atwood	$1,200
Baker	600
Calson	420
Dunlap	2,000
Ehen	800

10.4 LINE GRAPHS

A production manager recorded the total production at several times during an 8-hour shift. The shift started at 8:00 A.M. and ended at 5:00 P.M. with an hour off for lunch.

Total Production Until a Given Time in a Shift

Time	Production Units
8:00 A.M.	0
9:00 A.M.	220
10:00 A.M.	400
12:00 noon	630
1:00 P.M.	630
2:00 P.M.	730
4:00 P.M.	850

14. Use the data to construct a line graph of the total production at various times during the shift.

15. Read from the graph you constructed the total production at 11:00 A.M.

16. The process of approximating the production for 11:00 A.M. between the two known values of the production at 10:00 A.M. and noon is called _____ (interpolation or extrapolation).

17. Predict from your graph what the production will be at the end of the shift at 5:00 P.M.

18. The process of approximating the production at 5:00 P.M. beyond the known values is called

_____ (interpolation or extrapolation).

19. How could you explain the leveling off of the production from noon to 1:00 P.M.?

20. Is production increasing at a faster or slower rate at 9:00 A.M. than it is at 2:00 P.M.? Explain why this is reasonable.

10.5 RECTANGULAR COORDINATE SYSTEM

21. Match the letter from the figure to the right with the proper word.

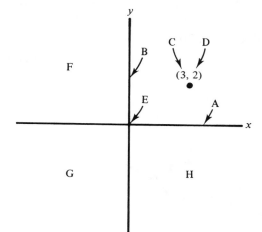

  a. second quadrant
  b. x axis
  c. x coordinate
  d. third quadrant
  e. fourth quadrant
  f. origin
  g. y axis
  h. y coordinate

22. Locate the points on the coordinate system shown:
(4, 0), (⁻4, ⁻2), (2, 1), (0, 2),
(0, 0), (⁻2, ⁻3), (4, ⁻3), (0, ⁻3),
(4, 5), (⁻1, 0)

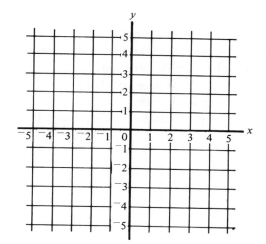

23. Name the coordinates of each of the points on the coordinate system shown:

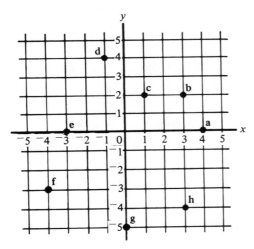

24. A man went on a combination diet and exercise program on day zero. The previous 7 days he had been exercising only and the 7 days before that he had been doing nothing but keeping track of his weight. A line graph of his weight changes in pounds relative to his weight at the beginning of the 3 week period is shown.

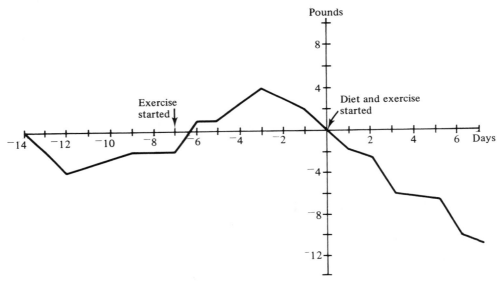

   a. What was the relative weight change over the first 2 weeks?
   b. How many days before he started his diet and exercise program did he weigh the most?
   c. What was his weight change at the start of his exercise program?
   d. What was his weight 3 days after he started both exercise and diet?
   e. How much weight was lost during the last one week period?

25. a. Use the equation $y = x + 2$ which tells how y is related to x to determine three other points besides the ones listed in the chart.

x	y
$^-2$	$^-2 + 2 = 0$
$^-1$	
0	
2	$2 + 2 = 4$
4	

b. Graph the 5 points and draw a line through them.

c. Use the graph to predict what y corresponds to $x = ^-4$.

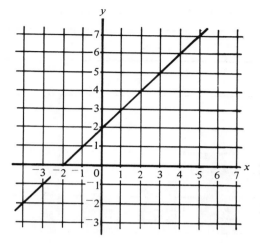

26. The intrathoracic pressure of the thorax which surrounds the lungs and heart is usually negative under spontaneous breathing. However, under assisted breathing with a mechanical ventilator using a driving pressure of 5 cm H_2O it has the accompanying curve.

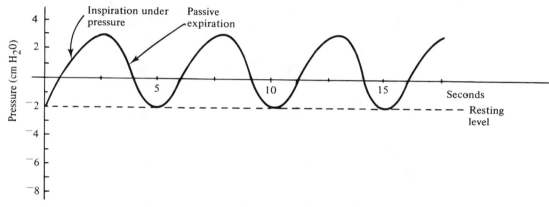

a. What is the name of the kind of graph which repeats the same pattern over and over?

b. How long is each cycle in the above graph?

c. How many cycles of assisted breathing are represented on the graph?

d. How many breaths per minute will the patient receive?

e. What is the intrathoracic pressure at the highest value in each cycle?

f. What is the resting intrathoracic pressure?

g. Is there more time of positive pressure in each cycle or more time of negative pressure?

CHAPTER 10 SAMPLE TEST ANSWERS

1. a. continuous   **b.** discrete   **c.** continuous   **d.** continuous

2. a. bar graph   **b.** circle graph   **c.** circle graph

3. a. bar graph   **b.** line graph   **c.** bar graph

4. 1.5 billion   **5.** 2.5 billion   **6.** 360°   **7.** 36°

8. 72°

9. 1. The vertical scale has been broken between 28,000 and 40,000.

    2. The vertical scale does not begin at zero.

10. $25,000   **11.** $21,500   **12.** 1 space = 20 million

13.

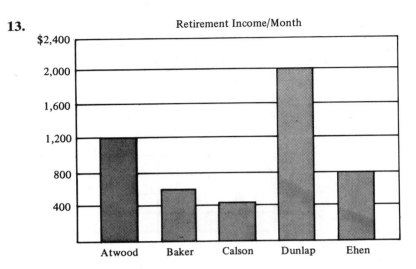

Retirement Income/Month

14.

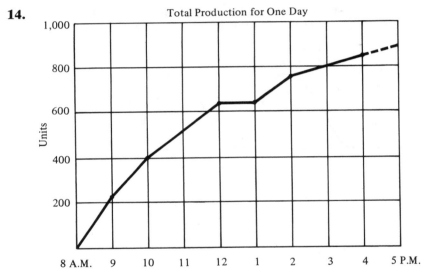

Total Production for One Day

15. 520   **16.** interpolation   **17.** 900   **18.** extrapolation

19. lunch break

20. faster rate; People are fresh in the morning and tired later in the day.

21. a. F   **b.** A   **c.** C   **d.** G

e. H   **f.** E   **g.** B   **h.** D

22.

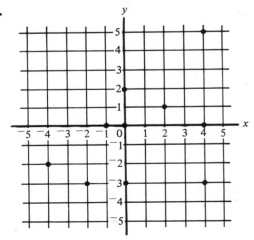

23. a. (4, 0)   **b.** (3, 2)   **c.** (1, 2)   **d.** ($^-$1, 4)

  e. ($^-$3, 0)   **f.** ($^-$4, $^-$3)   **g.** (0, $^-$5)   **h.** (3, $^-$4)

24. a. 0 lb   **b.** 3 days   **c.** $^-$2 lb   **d.** $^-$6 lb   **e.** 11 lb

25. a.

x	y
$^-$2	0
$^-$1	1
0	2
2	4
4	6

  c. $y = {}^-2$

b.

26. a. periodic   **b.** 5 sec   **c.** $3\frac{1}{2}$ cycles   **d.** 12 breaths/min

  e. 3 cm H_2O **f.** $^-$2 cm H_2O **g.** positive

CHAPTER 11

INTRODUCTION TO STATISTICS

Statistics has become a frequently used mathematical tool in the health sciences. One needs fundamental knowledge of statistics to read the journals, magazines, and textbooks in the field. The elementary notions of statistics will be presented in this chapter.

11.1 MEAN, MEDIAN, AND MODE

1	The field of statistics was developed to take sets of numbers called *data** and identify the important characteristics of them. One goal is to pick one number that is representative of a set of numbers. This number is called a *measure of central tendency*.
	Three different ways of deciding on the most representative number have been developed. These produce the mean, the median, and the mode. For some data (sets of numbers) the mean, median, and mode are equal; for others, they are different.
	The *mode* of a set of numbers is the number that occurs with the greatest frequency.
	Example: Find the mode of the following numbers:
	2, 7, 5, 3, 7, 4, 3, 3
	Solution: The number 3 occurs three times, 7 twice, and all other numbers once. Therefore, 3 is the mode.
	*The word "data" is considered plural.

Q1 The number of emergency patients per hour for 7 hours is 2, 5, 3, 2, 5, 4, 5. Find the mode of the data. _____

\# \# \# • \# \# \# • \# \# \# • \# \# \# • \# \# \# • \# \# \# • \# \# \# • \# \# \# • \# \# \#

A1 5 patients: 5 occurs three times which is more times than any other number from the data set.

Q2 The length of hospital stay in days is given for a particular hospital for 16 patients: 4, 3, 7, 4, 8, 6, 5, 7, 4, 2, 3, 4, 4, 8, 3, 2. Find the mode. _____

\# \# \# • \# \# \# • \# \# \# • \# \# \# • \# \# \# • \# \# \# • \# \# \# • \# \# \# • \# \# \#

A2 4 days: 4 occurs five times.

2	There are some potential problems in finding the mode: There may be no mode or there may be more than one.
	1. If each number occurs only once, there is *no mode*.

438

2. If *two* numbers occur with the same frequency and this frequency is greater than all other frequencies, they are *both* considered to be modes. The data are said to be *bimodal.*

Although it does not occur often, it is possible to have three modes, four modes, and so on. The data are said to be *multimodal.*

Example 1: Find the mode of the following data: 3, 5, 7, 2, 9, 8, 4, 6.

Solution: There is no mode.

Example 2: The number of years of survival after a kidney transplant is given for eleven patients: 3, 5, 7, 4, 5, 3, 2, 8, 7, 5, 3. Find the mode.

Solution: The modes are 5 years and 3 years. The distribution* is bimodal.

*Data are sometimes referred to as a *distribution,* because any data set forms a uniquely distributed pattern when arranged on a line.

Q3   Find the mode of each distribution:
   a. The number of permanent teeth decayed at age 40 for eleven people: 2, 5, 7, 4, 3, 12, 17, 7, 5, 8, 5. _____
   b. The weight loss in pounds in one week for eleven people: 5, 8, 3, 5, 7, 4, 5, 8, 2, 8, and 1. _____
   c. The measures of blood glucose in mg/100 ml for 9 people: 65, 80, 140, 95, 105, 120, 70, 100, and 75. _____

\# \# \# • \# \# \# • \# \# \# • \# \# \# • \# \# \# • \# \# \# • \# \# \# • \# \# \# • \# \# \#

A3   **a.** 5 teeth   **b.** 5 and 8 lb: bimodal   **c.** no mode

3   The second measure of central tendency is the *median.* To obtain the median do the following:

Step 1: Arrange the numbers from smallest to largest.

Step 2: Choose the middle number (for sets with an odd number of values).

Example: Find the median of the data: 5, 8, 3, 5, 7, 4, 5, 8, 2, 8, 1

Solution: Step 1: Arrange from smallest to largest:

1, 2, 3, 4, 5, 5, 5, 7, 8, 8, 8

Step 2: The median is 5, because there were an equal number above 5 as were below.

Q4   1. Arrange the data sets from smallest to largest, and
   2. determine the median.
   a. The number of immigrant MD's coming into the United States for seven years is 1,300, 2,200, 1,800, 6,200, 1,700, 3,000, 2,000.

   1. _____ 2. _____
   b. Nine males lived the following number of years over their life expectancy: 2, ⁻3, 7, 5, ⁻1, 4, 3, ⁻6, 7.

   1. _____ 2. _____

\# \# \# • \# \# \# • \# \# \# • \# \# \# • \# \# \# • \# \# \# • \# \# \# • \# \# \# • \# \# \#

A4   **a.** 1. 1,300, 1,700, 1,800, 2,000, 2,200, 3,000, 6,200
         2. 2,000 MD's
      b. 1. ⁻6, ⁻3, ⁻1, 2, 3, 4, 5, 7, 7
         2. 3 years: Notice that on a number line ⁻6 falls to the left of ⁻3 and therefore is smaller.

Q5   Eleven hospitals reported the following expenses per patient day: $45, $70, $60, $70, $120, $95, $70, $95, $110, $130, $90.
    a. Find the median.

    b. Find the mode.

\# \# \# • \# \# \# • \# \# \# • \# \# \# • \# \# \# • \# \# \# • \# \# \# • \# \# \# • \# \# \#

A5   **a.** $90   **b.** $70

---

4   Consider the numbers

    1, 5, 6, 9, 11

    The median or middle number (when they are arranged in order of size) is 6, because there are two numbers on each side. However, examine what happens when there are eight numbers in a set:

    1, 5, 5, 6, 8, 9, 9, 11

    There is no number that separates the set with the same number of numbers before it as after it. There are now two middle numbers. The *median* is the number one-half way between the two middle numbers. In the set above the two middle numbers are 6 and 8. The number one-half way between is $\dfrac{6+8}{2}$. The median is therefore 7. The median is found this way whenever there are an even number of numbers in the data.

Q6   Find the median of the data below:
    a. The number of examinees examined by the American Registry of Radiologic Technologists for 1969–1974 were 7,000, 7,400, 8,400, 9,700, 10,400, and 10,900.

    b. The number of personnel per 100 beds reported by 10 hospitals were 200, 230, 195, 250, 260, 222, 240, 207, 210, and 235.

\# \# \# • \# \# \# • \# \# \# • \# \# \# • \# \# \# • \# \# \# • \# \# \# • \# \# \# • \# \# \#

A6   **a.** 9,050 examinees: $\dfrac{8400+9700}{2}$

    b. 226: $\dfrac{222+230}{2}$

    If your answer is 241 you forgot to rearrange from smallest to largest.

---

5   The third measure of central tendency is the mean. The *mean* of a set of numbers is the result obtained when the numbers are added and the sum divided by the number of numbers in the data set. The mean is frequently called "the average." However, "average" is a very imprecise word, because the median and mode are also considered to be averages.

    Example: Find the mean of 5, 2, 7, 3, 3, 6.

    Solution: $\dfrac{5+2+7+3+3+6}{6}=\dfrac{26}{6}=4\dfrac{1}{3}$

    Therefore, the mean of the data is $4\dfrac{1}{3}$.

Q7   The radiation reported by five radiation workers for a 6-month period was 0.4 rad, 0.6 rad, 1.0 rad, 1.7 rad, and 1.8 rad. Find the mean.

•   # # #   •   # # #   •   # # #   •   # # #   •   # # #   •   # # #   •   # # #   •   # #

A7   1.1 rad: $\dfrac{0.4+0.6+1.0+1.7+1.8}{5} = \dfrac{5.5}{5} = 1.1$

Q8   The tidal volume of 10 female adults is 350 ml, 380 ml, 400 ml, 460 ml, 490 ml, 400 ml, 500 ml, 400 ml, 480 ml, and 460 ml.
      a. Find the mean.

      b. Find the median.

      c. Find the mode.

•   # # #   •   # # #   •   # # #   •   # # #   •   # # #   •   # # #   •   # # #   •   # #

A8   **a.** 432 ml   **b.** 430 ml   **c.** 400 ml

Q9   A small business consists of the president making $35,000 per year, a secretary making $6,000 per year, a custodian making $5,000 per year, and five "workers," each making $8,000 per year.
      a. Find the mean salary.

      b. Find the median salary.

      c. Find the mode salary.

•   # # #   •   # # #   •   # # #   •   # # #   •   # # #   •   # # #   •   # # #   •   # #

A9   **a.** $10,750: $\dfrac{86,000}{8}$ **b.** $8,000   **c.** $8,000

Q10   Answer yes or no. Which of the following would be affected if the president of the business in Q9 gave himself a $5,000 raise and left everyone else at the same salary?

      a. mean _____   **b.** median _____   **c.** mode _____

•   # # #   •   # # #   •   # # #   •   # # #   •   # # #   •   # # #   •   # # #   •   # #

A10   **a.** yes   **b.** no   **c.** no

---

6   One might wonder why there are three different ways of calculating an "average." This is because sometimes one method is more appropriate than the others. The mode is preferred when one wants to speak of the most popular choice or the result that occurs with the most frequency. The result chosen by more people than any other would be the mode. The mode does not even have to be a number as the median and mean must be.

      Example 1: The average person in the United States prefers to live in a small town.

Example 2: The average major surgical operation in the United States in a representative year is the tonsillectomy with adenoidectomy.

Q11   One sometimes sees a description of an "average" person in the United States. Such a description follows. Indicate yes if the description would be the result of finding a mode. Answer no, otherwise.
        The average man is married, has 2.43 children, owns his own home, drives a Chevrolet, makes $11,234 per year, and is not satisfied with his employment.

  a. is married _____   **b.** has 2.43 children _____

  c. owns his own home _____   **d.** drives a Chevrolet _____

  e. makes $11,234 _____   **f.** not satisfied with his employment _____

\# # # • # # # • # # # • # # # • # # # • # # # • # # # • # # # • # # #

A11   **a.** yes   **b.** no   **c.** yes   **d.** yes   **e.** no   **f.** yes

---

7   If one or a few values are so large (or small) that the mean is noticeably increased (or decreased) because of them, the most appropriate measure of central tendency is the median. In the business of Q9, the employees might not appreciate it if their president were to describe their company as paying an average salary of $10,750, when all the employees but himself make considerably less than that. The median of $8,000 seems to represent the salaries paid more accurately in this instance. In cases where there are a few very outstanding values, the median is most appropriate. The median is less affected by wide fluctuations of scores on the extremes of the distribution than the mean. Of course, if both median and mean are given, one has a better understanding of the data. If the median and mean are equal, the scores are "balanced" about the common value. On the other hand, if the mean is larger than the median, there are a few large values that caused the mean to be greater.

Q12   The absenteeism for an elementary school for a 12 week period is reported. At one time during the 12 weeks an epidemic of flu went through the school. Number of pupil absenteeism per week: 100, 105, 116, 75, 150, 1,055, 200, 160, 172, 140, 110, 95.
  a. Find the median.

  b. Find the mean.

  c. Would the mean or the median be the better representative of the "average" number of absentees? _____

\# # # • # # # • # # # • # # # • # # # • # # # • # # # • # # # • # # #

A12   **a.** 128   **b.** 206.5   **c.** median: The large fluctuation would affect the mean unduly.

Q13   If the mean height of a group of girls is 5 ft 1 in. and the median is 5 ft 4 in., does it indicate that there were a few very short or a few very tall girls? _____

\# # # • # # # • # # # • # # # • # # # • # # # • # # # • # # # • # # #

A13   a few very short girls: The mean is less than the median.

8 The mean is the most common measure of central tendency used and most people assume that the mean is meant when the word "average" is used. Do not be misled into thinking this way. *All three measures of central tendencies are averages.*

The mean is affected by each value of the data, is easily calculated, and is useful for more advanced statistical procedures. Since other statistical procedures are dependent upon the mean, almost every statistical description of data requires as a part of the analysis the calculation of the mean.

This completes the instruction for this section.

11.1 EXERCISE

Find the mean, median, and mode for the data sets in problems 1–5 (round off answers to 2 decimal places):

1. The nursing expense per patient day reported by five city hospitals were $40, $43, $43, $47, and $49.
2. The patient temperatures at 7:00 A.M. of each day of a 6-day illness were 39 °C, 40 °C, 40 °C, 38 °C, 38.5 °C, and 38 °C.
3. The systolic blood pressures of ten patients were 128, 120, 118, 120, 130, 125, 135, 120, 127, and 127, measured in mm Hg. (mm Hg symbolizes millimetres of mercury.)
4. The number of cases of meningitis among U.S. personnel between 1966 and 1972 were 90, 280, 320, 260, 60, and 0.
5. The amounts of pseudorenin in units/g found in a rat were adrenal 2.3, aorta 5.8, duodenum 6.2, kidney 1.7, liver 1.5, lung 3.2, pancreas 2.3, salivary gland 11.2, spleen 9.1, testis 1.0, and thymus 8.5.
6. In a data set with 10 numbers, not all the same, which measures of central tendency could be equal to the largest number in the data set?
7. Sometimes one of the measures of central tendency does not exist. Which one is it and under what circumstances does this happen?
8. When there is no middle number, how is the median found?
9. If a person wants to report an average score which is not unduly affected by one extremely large score, which measure of central tendency should be chosen?
10. What measure of central tendency is used for more advanced statistics?

11.1 EXERCISE ANSWERS

1. mean, $44.40; median, $43; mode, $43
2. mean, 38.92 °C; median, 38.75 °C: $\dfrac{38.5 + 39}{2}$; bimodal, 38 °C and 40 °C
3. mean, 125 mm Hg; median, 126 mm Hg; mode, 120 mm Hg (Remember to arrange the numbers from smallest to largest before finding the median.)
4. mean, 168.33; median, 175; no mode
5. mean, 4.8 units/g; median, 3.2 units/g; mode, 2.3 units/g
6. The mode if the largest number occurred more often than any other or the median if more than half the numbers were equal to the largest number.
7. The mode when all numbers occur only once.
8. The two middle numbers are added and the sum divided by two. (Alternatively, the mean of the two middle numbers is found.)
9. median   10. mean

11.2 FREQUENCY TABLES AND FREQUENCY POLYGONS

1   When given a large data set, it is helpful to construct a frequency table in order to more easily make computations. A *frequency table* lists all the possible values of the data with the number of times that value appears in the data listed beside it.

Example: Construct a frequency table for the following data: 15, 16, 12, 13, 15, 18, 17, 16, 14, 16, 14, 18, 17, 15, 17, 19, 14, 20, 16, 16, 17, 16, 14, 15, 13, 12, 14, 13.

Solution: The largest value in the data is 20 and the smallest is 12. These and all numbers between are listed in a column. A tally mark is made beside each value as you find it occurring in the data. Finally, the frequency of each value is listed beside it. The total frequency is listed below the frequency column.

Value	Tally	Frequency
12	||	2
13	|||	3
14	ﷻﾑ	5
15	||||	4
16	ﷻﾑ|	6
17	||||	4
18	||	2
19	|	1
20	|	1
		28

Q1   Answer the following questions about the frequency table constructed in Frame 1:

   a. How many times did the value 17 occur in the data? _____

   b. What value occurred most frequently? _____

   c. What would the value you gave for part **b** be called? _____

   d. How many times did a value of 15 or less occur? _____

   e. How many times did a value of 16 or larger occur? _____

•   # # #   •   # # #   •   # # #   •   # # #   •   # # #   •   # # #   •   # # #   •   # #

A1   **a.** 4   **b.** 16   **c.** mode   **d.** 14   **e.** 14

Q2   A patient had the following temperatures measured on the Celsius scale taken every 8 hours: 37.0, 37.5, 38.0, 38.0, 39.0, 39.0, 39.5, 39.5, 40.0, 39.5, 39.0, 38.0, 38.5, 39.0, 38.5, 38.0, 38.0, 38.5, 37.5, 38.0, 37.5. Construct a frequency table from the data.

Temperature (°C)	Tally	Frequency
37.0		

•   # # #   •   # # #   •   # # #   •   # # #   •   # # #   •   # # #   •   # # #   •   # #

A2

Temperature (°C)	Tally	Frequency
37.0	I	1
37.5	III	3
38.0	NI I	6
38.5	III	3
39.0	IIII	4
39.5	III	3
40.0	I	1
		21

Q3   Determine the mode of the data in Q2. _____

\# \# \#   •   \# \# \#   •   \# \# \#   •   \# \# \#   •   \# \# \#   •   \# \# \#   •   \# \# \#   •   \# \# \#   •   \# \# \#

A3   38.0 °C: It occurred 6 times.

2   The three measures of central tendency can be calculated by using the frequency table. The mode can be found as in Q1 or Q3 by finding the value with the greatest frequency. The median can be obtained from a frequency table by finding the middle or the mean of the two middle values. In the frequency table of Q2 there were 21 values. The eleventh score from each end would be the middle score since there would be ten values above and ten below it. The values must be arranged from smallest to largest. The frequencies are added until the eleventh value is obtained.

Temperature (°C)	Frequency
37.0	1
37.5	3 } 4 } 10 } 13
38.0	6
median → 38.5	3
39.0	4
39.5	3
40.0	1
	21

Since there were ten scores of thirty-eight or less, the eleventh score was one of the three 38.5's. Therefore, the median is 38.5 °C.

Q4   A man was fitted with a weight reduction program and his waist measurement was made to the nearest inch each week for twenty-five weeks. Find the median waist measurement.

Waist (inches)	Frequency
37	1
38	3
39	7
40	8
41	4
42	2
	25

\# \# \#   •   \# \# \#   •   \# \# \#   •   \# \# \#   •   \# \# \#   •   \# \# \#   •   \# \# \#   •   \# \# \#   •   \# \# \#

A4   40 inches:

Waist (inches)	Frequency
37	1
38	3 } 4 } 11 } 19
39	7
40	8
41	4
42	2
	25

The 13th score must be one of the scores of 40.

3   For large sets of data a system is needed to determine the position of the median in the data when the values are arranged from smallest to largest. The variable n is used to represent the number of values in the data set. If n is odd, there is a middle value. The position of that middle value may be obtained by adding 1 to n and taking half of it.

If n is odd, the middle value has position $\frac{1}{2}(n+1)$.

If n is even, there are two middle values. Their positions can be found by taking $\frac{1}{2}n$ and $\frac{1}{2}n+1$.

Example 1: The median has which position in a data set where $n = 405$?

Solution: middle number $= \frac{1}{2}(405+1) = 203$

The median is the 203rd number from the smallest.

Example 2: The median is computed from which positions in a data set where $n = 264$?

Solution: middle numbers are $\frac{1}{2}(264)$ and $\frac{1}{2}(264)+1$

The median is halfway between the 132nd and 133rd values.

Q5   Find the position of the median in a data set with each of the following values of n:
a. $n = 27$ **b.** $n = 94$

c. $n = 482$ **d.** $n = 507$

•   # # #   •   # # #   •   # # #   •   # # #   •   # # #   •   # # #   •   # # #   •   # #

A5   **a.** 14th from smallest: $\frac{1}{2}(27+1) = 14$

b. halfway between the 47th and 48th value from the smallest: $\frac{1}{2}(94)$ and $\frac{1}{2}(94)+1$

c. halfway between the 241st and 242nd from the smallest
d. 254th from the smallest

---

4   An example with an even number of values will be considered.

Example: Find the median and the mode.

Value	Frequency
24	10
25	15
26	17
27	19
28	24
29	20
30	12
31	5
	$n = 122$

25   42   61

Solution: Since there are 122 values (be careful *not* to count the values under the heading "value"), the two middle values are $\frac{1}{2}(122)$ and $\frac{1}{2}(122)+1$. Find the 61st and 62nd values. There are 61 values of 27 or below (found by adding the frequency column). Therefore, the 61st value is 27 and the 62nd value is 28. The median is $\frac{27+28}{2}=27.5$. The mode is 28, because it occurred 24 times, which was more frequent than any other value.

Q6 The frequency distribution in part **a** shows the number of deaths each year for the first six years of persons receiving a kidney transplant from a cadaver. The distribution in part **b** shows the same information for transplants from living, related donors. Find (1) the median and (2) the mode.

a.

Years since Transplant	Frequency
1	8
2	5
3	4
4	4
5	3
6	2
	$n = 26$

1. median _____ 2. mode _____

b.

Years since Transplant	Frequency
1	2
2	2
3	4
4	3
5	2
6	3
	$n = 16$

1. median _____ 2. mode _____

• # # # • # # # • # # # • # # # • # # # • # # # • # # # • # #

A6 **a.** 1. 2.5 years: The 13th value is 2, the 14th is 3.
2. 1 year

b. 1. 3.5 years: The 8th value is 3, the 9th is 4.
2. 3 years

5 When finding the mean of a data set with large *n*, it is easier to first make a frequency chart. Consider the data set below. If the mean was calculated from the original data set, 150 numbers would have to be added. Instead, follow this procedure:

Step 1: Multiply each value by its frequency.

Step 2: Add the products obtained in Step 1.

Step 3: Divide the sum of Step 2 by *n*.

Value	Frequency	Value × Frequency	
17	20	340 ⎫	
18	30	540 ⎪	
19	50	950 ⎬ ← Step 1	
20	40	800 ⎪	
21	10	210 ⎭	
	$n = 150$	2,840 ← Step 2	

$$\text{Step 3: mean} = \frac{2,840}{150} = 18.9\frac{1}{3}$$

Q7 The length of the hospital stay for 31 patients suffering from a particular disease is given in the table below. Find the mean, median, and mode. Round off to two decimal places.

Days	Frequency	Days × Frequency
25	2	
26	5	
27	10	
28	8	
29	3	
30	3	____
	$n = 31$	

mean = _____ median = _____ mode = _____

\# \# \#   •   \# \# \#   •   \# \# \#   •   \# \# \#   •   \# \# \#   •   \# \# \#   •   \# \# \#   •   \# \# \#   •   \# \# \#

A7   mean = 27.45 days   median = 27 days   mode = 27 days

Days	Frequency	Days × Frequency
25	2 ⎫ 7 ⎫	50
26	5 ⎬ ⎬ 17	130
27	10 - - ⎭	270
28	8	224
29	3	87
30	3	90
	$n = 31$	851

$$\text{mean} = \frac{851}{31} = 27.45 \quad \text{median is the 16th value} = 27$$

Q8 The highest temperature before treatment was recorded for 128 patients on a Fahrenheit scale. Find the mean, median, and mode of the following distribution. Round off to two decimal places.

Temperature (°F)	Frequency	Temperature × Frequency
100	10	
101	24	
102	30	
103	32	
104	22	
105	10	____
	$n = 128$	

mean _____ median _____ mode _____

\# \# \#   •   \# \# \#   •   \# \# \#   •   \# \# \#   •   \# \# \#   •   \# \# \#   •   \# \# \#   •   \# \# \#   •   \# \# \#

A8   mean = 102.48 °F   median = 102.5 °F   mode = 103 °F

6   Statisticians like to be able to look at a distribution of data graphically. Some characteristics of the data are more apparent in graphical form than in tabular form. The graph of a frequency table is called a *frequency polygon*. Shown here is a frequency table and its corresponding frequency polygon.

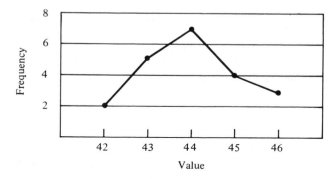

Value	Frequency
42	2
43	5
44	7
45	4
46	3
	$n = 21$

Notice that values are on the horizontal axis and frequencies on the vertical axis. Each point above a value represents the frequency of that value. After the points are plotted they are connected by line segments.

Q9   **a.**   The radiation per year in rads for 105 radiation workers is reported below. Use the frequency table to locate points and draw a frequency polygon.

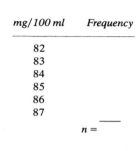

Rads	Frequency
24	10
25	15
26	25
27	30
28	20
29	5
	$n = 105$

b.   The number of people with a certain value of blood glucose in mg/100 ml of blood is given in a frequency polygon. Use the frequency polygon to fill in the frequency column in the frequency table.

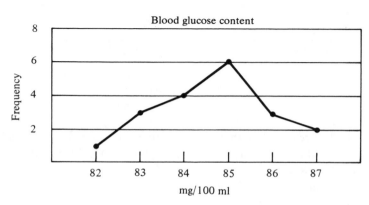

mg/100 ml	Frequency
82	
83	
84	
85	
86	
87	
$n =$	

•   # # #   •   # # #   •   # # #   •   # # #   •   # # #   •   # # #   •   # # #   •   # #

A9   **a.**

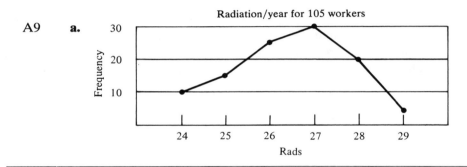

Radiation/year for 105 workers

b.

mg/100 ml	Frequency
82	1
83	3
84	4
85	6
86	3
87	2
	$n = 19$

This completes the instruction for this section.

11.2   EXERCISE

1. The number of x-ray films developed per hour for a 16-hour sample in an x-ray clinic: 23, 24, 25, 22, 23, 23, 24, 25, 21, 24, 23, 22, 26, 22, 24, 24. Construct a frequency table from the data.

2. The maximum temperature in degrees Fahrenheit associated with a disease for 28 people is recorded in the frequency table below. Find the mean, median, and mode of the frequency distribution. (Round off mean to nearest tenth.)

Maximum Temperature

Temperature (°F)	Frequency
101	1
102	3
103	10
104	7
105	4
106	3
	$n = 28$

3. Plot a frequency polygon corresponding to the frequency table of problem 2 above.

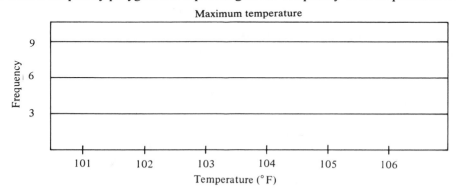

Maximum temperature

4. The respiratory therapy department in a hospital has had the following number of requests for assistance per day for the past 18 days: 47, 50, 52, 48, 49, 50, 49, 51, 50, 46, 48, 50, 48, 51, 53, 49, 48, 47.
   a. Construct a frequency table.
   b. Find the mode.
   c. Find the median.
   d. Find the mean (round off to nearest tenth).
   e. Construct a frequency polygon with the data.

5. Read the frequency polygon and fill in the frequency table.

Waist Sizes of 47 Boys at 16 years

Waist (inches)	Frequency
27	
28	
29	
30	
31	
32	

$n =$ _____

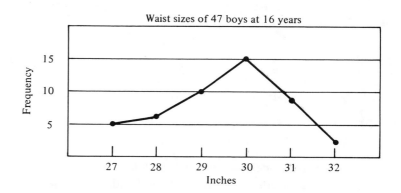

Waist sizes of 47 boys at 16 years

11.2   EXERCISE ANSWERS

1. Films Developed per Hour

# Films	Frequency
21	1
22	3
23	4
24	5
25	2
26	1
	$n = 16$

2.

Temperature (°F)	Frequency	Temperature × Frequency
101	1 ⎫ 4 ⎫	101
102	3 ⎬ ⎬ 14	306
103	10 -- ⎭	1030
104	7	728
105	4	420
106	3	318
	$n = 28$	2903

mean $= \dfrac{2903}{28} = 103.7\,°F$ (rounded off to tenths)

median $= 103.5\,°F$ (halfway between 14th and 15th value)

mode $= 103\,°F$

3.

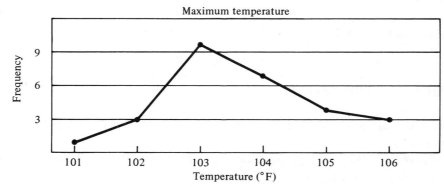

Maximum temperature

4.   Requests per Day of Respiratory Therapy Department

# Requests	Frequency	# Requests × Frequency
46	1	46
47	2	94
48	4	192
49	3	147
50	4	200
51	2	102
52	1	52
53	1	53
	$n = 18$	886

b. modes = 48 requests and 50 requests

c. median = 49 requests (9th and 10th values are both 49)

d. mean $= \dfrac{886}{18} = 49.2$ requests

e.

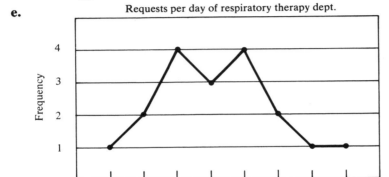

Requests per day of respiratory therapy dept.

5.   Waist sizes of 47 Boys at 16 Years

Value	Frequency
27	5
28	6
29	10
30	15
31	9
32	2
	$n = 47$

CHAPTER 11 SAMPLE TEST

At the completion of Chapter 11 you should be able to work the following problems.

11.1   MEAN, MEDIAN, AND MODE

Find the mean, median, and mode for each of the data sets in problems 1–3. (Round off answers to the nearest tenth.)

1. A sample of seven adults age 20 had the following number of teeth with decays or restorations: 8, 9, 11, 12, 13, 13, 17.

2. A major city in the United States reported the following number of suicides per week for a period of 8 weeks: 5, 3, 7, 3, 12, 6, 7, 2.

3. A walk-in clinic saw the following numbers of rubella cases per week for a six week period: 5, 1, 17, 49, 33, 11.

4. Choose the measure of central tendency that has been or should be used in each situation:

    a. The average registered nurse is female.

    b. The average score on the registry exam.

    c. The average length of the newborn babies born at a hospital during one year.

    d. The average yearly earnings per person in a clinic with one doctor, two nurses, two technicians, a secretary, and a custodian.

    e. The middle value.

    f. The most popular value.

    g. The average used for advanced statistics.

11.2 FREQUENCY TABLES AND FREQUENCY POLYGONS

5. The number of room calls to the nurses' station per hour for a 24 hour period is: 20, 22, 26, 24, 21, 23, 25, 23, 20, 24, 21, 22, 20, 23, 23, 22, 21, 20, 21, 24, 22, 23, 25, 23.

    a. Construct a frequency table.

    b. Construct a frequency polygon.

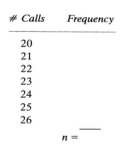

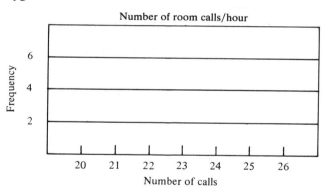

6. Use the frequency table below to complete a, b, and c.

Number of Units of Blood Used per Day by Blood Bank

# Units	Frequency	Frequency × # Units
40	5	
41	7	
42	6	
43	9	
44	5	
45	4	
	$n =$	___

    a. Find the mean of the data. (Round off to tenths.)

    b. Find the median of the data.

    c. Find the mode of the data.

CHAPTER 11 SAMPLE TEST ANSWERS

1. mean, 11.9; median, 12; mode, 13
2. mean, 5.6; median, 5.5; mode, 3 and 7
3. mean, 19.3; median, 14; mode, none
4. a. mode   **b.** mean or median   **c.** mean or median   **d.** median
    e. median   **f.** mode   **g.** mean

5. a.

# Calls	Frequency
20	4
21	4
22	4
23	6
24	3
25	2
26	1
	$n = \overline{24}$

b.

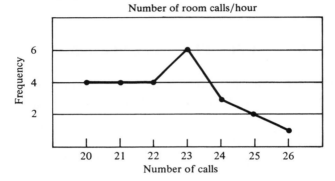

Number of room calls/hour

6. a. 42.4 units   **b.** 42.5 units   **c.** 43 units

CHAPTER 12

EXPONENTS AND LOGARITHMS

Many relationships in the health field can be described by using exponents. These relationships are also describable with logarithms, which the technician must be able to understand. This chapter will introduce logarithms by showing their relationships to exponents and will examine some applications of exponents and logarithms.

12.1 EXPONENTS AND SCIENTIFIC NOTATION

1	Exponents are used if a number, called the *base*, is to be multiplied times itself over and over. The expression 10^3 means to use 10, the base, as a factor three times in a multiplication problem; that is, $10^3 = 10 \cdot 10 \cdot 10 = 1000$. In this problem 10 is the base, 3 is the exponent, and the result of the operation, 1000, is called the 3rd power of 10.
	Example: Evaluate 5^4.
	Solution: $5^4 = 5 \cdot 5 \cdot 5 \cdot 5 = 625$

Q1 In the expression $4^3 = 64$:

    a. 4 is called the _____ .

    b. 3 is called the _____ .

    c. 64 is called the _____ .

\# \# \#　•　\# \# \#　•　\# \# \#　•　\# \# \#　•　\# \# \#　•　\# \# \#　•　\# \# \#　•　\# \# \#　•　\# \# \#

A1 **a.** base　　　　　　**b.** exponent　　　　　　**c.** third power of 4

Q2 Evaluate each power:

    a. 3^4 _____　　　**b.** 2^6 _____　　　**d.** 5^2 _____

    d. 10^4 _____　　　**e.** 100^2 _____　　　**f.** 6^3 _____

\# \# \#　•　\# \# \#　•　\# \# \#　•　\# \# \#　•　\# \# \#　•　\# \# \#　•　\# \# \#　•　\# \# \#　•　\# \# \#

A2 **a.** 81　　**b.** 64　　**c.** 25　　**d.** 10,000　　**e.** 10,000　　**f.** 216

Q3 Answer the following:

    a. What is the base of 4^3? _____

    b. What is the exponent in 2^5? _____

c. What is the 4th power of 2? _____

d. What is the 3rd power of 5? _____

e. What is the 2nd power of 2? _____

• # # # • # # # • # # # • # # # • # # # • # # # • # # # • # #

A3   **a.** 4   **b.** 5   **c.** 16   **d.** 125   **e.** 4

2	When logarithms are introduced in Section 12.2, they will be based on the powers of 10. The first three powers of 10 are

$$10^1 = 10 \qquad 10^2 = 100 \qquad 10^3 = 1000$$

Numbers of the form 10^1, 10^2, 10^3, etc. are said to be written in *exponential notation*.

10^1 says "10 raised to the first power" or "10 to the first."
10^2 says "10 squared" or "10 raised to the second power."
10^3 says "10 cubed" or "10 raised to the third power."

Q4   Determine the first 8 powers of 10:

a. $10^1 =$ _____   **b.** $10^2 =$ _____   **c.** $10^3 =$ _____

d. $10^4 =$ _____   **e.** $10^5 =$ _____   **f.** $10^6 =$ _____

g. $10^7 =$ _____   **h.** $10^8 =$ _____

• # # # • # # # • # # # • # # # • # # # • # # # • # # # • # #

A4   **a.** 10   **b.** 100   **c.** 1,000   **d.** 10,000
      e. 100,000   **f.** 1,000,000   **g.** 10,000,000   **h.** 100,000,000

Q5   From the results of Q4 what is the relationship in a power of 10 between the exponent and the

number of zeros? _____

• # # # • # # # • # # # • # # # • # # # • # # # • # # # • # #

A5   They are equal.

Q6   How many zeros would 10^{16} have if it were to be multiplied out? _____

• # # # • # # # • # # # • # # # • # # # • # # # • # # # • # #

A6   16

Q7   Write each of the following in exponential notation:

a. $10,000 =$ _____   **b.** $100 =$ _____   **c.** $100,000 =$ _____

d. $1,000,000,000 =$ _____   **e.** $10 =$ _____   **f.** $1,000 =$ _____

• # # # • # # # • # # # • # # # • # # # • # # # • # # # • # #

A7   **a.** 10^4 **b.** 10^2 **c.** 10^5 **d.** 10^9 **e.** 10^1 **f.** 10^3

3	Negative exponents can be changed to positive exponents if the bases are reciprocals, that is,

$$10^{-3} = \left(\frac{1}{10}\right)^3 = \frac{1}{10^3}.$$

Example 1: Write 3^{-4} with a positive exponent.

Solution: $3^{-4} = \left(\frac{1}{3}\right)^4 = \frac{1}{3^4}$

Example 2: Write 10^{-3} with a positive exponent in decimal form.

Solution: $10^{-3} = \left(\dfrac{1}{10}\right)^3 = \dfrac{1}{10^3} = \dfrac{1}{1000} = 0.001$

In general, we can say $a^{-n} = \left(\dfrac{1}{a}\right)^n = \dfrac{1}{a^n}$ for any integer n, and a is a positive number.

Q8   Write each number as a fraction with positive exponents:

    a. $3^{-4} = $ _____   **b.** $5^{-2} = $ _____   **c.** $3^{-1} = $ _____

    d. $4^{-3} = $ _____   **e.** $6^{-5} = $ _____   **f.** $10^{-3} = $ _____

\# \# \# • \# \# \# • \# \# \# • \# \# \# • \# \# \# • \# \# \# • \# \# \# • \# \# \# • \# \# \#

A8   **a.** $\dfrac{1}{3^4}$ **b.** $\dfrac{1}{5^2}$ **c.** $\dfrac{1}{3}$ **d.** $\dfrac{1}{4^3}$ **e.** $\dfrac{1}{6^5}$ **f.** $\dfrac{1}{10^3}$

Q9   Write each number in decimal form:

    a. $10^{-4} = $ _____   **b.** $10^{-2} = $ _____

    c. $10^{-1} = $ _____   **d.** $10^{-6} = $ _____

\# \# \# • \# \# \# • \# \# \# • \# \# \# • \# \# \# • \# \# \# • \# \# \# • \# \# \# • \# \# \#

A9   **a.** 0.0001   **b.** 0.01   **c.** 0.1   **d.** 0.000001

4   The exponent zero requires a special definition. Any nonzero base raised to the exponent zero is defined to be equal to 1. Thus, we have the following examples: $3^0 = 1$, $4^0 = 1$, $100^0 = 1$, $\left(\dfrac{1}{10}\right)^0 = 1$, $1^0 = 1$. The expression 0^0 is left undefined. It is not equal to 1.

Q10   Write each number in decimal form:

    a. $2^{-2} = $ _____   **b.** $5^2 = $ _____   **c.** $10^{-3} = $ _____

    d. $10^0 = $ _____   **e.** $3^0 = $ _____   **f.** $10^{-7} = $ _____

    g. $0^0 = $ _____

\# \# \# • \# \# \# • \# \# \# • \# \# \# • \# \# \# • \# \# \# • \# \# \# • \# \# \# • \# \# \#

A10   **a.** 0.25   **b.** 25   **c.** 0.001   **d.** 1

             e. 1   **f.** 0.0000001   **g.** undefined

5   The product of numbers written as powers of the same base can be obtained by adding exponents.

Example 1: Show that $3^2 \cdot 3^4 = 3^{2+4}$

Solution: $3^2 \cdot 3^4 = (3 \cdot 3)(3 \cdot 3 \cdot 3 \cdot 3) = 3^6$; also,
           $3^{2+4} = 3^6$, so therefore $3^2 \cdot 3^4 = 3^{2+4}$.

Example 2: Show that $4^{-2} \cdot 4^5 = 4^{-2+5}$.

Solution: $4^{-2} \cdot 4^5 = \dfrac{1}{4^2} \cdot 4^5 = \dfrac{\cancel{4} \cdot \cancel{4} \cdot 4 \cdot 4 \cdot 4}{\cancel{4} \cdot \cancel{4}} = 4^3$;
           $4^{-2+5} = 4^3$; therefore, $4^{-2} \cdot 4^5 = 4^{-2+5}$.

Example 3: Simplify $2^{-3} \cdot 2^4 \cdot 2^1 \cdot 2^5$

Solution: $2^{-3} \cdot 2^4 \cdot 2^1 \cdot 2^5 = 2^{-3+4+1+5} = 2^7$

The principle which is illustrated can be generalized as $a^m \cdot a^n = a^{m+n}$ for any integers m and n and positive number a. Notice that it states that the *product* of powers of the same base is found by *adding* the exponents.

Q11 Multiply (leave answer in exponential notation):

a. $2^3 \cdot 2^4 =$ _____   **b.** $3^2 \cdot 3^4 =$ _____   **c.** $4^5 \cdot 4^3 =$ _____

d. $10^2 \cdot 10^3 =$ _____   **e.** $10^4 \cdot 10 =$ _____   **f.** $10 \cdot 10 \cdot 10^3 =$ _____

\# \# \# • \# \# \# • \# \# \# • \# \# \# • \# \# \# • \# \# \# • \# \# \# • \# \# \# • \# \# \#

A11   **a.** 2^7 **b.** 3^6 **c.** 4^8 **d.** 10^5 **e.** 10^5 **f.** 10^5

Q12 Multiply (leave answer in exponential notation):

a. $2^4 \cdot 2^{-3} =$ _____   **b.** $2^{-4} \cdot 2^{-5} =$ _____

c. $10^3 \cdot 10^4 \cdot 10^{-2} =$ _____   **d.** $10 \cdot 10^{-1} \cdot 10^3 =$ _____

e. $10^3 \cdot 10^4 \cdot 10^0 =$ _____   **f.** $10^{-3} \cdot 10^3 =$ _____

\# \# \# • \# \# \# • \# \# \# • \# \# \# • \# \# \# • \# \# \# • \# \# \# • \# \# \# • \# \# \#

A12   **a.** 2: $2^4 \cdot 2^{-3} = 2^{4+-3} = 2^1 = 2$ **b.** 2^{-9}

     c. 10^5 **d.** 10^3: $10 \cdot 10^{-1} \cdot 10^3 = 10^{1+-1+3} = 10^3$

     e. 10^7 **f.** 1: $10^{-3} \cdot 10^3 = 10^{-3+3} = 10^0 = 1$

---

6   Dividing can also be done easily with powers of the same base. The quotient of powers of the same base is found by subtracting exponents.

Example 1: Show that $\dfrac{2^5}{2^3} = 2^{5-3}$.

Solution: $\dfrac{2^5}{2^3} = \dfrac{\not2 \cdot \not2 \cdot \not2 \cdot 2 \cdot 2}{\not2 \cdot \not2 \cdot \not2} = 2^2 = 2^{5-3}$

Example 2: Show that $\dfrac{3^2}{3^6} = 3^{2-6}$.

Solution: $\dfrac{3^2}{3^6} = \dfrac{\not3 \cdot \not3}{\not3 \cdot \not3 \cdot 3 \cdot 3 \cdot 3 \cdot 3} = \dfrac{1}{3^4} = 3^{-4} = 3^{2-6}$

Example 3: Simplify $\dfrac{5^2 \cdot 5^3}{5^4}$.

Solution: $\dfrac{5^2 \cdot 5^3}{5^4} = \dfrac{5^{2+3}}{5^4} = \dfrac{5^5}{5^4} = 5^{5-4} = 5^1 = 5$

Example 4: Simplify $\dfrac{2^{42}}{2^{14}}$.

Solution: $\dfrac{2^{42}}{2^{14}} = 2^{42-14} = 2^{28}$

The principle that is illustrated above can be stated as $\dfrac{a^m}{a^n} = a^{m-n}$, where m and n are natural numbers, and a is positive, which says that the *quotient* of powers with the same base is found by *subtracting* exponents.

Q13   Simplify (leave answer in exponential notation):

a. $\dfrac{2^5}{2^3} =$ _____

b. $\dfrac{2^{17}}{2^{12}} =$ _____

c. $\dfrac{10^6}{10^2} =$ _____

d. $\dfrac{10^8}{10^0} =$ _____

e. $\dfrac{10^7}{10} =$ _____

f. $\dfrac{10^4 \cdot 10^3}{10^5} =$ _____

\# \# \# • \# \# \# • \# \# \# • \# \# \# • \# \# \# • \# \# \# • \# \# \# • \# \# \# • \# \# \#

A13   a. 2^2: 2^{5-3} b. 2^5: 2^{17-12} c. 10^4: 10^{6-2}

d. 10^8: 10^{8-0} e. 10^6: 10^{7-1} f. 10^2: $10^{4+3-5} = 10^2$

Q14   Simplify (leave answer in exponential notation):

a. $\dfrac{3^2}{3^5} =$ _____

b. $\dfrac{2^4}{2^7} =$ _____

c. $\dfrac{10^7}{10^{12}} =$ _____

d. $\dfrac{10^3 \cdot 10^2}{10^7} =$ _____

\# \# \# • \# \# \# • \# \# \# • \# \# \# • \# \# \# • \# \# \# • \# \# \# • \# \# \# • \# \# \#

A14   a. 3^{-3}: $3^{2-5} = 3^{-3}$ b. 2^{-3}: $2^{4-7} = 2^{-3}$

c. 10^{-5} d. 10^{-2}

Q15   Simplify (leave answer in exponential notation):

a. $\dfrac{2^3 \cdot 2}{2^4} =$ _____

b. $\dfrac{10^7}{10} =$ _____

c. $\dfrac{10^6 \cdot 10^{-3}}{10^2} =$ _____

d. $\dfrac{10^4 \cdot 10}{10^6} =$ _____

\# \# \# • \# \# \# • \# \# \# • \# \# \# • \# \# \# • \# \# \# • \# \# \# • \# \# \# • \# \# \#

A15   a. 1: $2^{3+1-4} = 2^0 = 1$ b. 10^6: 10^{7-1}

c. 10: $10^{6-3-2} = 10^1$ d. 10^{-1}: $10^{4+1-6} = 10^{-1}$

Q16   Complete the statement of the properties of the exponents that we have been using:

a. $a^m \cdot a^n =$ _____

b. $a^{-n} = ($____$)^n$

c. $\dfrac{a^m}{a^n} =$ _____

\# \# \# • \# \# \# • \# \# \# • \# \# \# • \# \# \# • \# \# \# • \# \# \# • \# \# \# • \# \# \#

A16   a. a^{m+n} b. $\dfrac{1}{a}$ c. a^{m-n}

---

7   Exponents are used to write numbers in *scientific notation*. A number in scientific notation is written as a number greater than or equal to 1 but less than 10, times a power of 10. Examples of numbers written in scientific notation are:

$$2.45 \times 10^5$$
$$3 \times 10^{-3}$$
$$9.98 \times 10^2$$
$$\underbrace{2.6} \times \underbrace{10}$$

number greater than or   power of 10
equal to 1 but less than 10

Examples of numbers which are not in scientific notation are:

2,460,000 (not proper form)
0.34 (not proper form)
75.3×10^4 (75.3 is not between 1 and 10)
0.006×10^5 (0.006 is not between 1 and 10)

Q17 Write yes if the number is written in scientific notation; otherwise, indicate no.

a. 3.46×10^5 _____ **b.** 3,460 _____ **c.** 0.24×10^3 _____

d. 4×10^{-3} _____ **e.** 720×10^{-2} _____ **f.** $7.9 \cdot 10^{-3}$ _____

\# \# \# • \# \# \# • \# \# \# • \# \# \# • \# \# \# • \# \# \# • \# \# \# • \# \# \# • \# \# \#

A17 **a.** yes **b.** no **c.** no **d.** yes **e.** no **f.** yes

---

8 In order to work with logarithms, you must be able to perform conversions between scientific notation and decimal notation. Recall that multiplying a number by a positive power of 10 moves the decimal point to the right the same number of places as there are zeros in the power of 10.

Example 1: Write 2.62×10^3 in decimal notation.

Solution: $2.62 \times 10^3 = 2.62 \times 1000$
$= 2,620$

Example 2: Write 4.6×10^6 in decimal notation.

Solution: $4.6 \times 10^6 = 4.6 \times 1,000,000$
$= 4,600,000$

Note that the decimal is moved the same number of positions that appears as the exponent of 10. With this in mind the middle step need not be included and the decimal point is moved the appropriate number of places to the *right*.

Example 3: Write 4.7×10^3 in decimal notation.

Solution: $4.7 \times 10^3 = 4,700.$

Q18 Write in decimal notation:

a. $5.72 \times 10^4 =$ _____ **b.** $6.24 \times 10 =$ _____ **c.** $7 \times 10^7 =$ _____

\# \# \# • \# \# \# • \# \# \# • \# \# \# • \# \# \# • \# \# \# • \# \# \# • \# \# \# • \# \# \#

A18 **a.** 57,200 **b.** 62.4 **c.** 70,000,000 (remember 7 means 7. not 0.7)

---

9 Numbers that include negative exponents can be converted from scientific notation to decimal notation by means of division by a power of 10. Division moves the decimal to the *left*.

Example 1: Write 8.2×10^{-2} in decimal notation.

Solution: $8.2 \times 10^{-2} = 8.2 \times \dfrac{1}{10^2} = \dfrac{8.2}{100} = 0.082$

The intermediate steps may be omitted and the decimal point moved the appropriate number of places to the *left*.

Example 2: Convert 5.34×10^{-4} to decimal notation.

Solution: $5.34 \times 10^{-4} = 0.000534$

Q19   Convert to decimal notation:

   a. $4.6 \times 10^{-2} =$ _____

   b. $9.804 \times 10^{-4} =$ _____

   c. $4.7 \times 10^{0} =$ _____

\# \# \#   •   \# \# \#   •   \# \# \#   •   \# \# \#   •   \# \# \#   •   \# \# \#   •   \# \# \#   •   \# \# \#   •   \# \# \#

A19   **a.** 0.046   **b.** 0.0009804   **c.** 4.7 (recall that $10^{0} = 1$)

---

10   A number, N, is written in scientific notation by writing N as the product of a decimal m (where m is greater than or equal to 1 but less than 10), times a power of 10, 10^{c}, where c is an integer. That is, $N = m \times 10^{c}$.

   Example 1: Write 2,420 in scientific notation.

   Solution: $2{,}420 = 2.420 \times 10^{3}$

   Example 2: Write 0.00402 in scientific notation.

   Solution: $0.00402 = 4.02 \times 10^{-3}$

Q20   Write in scientific notation:

   a. $42{,}640 =$ _____   **b.** $8{,}000{,}000 =$ _____

   c. $53 =$ _____   **d.** $0.046 =$ _____

   e. $0.0009 =$ _____

\# \# \#   •   \# \# \#   •   \# \# \#   •   \# \# \#   •   \# \# \#   •   \# \# \#   •   \# \# \#   •   \# \#·\#   •   \# \# \#

A20   **a.** 4.264×10^{4} **b.** 8.0×10^{6} **c.** 5.3×10 **d.** 4.6×10^{-2}
       e. $9 \times 10^{-4}\, (9.0 \times 10^{-4})$

---

11   Sometimes a number is written in a form that is similar to scientific notation, but the first number is not between 1 and 10. Such a number may be converted to scientific notation.

   Example 1: Write 28×10^{4} in scientific notation.

   Solution: 28×10^{4}
                 $2.8 \times 10^{1} \times 10^{4}$
                 2.8×10^{5}

   Notice that 28 is first converted to scientific notation and then multiplied by 10^{4}.

   Example 2: Write 4280×10^{-2} in scientific notation.

   Solution: 4280×10^{-2}
                 $4.28 \times 10^{3} \times 10^{-2}$
                 4.28×10

   Example 3: Write 0.024×10^{-4} in scientific notation.

   Solution: 0.024×10^{-4}
                 $2.4 \times 10^{-2} \times 10^{-4}$
                 2.4×10^{-6}

Q21   Convert to scientific notation:
    a. 46×10^3 **b.** 522×10^2 **c.** 0.420×10^{-5}

•   # # #   •   # # #   •   # # #   •   # # #   •   # # #   •   # # #   •   # # #   •   # #

A21   **a.** 4.6×10^4 **b.** 5.22×10^4 **c.** 4.20×10^{-6}

---

12   Another property of exponents allows a power of a number to be further raised to a power. For example, $(2^3)^4 = (2^3)(2^3)(2^3)(2^3) = 2^{12}$ but a quicker way to simplify would be $(2^3)^4 = 2^{3 \cdot 4} = 2^{12}$.

Example 1: Show that $(2^4)^2 = 2^{4 \cdot 2}$.

Solution: $(2^4)^2 = (2^4)(2^4) = 2^8$ also $2^{4 \cdot 2} = 2^8$ so, $(2^4)^2 = 2^{4 \cdot 2}$

Example 2: Simplify $(3^2)^5$ (leave answer in exponential notation).

Solution: $(3^2)^5 = 3^{2 \cdot 5} = 3^{10}$

Example 3: Simplify $\dfrac{(3^2)^4(3^3)}{3^2}$ (leave answer in exponential notation).

Solution: $\dfrac{(3^2)^4(3^3)}{3^2} = \dfrac{3^8 \cdot 3^3}{3^2} = 3^{8+3-2} = 3^9$

The principle that is illustrated above can be generalized as $(a^m)^n = a^{mn}$ for any integers, m and n.

Q22   Simplify (leave answer in exponential notation in this and the remaining portion of this section).
    a. $(3^2)^3 = $_____   **b.** $(5^2)^5 = $_____   **c.** $(2^{-1})^{-5} = $_____
    d. $(3^3)^3 = $_____   **e.** $(10^2)^{-2} = $_____   **f.** $(10^3)^2 = $_____

•   # # #   •   # # #   •   # # #   •   # # #   •   # # #   •   # # #   •   # # #   •   # #

A22   **a.** 3^6 **b.** 5^{10} **c.** 2^5 **d.** 3^9 **e.** 10^{-4} **f.** 10^6

Q23   Simplify $\dfrac{(2^3)^2(2^5)}{2}$.

•   # # #   •   # # #   •   # # #   •   # # #   •   # # #   •   # # #   •   # # #   •   # #

A23 2^{10}: $\dfrac{(2^3)^2(2^5)}{2} = \dfrac{2^6 \cdot 2^5}{2} = 2^{6+5-1} = 2^{10}$

Q24   Simplify $\dfrac{10^2(10^{-5})^2}{10^5}$.

•   # # #   •   # # #   •   # # #   •   # # #   •   # # #   •   # # #   •   # # #   •   # #

A24 10^{-13}: $\dfrac{10^2(10^{-5})^2}{10^5} = \dfrac{10^2 \cdot 10^{-10}}{10^5} = 10^{2-10-5} = 10^{-13}$

13   Square roots can be written by using fractional exponents. The square root of a nonnegative number is equal to that number to the $\frac{1}{2}$ power. That is, $\sqrt{a} = a^{1/2}$. This property is useful for finding square roots of nonnegative numbers written as powers.

Example 1: Simplify $\sqrt{10^4}$.

Solution: $\sqrt{10^4} = (10^4)^{1/2} = 10^{4 \cdot 1/2} = 10^2$

Example 2: Simplify $\sqrt{2^8}$.

Solution: $\sqrt{2^8} = (2^8)^{1/2} = 2^{8 \cdot 1/2} = 2^4$

Q25   Simplify

    a. $\sqrt{10^6}$ **b.** $\sqrt{3^{10}}$ **c.** $\sqrt{5^4}$ **d.** $\sqrt{2^{-8}}$

\# \# \#   •   \# \# \#   •   \# \# \#   •   \# \# \#   •   \# \# \#   •   \# \# \#   •   \# \# \#   •   \# \# \#   •   \# \# \#

A25   **a.** 10^3: $\sqrt{10^6} = (10^6)^{1/2} = 10^{6 \cdot 1/2} = 10^3$
      b. 3^5 **c.** 5^2
      d. 2^{-4}: $\sqrt{2^{-8}} = (2^{-8})^{1/2} = 2^{-8 \cdot 1/2} = 2^{-4}$

14   Other roots may be interpreted similarly. Hence, the cube root of a number is the number raised to the $\frac{1}{3}$ power. The fourth root of a nonnegative number is the number raised to the $\frac{1}{4}$ power, etc. For our purposes, we will assume that the number a under the radical sign, $\sqrt[n]{a}$, is always nonnegative.

$\sqrt[3]{a} = a^{1/3}$
$\sqrt[4]{a} = a^{1/4}$
$\sqrt[n]{a} = a^{1/n}$

Example 1: Simplify $\sqrt[3]{2^9}$.

Solution: $\sqrt[3]{2^9} = (2^9)^{1/3} = 2^{9 \cdot 1/3} = 2^3$

Example 2: Simplify $\sqrt{10^4} \cdot \sqrt[3]{10^{15}}$.

Solution: $\sqrt{10^4} \cdot \sqrt[3]{10^{15}} = (10^4)^{1/2} \cdot (10^{15})^{1/3}$
                          $= 10^2 \cdot 10^5$
                          $= 10^7$

Q26   Simplify:

    a. $\sqrt[3]{2^6}$ **b.** $\sqrt[4]{2^{12}}$

    c. $\sqrt[3]{10^6}$ **d.** $\sqrt{10^{-6}}$

\# \# \#   •   \# \# \#   •   \# \# \#   •   \# \# \#   •   \# \# \#   •   \# \# \#   •   \# \# \#   •   \# \# \#   •   \# \# \#

A26   **a.** 2^2: $\sqrt[3]{2^6} = (2^6)^{1/3} = 2^{6 \cdot 1/3} = 2^2$
      b. 2^3: $\sqrt[4]{2^{12}} = (2^{12})^{1/4} = 2^{12 \cdot 1/4} = 2^3$
      c. 10^2: $\sqrt[3]{10^6} = (10^6)^{1/3} = 10^{6 \cdot 1/3} = 10^2$
      d. 10^{-3}: $\sqrt{10^{-6}} = (10^{-6})^{1/2} = 10^{-6 \cdot 1/2} = 10^{-3}$

Q27   Simplify:

a. $\dfrac{\sqrt[3]{10^6} \cdot \sqrt[5]{10^{10}}}{\sqrt{10^4}}$

b. $\dfrac{\sqrt{10^8} \cdot \sqrt[3]{10^9}}{\sqrt[5]{10^{15}}}$

\# \# \#   •   \# \# \#   •   \# \# \#   •   \# \# \#   •   \# \# \#   •   \# \# \#   •   \# \# \#   •   \# \# \#   •   \# \# \#

A27   **a.** 10^2: $\dfrac{\sqrt[3]{10^6} \cdot \sqrt[5]{10^{10}}}{\sqrt{10^4}} = \dfrac{(10^6)^{1/3} \cdot (10^{10})^{1/5}}{(10^4)^{1/2}} = \dfrac{\cancel{10^2} \cdot 10^2}{\cancel{10^2}} = 10^2$

b. 10^4: $\dfrac{\sqrt{10^8} \cdot \sqrt[3]{10^9}}{\sqrt[5]{10^{15}}} = \dfrac{(10^8)^{1/2} \cdot (10^9)^{1/3}}{(10^{15})^{1/5}} = \dfrac{10^4 \cdot \cancel{10^3}}{\cancel{10^3}} = 10^4$

This completes the instruction for this section.

12.1   EXERCISE

1. In the statement $2^3 = 8$:
    a. What is the base?
    b. What is the exponent?
    c. What is the third power of 2?
2. Evaluate each power:
    a. 3^3 b. 4^2 c. 10^5 d. 5^0
3. The number 10^{23} would be written with a 1 followed by how many zeros?
4. Write the following in exponential notation:

    a. 10,000   b. 1,000,000   c. $\dfrac{1}{1000}$

    d. $\dfrac{1}{10,000}$ e. 1   f. 10
5. Write each number using positive exponents:
    a. 3^{-3} b. 4^{-2} c. 10^{-5} d. 10^{-1}
6. Write each number in decimal form:
    a. 10^{-2} b. 10^{-4} c. 10^{-1} d. 10^{-6}
7. Simplify (leave in exponential notation):
    a. $2^4 \cdot 2^6$ b. $3^2 \cdot 3 \cdot 3^0$ c. $10^2 \cdot 10^5 \cdot 10$ d. $10 \cdot 10 \cdot 10$
8. Simplify (leave in exponential notation):
    a. $10^{-3} \cdot 10^5$ b. $3^2 \cdot 3 \cdot 3^{-3}$ c. $4^5 \cdot 4^{-1} \cdot 4^{-3}$ d. $4^0 \cdot 4^{-3} \cdot 4^5$
9. Simplify (leave in exponential notation):

    a. $\dfrac{2^5}{2^3}$ b. $\dfrac{10^6}{10^4}$ c. $\dfrac{10^5}{10^7}$ d. $\dfrac{10^3}{10^0}$
10. Simplify (leave in exponential notation):

    a. $\dfrac{10^5 \cdot 10^{-2}}{10^2}$ b. $\dfrac{3^4 \cdot 3 \cdot 3^2}{3^5}$
11. Complete the statements of the properties of exponents where a is a positive number and m and n are integers:

    a. $a^m \cdot a^n =$ _____   b. $\dfrac{a^m}{a^n} =$ _____   c. $a^{-n} =$ _____

    d. $(a^m)^n =$ _____   e. $\sqrt[n]{a} =$ _____ where n is nonnegative.

12. Write the numbers given below in decimal notation:

    a. 3.6×10^5 **b.** 4.0×10^3 **c.** 1.7×10^2 **d.** 9.862×10

13. Write in decimal notation:

    a. 3.6×10^{-2} **b.** 4.0×10^{-1} **c.** 4.60×10^0 **d.** 9×10^{-5}

14. Write in scientific notation:

    a. 4,200,000   **b.** 528   **c.** 4,290

    d. 0.0032   **e.** 96.42   **f.** 0.0005

15. Convert to scientific notation:

    a. $2,400 \times 10^2$ **b.** 27.6×10^{-2} **c.** 0.24×10^3 **d.** 0.06×10^{-3}

16. Simplify (leave in exponential notation):

    a. $(10^2)^5$ **b.** $(2^3)^5$ **c.** $(2^{-3})^{-2}$ **d.** $(10^{-2})^{-3}(10^5)^2$

17. Simplify (leave in exponential notation):

    a. $\sqrt{10^4}$ **b.** $\sqrt{10^8}$ **c.** $\sqrt[3]{2^6}$ **d.** $\sqrt[4]{10^{12}}$

12.1 EXERCISE ANSWERS

1. a. 2   **b.** 3   **c.** 8

2. a. 27   **b.** 16   **c.** 100,000   **d.** 1

3. 23 zeros

4. a. 10^4 **b.** 10^6 **c.** 10^{-3} **d.** 10^{-4}

    e. 10^0 **f.** 10^1

5. a. $\frac{1}{3^3}$ **b.** $\frac{1}{4^2}$ **c.** $\frac{1}{10^5}$ **d.** $\frac{1}{10}$

6. a. 0.01   **b.** 0.0001   **c.** 0.1   **d.** 0.000001

7. a. 2^{10} **b.** 3^3 **c.** 10^8 **d.** 10^3

8. a. 10^2 **b.** 3^0 or 1   **c.** 4   **d.** 4^2

9. a. 2^2 **b.** 10^2 **c.** 10^{-2} **d.** 10^3

10. a. 10   **b.** 3^2

11. a. a^{m+n} **b.** a^{m-n} **c.** $\left(\frac{1}{a}\right)^n$ **d.** a^{mn}

    e. $a^{1/n}$

12. a. 360,000   **b.** 4,000   **c.** 170   **d.** 98.62

13. a. 0.036   **b.** 0.40   **c.** 4.60   **d.** 0.00009

14. a. 4.2×10^6 **b.** 5.28×10^2 **c.** 4.29×10^3 **d.** 3.2×10^{-3}

    e. 9.642×10 **f.** 5×10^{-4}

15. a. 2.4×10^5 **b.** 2.76×10^{-1} **c.** 2.4×10^2 **d.** 6.0×10^{-5}

16. a. 10^{10} **b.** 2^{15} **c.** 2^6 **d.** 10^{16}

17. a. 10^2 **b.** 10^4 **c.** 2^2 **d.** 10^3

12.2 LOGARITHMS

1   It is possible to represent any positive number as a power of 10. You know how to do this with a few numbers. You will learn how to do it with others. Many examples follow:

$$0.01 = 10^{-2}$$
$$1.00 = 10^0$$
$$10 = 10^1$$
$$1000 = 10^3$$
$$1,000,000 = 10^6$$

When a number is written as a power of 10, the exponent used is called the *logarithm* of the number to the base 10.

Example 1: What is the logarithm of 100?

Solution: Since $100 = 10^2$, the exponent 2 is the logarithm of 100.

Example 2: What is the logarithm of 0.001?

Solution: Since $0.001 = 10^{-3}$, the logarithm of 0.001 is $^-3$.

Q1   Determine the logarithm of each number:

a. 1000 _____   b. 10 _____

c. 1,000,000 _____   d. 0.01 _____

•   # # #   •   # # #   •   # # #   •   # # #   •   # # #   •   # # #   •   # # #   •   # #

A1   a. 3: $1000 = 10^3$ b. 1: $10 = 10^1$
     c. 6: $1,000,000 = 10^6$ d. $^-2$: $0.01 = 10^{-2}$

---

2   The notation that is used to represent the logarithm of a number n to the base 10 is $\log_{10} n$. Therefore, $\log_{10} 1000 = 3$ since $10^3 = 1000$. Any equation in exponential form may be converted to logarithmic form.

Examples: $10^2 = 100$ becomes $\log_{10} 100 = 2$
        $10^{-3} = 0.001$ becomes $\log_{10} 0.001 = ^-3$
        $10^6 = 1,000,000$ becomes $\log_{10} 1,000,000 = 6$

Q2   Find each logarithm by finding the proper exponent:

a. $\log_{10} 0.01 =$ _____   b. $\log_{10} 0.1 =$ _____   c. $\log_{10} 1 =$ _____

d. $\log_{10} 10 =$ _____   e. $\log_{10} 100 =$ _____   f. $\log_{10} 1000 =$ _____

•   # # #   •   # # #   •   # # #   •   # # #   •   # # #   •   # # #   •   # # #   •   # #

A2   a. $^-2$ b. $^-1$ c. 0   d. 1   e. 2   f. 3

---

3   Notice in Q2 as the number increased from 0.01 to 1000 the logarithms increased from $^-2$ to 3. This relationship can be shown on a line graph by locating the numbers on the horizontal axis and the logarithms of them on the vertical axis. The graph is a fast-rising graph from zero to 1 but then the logarithms increase very slowly as the values of n get larger.

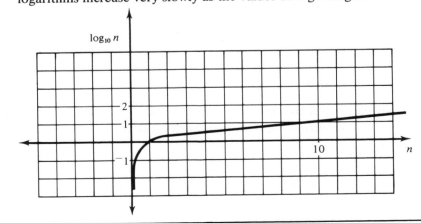

Q3 Use the graph in Frame 3 to answer the questions:

    a. Are the logarithms of numbers between 0 and 1 positive or negative? _____

    b. The logarithms of numbers between 1 and 10 fall between what two numbers? _____

    c. Are there any logarithms of negative values of n? _____

\# \# \# • \# \# \# • \# \# \# • \# \# \# • \# \# \# • \# \# \# • \# \# \# • \# \# \# • \# \# \#

A3   **a.** negative   **b.** 0 and 1   **c.** no: Logarithms of negative numbers do not exist.

---

4 We have been considering logarithms of numbers which could be obtained by changing to exponential form. Many logarithms cannot be found this way. For these numbers, tables of logarithms will allow you to obtain their value. Such a table is found in the appendix of this text (see Table XI).

    The number N is located on the left column and the decimal value of the logarithm is in the body of the table. For example, to find log 2.00 locate 2.0 in the left column. $\log_{10} 2.00$ is under the heading "0" opposite 2.0. Therefore, $\log_{10} 2.00 = 0.3010$. Notice you must place the decimal point yourself in the logarithm.

Example 1: Find $\log_{10} 2.04$.

Solution: $\text{Log}_{10} 2.04$ is on the same line in the table as $\log_{10} 2.00$, but the value is under the column headed 4. Therefore, $\log_{10} 2.04 = 0.3096$. Because 2.04 is between 1 and 10, its logarithm is between 0 and 1.

Example 2: Find $\log_{10} 6.38$.

Solution: Looking in the table where $N = 6.3$ and under the column 8 we find $\log_{10} 6.38 = 0.8048$.

Q4 Look up the values in the table:

    a. $\log_{10} 5.72 =$ _____   **b.** $\log_{10} 2.43 =$ _____

    c. $\log_{10} 1.72 =$ _____   **d.** $\log_{10} 9.10 =$ _____

\# \# \# • \# \# \# • \# \# \# • \# \# \# • \# \# \# • \# \# \# • \# \# \# • \# \# \# • \# \# \#

A4   **a.** 0.7574   **b.** 0.3856   **c.** 0.2355   **d.** 0.9590

---

5 We have changed an exponential equation into an equivalent logarithmic equation. For example, $10^3 = 1{,}000$ becomes $\log_{10} 1{,}000 = 3$. We now change logarithmic equations into exponential equations in the same way.

Example 1: Convert $\log_{10} 4.5 = 0.6532$ into an exponential equation.

Solution: The base is 10. The logarithm is the exponent. The equation is $10^{0.6532} = 4.5$.

Example 2: Convert $\log_{10} 6 = 0.7782$ to an exponential equation.

Solution: $10^{0.7782} = 6$.

Example 3: Write 7 as a power of 10.

Solution: Looking up $\log_{10} 7$ in the table, we get $\log_{10} 7 = 0.8451$. Therefore, $7 = 10^{0.8451}$.

Q5 Convert each logarithmic equation to an exponential equation:

    a. $\log_{10} 1.5 = 0.1761$ **b.** $\log_{10} 4 = 0.6021$

\# \# \# • \# \# \# • \# \# \# • \# \# \# • \# \# \# • \# \# \# • \# \# \# • \# \# \# • \# \# \#

A5   **a.** $10^{0.1761} = 1.5$ **b.** $10^{0.6021} = 4$

Q6   Write each number as a power of 10:
    a. $5.3 =$ _____   **b.** $8.7 =$ _____

\# \# \# • \# \# \# • \# \# \# • \# \# \# • \# \# \# • \# \# \# • \# \# \# • \# \# \# • \# \# \#

A6   **a.** $10^{0.7243}$: Since $\log_{10} 5.3 = 0.7243$ **b.** $10^{0.9395}$

---

6   Although only logarithms of numbers between 1 and 9.99 are located in the table, properties of exponents can be used to extend the table.

The logarithm of 732 can be found by converting to scientific notation and using properties of exponents.

$$732 = 7.32 \times 10^2 \quad \text{(converting to scientific notation)}$$
$$= 10^{0.8645} \times 10^2 \quad \text{(looking up } \log_{10} 7.32\text{)}$$
$$= 10^{0.8645+2} \quad \text{(adding exponents)}$$
$$= 10^{2.8645}$$

Since 2.8645 is the exponent which must be used to the base 10 to equal 732 we say $\log_{10} 732 = 2.8645$.

The logarithms of numbers between 0 and 1 or larger than 10 will be found in a similar manner. The part of the logarithm that follows the decimal is always located in a table and is called the *mantissa*. The integer portion of the logarithm is called the *characteristic*. The characteristic is always the integer exponent of the power of 10 when the number is written in scientific notation.

Example 1: Find $\log_{10} 862$.

Solution: $862 = 8.62 \times 10^2$. Look up $\log_{10} 8.62 = 0.9355$ (mantissa). The characteristic is 2. Therefore, $\log_{10} 862 = 2.9355$.

Example 2: Find $\log_{10} 9{,}240{,}000$.

Solution: $9{,}240{,}000 = 9.24 \times 10^6$. The mantissa is $\log_{10} 9.24 = 0.9657$. The characteristic is 6. Therefore, $\log_{10} 9{,}240{,}000 = 6.9657$.

Q7   Find the logarithm of 2,300 by completing these steps:

    a. Write 2,300 in scientific notation. _____

    b. What is the mantissa? _____

    c. What is the characteristic? _____

    d. $\log_{10} 2300 =$ _____

\# \# \# • \# \# \# • \# \# \# • \# \# \# • \# \# \# • \# \# \# • \# \# \# • \# \# \# • \# \# \#

A7   **a.** 2.3×10^3 **b.** 0.3617   **c.** 3   **d.** 3.3617

Q8   Find the logarithm of 42.7 by completing these steps:

    a. Write 42.7 in scientific notation. _____

    b. What is the mantissa? _____

    c. What is the characteristic? _____

    d. $\log_{10} 42.7 =$ _____

\# \# \# • \# \# \# • \# \# \# • \# \# \# • \# \# \# • \# \# \# • \# \# \# • \# \# \# • \# \# \#

A8   **a.** 4.27×10^1 **b.** 0.6304   **c.** 1   **d.** 1.6304

Q9   Evaluate the following by using the logarithm table and the procedure from Frame 6:

    a. $\log_{10} 279 = $ _____

    b. $\log_{10} 1{,}760 = $ _____

    c. $\log_{10} 50{,}000 = $ _____

\# \# \#　•　\# \# \#　•　\# \# \#　•　\# \# \#　•　\# \# \#　•　\# \# \#　•　\# \# \#　•　\# \# \#　•　\# \# \#

A9   **a.** 2.4456　　　　　　**b.** 3.2455　　　　　　**c.** 4.6990

Q10   Find the following:

    a. $\log_{10} 8.00 = $ _____　　　　　**b.** $\log_{10} 147 = $ _____

    c. $\log_{10} 248.0 = $ _____　　　　**d.** $\log_{10} 9070 = $ _____

\# \# \#　•　\# \# \#　•　\# \# \#　•　\# \# \#　•　\# \# \#　•　\# \# \#　•　\# \# \#　•　\# \# \#　•　\# \# \#

A10   **a.** 0.9031　　　**b.** 2.1673　　　**c.** 2.3945　　　**d.** 3.9576

---

7   Recall from Frame 3 that the logarithms of numbers between 0 and 1 are negative. To find the numerical value of these logarithms the same procedure is employed. The procedure will be illustrated for $\log_{10} 0.0046$.

Step 1: Convert 0.0046 to scientific notation. $0.0046 = 4.6 \times 10^{-3}$.

Step 2: Find the mantissa which is $\log_{10} 4.6$. $\log_{10} 4.6 = 0.6628$.

Step 3: Determine the characteristic which in this case is $^{-}3$.

Step 4: Add the mantissa and characteristic. $0.6628 + {}^{-}3$ or $0.6628 - 3$.

    The mantissa and characteristic could be combined to obtain $^{-}2.3372$ which would be correct but is very seldom useful. Therefore, logarithms of numbers between 0 and 1 are represented as the positive mantissa plus the negative characteristic.

Q11   Determine the $\log_{10} 0.00024$ by completing these steps:

    a. Write 0.00024 in scientific notation. _____

    b. What is the mantissa? _____

    c. What is the characteristic? _____

    d. $\log_{10} 0.00024 = $ _____

\# \# \#　•　\# \# \#　•　\# \# \#　•　\# \# \#　•　\# \# \#　•　\# \# \#　•　\# \# \#　•　\# \# \#　•　\# \# \#

A11   **a.** 2.4×10^{-4}　　　**b.** 0.3802　　　**c.** $^{-}4$　　　**d.** $0.3802 - 4$

Q12   Determine the logarithms:

    a. $\log_{10} 0.0093 = $ _____

    b. $\log_{10} 0.0263 = $ _____

    c. $\log_{10} 0.431 = $ _____

\# \# \#　•　\# \# \#　•　\# \# \#　•　\# \# \#　•　\# \# \#　•　\# \# \#　•　\# \# \#　•　\# \# \#　•　\# \# \#

A12   **a.** $0.9685 - 3$　　　　　**b.** $0.4200 - 2$　　　　　**c.** $0.6345 - 1$

---

8   You must be able to determine the number if you know the logarithm of the number. If the characteristic of the logarithm is zero you know the number falls between 1 and 10. To obtain its numerical value find the mantissa in the body of the table and read the number whose logarithm equals that mantissa.

Example: If $\log_{10} N = 0.8768$, find N.

Solution: We look up 8768 in the body of the logarithm table. It is located opposite 7.5 and below 3. Therefore, $N = 7.53$.

The number 7.53 is called the *antilogarithm* of 0.8768.

Q13   Use Table XI in the Appendix to find antilogarithms:

    a. If $\log_{10} N = 0.8751$, $N =$ _____   **b.** If $\log_{10} N = 0.7818$, $N =$ _____

    c. If $\log_{10} N = 0.2253$, $N =$ _____   **d.** If $\log_{10} N = 0.6637$, $N =$ _____

• # # # • # # # • # # # • # # # • # # # • # # # • # # # • # #

A13   **a.** 7.50   **b.** 6.05   **c.** 1.68   **d.** 4.61

---

9   If the mantissa is not found exactly in the body of the table we will choose the closest number to it.

Example: If $\log_{10} N = 0.3642$, find N.

Solution: Since 0.3642 falls between the values of 0.3636 and 0.3655 but is closer to 0.3636 we say N is the antilogarithm of 0.3636. Therefore $N = 2.31$.

If the mantissa falls half way between two numbers, choose the larger number.

Q14   Find antilogarithms to determine N:

    a. $\log_{10} N = 0.1692$, $N =$ _____   **b.** $\log_{10} N = 0.4872$, $N =$ _____

    c. $\log_{10} N = 0.9241$, $N =$ _____   **d.** $\log_{10} N = 0.3988$, $N =$ _____

• # # # • # # # • # # # • # # # • # # # • # # # • # # # • # #

A14   **a.** 1.48   **b.** 3.07   **c.** 8.40
    d. 2.51:   We choose the larger number if it is half-way between two numbers.

---

10   For numbers whose logarithms have a nonzero characteristic, the antilogarithm is found by first finding the antilogarithm of the mantissa and then writing the number in scientific notation. The number is then converted to decimal form.

Example 1: If $\log_{10} N = 3.6821$, find N.

Solution: Find the antilogarithm of the mantissa 0.6821 which is 4.81. Locate the characteristic which is 3. Write the number N in scientific notation: $N = 4.81 \times 10^3$. Therefore, $N = 4,810$.

Example 2: If $N = 0.3075 - 4$, find N.

Solution: The mantissa is 0.3075 and the characteristic is $^-4$. The antilogarithm of 0.3075 is 2.03. The number N is therefore 2.03×10^{-4} or 0.000203.

Q15   Find the antilogarithm of 3.6503 by following these steps:

    a. What is the mantissa? _____

    b. What is the antilogarithm of the mantissa? _____

    c. What is the characteristic? _____

d. Write the antilogarithm in scientific notation. _____

e. Write the antilogarithm in decimal notation. _____

\# \# \# • \# \# \# • \# \# \# • \# \# \# • \# \# \# • \# \# \# • \# \# \# • \# \# \# • \# \# \#

A15 **a.** 0.6503 **b.** 4.47 **c.** 3 **d.** 4.47×10^3 **e.** 4,470

Q16 Find the antilogarithm of 1.8603, that is, find N if $\log_{10} N = 1.8603$.

\# \# \# • \# \# \# • \# \# \# • \# \# \# • \# \# \# • \# \# \# • \# \# \# • \# \# \# • \# \# \#

A16 72.5: The mantissa is 8603 whose antilog is 7.25. The characteristic is 1. Therefore, $N = 7.25 \times 10^1$.

Q17 Find the antilogarithms of the following:
a. 5.8414 **b.** 2.7427

\# \# \# • \# \# \# • \# \# \# • \# \# \# • \# \# \# • \# \# \# • \# \# \# • \# \# \# • \# \# \#

A17 **a.** 694,000 **b.** 553

Q18 Find the antilogarithm of $0.8669 - 4$ following these steps:

a. What is the mantissa? _____

b. Find the antilogarithm of the mantissa. _____

c. What is the characteristic? _____

d. Write the antilogarithm in scientific notation. _____

e. Write the antilogarithm in decimal notation. _____

\# \# \# • \# \# \# • \# \# \# • \# \# \# • \# \# \# • \# \# \# • \# \# \# • \# \# \# • \# \# \#

A18 **a.** 0.8669 **b.** 7.36 **c.** $^-4$ **d.** 7.36×10^{-4} **e.** 0.000736

Q19 Find the antilogarithm of $0.7796 - 3$.

\# \# \# • \# \# \# • \# \# \# • \# \# \# • \# \# \# • \# \# \# • \# \# \# • \# \# \# • \# \# \#

A19 0.00602: The mantissa is 0.7796 whose antilogarithm is 6.02. Therefore, the antilogarithm of $0.7796 - 3 = 6.02 \times 10^{-3}$.

Q20 Find the antilogarithms of the following:
a. $0.4762 - 5$ **b.** $0.1672 - 1$

\# \# \# • \# \# \# • \# \# \# • \# \# \# • \# \# \# • \# \# \# • \# \# \# • \# \# \# • \# \# \#

A20 **a.** 0.0000299 **b.** 0.147

11 Sometimes a logarithm such as $0.9786 - 2$ is written as $8.9786 - 10$. Notice that the mantissa of each is identical. The characteristic of $0.9786 - 2$ is $^-2$. If the integer parts of $8.9786 - 10$ are combined you obtain $8-10$ or $^-2$ also. Therefore, the logarithms are the same. Remember that the characteristic of a logarithm is the sum of the integer parts of the logarithm.

Example: Choose the logarithms which have the same characteristic as $0.0692-3$.
$7.0692-10$, $6.0692-10$, $4.0692-7$, $1.0692-4$

Solution: $7.0692-10$, $4.0692-7$, and $1.0692-4$, since the sum of the integer parts is $^-3$ in all cases.

Q21   Circle the logarithms whose characteristic is the same as the characteristic of $0.2346-2$.

$3.2346-4$, $5.2346-7$, $9.2346-10$, $8.2346-10$

\# \# \#   •   \# \# \#   •   \# \# \#   •   \# \# \#   •   \# \# \#   •   \# \# \#   •   \# \# \#   •   \# \# \#   •   \# \# \#

A21 $5.2346-7$ and $8.2346-10$

Q22   Write the characteristic of each of the following logarithms:

    a. $4.0923-5$ _____

    b. $0.7623-5$ _____

    c. $9.0658-10$ _____

    d. $21.7892-24$ _____

\# \# \#   •   \# \# \#   •   \# \# \#   •   \# \# \#   •   \# \# \#   •   \# \# \#   •   \# \# \#   •   \# \# \#   •   \# \# \#

A22   **a.** $^-1$ **b.** $^-5$ **c.** $^-1$ **d.** $^-3$

Q23   Find N if $\log_{10} N = 8.9053-10$

\# \# \#   •   \# \# \#   •   \# \# \#   •   \# \# \#   •   \# \# \#   •   \# \# \#   •   \# \# \#   •   \# \# \#   •   \# \# \#

A23 0.0804:   The mantissa is 0.9053 and the characteristic is $^-2$.

This completes the instruction for this section.

12.2   EXERCISE

1. Determine the logarithms by first writing the number as a power of 10:
    a. $\log_{10} 100,000$ **b.** $\log_{10} 100$ **c.** $\log_{10} 0.001$ **d.** $\log_{10} 0.01$

2. As N increases from 1 to 100, $\log_{10} N$ increases from _____ to _____.

3. Use the table of logarithms to find the following logarithms:
    a. $\log_{10} 4.25$ **b.** $\log_{10} 1.72$ **c.** $\log_{10} 1.09$
    d. $\log_{10} 7.37$ **e.** $\log_{10} 27.6$ **f.** $\log_{10} 42,100$
    g. $\log_{10} 1,490,000$ **h.** $\log_{10} 1,090$ **i.** $\log_{10} 0.042$
    j. $\log_{10} 0.0007$ **k.** $\log_{10} 0.571$ **l.** $\log_{10} 0.9$

4. Find the antilogarithms of the following numbers:
    a. 0.8149 **b.** 0.9435 **c.** 0.0086
    d. 0.7767 **e.** 2.1492 **f.** 3.5999
    g. 6.6505 **h.** 1.9867 **i.** $0.9154-2$
    j. $0.9427-4$ **k.** $6.8102-10$ **l.** $2.3784-4$

5. Name the characteristic of the following logarithms:
    a. $\log_{10} N = 4.6234$ **b.** $\log_{10} N = 8.0692-10$
    c. $\log_{10} N = 0.4321-7$ **d.** $\log_{10} N = 2.4624-5$

12.2   EXERCISE ANSWERS

1. a. 5   **b.** 2   **c.** ⁻3   **d.** ⁻2

2. 0 to 2

3. a. 0.6284   **b.** 0.2355   **c.** 0.0374   **d.** 0.8675

    e. 1.4409   **f.** 4.6243   **g.** 6.1732   **h.** 3.0374

    i. 0.6232−2   **j.** 0.8451−4   **k.** 0.7566−1   **l.** 0.9542−1

4. a. 6.53   **b.** 8.78   **c.** 1.02   **d.** 5.98

    e. 141   **f.** 3980   **g.** 4,470,000   **h.** 97.0

    i. 0.0823   **j.** 0.000876   **k.** 0.000646   **l.** 0.0239

5. a. 4   **b.** ⁻2   **c.** ⁻7   **d.** ⁻3

12.3   CALCULATIONS WITH LOGARITHMS

1   Logarithms can be used to simplify the calculation of products and quotients, finding powers, and the taking of roots. They are of no use for calculation of addition and subtraction problems.

Q1   **a.** Name four operations which can be performed by the use of logarithms.

_____

b. Name two operations that cannot be performed with logarithms.

_____

\# # # • # # # • # # # • # # # • # # # • # # # • # # # • # # # • # # #

A1   **a.** multiplication, division, finding powers, taking roots

    b. addition, subtraction

2   We will first consider multiplication. The procedure will be illustrated for the product of 8.62×17.9.

Step 1: Find $\log_{10} 8.62$ and $\log_{10} 17.9$. These are 0.9355 and 1.2529.

Step 2: Add the logarithms. $0.9355 + 1.2529 = 2.1884$.

Step 3: Find the antilogarithm of the sum. The antilogarithm of 2.1884 is 154. Therefore, $8.62 \times 17.9 = 154$.

The accuracy of the product will be correct to three figures. In this case if 8.62 and 17.9 are multiplied without using logarithms the product is 154.298.

Q2   Use the steps below to find the product of 253×10.3:

a. Find $\log_{10} 253$ and $\log_{10} 10.3$. _____

b. Add the logarithms. _____

c. Find the antilogarithm of the sum. _____

\# # # • # # # • # # # • # # # • # # # • # # # • # # # • # # # • # # #

A2   **a.** 2.4031 and 1.0128   **b.** 3.4159   **c.** 2,610

Q3   Find the product of 1,290 and 24.7 using logarithms.

$$\# \# \# \quad \bullet \quad \# \# \# \quad \bullet \quad \# \# \# \quad \bullet \quad \# \# \# \quad \bullet \quad \# \# \# \quad \bullet \quad \# \# \# \quad \bullet \quad \# \# \# \quad \bullet \quad \# \# \# \quad \bullet \quad \# \# \#$$

A3   31,900: $\log_{10} 1290 + \log_{10} 24.7 = 3.1106 + 1.3927 = 4.5033$

---

3   The reason that this method gives the correct product is based on the properties of exponents. The explanation will be shown for the product 8.62×17.9 of Frame 2.

$$8.62 \times 17.9 = 10^{0.9355} \times 10^{1.2529} \quad \text{(finding logarithms)}$$
$$= 10^{0.9355+1.2529} \quad \text{(adding exponents)}$$
$$= 10^{2.1884}$$
$$= 154 \quad \text{(finding the antilogarithm)}$$

This illustration shows that the procedure of Frame 2 is justified because of the fact that a logarithm is actually an exponent.

The procedure can be extended to find the product of any number of numbers.

Example: Find the product of $126 \times 127 \times 128 \times 129$.

Solution:

Step 1: Find the logarithms. $2.1004 + 2.1038 + 2.1072 + 2.1106$.

Step 2: Add. The sum is 8.4220.

Step 3: Find the antilogarithm. The antilogarithm of 8.4220 is 264,000,000. Thus, $126 \times 127 \times 128 \times 129 = 264,000,000$.

Q4   Find the product of $4.68 \times 24.7 \times 10,900$ using logarithms.

$$\# \# \# \quad \bullet \quad \# \# \# \quad \bullet \quad \# \# \# \quad \bullet \quad \# \# \# \quad \bullet \quad \# \# \# \quad \bullet \quad \# \# \# \quad \bullet \quad \# \# \# \quad \bullet \quad \# \# \# \quad \bullet \quad \# \# \#$$

A4   1,260,000:   The logarithms are 0.6702, 1.3927, and 4.0374. Their sum is 6.1003.

---

4   To find the product of numbers where one or more are less than 1, use the same procedure but keep the negative characteristics separate and combine with the positive characteristics for the final sum.

Example: Find the product $0.07 \times 126 \times 0.00243$.

Solution: $\log_{10} 0.07 + \log_{10} 126 + \log_{10} 0.00243$
$$= 0.8451 - 2 + 2.1004 + 0.3856 - 3$$
$$= 3.3311 - 5$$
$$= 0.3311 - 2 \text{ since } 3 - 5 = {}^{-}2$$

The antilogarithm of $0.3311 - 2$ is 0.0214. Thus, $0.07 \times 126 \times 0.00243 = 0.0214$.

Q5   Find the product $0.029 \times 0.00872 \times 46.2$ using logarithms.

$$\# \# \# \quad \bullet \quad \# \# \# \quad \bullet \quad \# \# \# \quad \bullet \quad \# \# \# \quad \bullet \quad \# \# \# \quad \bullet \quad \# \# \# \quad \bullet \quad \# \# \# \quad \bullet \quad \# \# \# \quad \bullet \quad \# \# \#$$

A5   0.0117: $\log 0.029 + \log 0.00872 + \log 46.2$
      $= 0.4624 - 2 + 0.9405 - 3 + 1.6646$
      $= 3.0675 - 5$
      $= 0.0675 - 2$
The antilogarithm of $0.0675 - 2$ is 0.0117.

---

5   Quotients can be found by using logarithms following the procedure below.

Example: Find the quotient of $2,490 \div 17.5$.

Solution:

Step 1: Find $\log_{10} 2,490$ and $\log_{10} 17.5$. These are 3.3962 and 1.2430.

Step 2: Subtract $3.3962 - 1.2430$. The difference is 2.1532.

Step 3: Find the antilogarithm of the difference. The antilogarithm of 2.1532 is 142. Thus, $2,490 \div 17.5 = 142$.

Q6   Find the quotient $24.6 \div 1.83$ by completing these steps:

   a. $\log_{10} 24.6 - \log_{10} 1.83 = $ _____ $-$ _____ .

   b. The difference is _____ .

   c. The antilogarithm is _____ .

   d. Thus, $24.6 \div 1.83 = $ _____ .

•   # # #   •   # # #   •   # # #   •   # # #   •   # # #   •   # # #   •   # # #   •   # #

A6   **a.** $1.3909 - 0.2625$ **b.** 1.1284 **c.** 13.4 **d.** 13.4

Q7   Find the quotient $48,700 \div 2,680$ using logarithms.

•   # # #   •   # # #   •   # # #   •   # # #   •   # # #   •   # # #   •   # # #   •   # #

A7   18.2: $\log 48,700 - \log 2,680 = 4.6875 - 3.4281 = 1.2594$. The antilogarithm of 1.2594 is 18.2.

---

6   You must be careful when dividing numbers less than 1 or when the quotient is less than 1. These problems are the source of many errors. Follow the example below.

Example: Find $24.6 \div 0.028$.

Solution: $\log_{10} 24.6 - \log_{10} 0.028$
      $= 1.3909 - (0.4472 - 2)$
      $= 1.3909 - 0.4472 + 2$ (notice the change of signs)
      $= 2.9437$

The antilogarithm of 2.9437 is 878. Thus, $24.6 \div 0.028 = 878$.

Q8   Find $4.78 \div 0.43$ using logarithms.

•   # # #   •   # # #   •   # # #   •   # # #   •   # # #   •   # # #   •   # # #   •   # #

A8   11.1: $\log_{10} 4.78 - \log_{10} 0.43$
$= 0.6794 - (0.6335 - 1)$
$= 0.6794 - 0.6335 + 1$
$= 0.0459 + 1$
$= 1.0459$

The antilogarithm of 1.0459 is 11.1.

Q9   Find $0.792 \div 0.0024$ using logarithms.

\# \# \#   •   \# \# \#   •   \# \# \#   •   \# \# \#   •   \# \# \#   •   \# \# \#   •   \# \# \#   •   \# \# \#   •   \# \# \#

A9   330: $\log_{10} 0.792 - \log_{10} 0.0024$
$= 0.8987 - 1 - (0.3802 - 3)$
$= 0.8987 - 1 - 0.3802 + 3$
$= 0.5185 + 2$
$= 2.5185$

The logarithm of 2.5185 is 330.

7   The mantissas that are in the logarithm table are all positive values. Care should therefore be taken to keep the decimal values positive throughout your calculations. If the divisor is larger than the dividend this presents a problem. A method of solving this problem is presented in the next example.

Example: Find $0.017 \div 47$.

Solution: $\log_{10} 0.017 - \log_{10} 47 = (0.2304 - 2) - (1.6721)$

At this point in the solution there is a problem. If 0.2304 and -1.6721 were combined, a negative mantissa would result. This would do us no good since we could not look it up in the table. We therefore rewrite $0.2304 - 2$ in such a way that 1.6721 can be subtracted from it and a positive mantissa will result. If we "add and subtract 2" to $0.2304 - 2$, the result has the same value.

$$0.2304 - 2$$
$$\underline{2 \quad\quad -2}$$
$$2.2304 - 4$$

At the same time, 2.2304 is greater than 1.6721. We can now proceed as follows:

$$0.2304 - 2 - (1.6721) = 2.2304 - 4 - (1.6721) = 0.5583 - 4$$

The antilogarithm of $0.5583 - 4$ is 0.000362. Thus, $0.017 \div 47 = 0.000362$.

Q10   Find $47.9 \div 247$ using logarithms.

\# \# \#   •   \# \# \#   •   \# \# \#   •   \# \# \#   •   \# \# \#   •   \# \# \#   •   \# \# \#   •   \# \# \#   •   \# \# \#

A10   0.194: $\log_{10} 47.9 - \log_{10} 247$
$$= 1.6803 - 2.3927$$
$$= 2.6803 - 1 - 2.3927 \quad \text{(adding and subtracting 1 to 1.6803)}$$
$$= 0.2876 - 1$$

The antilogarithm of $0.2876 - 1$ is 0.194.

Q11   Find the quotient of 0.0462 and 48.2.

\# \# \# • \# \# \# • \# \# \# • \# \# \# • \# \# \# • \# \# \# • \# \# \# • \# \# \# • \# \# \#

A11   0.000959: $\log_{10} 0.0462 - \log_{10} 48.2$
$$= 0.6646 - 2 - 1.6830$$
$$= 2.6646 - 4 - 1.6830 \quad \text{(adding and subtracting 2 to } 0.6646 - 2)$$
$$= 0.9816 - 4$$

---

8   Problems involving both multiplication and division can be completed with logarithms.

Example: Find $48.6 \div 27.3 \times 242$.

Solution: $\log_{10} 48.6 - \log_{10} 27.3 + \log_{10} 242$
$$= 1.6866 - 1.4362 + 2.3838$$
$$= 2.6342$$

The antilogarithm of 2.6342 is 431. Thus, $48.6 \div 27.3 \times 242 = 431$.

Q12   Use logarithms to find $24{,}600 \div 27.8 \times 62.7$.

\# \# \# • \# \# \# • \# \# \# • \# \# \# • \# \# \# • \# \# \# • \# \# \# • \# \# \# • \# \# \#

A12   55,500: $\log_{10} 24{,}600 - \log_{10} 27.8 + \log_{10} 62.7$
$$= 4.3909 - 1.4440 + 1.7973$$
$$= 4.7442$$

The antilogarithm of 4.7442 is 55,500.

Q13   Use logarithms to find $0.48 \times 98.3 \times 26.5 \div 0.028$.

\# \# \# • \# \# \# • \# \# \# • \# \# \# • \# \# \# • \# \# \# • \# \# \# • \# \# \# • \# \# \#

A13   44,700: $\log_{10} 0.48 + \log_{10} 98.3 + \log_{10} 26.5 - \log_{10} 0.028$
$$= 0.6812 - 1 + 1.9926 + 1.4232 - (0.4472 - 2)$$
$$= 0.6812 - 1 + 1.9926 + 1.4232 - 0.4472 + 2$$
$$= 3.6498 + 1$$
$$= 4.6498 \quad \text{(comment at top of next page)}$$

The antilogarithm of 4.6498 is exactly half-way between 44,600 and 44,700. It is rounded up to 44,700.

---

9 Logarithms can be used to raise a number to a power by multiplying the exponent times the logarithm of the base and then finding the antilogarithm. The method is illustrated below.

Example: Find $(2.73)^7$ using logarithms.

Solution: $7\,(\log_{10} 2.73) = 7(0.4362)$
$$= 3.0534$$

The antilogarithm of 3.0534 is 1,130. Thus, $(2.73)^7 = 1,130$.

Q14 Find $(8.63)^5$ by using logarithms.

• # # # • # # # • # # # • # # # • # # # • # # # • # # # • # #

A14 47,900: $5\,(\log_{10} 8.63) = 5(0.9360)$
$$= 4.6800$$

The antilogarithm of 4.6800 is 47,900.

---

10 The method for raising to powers with logarithms can again be justified by referring to properties of exponents. Consider $(2.73)^7$ as an example.

$(2.73)^7 = (10^{0.4362})^7$ (looking up $\log_{10} 2.73$)
$= 10^{0.4362 \times 7}$ (multiplying exponents)
$= 10^{3.0534}$
$= 1,130$ (finding the antilogarithm of 3.0534)

Consider an example with a number less than 1 as the base.

Example: Find $(0.896)^6$.

Solution: $6(\log_{10} 0.896) = 6(0.9523 - 1)$
$$= 5.7138 - 6$$
$$= 0.7138 - 1$$

The antilogarithm of $0.7138 - 1$ is 0.517.

Q15 Find $(0.525)^4$ using logarithms.

• # # # • # # # • # # # • # # # • # # # • # # # • # # # • # #

A15 0.0760: $4(\log_{10} 0.525) = 4(0.7202 - 1)$
$$= 2.8808 - 4$$
$$= 0.8808 - 2$$

The antilogarithm of $0.8808 - 2$ is 0.0760.

---

11 Roots are calculated using logarithms by converting them to equivalent problems stated with fractional exponents.

Example 1: Calculate $\sqrt{296}$.

Solution: $\sqrt{296} = (296)^{1/2}$

Therefore, use the procedure for finding powers.

$$\frac{1}{2}\log_{10} 296 = \frac{1}{2}(2.4713)$$

$$= 1.23565$$

The antilogarithm of 1.23565 is 17.2. Thus, $\sqrt{296} = 17.2$.

Example 2: Calculate $\sqrt[3]{0.026}$.

Solution: $\sqrt[3]{0.026} = (0.026)^{1/3}$

$$\frac{1}{3}\log_{10}(0.026) = \frac{1}{3}(0.4150 - 2)$$

At this point we must divide both the mantissa and characteristic by 3. However, we want to keep the characteristic an integer so we change $0.4150 - 2$ to $1.4150 - 3$ by adding and subtracting 1, so the negative number is evenly divisible by 3. Then $\frac{1}{3}(0.4150 - 2) = \frac{1}{3}(1.4150 - 3) = 0.4717 - 1$. The antilogarithm of $0.4717 - 1$ is 0.296. Therefore, $\sqrt[3]{0.026} = 0.296$.

Q16   Use logarithms to find $\sqrt{42.6}$.

\# \# \# · • \# \# \# • \# \# \# • \# \# \# • \# \# \# • \# \# \# • \# \# \# • \# \# \# • \# \# \#

A16   6.53: $\sqrt{42.6} = (42.6)^{1/2}$

$$\frac{1}{2}\log_{10} 42.6 = \frac{1}{2}(1.6294)$$

$$= 0.8147$$

The antilogarithm of 0.8147 is 6.53.

Q17   Find $\sqrt{0.078}$ using logarithms.

\# \# \# • \# \# \# • \# \# \# • \# \# \# • \# \# \# • \# \# \# • \# \# \# • \# \# \# • \# \# \#

A17   0.279: $\frac{1}{2}\log_{10} 0.078 = \frac{1}{2}(0.8921 - 2)$

$$= 0.4461 - 1 \quad \text{(rounded off to ten-thousandths)}$$

The antilogarithm of $0.4461 - 1$ is 0.279.

Q18   Find $\sqrt[3]{0.0013}$.

\# \# \# • \# \# \# • \# \# \# • \# \# \# • \# \# \# • \# \# \# • \# \# \# • \# \# \# • \# \# \#

A18   0.109: $\frac{1}{3}\log_{10} 0.0013 = \frac{1}{3}(0.1139 - 3)$

$$= 0.0380 - 1$$

The antilogarithm of $0.0380 - 1$ is 0.109.

Q19   Sometimes you must adjust the characteristic to make the negative term divisible by some number. How would you rewrite $0.1247-2$ as an equivalent number whose negative term is divisible by 3?

\# \# \#   •   \# \# \#   •   \# \# \#   •   \# \# \#   •   \# \# \#   •   \# \# \#   •   \# \# \#   •   \# \# \#   •   \# \# \#

A19 $1.1247-3$:   Add and subtract 1.

Q20   Find $\sqrt[3]{0.476}$ using logarithms.

\# \# \#   •   \# \# \#   •   \# \# \#   •   \# \# \#   •   \# \# \#   •   \# \# \#   •   \# \# \#   •   \# \# \#   •   \# \# \#

A20 0.781: $\frac{1}{3}\log_{10}0.476=\frac{1}{3}(0.6776-1)$

$$=\frac{1}{3}(2.6776-3)\quad\text{(adding and subtracting 2)}$$

$$=0.8925-1$$

The antilogarithm of $0.8925-1$ is 0.781.

Q21   Find $(\sqrt[5]{2.71})(\sqrt[3]{42.7})$.

\# \# \#   •   \# \# \#   •   \# \# \#   •   \# \# \#   •   \# \# \#   •   \# \# \#   •   \# \# \#   •   \# \# \#   •   \# \# \#

A21 4.27: $\frac{1}{5}\log_{10}2.71+\frac{1}{3}\log_{10}42.7$

$$=\frac{1}{5}(0.4330)+\frac{1}{3}(1.6304)$$

$$=0.0866+0.5435$$

$$=0.6301$$

The antilogarithm of 0.6301 is 4.27.

*Q22   Find $\dfrac{(2.78)^7\times(\sqrt{46.8})}{47.8}$.

\# \# \#   •   \# \# \#   •   \# \# \#   •   \# \# \#   •   \# \# \#   •   \# \# \#   •   \# \# \#   •   \# \# \#   •   \# \# \#

*A22 184: $7\log_{10}2.78+\frac{1}{2}\log_{10}46.8-\log_{10}47.8$

$$=7(0.4440)+\frac{1}{2}(1.6702)-1.6794$$

$$=3.1080+0.8351-1.6794$$

$$=2.2637$$

The antilogarithm of 2.2637 is 184.

This completes the instruction for this section.

12.3 EXERCISE

Perform the following calculations by using logarithms:
1. **a.** 2.78×4.86 **b.** $9,280 \times 42$ **c.** 0.078×92.4 **d.** 0.0036×0.0792
2. **a.** $462 \div 2.48$ **b.** $2.71 \div 0.082$ **c.** $0.029 \div 0.012$ **d.** $420 \div 9,720$
3. **a.** $(4.96)^5$ **b.** $(206)^4$ **c.** $(0.037)^4$ **d.** $(0.988)^{10}$
4. **a.** $\sqrt{24.6}$ **b.** $\sqrt{1.92}$ **c.** $\sqrt[5]{0.00211}$ **d.** $\sqrt[3]{0.191}$
5. **a.** $\dfrac{246 \times 5.32}{261}$ **b.** $\dfrac{423\sqrt{2.36}}{2}$ **c.** $\dfrac{432 \times 521 \times 0.0031}{42.7 \times 21.6}$

12.3 EXERCISE ANSWERS

1. **a.** 13.5 **b.** 390,000 **c.** 7.21 **d.** 0.000285
2. **a.** 186 **b.** 33.1 **c.** 2.42 **d.** 0.0432
3. **a.** 3000 **b.** 1,800,000,000 **c.** 0.00000187 **d.** 0.887
4. **a.** 4.96 **b.** 1.39 **c.** 0.128 **d.** 0.576
5. **a.** 5.01 **b.** 325 **c.** 0.757

12.4 APPLICATIONS

1 Many of the applications of logarithms and exponents in medicine result from the necessity to deal with the molecular structure of substances. You will, in the following problems, occasionally see some unfamiliar words. Do not worry if you do not understand them. Your knowledge of mathematics should be sufficient for you to solve the problems.

Q1 Some properties of the helium atom are: mass = 0.00000000000000000000000665 g; radius = 0.0000000093 cm. Express these quantities in scientific notation.

mass = _____   radius = _____

• # # # • # # # • # # # • # # # • # # # • # # # • # # # • # #

A1 mass $= 6.65 \times 10^{-24}$ g   radius $= 9.3 \times 10^{-9}$ cm

2 When carbon burns it combines with oxygen to form carbon dioxide. In the process heat is produced. When one gram of carbon burns, 7.86×10^3 calories of heat are produced.

Example: Find the amount of heat produced when 14.7 g of carbon are burned. Use logarithms to calculate.

Solution: Since 7.86×10^3 calories are produced when 1 g is burned, 14.7 g will produce $(14.7) \times (7.86 \times 10^3)$ calories. To calculate this product, proceed as follows:

$\log_{10} 14.7 + \log_{10} (7.86 \times 10^3)$
$= 1.1673 + 3.8954$
$= 5.0627$

The antilogarithm of 5.0627 is 1.16×10^5. Therefore, $(14.7) \times (7.86 \times 10^3) = 1.16 \times 10^5$. Hence, there are 1.16×10^5 calories.

Q2   If there are 7.86×10^3 calories produced when 1 g of carbon is burned, use logarithms to find the number of calories formed when:
a. 93.7 g are burned.

b. 0.082 g are burned.

\# \# \# • \# \# \# • \# \# \# • \# \# \# • \# \# \# • \# \# \# • \# \# \# • \# \# \# • \# \# \#

A2   **a.** 7.36×10^5 calories: $\log_{10} 93.7 + \log_{10}(7.86 \times 10^3) = 1.9717 + 3.8954 = 5.8671$
b. 6.44×10^2 calories: $\log_{10} 0.082 + \log_{10}(7.86 \times 10^3) = 0.9138 - 2 + 3.8954 = 2.8092$

---

3   The half-life, $t_{1/2}$, of a substance is the time required for one half of the substance to decay radioactively.

Example: Calculate using logarithms the half-life of radium in days if

$$t_{1/2} = \frac{(0.693)(365)}{4.33 \times 10^{-4}}$$

Solution: The solution is obtained by using the fact that if two numbers are equal their logarithms are equal.

$$\log_{10} t_{1/2} = \log_{10} \left[\frac{(0.693)(365)}{4.33 \times 10^{-4}} \right]$$
$$\log_{10} t_{1/2} = \log_{10} 0.693 + \log_{10} 365 - \log_{10}(4.33 \times 10^{-4})$$
$$\log_{10} t_{1/2} = (0.8407 - 1) + 2.5623 - (0.6365 - 4)$$
$$\log_{10} t_{1/2} = 0.8407 - 1 + 2.5623 - 0.6365 + 4$$
$$\log_{10} t_{1/2} = 3 + 0.8407 + 2.5623 - 0.6365$$
$$\log_{10} t_{1/2} = 3.8407 + 2.5623 - 0.6365$$
$$\log_{10} t_{1/2} = 5.7665$$
$$t_{1/2} = 584,000$$

(Recall that $t_{1/2}$ is the antilogarithm of 5.7665). Therefore, the half-life of radium is 584,000 days.

Q3   Calculate the half-life of radium in years using logarithms if $t_{1/2} = \dfrac{0.693}{4.33 \times 10^{-4}}$.

\# \# \# • \# \# \# • \# \# \# • \# \# \# • \# \# \# • \# \# \# • \# \# \# • \# \# \# • \# \# \#

A3   1,600 yr: $\log_{10} t_{1/2} = \log_{10} 0.693 - \log_{10}(4.33 \times 10^{-4})$
$\log_{10} t_{1/2} = (0.8407 - 1) - (0.6365 - 4)$
$\log_{10} t_{1/2} = 0.8407 - 1 - 0.6365 + 4$
$\log_{10} t_{1/2} = 3.2042$
$t_{1/2} = 1,600$ (antilogarithm of 3.2042)

Q4 Calculate the half-life of radium in hours if $t_{1/2} = \dfrac{(0.693)(8760)}{4.33 \times 10^{-4}}$.

• # # # • # # # • # # # • # # # • # # # • # # # • # # # • # #

A4 1.40×10^7 hr: $\log_{10} t_{1/2} = \log_{10} 0.693 + \log_{10} 8760 - \log_{10}(4.33 \times 10^{-4})$

$\log_{10} t_{1/2} = 0.8407 - 1 + 3.9425 - (0.6365 - 4)$

$\log_{10} t_{1/2} = 0.8407 - 1 + 3.9425 - 0.6365 + 4$

$\log_{10} t_{1/2} = 7.1467$

$t_{1/2} = 1.40 \times 10^7$ (antilogarithm of 7.1467)

---

4   The solubility of the compound PbF_2 is given by

$$s = \sqrt[3]{\frac{4.0 \times 10^{-8}}{4}}$$

Example: Calculate s using logarithms.

Solution: $\log_{10} s = \log_{10} \sqrt[3]{\dfrac{4.0 \times 10^{-8}}{4}}$

$\log_{10} s = \log_{10}(1.0 \times 10^{-8})^{1/3}$

$\log_{10} s = \dfrac{1}{3} \log_{10}(1.0 \times 10^{-8})$

$\log_{10} s = \dfrac{1}{3}(0.0000 - 8)$

$\log_{10} s = \dfrac{1}{3}(1.0000 - 9)$ (1 is added and subtracted so 3 will divide 9.)

$\log_{10} s = (0.3333 - 3)$

$s = 2.15 \times 10^{-3}$

$s = 0.00215$ (antilogarithm of 0.3333 - 3).

Q5   Find the solubility of $Fe(OH)_3$ by using logarithms if $s = \sqrt[4]{0.185 \times 10^{-38}}$.

• # # # • # # # • # # # • # # # • # # # • # # # • # # # • # #

A5   0.000000000207: $\log_{10} s = \log_{10}(0.185 \times 10^{-38})^{1/4}$

$\log_{10} s = \log_{10}(1.85 \times 10^{-39})^{1/4}$

$\log_{10} s = \dfrac{1}{4} \log_{10}(1.85 \times 10^{-39})$

$\log_{10} s = \dfrac{1}{4}(0.2672 - 39)$

$\log_{10} s = \dfrac{1}{4}(1.2672 - 40)$

$\log_{10} s = 0.3168 - 10$

$s = 2.07 \times 10^{-10}$

5 The concept of pH is used to measure the acidity or alkalinity of a solution. The term pH is defined as the opposite of the logarithm of the concentration of hydrogen ions, H^+. Concentration of H^+ is measured in moles per litre and symbolized by capital M or moles/litre.

pH = $^-\log_{10}$ [concentration of H^+]

We will use cH^+ to represent the concentration of H^+. Therefore

pH = $^-\log_{10}$ [cH^+]

The concentration of H^+ of water is $1 \times 10^{-7} M$ so the pH of water is

pH = $^-\log_{10} (1 \times 10^{-7})$
    = $^-(^-7)$
    = 7

A pH of 7 is said to be neutral. A pH larger than 7 is *alkaline*, while a pH below 7 is *acid*.

Example 1: Find the pH of a solution with a concentration of H^+ of $5.5 \times 10^{-8} M$.

Solution: pH = $^-\log_{10}[cH^+]$
pH = $^-\log_{10} (5.5 \times 10^{-8})$
pH = $^-(0.7404 - 8)$
pH = $^-0.7404 + 8$
pH = $^-0.7404 + 8.0000$
pH = 7.2596

Example 2: Is the solution of Example 1 acid or alkaline?

Solution: Alkaline since its pH is above 7.

Q6 **a.** Calculate the pH for a solution with a concentration of $2.61 \times 10^{-5} M$ of H^+.

b. Is the solution acid or alkaline? _____

\# \# \# • \# \# \# • \# \# \# • \# \# \# • \# \# \# • \# \# \# • \# \# \# • \# \# \# • \# \# \#

A6 **a.** 4.5834: pH = $^-\log (2.61 \times 10^{-5})$ **b.** acid
pH = $^-(0.4166 - 5)$
pH = $^-0.4166 + 5$
pH = $^-0.4166 + 5.0000$
pH = 4.5834

Q7 **a.** Calculate the pH for a solution with a concentration of $5.16 \times 10^{-12} M$ of H^+.

b. Is the solution acid or alkaline? _____

\# \# \# • \# \# \# • \# \# \# • \# \# \# • \# \# \# • \# \# \# • \# \# \# • \# \# \# • \# \# \#

A7 **a.** 11.2874: pH = $^-\log_{10} (5.16 \times 10^{-12})$ **b.** alkaline
pH = $^-(0.7127 - 12)$
pH = $^-0.7127 + 12$
pH = 11.2874

6   The same equation used for calculating pH can be used to calculate the concentration of H^+ if the pH is known.

Example: Suppose the pH of an acid solution is 5.4. Find the concentration of H^+.

Solution: $pH = ^-\log_{10}[cH^+]$
$^-pH = \log_{10}[cH^+]$ (multiplying both sides by $^-1$)
$^-5.4 = \log_{10}[cH^+]$

At this point the antilogarithm must be found. However, the mantissa (the decimal part) of the logarithm must be written as a positive number before the antilogarithm can be found in the table. We therefore add and subtract the number 6 to $^-5.4$ causing the decimal to be positive.

$^-5.4 + 6 - 6 = \log_{10}[cH^+]$
$0.6000 - 6 = \log_{10}[cH^+]$
$3.98 \times 10^{-6} = cH^+$

Therefore, concentration of H^+ is 0.00000398 *M*. Recall that *M* stands for moles/litre.

Q8   Find the concentration of H^+ if the pH is 3.7.

\# \# \# • \# \# \# • \# \# \# • \# \# \# • \# \# \# • \# \# \# • \# \# \# • \# \# \# • \# \# \#

A8   0.0002 *M*: $pH = ^-\log_{10}[cH^+]$
$^-pH = \log_{10}[cH^+]$
$^-3.7 = \log_{10}[cH^+]$
$^-3.7 + 4 - 4 = \log_{10}[cH^+]$
$0.3000 - 4 = \log_{10}[cH^+]$
$2.00 \times 10^{-4} = cH^+$

Q9   Find the concentration of H^+ if the pH is 3.

\# \# \# • \# \# \# • \# \# \# • \# \# \# • \# \# \# • \# \# \# • \# \# \# • \# \# \# • \# \# \#

A9   0.001 *M*: $pH = ^-\log_{10}[cH^+]$
$^-pH = \log_{10}[cH^+]$
$^-3 = \log_{10}[cH^+]$
$1 \times 10^{-3} = cH^+$ (Notice that the mantissa is 0 and the characteristic is $^-3$.)

Q10   Find the concentration of H^+ if the pH is 6.71.

\# \# \# • \# \# \# • \# \# \# • \# \# \# • \# \# \# • \# \# \# • \# \# \# • \# \# \# • \# \# \#

A10   0.000000195 M:

$$pH = {}^{-}\log_{10}[cH^{+}]$$
$$^{-}pH = \log_{10}[cH^{+}]$$
$$^{-}6.71 = \log_{10}[cH^{+}]$$
$$^{-}6.71 + 7 - 7 = \log_{10}[cH^{+}]$$
$$0.2900 - 7 = \log_{10}[cH^{+}]$$
$$1.95 \times 10^{-7} = cH^{+}$$

---

7   Equations involving logarithms occur frequently in the health sciences. An example is a formula called the 1st order rate law which shows the relationship of the original concentration of reactant, x_o, the time, t, since the experiment started, and the concentration, x, at time t.

$$t = \frac{2.303}{k}\log_{10}\left(\frac{[x_o]}{[x]}\right)$$

Example: Find the time to the nearest minute required for the concentration of reactant to drop from 1.5 mole/litre to 0.1 mole/litre when $k = 2.0 \times 10^{-3}$ per minute.

Solution: $x_o = 1.5$ $x = 0.1$ $k = 2.0 \times 10^{-3}$

$$t = \frac{2.303}{2.0 \times 10^{-3}}\log_{10}\left(\frac{1.5}{0.1}\right)$$

$$t = \frac{2.303}{0.002}\log_{10}(15)$$

$$t = 1151.5\log_{10}15$$
$$t = 1151.5 \times 1.1761$$
$$t = 1{,}354 \quad \text{(rounded off to whole minutes)}$$

Therefore, the time is 1,354 minutes.

Q11   Find the time required for the concentration of reactant to drop from 1.2 mole/litre to 0.2 mole/litre when $k = 2.0 \times 10^{-3}$ per min. Round off to a whole number of minutes.

$$t = \frac{2.303}{k}\log_{10}\left(\frac{[x_o]}{[x]}\right)$$

•   # # #   •   # # #   •   # # #   •   # # #   •   # # #   •   # # #   •   # # #   •   # #

A11   896 min: $t = \dfrac{2.303}{2.0 \times 10^{-3}}\log_{10}\left(\dfrac{1.2}{0.2}\right)$

$$= \frac{2.303}{0.002}\log_{10}6$$

$$= 1151.5 \times 0.7782$$

$$= 896$$

Q12 Find the time required for the concentration of reactant to be cut in half if it begins at 3.4 mole/litre when $k = 2.0 \times 10^{-3}$ per min. Round off to a whole number of minutes. $t = \dfrac{2.303}{k} \log_{10}\left(\dfrac{[x_o]}{[x]}\right)$

\# \# \# • \# \# \# • \# \# \# • \# \# \# • \# \# \# • \# \# \# • \# \# \# • \# \# \# • \# \# \#

A12 347 min: $t = \dfrac{2.303}{2.0 \times 10^{-3}} \log_{10}\left(\dfrac{3.4}{1.7}\right)$

$t = \dfrac{2.303}{0.002} \log_{10} 2$

$t = 1151.5 \times 0.3010$

$t = 347$

---

8 One of the most important formulas for people working with respiratory therapy is the Henderson–Hasselbach equation (H–H equation). The formula will give the pH of arterial blood if the blood bicarbonate and the dissolved carbon dioxide (CO_2) are given. These are measured in milliequivalents/litre (mEq/l). The H–H equation is

$$pH = 6.1 + \log_{10}\left(\frac{[\text{bicarbonate}]}{[\text{dissolved } CO_2]}\right)$$

The normal range of arterial blood pH is slightly alkaline, being between 7.35 and 7.45. If the pH varies outside the range of 7.00 to 7.80, survival is unlikely. The condition of having blood pH below the normal range is called *acidemia*. If the pH is above the normal range the patient is said to have *alkalemia*.

Example: Find the pH of arterial blood whose bicarbonate level is 24 mEq/l and the dissolved carbon dioxide is 1.2 mEq/l.

Solution: $pH = 6.1 + \log_{10}\left(\dfrac{[\text{bicarbonate}]}{[\text{dissolved } CO_2]}\right)$

$pH = 6.1 + \log_{10}\left(\dfrac{24}{1.2}\right)$

$pH = 6.1 + \log_{10} 20$

$pH = 6.1 + 1.3010$

$pH = 7.4010$

Therefore, the pH is 7.4010.

Q13 **a.** Find the blood pH if the bicarbonate is 27 mEq/l and the dissolved carbon dioxide is 1.5 mEq/l.

b. Does this pH fall within the normal range of arterial blood pH? _____

\# \# \#　•　\# \# \#　•　\# \# \#　•　\# \# \#　•　\# \# \#　•　\# \# \#　•　\# \# \#　•　\# \# \#　•　\# \# \#

A13　**a.** 7.3553:　$pH = 6.1 + \log_{10}\left(\dfrac{27}{1.5}\right)$　**b.** yes

$pH = 6.1 + \log_{10}(18)$
$pH = 6.1 + 1.2553$
$pH = 7.3553$

Q14　**a.** Suppose the bicarbonate stays at 27 mEq/l as in Q13 but the dissolved carbon dioxide goes up to 2.0 mEq/l. Find the pH.

b. Does increasing the dissolved CO_2 increase or decrease the pH? _____

c. Is the new pH in the normal range for arterial blood? _____

\# \# \#　•　\# \# \#　•　\# \# \#　•　\# \# \#　•　\# \# \#　•　\# \# \#　•　\# \# \#　•　\# \# \#　•　\# \# \#

A14　**a.** 7.2303:　$pH = 6.1 + \log_{10}\left(\dfrac{27}{2.0}\right)$

$pH = 6.1 + \log_{10}(13.5)$
$pH = 6.1 + 1.1303.$
$pH = 7.2303$

b. decreases the pH

c. no:　It is below 7.35. The patient has acidemia.

Q15　Suppose a stimulation of ventilation causes the dissolved carbon dioxide to be reduced from the 2.00 mEq/l in Q14 to 0.8 mEq/l. The bicarbonate remains at 27 mEq/l.
a. Calculate the pH.

b. Does the pH now fall in the normal range? _____

\# \# \#　•　\# \# \#　•　\# \# \#　•　\# \# \#　•　\# \# \#　•　\# \# \#　•　\# \# \#　•　\# \# \#　•　\# \# \#

A15　**a.** 7.6289:　$pH = 6.1 + \log_{10}\left(\dfrac{27}{0.8}\right)$

$pH = 6.1 + \log_{10}(33.8)$
$pH = 6.1 + 1.5289$
$pH = 7.6289$

b. no:　The pH now falls above 7.45. The patient has alkalemia.

9   A second form of the Henderson–Hasselbach equation can be used to find the partial pressure of CO_2 gas (P_{CO_2}) in the arterial blood. P_{CO_2} is measured in millimetres of mercury (mm Hg). In order to use the equation you need to know the pH and the total CO_2 in the blood. The total CO_2 in arterial blood is the sum of the bicarbonate and the dissolved CO_2 which appeared in the previous form of the H–H equation. The equation is

$$P_{CO_2} = \frac{[\text{total } CO_2]}{0.03 \times [1 + \text{antilog } (\text{pH} - 6.1)]}$$

Example: Find the partial pressure of CO_2 in arterial blood if the total CO_2 is 25 mEq/l and the pH is 7.4.

Solution:
$$P_{CO_2} = \frac{[\text{total } CO_2]}{0.03 \times [1 + \text{antilog } (\text{pH} - 6.1)]}$$
$$P_{CO_2} = \frac{25}{0.03 \times [1 + \text{antilog } (7.4 - 6.1)]}$$
$$P_{CO_2} = \frac{25}{0.03 \times [1 + \text{antilog } (1.3000)]}$$
$$P_{CO_2} = \frac{25}{0.03 \times (1 + 20.0)}$$
$$P_{CO_2} = \frac{25}{0.03 \times 21}$$
$$P_{CO_2} = \frac{25}{0.63}$$
$$P_{CO_2} = 39.7 \quad \text{(rounded off to tenths)}$$

Therefore, $P_{CO_2} = 39.7$ mm Hg.

Q16   Use the example of Frame 9 as a guide to find the partial pressure of CO_2 if the total CO_2 is 30 mEq/l and the pH is 7.44. Round off your answer to tenths.

\# \# \#   •   \# \# \#   •   \# \# \#   •   \# \# \#   •   \# \# \#   •   \# \# \#   •   \# \# \#   •   \# \# \#   •   \# \# \#

A16   43.7 mm Hg:
$$P_{CO_2} = \frac{30}{0.03 \times [1 + \text{antilog } (7.44 - 6.1)]}$$
$$P_{CO_2} = \frac{30}{0.03 \times [1 + \text{antilog } (1.34)]}$$
$$P_{CO_2} = \frac{30}{0.03 \times (1 + 21.9)}$$
$$P_{CO_2} = \frac{30}{0.03 \times 22.9}$$
$$P_{CO_2} = \frac{30}{0.687}$$
$$P_{CO_2} = 43.7$$

Q17   Find the partial pressure of CO_2 if the total CO_2 is 19.7 mEq/l and the pH is 7.55.

＃＃＃ · ＃＃＃ · ＃＃＃ · ＃＃＃ · ＃＃＃ · ＃＃＃ · ＃＃＃ · ＃＃＃ · ＃＃＃ · ＃＃＃

A17   22.5 mm Hg: $P_{CO_2} = \dfrac{19.7}{0.03 \times [1 + \text{antilog}\,(7.55 - 6.1)]}$

$P_{CO_2} = \dfrac{19.7}{0.03 \times (1 + 28.2)}$

$P_{CO_2} = \dfrac{19.7}{0.876}$

$P_{CO_2} = 22.5$

10   The examples of this section are authentic formulas which occur in medicine. However, there are many other places where logarithms are used in medicine. Space does not allow us to consider these. Be assured that mathematical procedures you have learned in this chapter will allow you to understand other formulas involving logarithms.

This completes the instruction for this section.

12.4   EXERCISE

1. The number of atoms in one gram of the element carbon is 50,150,000,000,000,000,000,000. Express this in scientific notation.
2. If burning 1 g of carbon produces 7.86×10^3 calories, use logarithms to calculate how many calories of heat are produced when 1.70×10^5 g are burned.
3. When calcium crystallizes a cubic structure is formed with the diagonal of one face, d, being 7.88×10^{-8} cm. Calculate the length of one side of the cube using logarithms if the length, l, is given by $l = \sqrt{\dfrac{d^2}{2}}$.
4. Find the pH of the solutions below if $pH = {}^-\log_{10}(cH^+)$:
   a. $cH^+ = 4.6 \times 10^{-5}\,M$ b. $cH^+ = 2.7 \times 10^{-8}\,M$
5. Consider your answers for problem 4 and determine if each solution is acid or alkaline (see Frame 5).
6. Use $pH = {}^-\log_{10}(cH^+)$ to determine the concentration of hydrogen ions if:
   a. $pH = 5.7$ b. $pH = 10.2$
7. a. Use the Henderson–Hasselbach equation to find the pH if the arterial blood bicarbonate is 30 mEq/l and the dissolved carbon dioxide is 1.2 mEq/l. Round off to tenths.

   $pH = 6.1 + \log_{10}\left(\dfrac{[\text{bicarbonate}]}{[\text{dissolved } CO_2]}\right)$

   b. Is this pH in its normal range (see Frame 8)?

8. Find the partial pressure of CO_2 if the total CO_2 is 27 mEq/l and the pH is 7.5. Round off to tenths.

$$P_{CO_2} = \frac{[\text{total } CO_2]}{0.03 \times [1 + \text{antilog} (pH - 6.1)]}$$

12.4   EXERCISE ANSWERS

1. 5.015×10^{22} **2.** 1.34×10^9 **3.** 5.57×10^{-8}

4. a. 4.3372   **b.** 7.5686   **5. a.** acid   **b.** alkaline

6. a. $2.00 \times 10^{-6} M$ **b.** $6.31 \times 10^{-11} M$ **7. a.** 7.5   **b.** No   **8.** 34.5 mm Hg

CHAPTER 12 SAMPLE TEST

At the completion of Chapter 12 you should be able to work the following problems.

12.1   EXPONENTS AND SCIENTIFIC NOTATION

1. In the expression $5^3 = 125$:

  a. the exponent is _____ .

  b. the base is _____ .

  c. _____ is the 3rd power of 5.

2. Evaluate:
  a. 10^4 **b.** 10^0 **c.** 10^{-1}

3. Write each number in exponential notation:

  a. 100,000   **b.** $\dfrac{1}{10,000}$

4. Write with positive exponents:
  a. 10^{-3} **b.** 10^{-5}

5. Write in decimal form:
  a. 10^{-2} **b.** 10^{-5}

6. Simplify (leave in exponential notation):
  a. $2^4 \cdot 2^5 \cdot 2$ **b.** $10^{-3} \cdot 10^4$ **c.** $3 \cdot 3^4 \cdot 3^0$ **d.** $5^{-3} \cdot 5^3$
  e. $\dfrac{2^5}{2^2}$ **f.** $\dfrac{10^3}{10^6}$ **g.** $(10^2)^5$ **h.** $(3^2)(3^3)^2$

7. Write in decimal form:
  a. 4.7×10^4 **b.** 1.6×10^2 **c.** 4.3×10^{-2} **d.** 8×10^{-4}

8. Write in scientific notation:
  a. 4,240,000   **b.** 0.024   **c.** 34.6×10^2 **d.** 0.002×10^{-5}

9. Simplify (leave in exponential notation):
  a. $\sqrt{10^8}$ **b.** $\sqrt[3]{5^6}$

12.2 LOGARITHMS

10. Determine the logarithm by first writing the number as a power of 10:
    a. $\log_{10} 10{,}000$ **b.** $\log_{10} 0.001$

11. Use the table of logarithms in the appendix to find the following:
    a. $\log_{10} 4.76$ **b.** $\log_{10} 986$ **c.** $\log_{10} 0.062$ **d.** $\log_{10} 0.7$

12. Use the table of logarithms in the appendix to find the antilogarithms of the following numbers:
    a. 0.9047 **b.** 5.7931 **c.** $6.6107-8$ **d.** $0.1903-4$

12.3 CALCULATIONS WITH LOGARITHMS

Perform the following calculations by using logarithms:

13. a. 5.72×3.42 **b.** $9{,}600 \times 553$

14. a. $47 \div 2.73$ **b.** $4.17 \div 0.017$

15. a. $(5.73)^7$ **b.** $\sqrt{4.73}$

16. $\dfrac{243 \times \sqrt{32}}{2.73}$

12.4 APPLICATIONS

17. The mass of a carbon atom is $0.00000000000000000000001994$ g. Write this in scientific notation.

18. Find the pH if the concentration of hydrogen ions is 4.6×10^{-6} and $pH = {}^-\log_{10}(cH^+)$.

19. Find cH^+ if pH is 3.7 and $pH = {}^-\log_{10}(cH^+)$.

20. In a one-tenth Mole solution of acetic acid, the concentration of H^+ is given by the equation $cH^+ = \sqrt{1.80 \times 10^{-6}}$. Find cH^+.

21. Use the Henderson–Hasselbach equation to find the pH if the bicarbonate in arterial blood is 25.6 mEq/l and the dissolved CO_2 is 1.6 mEq/l. Round off to tenths.

$$pH = 6.1 + \log_{10}\left(\frac{[\text{bicarbonate}]}{[\text{dissolved } CO_2]}\right)$$

22. Find the partial pressure of CO_2 if the total CO_2 is 34 mEq/l and the pH is 8.0. Round off to tenths.

$$P_{CO_2} = \frac{[\text{total } CO_2]}{0.03 \times [1 + \text{antilog}(pH - 6.1)]}$$

CHAPTER 12 SAMPLE TEST ANSWERS

1. a. 3   **b.** 5   **c.** 125

2. a. 10,000   **b.** 1   **c.** 0.1 or $\dfrac{1}{10}$

3. a. 10^5 **b.** 10^{-4}

4. a. $\dfrac{1}{10^3}$ **b.** $\dfrac{1}{10^5}$ **5. a.** 0.01   **b.** 0.00001

6. a. 2^{10} **b.** 10   **c.** 3^5 **d.** 1
   e. 2^3 **f.** 10^{-3} **g.** 10^{10} **h.** 3^8
7. a. 47,000   **b.** 160   **c.** 0.043   **d.** 0.0008
8. a. 4.24×10^6 **b.** 2.4×10^{-2} **c.** 3.46×10^3 **d.** 2×10^{-8}
9. a. 10^4 **b.** 5^2 **10. a.** 4   **b.** $^-3$
11. a. 0.6776   **b.** 2.9939   **c.** $0.7924 - 2$ **d.** $0.8451 - 1$
12. a. 8.03   **b.** 621,000   **c.** 0.0408   **d.** 0.000155
13. a. 19.6   **b.** 5,310,000   **14. a.** 17.2   **b.** 245
15. a. 203,000   **b.** 2.18
16. 504   **17.** 1.994×10^{-23} **18.** 5.3372   **19.** $2.00 \times 10^{-4}\,M$
20. 0.00134 M **21.** 7.3   **22.** 14.1 mm Hg

APPENDIX

Table I   Multiplication Facts

1	2	3	4	5	6	7	8	9	10	11	12	13	14	15	16	17	18	19	20	21	22	23	24	25
2	4	6	8	10	12	14	16	18	20	22	24	26	28	30	32	34	36	38	40	42	44	46	48	50
3	6	9	12	15	18	21	24	27	30	33	36	39	42	45	48	51	54	57	60	63	66	69	72	75
4	8	12	16	20	24	28	32	36	40	44	48	52	56	60	64	68	72	76	80	84	88	92	96	100
5	10	15	20	25	30	35	40	45	50	55	60	65	70	75	80	85	90	95	100	105	110	115	120	125
6	12	18	24	30	36	42	48	54	60	66	72	78	84	90	96	102	108	114	120	126	132	138	144	150
7	14	21	28	35	42	49	56	63	70	77	84	91	98	105	112	119	126	133	140	147	154	161	168	175
8	16	24	32	40	48	56	64	72	80	88	96	104	112	120	128	136	144	152	160	168	176	184	192	200
9	18	27	36	45	54	63	72	81	90	99	108	117	126	135	144	153	162	171	180	189	198	207	216	225
10	20	30	40	50	60	70	80	90	100	110	120	130	140	150	160	170	180	190	200	210	220	230	240	250
11	22	33	44	55	66	77	88	99	110	121	132	143	154	165	176	187	198	209	220	231	242	253	264	275
12	24	36	48	60	72	84	96	108	120	132	144	156	168	180	192	204	216	228	240	252	264	276	288	300
13	26	39	52	65	78	91	104	117	130	143	156	169	182	195	208	221	234	247	260	273	286	299	312	325
14	28	42	56	70	84	98	112	126	140	154	168	182	196	210	224	238	252	266	280	294	308	322	336	350
15	30	45	60	75	90	105	120	135	150	165	180	195	210	225	240	255	270	285	300	315	330	345	360	375
16	32	48	64	80	96	112	128	144	160	176	192	208	224	240	256	272	288	304	320	336	352	368	384	400
17	34	51	68	85	102	119	136	153	170	187	204	221	238	255	272	289	306	323	340	357	374	391	408	425
18	36	54	72	90	108	126	144	162	180	198	216	234	252	270	288	306	324	342	360	378	396	414	432	450
19	38	57	76	95	114	133	152	171	190	209	228	247	266	285	304	323	342	361	380	399	418	437	456	475
20	40	60	80	100	120	140	160	180	200	220	240	260	280	300	320	340	360	380	400	420	440	460	480	500
21	42	63	84	105	126	147	168	189	210	231	252	273	294	315	336	357	378	399	420	441	462	483	504	525
22	44	66	88	110	132	154	176	198	220	242	264	286	308	330	352	374	396	418	440	462	484	506	528	550
23	46	69	92	115	138	161	184	207	230	253	276	299	322	345	368	391	414	437	460	483	506	529	552	575
24	48	72	96	120	144	168	192	216	240	264	288	312	336	360	384	408	432	456	480	504	528	552	576	600
25	50	75	100	125	150	175	200	225	250	275	300	325	350	375	400	425	450	475	500	525	550	575	600	625

Table II   English Weights and Measures

Units of Length

1 foot (ft or ′) = 12 inches (in. or ″)
    1 yard (yd) = 3 feet
    1 rod (rd) = $5\frac{1}{2}$ yards = $16\frac{1}{2}$ feet
    1 mile(mi) = 1,760 yards = 5,280 feet

Units of Area

1 square foot = 144 square inches
1 square yard = 9 square feet
    1 acre = 43,560 square feet
1 square mile = 640 acres

Units of Weight

1 pound (lb) = 16 ounces (oz)
    1 ton = 2,000 pounds

Units of Capacity (Volume)
Liquid

1 pint (pt) = 16 fluid ounces (fl oz)
1 quart (qt) = 2 pints
1 gallon (gal) = 4 quarts = 8 pints

Dry

1 quart (qt) = 2 pints (pt)
1 peck (pk) = 8 quarts
1 bushel (bu) = 4 pecks = 32 quarts

Units of Capacity

1 cubic foot = 1,728 cubic inches
1 cubic yard = 27 cubic feet
    1 gallon = 231 cubic inches
1 cubic foot = 7.48 gallons

TABLE III   Metric Weights and Measures   **495**

Table III   Metric Weights and Measures

Units of Length
1 millimetre (mm) = 1000 micrometres (μm)
1 centimetre (cm) = 10 millimetres
1 decimetre (dm) = 10 centimetres
1 metre (m) = 10 decimetres
1 dekametre (dam) = 10 metres
1 hectometre (hm) = 10 dekametres
1 kilometre (km) = 10 hectometres

Units of Weight

1 milligram (mg) = 1000 micrograms (μg)
1 centigram (cg) = 10 milligrams
1 decigram (dg) = 10 centigrams
1 gram (g) = 10 decigrams
1 dekagram (dag) = 10 grams
1 hectogram (hg) = 10 deckagrams
1 kilogram (kg) = 10 hectograms
1 megagram (Mg) = 1000 kilograms
(metric ton)

Units of Area
1 square centimetre = 100 square millimetres
1 square decimetre = 100 square centimetres
1 square metre = 100 square decimetres
1 square kilometre = 1 000 000 square metres
1 hectare (ha) = 10 000 square metres
1 are (a) = 100 square metres

Units of Capacity (Volume)

1 millilitre (ml) = 1 cubic
centimetre (cc or cm^3)
1 centilitre (cl) = 10 millilitres
1 decilitre (dl) = 10 centilitres
1 litre (l) = 10 decilitres
= 1000 cubic centimetres
1 deckalitre (dal) = 10 litres
1 hectolitre (hl) = 10 dekalitres
1 kilolitre (kl) = 10 hectolitres
1 megalitre (Ml) = 1000 kilolitres

Table IV   Metric and English Conversion

Length

English   Metric

1 inch = 2.54 cm
1 foot = 30.5 cm
1 yard = 91.4 cm
1 mile = 1610 m
1 mile = 1.61 km
0.0394 in. = 1 mm
0.394 in. = 1 cm
39.4 in. = 1 m
3.28 ft = 1 m
1.09 yd = 1 m
0.621 mi = 1 km

Capacity

English   Metric

1 gallon = 3.79 l
1 quart = 0.946 l
0.264 gal = 1 l
1.05 qt = 1 l

Weight

English   Metric

1 ounce = 28.3 g
1 pound = 454 g
1 pound = 0.454 kg
0.0353 oz = 1 g
0.00220 lb = 1 g
2.20 lb = 1 kg

Area

English   Metric

1 square inch = 6.45 square centimetres
1 square foot = 929 square centimetres
1 square yard = 8361 square centimetres
1 square rod = 25.3 square metres
1 acre = 4047 square metres
1 square mile = 2.59 square kilometres
10.76 square feet = 1 square metre
1,550 square inches = 1 square metre
0.0395 square rod = 1 square metre
1.196 square yards = 1 square metre
0.155 square inch = 1 square centimetre
247.1 acres = 1 square kilometre
0.386 square mile = 1 square kilometre

Volume

English   Metric

1 cubic inch = 16.39 cubic centimetres
1 cubic foot = 28.317 cubic centimetres
1 cubic yard = 0.7646 cubic metres
0.06102 cubic inch = 1 cubic centimetre
35.3 cubic feet = 1 cubic metre

TABLE V   Apothecary, Household, and Metric Conversion   **497**

Table V   Apothecary, Household, and Metric Conversion

The Apothecaries' System

gr	grain
ʒ	dram
℥	ounce
lb	pound
m	minim
fʒ	fluidram
f℥	fluidounce
pt	pint
O	
qt	quart
gal	gallon
C	

Weight

1 dram = 60 grains
1 ounce = 8 drams
1 pound = 12 ounces

Liquid Volume

1 fluidram = 60 minims
1 fluidounce = 8 fluidrams
1 pint = 16 fluidounces
1 quart = 2 pints
1 gallon = 4 quarts

The Household System

gtt	drop
tsp	teaspoon
tbsp	tablespoon

60 drops = 1 teaspoon
3 teaspoons = 1 tablespoon
2 tablespoons = 1 ounce
6 ounces = 1 teacup
8 ounces = 1 glass

Household–Apothecary

1 drop = 1 minim
1 teaspoon = 1 fluidram
1 tablespoon = 4 fluidrams
1 glass = 8 fluidounces
1 teacup = 6 fluidounces

Metric–Apothecary

g	gram
mg	milligram

Weight

1 gram = 15 grains
4 grams = 1 dram
30 grams = 1 ounce
60 milligrams = 1 grain

Metric–Apothecary

ml	millilitre
l	litre

Liquid Volume

1 milliliter* = 15 or 16 minims
4 millilitres = 1 fluidram
30 millilitres = 1 fluidounce
500 millilitres = 1 pint
1000 millilitres = 1 quart
1 litre = 1 quart

*1 ml = 1 cm^3 = 1 cc

Household–Metric

1 drop = 0.06 millilitres
1 teaspoon = 5 millilitres
1 tablespoon = 15 millilitres
1 fluidounce = 30 millilitres
1 teacup = 180 millilitres
1 glass = 240 millilitres

TABLE VI   Decimal Fraction and Common Fraction Equivalents   **499**

Table VI   Decimal Fraction and Common Fraction Equivalents

$\frac{1}{64} = 0.015625$	$\frac{9}{32} = 0.28125$	$\frac{17}{32} = 0.53125$	$\frac{25}{32} = 0.78125$
$\frac{1}{32} = 0.03125$	$\frac{19}{64} = 0.296875$	$\frac{35}{64} = 0.546875$	$\frac{51}{64} = 0.796875$
$\frac{3}{64} = 0.046875$	$\frac{5}{16} = 0.3125$	$\frac{9}{16} = 0.5625$	$\frac{4}{5} = 0.8$
$\frac{1}{16} = 0.0625$	$\frac{21}{64} = 0.328125$	$\frac{37}{64} = 0.578125$	$\frac{13}{16} = 0.8125$
$\frac{5}{64} = 0.078125$	$\frac{1}{3} = 0.333$	$\frac{19}{32} = 0.59375$	$\frac{53}{64} = 0.828125$
$\frac{3}{32} = 0.09375$	$\frac{11}{32} = 0.34375$	$\frac{3}{5} = 0.6$	$\frac{27}{32} = 0.84375$
$\frac{7}{64} = 0.109375$	$\frac{23}{64} = 0.359375$	$\frac{39}{64} = 0.609375$	$\frac{55}{64} = 0.859375$
$\frac{1}{8} = 0.125$	$\frac{3}{8} = 0.375$	$\frac{5}{8} = 0.625$	$\frac{7}{8} = 0.875$
$\frac{9}{64} = 0.140625$	$\frac{25}{64} = 0.390625$	$\frac{41}{64} = 0.640625$	$\frac{57}{64} = 0.890625$
$\frac{5}{32} = 0.15625$	$\frac{2}{5} = 0.4$	$\frac{21}{32} = 0.65625$	$\frac{29}{32} = 0.90625$
$\frac{11}{64} = 0.171875$	$\frac{13}{32} = 0.40625$	$\frac{2}{3} = 0.66\overline{6}$	$\frac{59}{64} = 0.921875$
$\frac{3}{16} = 0.1875$	$\frac{27}{64} = 0.421875$	$\frac{43}{64} = 0.671875$	$\frac{15}{16} = 0.9375$
$\frac{1}{5} = 0.2$	$\frac{7}{16} = 0.4375$	$\frac{11}{16} = 0.6875$	$\frac{61}{64} = 0.953125$
$\frac{13}{64} = 0.203125$	$\frac{29}{64} = 0.453125$	$\frac{45}{64} = 0.703125$	$\frac{31}{32} = 0.96875$
$\frac{7}{32} = 0.21875$	$\frac{15}{32} = 0.46875$	$\frac{23}{32} = 0.71875$	$\frac{63}{64} = 0.984375$
$\frac{15}{64} = 0.234375$	$\frac{31}{64} = 0.484375$	$\frac{47}{64} = 0.734375$	
$\frac{1}{4} = 0.25$	$\frac{1}{2} = 0.5$	$\frac{3}{4} = 0.75$	
$\frac{17}{64} = 0.265625$	$\frac{33}{64} = 0.515625$	$\frac{49}{64} = 0.765625$	

Table VII   Fraction, Decimal, and Percent Equivalents

$\frac{1}{16} = 0.06\frac{1}{4}$ or $0.0625 = 6\frac{1}{4}\%$ or 6.25%

$\frac{1}{12} = 0.08\frac{1}{3} = 8\frac{1}{3}\%$

$\frac{1}{10} = 0.1 = 10\%$

$\frac{1}{9} = 0.11\frac{1}{9} = 11\frac{1}{9}\%$

$\frac{1}{8} = 0.12\frac{1}{2}$ or $0.125 = 12\frac{1}{2}\%$ or 12.5%

$\frac{1}{7} = 0.14\frac{2}{7} = 14\frac{2}{7}\%$

$\frac{1}{6} = 0.16\frac{2}{3} = 16\frac{2}{3}\%$

$\frac{1}{5} = 0.2 = 20\%$

$\frac{1}{4} = 0.25 = 25\%$

$\frac{3}{10} = 0.3 = 30\%$

$\frac{1}{3} = 0.33\frac{1}{3} = 33\frac{1}{3}\%$

$\frac{3}{8} = 0.37\frac{1}{2}$ or $0.375 = 37\frac{1}{2}\%$ or 37.5%

$\frac{2}{5} = 0.4 = 40\%$

$\frac{1}{2} = 0.5 = 50\%$

$\frac{3}{5} = 0.6 = 60\%$

$\frac{5}{8} = 0.62\frac{1}{2}$ or $0.625 = 62\frac{1}{2}\%$ or 62.5%

$\frac{2}{3} = 0.66\frac{2}{3} = 66\frac{2}{3}\%$

$\frac{7}{10} = 0.7 = 70\%$

$\frac{3}{4} = 0.75 = 75\%$

$\frac{4}{5} = 0.8 = 80\%$

$\frac{5}{6} = 0.83\frac{1}{3} = 83\frac{1}{3}\%$

$\frac{7}{8} = 0.87\frac{1}{2}$ or $0.875 = 87\frac{1}{2}\%$ or 87.5%

TABLE VIII   Formulas from Geometry   **501**

Table VIII   Formulas from Geometry

		PERIMETER	AREA
Rectangle		$p = 2l + 2w$	$A = lw$
Square		$p = 4s$	$A = s^2$
Parallelogram		$p = 2a + 2b$	$A = bh$
Trapezoid			$A = \frac{1}{2}h(b_1 + b_2)$
Triangle		$p = a + b + c$	$A = \frac{1}{2}bh$

The sum of the measures of the angles of a triangle $= 180°$. In a right triangle:

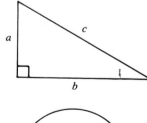

$c^2 = a^2 + b^2$
(Pythagorean theorem)

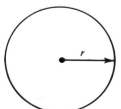

	CIRCUMFERENCE	AREA
Circle	$C = 2\pi r$ $C = \pi d$	$A = \pi r^2 \; (d = 2r)$

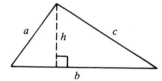

VOLUME

Triangular prism

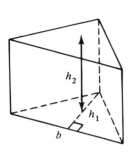

$$V = \frac{1}{2}bh_1h_2$$

or

$V = Bh$, where B is the area of the base

Cube

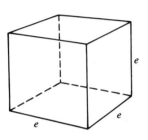

$$V = e^3$$

Rectangular prism

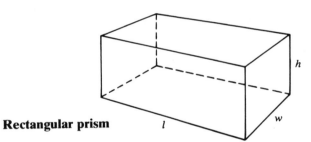

$V = lwh$

or

$V = Bh$, where B is the area of the base

Cylinder

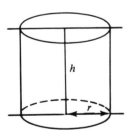

$$V = \pi r^2 h$$

Pyramid

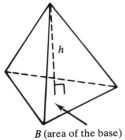

B (area of the base)

$$V = \frac{1}{3}Bh$$

TABLE VIII   Formulas from Geometry   **503**

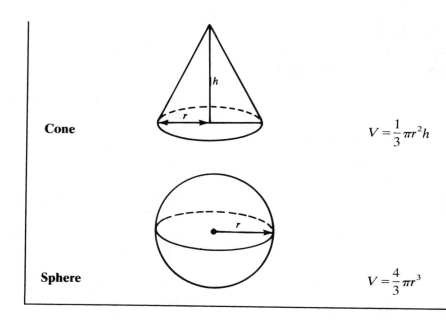

Cone

$$V = \frac{1}{3}\pi r^2 h$$

Sphere

$$V = \frac{4}{3}\pi r^3$$

Table IX Symbols

The section number indicates the first use of the symbol.

1.1	$+$	"plus"	Indicates addition (sum) of two numbers
1.1	$=$	"is equal to"	
1.1	$-$	"minus"	Indicates subtraction (difference) of two numbers
1.1	$\times$	"times"	Indicates multiplication (product) of two numbers
1.1	$\div$	"divided by"	Indicates division (quotient) between two numbers
1.2	$\dfrac{a}{b}$	"a over b"	Fraction indicating a of b equal parts
1.3	$.$	"point" or "and"	Decimal point used to separate the whole-number part of a number from the decimal (fraction) part of the number
2.1	$0 \cdot \overline{ab}$	"bar"	Indicates that the group of numbers under the bar repeats endlessly
2.1	$\%$	"percent"	Abbreviation for the word "percent"
3.1	$\neq$	"is not equal"	
3.1	$l_1 \perp l_2$		Indicates that l_1 and l_2 are perpendicular (l_1 reads as l sub-one)
3.1	$\parallel$	"is parallel to"	
3.1	$\perp$	"is perpendicular to"	
3.1	$\overleftrightarrow{AB}$	"line AB"	
3.1	$\overline{AB}$	"line segment AB"	
3.1	$\overrightarrow{AB}$	"ray AB"	
3.1	$\angle$	"angle"	
3.1	$\circ$	"degree"	Unit of measure of an angle
3.1	$m\angle A$	"measure of angle A"	
3.2	$\doteq$	"is approximately equal to"	
3.2	π	"pi"	Constant whose value is generally given as approximately equal to 3.14 or $\dfrac{22}{7}$
3.2	$a(b)=(a)(b)$ $=(a)b=ab$		Product of a and b
3.2	$a \cdot b$	"times"	Raised dot to indicate the product of a and b

TABLE IX Symbols **505**

3.2	a^b	"a to the bth power"	Exponential notation
6.1	$^+$	"positive"	Raised plus sign to denote a positive number
6.2	^-a	"opposite of a"	Raised minus sign to indicate the opposite of a number
6.1	$^-$	"negative"	Raised minus sign to denote a negative number
6.1	$,\ldots$	"and so forth"	Indicates the list continues
6.2	( )	"quantity"	Parentheses used as a grouping symbol
6.6	LCD	"least common denominator"	
7.4	b_1 and b_2	"b sub-one and b sub-two"	Subscripts used to distinguish between two different values of the same quantity
8.1	$a : b$	"a to b" or "a is to b"	Colon used in expressing a ratio of two numbers or quantities
9.1	/	"per"	
10.5	(a, b)	"the ordered pair a, b"	
12.1	$\sqrt{\ }$	"radical" or "square root of"	
12.2	log	abbreviation of "logarithm"	
12.2	$\log_{10} n$	"the log of n, base 10"	
12.2	$y = \log_b x$	"y equals the log of x to the base b"	Equivalent to $x = b^y$
12.2	$\sqrt[n]{x}$	"the nth root of x"	

Table X   Squares and Square Roots

Number	Square	Square Root	Number	Square	Square Root	Number	Square	Square Root
1	1	1.000	51	26 01	7.141	101	1 02 01	10.050
2	4	1.414	52	27 04	7.211	102	1 04 04	10.100
3	9	1.732	53	28 09	7.280	103	1 06 09	10.149
4	16	2.000	54	29 16	7.348	104	1 08 16	10.198
5	25	2.236	55	30 25	7.416	105	1 10 25	10.247
6	36	2.449	56	31 36	7.483	106	1 12 36	10.296
7	49	2.646	57	32 49	7.550	107	1 14 49	10.344
8	64	2.828	58	33 64	7.616	108	1 16 64	10.392
9	81	3.000	59	34 81	7.681	109	1 18 81	10.440
10	1 00	3.162	60	36 00	7.746	110	1 21 00	10.488
11	1 21	3.317	61	37 21	7.810	111	1 23 21	10.536
12	1 44	3.464	62	38 44	7.874	112	1 25 44	10.583
13	1 69	3.606	63	36 69	7.937	113	1 27 69	10.630
14	1 96	3.742	64	40 96	8.000	114	1 29 96	10.677
15	2 25	3.873	65	42 25	8.062	115	1 32 25	10.724
16	2 56	4.000	66	43 56	8.124	116	1 34 56	10.770
17	2 89	4.123	67	44 89	8.185	117	1 36 89	10.817
18	3 24	4.243	68	46 24	8.246	118	1 39 24	10.863
19	3 61	4.359	69	47 61	8.307	119	1 41 61	10.909
20	4 00	4.472	70	49 00	8.367	120	1 44 00	10.954
21	4 41	4.583	71	50 41	8.426	121	1 46 41	11.000
22	4 84	4.690	72	51 84	8.485	122	1 48 84	11.045
23	5 29	4.796	73	53 29	8.544	123	1 51 29	11.091
24	5 76	4.899	74	54 76	8.602	124	1 53 76	11.136
25	6 25	5.000	75	56 25	8.660	125	1 56 25	11.180
26	6 76	5.099	76	57 76	8.718	126	1 58 76	11.225
27	7 29	5.196	77	59 29	8.775	127	1 61 29	11.269
28	7 84	5.292	78	60 84	8.832	128	1 63 84	11.314
29	8 41	5.385	79	62 41	8.888	129	1 66 41	11.358
30	9 00	5.477	80	64 00	8.944	130	1 69 00	11.402
31	9 61	5.568	81	65 61	9.000	131	1 71 61	11.446
32	10 24	5.657	82	67 24	9.055	132	1 74 24	11.489
33	10 89	5.745	83	68 89	9.110	133	1 76 89	11.533
34	11 56	5.831	84	70 56	9.165	134	1 79 56	11.576
35	12 25	5.916	85	72 25	9.220	135	1 82 25.	11.619
36	12 96	6.000	86	73 96	9.274	136	1 84 96	11.662
37	13 69	6.083	87	75 69	9.327	137	1 87 69	11.705
38	14 44	6.164	88	77 44	9.381	138	1 90 44	11.747
39	15 21	6.245	89	79 21	9.434	139	1 93 21	11.790
40	16 00	6.325	90	81 00	9.487	140	1 96 00	11.832
41	16 81	6.403	91	82 81	9.539	141	1 98 81	11.874
42	17 64	6.481	92	84 64	9.592	142	2 01 64	11.916
43	18 49	6.557	93	86 49	9.644	143	2 04 49	11.958
44	19 36	6.633	94	88 36	9.695	144	2 07 36	12.000
45	20 25	6.708	95	90 25	9.747	145	2 10 25	12.042
46	21 16	6.782	96	92 16	9.798	146	2 13 16	12.083
47	22 09	6.856	97	94 09	9.849	147	2 16 09	12.124
48	23 04	6.982	98	96 04	9.899	148	2 19 04	12.166
49	24 01	7.000	99	98 01	9.950	149	2 22 01	12.207
50	25 00	7.071	100	1 00 00	10.000	150	2 25 00	12.247

TABLE XI   Common Logarithms   **507**

Table XI   Common Logarithms

N	0	1	2	3	4	5	6	7	8	9
1.0	0000	0043	0086	0128	0170	0212	0253	0294	0334	0374
1.1	0414	0453	0492	0531	0569	0607	0645	0682	0719	0755
1.2	0792	0828	0864	0899	0934	0969	1004	1038	1072	1106
1.3	1139	1173	1206	1239	1271	1303	1335	1367	1399	1430
1.4	1461	1492	1523	1553	1584	1614	1644	1673	1703	1732
1.5	1761	1790	1818	1847	1875	1903	1931	1959	1987	2014
1.6	2041	2068	2095	2122	2148	2175	2201	2227	2253	2279
1.7	2304	2330	2355	2380	2405	2430	2455	2480	2504	2529
1.8	2553	2577	2601	2625	2648	2672	2695	2718	2742	2765
1.9	2788	2810	2833	2856	2878	2900	2923	2945	2967	2989
2.0	3010	3032	3054	3075	3096	3118	3139	3160	3181	3201
2.1	3222	3243	3263	3284	3304	3324	3345	3365	3385	3404
2.2	3424	3444	3464	3483	3502	3522	3541	3560	3579	3598
2.3	3617	3636	3655	3674	3692	3711	3729	3747	3766	3784
2.4	3802	3820	3838	3856	3874	3892	3909	3927	3945	3962
2.5	3979	3997	4014	4031	4048	4065	4082	4099	4116	4133
2.6	4150	4166	4183	4200	4216	4232	4249	4265	4281	4298
2.7	4314	4330	4346	4362	4378	4393	4409	4425	4440	4456
2.8	4472	4487	4502	4518	4533	4548	4564	4579	4594	4609
2.9	4624	4639	4654	4669	4683	4698	4713	4728	4742	4757
3.0	4771	4786	4800	4814	4829	4843	4857	4871	4886	4900
3.1	4914	4928	4942	4955	4969	4983	4997	5011	5024	5038
3.2	5051	5065	5079	5092	5105	5119	5132	5145	5159	5172
3.3	5185	5198	5211	5224	5237	5250	5263	5276	5289	5302
3.4	5315	5328	5340	5353	5366	5378	5391	5403	5416	5428
3.5	5441	5453	5465	5478	5490	5502	5514	5527	5539	5551
3.6	5563	5575	5587	5599	5611	5623	5635	5647	5658	5670
3.7	5682	5694	5705	5717	5729	5740	5752	5763	5775	5786
3.8	5798	5809	5821	5832	5843	5855	5866	5877	5888	5899
3.9	5911	5922	5933	5944	5955	5966	5977	5988	5999	6010
4.0	6021	6031	6042	6053	6064	6075	6085	6096	6107	6117
4.1	6128	6138	6149	6160	6170	6180	6191	6201	6212	6222
4.2	6232	6243	6253	6263	6274	6284	6294	6304	6314	6325
4.3	6335	6345	6355	6365	6375	6385	6395	6405	6415	6425
4.4	6435	6444	6454	6464	6474	6484	6493	6503	6513	6522
4.5	6532	6542	6551	6561	6571	6580	6590	6599	6609	6618
4.6	6628	6637	6646	6656	6665	6675	6684	6693	6702	6712
4.7	6721	6730	6739	6749	6758	6767	6776	6785	6794	6803
4.8	6812	6821	6830	6839	6848	6857	6866	6875	6884	6893
4.9	6902	6911	6920	6928	6937	6946	6955	6964	6972	6981
5.0	6990	6998	7007	7016	7024	7033	7042	7050	7059	7067
5.1	7076	7084	7093	7101	7110	7118	7126	7135	7143	7152
5.2	7160	7168	7177	7185	7193	7202	7210	7218	7226	7235
5.3	7243	7251	7259	7267	7275	7284	7292	7300	7308	7316
5.4	7324	7332	7340	7348	7356	7364	7372	7380	7388	7396
5.5	7404	7412	7419	7427	7435	7443	7451	7459	7466	7474
5.6	7482	7490	7497	7505	7513	7520	7528	7536	7543	7551
5.7	7559	7566	7574	7582	7589	7597	7604	7612	7619	7627
5.8	7634	7642	7649	7657	7664	7672	7679	7686	7694	7701
5.9	7709	7716	7723	7731	7738	7745	7752	7760	7767	7774

N	0	1	2	3	4	5	6	7	8	9
6.0	7782	7789	7796	7803	7810	7818	7825	7832	7839	7846
6.1	7853	7860	7868	7875	7882	7889	7896	7903	7910	7917
6.2	7924	7931	7938	7945	7952	7959	7966	7973	7980	7987
6.3	7993	8000	8007	8014	8021	8028	8035	8041	8048	8055
6.4	8062	8069	8075	8082	8089	8096	8102	8109	8116	8122
6.5	8129	8136	8142	8149	8156	8162	8169	8176	8182	8189
6.6	8195	8202	8209	8215	8222	8228	8235	8241	8248	8254
6.7	8261	8267	8274	8280	8287	8293	8299	8306	8312	8319
6.8	8325	8331	8338	8344	8351	8357	8363	8370	8376	8382
6.9	8388	8395	8401	8407	8414	8420	8426	8432	8439	8445
7.0	8451	8457	8463	8470	8476	8482	8488	8494	8500	8506
7.1	8513	8519	8525	8531	8537	8543	8549	8555	8561	8567
7.2	8573	8579	8585	8591	8597	8603	8609	8615	8621	8627
7.3	8633	8639	8645	8651	8657	8663	8669	8675	8681	8686
7.4	8692	8698	8704	8710	8716	8722	8727	8733	8739	8745
7.5	8751	8756	8762	8768	8774	8779	8785	8791	8797	8802
7.6	8808	8814	8820	8825	8831	8837	8842	8848	8854	8859
7.7	8865	8871	8876	8882	8887	8893	8899	8904	8910	8915
7.8	8921	8927	8932	8938	8943	8949	8954	8960	8965	8971
7.9	8976	8982	8987	8993	8998	9004	9009	9015	9020	9025
8.0	9031	9036	9042	9047	9053	9058	9063	9069	9074	9079
8.1	9085	9090	9096	9101	9106	9112	9117	9122	9128	9133
8.2	9138	9143	9149	9154	9159	9165	9170	9175	9180	9186
8.3	9191	9196	9201	9206	9212	9217	9222	9227	9232	9238
8.4	9243	9248	9253	9258	9263	9269	9274	9279	9284	9289
8.5	9294	9299	9304	9309	9315	9320	9325	9330	9335	9240
8.6	9345	9350	9355	9360	9365	9370	9375	9380	9385	9390
8.7	9395	9400	9405	9410	9415	9420	9425	9430	9435	9440
8.8	9445	9450	9455	9460	9465	9469	9474	9479	9484	9489
8.9	9494	9499	9504	9509	9513	9518	9523	9528	9533	9538
9.0	9542	9547	9552	9557	9562	9566	9571	9576	9581	9586
9.1	9590	9595	9600	9605	9609	9614	9619	9624	9628	9633
9.2	9638	9643	9647	9652	9657	9661	9666	9671	9675	9680
9.3	9685	9689	9694	9699	9703	9708	9713	9717	9722	9727
9.4	9731	9736	9741	9745	9750	9754	9759	9763	9768	9773
9.5	9777	9782	9786	9791	9795	9800	9805	9809	9814	9818
9.6	9823	9827	9832	9836	9841	9845	9850	9854	9859	9863
9.7	9868	9872	9877	9881	9886	9890	9894	9899	9903	9908
9.8	9912	9917	9921	9926	9930	9934	9939	9943	9948	9952
9.9	9956	9961	9965	9969	9974	9978	9983	9987	9991	9996

GLOSSARY

1. When a bar is placed over a vowel, the vowel says its own name.
2. A curved mark over a vowel indicates the following sounds:
  a. ă as in at
  b. ĕ as in bed
  c. ĭ as in it
  d. ŏ as in ox
  e. ŭ as in rug

Acute (ŭ kūt′)
  (angle)   Angle whose measure is less than 90°.
  (triangle)   Triangle with three angles less than 90°.

Add (ăd)   To combine into a sum.

Addend (ăd′ ĕnd)   Value to be added to another.

Addition (ă dĭ′ shŭn)   Act of adding.

Adjacent (ŭ jā′ sĕnt) **(sides of a quadrilateral)**   Any two sides that intersect at a vertex.

Algebraic (ăl′ jŭ brā′ ĭk) . **(open expression)**   Expression in which the position of an unknown number is held by a letter (variable).

Altitude (ăl′ tĭ tōōd)
  (of a parallelogram)   Perpendicular distance between two parallel sides.
  (of a pyramid)   Line segment from the apex perpendicular to the base.
  (of a right-circular cone)   Length of the axis.
  (of a right-circular cylinder)   Length of the axis.
  (of a trapezoid)   Perpendicular distance between the two parallel sides.
  (of a triangle)   Line segment from the vertex perpendicular to the base.

Ampere (ăm′ pēr)   Unit of intensity of electrical current, produced by one volt acting through a resistance of one ohm.

Ampul (ăm′ pūl)   Small sealed glass vessel used to hold sufficient solution for a single hypodermic injection.

Angle (ăng′ g′l)   Two rays with a common endpoint.

Antilogarithm (ăn tĭ log′ rĭth ŭm)   Where $\log_{10} N = b$, N is the antilogarithm of b, base 10.

Apex (ā′ pĕx) **(of a pyramid)**   Common vertex of the faces which is not part of the base.

Apophysial (ah pŏf′ ĭ sē al) **(joint)**   Pertaining to outgrowth or swelling.

Apothecaries' (ah pŏth′ ŭ kĕr eez) **(system)**   System of liquid weight and volume measure used in pharmacy.

Area (air′ ē ŭ)   Measure (in square units) of the region within a closed curve (including polygons) in a plane.

Associative (ŭ sō′ shŭ tĭv)   Indicates that the grouping of three numbers in an addition or multiplication can be changed without affecting the sum or product.

Asthma (ăz′mah)   Chronic respiratory disease, often arising from allergies, and accompanied by labored breathing, chest constriction, and coughing.

Atmosphere (ăt′ mah sfĭr)   Unit of pressure.

Atrial (ā′ trē ăl)   Pertaining to an atrium (upper chamber on either side of the heart).

Axis (ăk′ sĭs)
   (of a cone)   Line segment connecting the vertex to the center of the base.
   (of a cylinder)   Line sement connecting the centers of the bases.

Base (bās)   Value that is being multiplied by a percent. That is, in $5\% \times 30$, 30 is the base.
   (of a logarithm)   In $\log_{10} N = b$, 10 is the base.
   (of a power)   Number being raised to a power.
   of a triangle)   Side opposite a vertex.

Bases (bās′ ĭz)
   (of a cylinder)   Two circular regions that are parallel.
   (of a prism)   Parallel faces.
   (of a trapezoid)   Parallel sides.

Biparietal (bī pah rī′ ah tăl) **(diameter)**   Diameter across skull by prominent, bulging bones behind frontal bone. Parietal bones form topsides of cranial cavity.

Bronchi (brŏng′ kī)   Plural of bronchus (either of two main branches of the trachea).

Calorie (kăl′ ahr ē)   Unit of energy.

Celsius (sĕl′ sē ŭs) **(scale)**   Temperature scale on which the interval between the freezing point and boiling point of water is divided into 100 parts or degrees, so that 0 °Celsius corresponds to 32 °Fahrenheit and 100 °Celsius to 212 °Fahrenheit.

Centi (sĕn′ tĭ)   Latin prefix indicating one-hundredth.

Central (sĕn′ trăl) **(angle)**   Angle with its vertex at the center of a circle.

Characteristic (kăr ĭk tah rĭs′ tĭk)   Integer portion of the logarithm.

Circle (sur′ kŭl)   Set of all points in a plane whose distance from a given point (center) is equal to a positive number, r (radius).

Circumference (sur kŭm′ fur ĕns) **(of a circle)**   Distance around.

Cofficient (kō ĕ fĭsh′ ŭnt)   Any numeral or literal symbol placed before another symbol or combination of symbols as a multiplier.

Commutative (kŭ mū′ tŭ tĭv)   Indicates that the order of two numbers in an addition or multiplication can be changed without affecting the sum or product.

Compass (kŭm′ pŭs)   Instrument to draw circles and compare distances.

Complementary (kŭm plŭ mĕn′ tŭ rē) **(angles)**   Two angles whose measures added together result in a sum of 90°.

Compliance (kŏm plī′ ans)   Measure of elasticity.

Composite (kŏm pŏz′ ĭt) **(number)** Whole number greater than 0 that has more than two whole-number factors.

Cone (kōn) **(right-circular)** Circular region (base) and the surface made up of line segments connecting the circle with a point (vertex) located on a line through the center of the circle and perpendicular to the plane of the circle.

Constant (kŏn′ stănt) Numbers without a literal coefficient (numbers that do not vary in value).

Continuous (kŭn tĭn′ ū ŭs) **(data)** Measurements that can be made more precise if a person chooses, such as the length of a line.

Cube (kūb) Regular hexahedron (polyhedron of six equal faces).

Cylinder (sĭl′ ĭn dur) **(right-circular)** Two circular regions with the same radius in parallel planes (bases) connected by line segments perpendicular to the planes of the two circles.

Data (dā′ tŭ) Something, actual or assumed, used as a basis for reckoning, such as sets of numbers.

Decagon (dĕk′ ŭ gŏn) Polygon with 10 sides.

Deci (dĕs′ ĭ) Latin prefix indicating one-tenth (the decimal number system is a system based on the use of 10 digits, where each position in a numeral has a value one-tenth the position to its left).

Decimal (dĕs′ ĭ măl) **(fraction)** Fraction whose denominator is a power (multiple) of 10; such as $0.5 = \dfrac{5}{10}$, $2.67 = \dfrac{267}{100}$, etc.

Degree (dŭ grē′) **(of angular measure)** $\dfrac{1}{360}$ of a complete revolution of a ray around its endpoint.

Deka (dĕk′ ŭ) Greek prefix indicating a multiple of 10.

Denominate (dē nŏm′ ĭ nāt) **(number)** Number expressed in terms of a standard unit of measure, such as 15 inches.

Denominator (dŭ nŏm′ ĭ nā tur) Bottom number in a fraction, such as 3 in $\dfrac{2}{3}$.

Dial (dī′ ăl) Graduated plate or face with a pointer for indicating something, as steam pressure.

Diameter (dī ăm′ ŭ tur) **(of a circle)** Twice the radius (of the circle).

Diastolic (dī ah stŏl′ ĭk) **(pressure)** Normal rhythmically occurring relaxation and dilatation of the heart cavities during which the cavities are filled with blood.

Difference (dĭf′ ur ĕns) Result of a subtraction of two numbers, such as 5 in $7 - 2 = 5$.

Digit (dĭj′ ĭt) Any one of the symbols 0, 1, 2, 3, 4, 5, 6, 7, 8, or 9.

Discrete (dĭs krēt′) **(data)** Allows no interpretation between the values of the data, such as the number of people in a room.

Divide (dĭ vīd′)

Dividend (dĭv′ ĭ dĕnd) Number being divided, such as 15 in $15 \div 3$.

Divisibility (dĭ vĭz′ ĭ bĭl′ ĭ tē)

Divisible (dĭ vĭz′ ĭ b′l)

Division (dĭ vĭ′ zhŭn) Act of dividing.

Divisor (dĭ vĭ′ zur) Number by which another number (dividend) is divided, such as 3 in $15 \div 3$.

Dodecagon (dō dĕk′ ŭ gŏn) Polygon with twelve sides.

Dodecahedron (dō′ dĕk ŭ hē′ drŭn) Polyhedron that has twelve faces.

Dosage (dō′ sĭj) Amount administered.

Dram (drăm)   Unit of weight in the apothecaries' system (1 dram = 60 grains).

Edges (ĕ' jĕz) **(of a polyhedron)**   Sides of the faces of a polyhedron.

Electrocardiogram (ĭ lĕk trō kar' dē oh grăm)   **EKG**   Curve traced by an electrocardiograph used to diagnose heart disease.

Elements (ĕl' ŭ mĕnts)   Things that make up a set.

Encephalitis (ĕn sĕf ah lī' tĭs) **lethargica** (lah thăr' jĭ kah)   Sleeping sickness.

Equation (ē kwā' zhŭn)   Statement of equality between two values or quantities.

Equilateral (ē' kwĭ lăt' ur ŭl) **(triangle)**   Triangle with three equal sides.

Equivalent (ŭ kwĭv' ŭ lĕnt) **(expressions)**   Two or more expressions that have the same evaluation for all replacements of the variable.

Exhalation (ĕks hah lā' shun)   Act of breathing out.

Exponent (ĕks'pō nŭnt)   Indicates the number of times the base is used as a factor. For example, in 2^3, 3 is the exponent and indicates that 2 (base) is being used three times as a factor. That is, $2^3 = 2 \cdot 2 \cdot 2$.

Extrapolation (ĕks' tră pŭ lā' shŭn)   Approximating beyond the available data.

Extremes (ĕks trēmz') **(of a proportion)**   First and fourth terms of a proportion, such as 2 and 35 in $2:5 = 14:35$.

Faces (fās' ĭz) **(of a polyhedron)**   Polygonal regions that form the surface of the polyhedron.

Factor (făk' tur)   One of the values in a multiplication expression.

Fahrenheit (făr' ĕn hīt) **(scale)**   Temperature scale on which the interval between the freezing point and boiling point of water is divided into 180 parts or degrees, so that 32 °Fahrenheit corresponds to 0 °Celsius and 212 °Fahenheit to 100 °Celsius.

Femur (fē' mur)   Thigh bone.

Fibia (fĭb' ē ah)   Long slender bone of lateral side of lower leg.

Finite (fī' nīt) **(set)**   Set in which the elements can be counted and the count has a last number.

Fluidounce (flōō' ĭd ouns)   Unit of liquid volume in the apothecaries' system (1 fluidounce = 8 fluidrams).

Fluidram (flōō'ĭd drăm)   Unit of liquid volume in the apothecaries' system (volume of one teaspoon of water).

Fraction (frăk' shŭn)   Number which indicates that some whole has been divided into a number of equal parts and that a portion of the equal parts are represented.

Gauge (gāj)   Instrument for or means of measuring.

Gonorrhea (gŏn ah rē' ah)   Infectious disease of the genitourinary tract, rectum, and cervix.

Grain (grān)   Smallest unit of weight in the apothecaries' system (1 gram = 15 grains).

Great circle (of a sphere)   Intersection of the sphere and a plane containing the center of the sphere.

Gross (grōs)   Twelve dozen; that is, 144.

Hectare (hĕk' tair)   10 000 square metres.

Hecto (hĕk' tŭ)   Greek prefix indicating a multiple of 100.

Hemocytometer (hē' mah sīt ō mē tur)   Glass instrument used to hold diluted blood in order to count blood cells under a microscope.

Hexagon (hĕk′ sŭ gŏn)   Polygon with six sides.

Hexahedron (hĕk′ sŭ hē′ drŭn)   Polyhedron that has six faces.

Hindu-Arabic (hĭn′ dōō-ăr′ ah bĭk) **(numerals)**   Numbers formed by arrangement of the digits 0, 1, 2, 3, 4, 5, 6, 7, 8, and 9.

Histogram (hĭs′ tah grăm)   Graph in which values found in a statistical study are represented by lines (bars) placed horizontally, or vertically, to indicate frequency distribution.

Horizontal (hŏr ĭ zŏn′ tăl) **axis** (ăk′ sĭs) **(x axis)**   Number line that runs from left to right in a rectangular coordinate system.

Horizontal (hŏr ĭ zŏn′ tăl) **(line)**   Line parallel to the horizon.

Hypodermically (H) (hī pah dur′ mĭ kăl lē)   Injection beneath the skin.

Hypotenuse (hī pŏt′ ŭ nōōs)   Side opposite the right angle in a right triangle.

Icosahedron (ī′ kō sŭ hē′ drŭn)   Polyhedron that has twenty faces.

Improper (ĭm prŏp′ ur) **(fraction)**   Fraction that has a value greater than or equal to 1.

Infectious (ĭn fĕk′ shus) **mononucleosis** (mon ō nŭ klē ō′ sĭs)   Excess of mononuclear leukocytes in the blood.

Infinite (ĭn′ fĭ nĭt) **(set)**   Set whose count is unending.

Inhalation (ĭn hah lā′ shun)   Drawing of air into the lungs.

Inspiration (ĭn spah rā′ shun)   Act of breathing in, inhalation.

Integer (ĭn′ tŭ jur)   Any number that is in the following list: . . . , ⁻2, ⁻1, 0, 1, 2, ...

Interpolation (ĭn tur′ pŭ lā′ shun)   Approximation between two known values.

Intersecting (ĭn′ tur sĕkt′ ĭng) **(lines)**   Two (or more) lines that have one point in common.

Intra-alveolar (ĭn trah-ăl vē′ ō lăr) **(pressure)**   Pertaining to the jaw section containing the tooth sockets or the alveoli (air sac) of the lungs.

Intramuscularly (IM) (ĭn trah mŭs′ kyah lăr lē)   Injection within a muscle.

Intravenously (IV) (ĭn trah vē′ nahs lē)   Injection within a vein or veins.

Isosceles (ī sŏs′ ĕ lēz) **(triangle)**   Triangle with at least two sides equal.

Kelvin (kĕl′ vĭn) **(scale)**   Scale of absolute temperature, in which the zero is approximately ⁻273.15 °Celsius. The interval between the freezing point and boiling point of water is divided into 100 parts or degrees, so 273.15 Kelvin corresponds to 0 °Celsius and 373.15 Kelvin to 100 °Celsius.

Kilo (kĭl′ ŭ)   Greek prefix indicating a multiple of 1000.

Kilogram (kĭl′ ŭ grăm)   Base unit of weight in the metric system (1 kilogram = 1000 grams).

Lateral (lăt′ ur ŭl) **(surface of a cylinder)**   Curved surface connecting the bases.

Least common denominator   Smallest number that is exactly divisible by each of the original denominators of two or more fractions.

Leukemia (lu kē′ mē ah)   Malignant disease of the tissues in the bone marrow, spleen, and lymph nodes.

Like terms   Terms of an algebraic expression which have exactly the same literal coefficients (including exponents).

Line (līn)   Set of points represented with a picture such as ←——————————→ (a line is always straight, has no thickness, and extends forever in both directions).

Linear (lĭn′ ē ur) **(measurement)**   Measurement along a (straight) line.

(line) segment (sĕg′ mĕnt)   Portion of a line between two points (including its end points).

Literal (lĭt′ ŭr ŭl) **coefficient** (kō′ ĕ fĭsh′ ŭnt)   Letter factor of an indicated product of a number and one or more variables.

Literal (lĭt′ ur ŭl) **(equation)**   Equation having more than one letter or variable.

Litre (lē′ tur)   Base unit of volume or capacity in the metric system.

Logarithm (log′ ah rith ŭm)   Exponent used when a number is written as a power of 10. In this case the base is 10. That is, the logarithm of 100 is 2 because $10^2 = 100$.

Lymphocytic (lĭm fō sīt′ ĭk)   Pertaining to white blood cells formed in lymphoid tissue.

Mantissa (măn tĭs′ ah)   Part of a logarithm that follows the decimal point.

Mean (mēn) **(of a set of numbers)**   Result obtained when all numbers of the set are added and the sum is divided by the number of numbers.

Means (mēnz) **(of a proportion)**   Second and third terms of a proportion, such as 5 and 14 in $2 : 5 = 14 : 35$.

Median (mē′ dē ăn) **(of a set of numbers)**   Middle number of a set of numbers that have been arranged from smallest to largest; in a set with an even number of numbers, the median is one-half way between the two middle numbers.

Metre (mē′ tŭr)   Base unit of length in the metric system.

Micrometre (mī′ krō mē′ tŭr)   0.000 001 metre or $\dfrac{1}{1\ 000\ 000}$ metre.

Midpoint   Point on a line segment that divides its length by 2.

Milli (mĭl′ ĭ)   Latin prefix indicating one-thousandth.

Minim (mĭn′ im)   Unit of liquid volume in the apothecaries′ system (volume of one drop of water).

Mixed number   Understood sum of a whole number and a proper fraction.

Mode (mōd) **(of a set of numbers)**   Number that occurs with the greatest frequency.

Multiple (mŭl′ tĭ p′l)   Product of a quantity by a whole number.

Multiplication (mŭl′ tĭ plī kā′ shun)   Act of multiplying.

Multiply (mŭl′ tĭ plī)

Myelogenous (mī ĕ lōj′ ĕ nus)   Produced in or by the bone marrow.

Natural (năt′ yū răl) **(number)**   Any number that is in the following list: 1, 2, 3, ...

Negative (nĕg′ ŭ tĭv) **(number)**   Any number that is located to the left of zero on a horizontal number line.

Nomogram (nŏm′ ah gram) **(nomograph)**   Three or more parallel and equally spaced scales constructed to relate the variables that each scale represents.

Numeral (nōō′ mur ŭl)   A symbol that represents a number such as V, ⊬⊬, and 5, which are all numerals naming the number five.

Numerator (nōō′ mur ā′ tur)   Top number in a fraction, such as 2 in $\dfrac{2}{3}$.

Numerical (nōō′ mēr′ ĭ kŭl) **(coefficient)**   Number factor of an indicated product of a number and a variable.

Obtuse (ŏb tōos′)
    (angle)   Angle whose measure is between 90° and 180°.
    (triangle)   Triangle that has one angle greater than 90°.

Octagon (ŏk′ tŭ gŏn)   Polygon with eight sides.

Octahedron (ŏk′ tŭ hē′ drŭn)   Polyhedron that has eight faces.

Ohm (ōm)   Unit of electrical resistance of a circuit in which a potential difference of one volt produces a current of one ampere.

Open sentence   Equation that does not contain enough information to be judged as either true or false, such as $x + 2 = 7$.

Opposite (ŏp′ ŭ zĭt) **(sides of a quadrilateral)**   Pairs of sides that do not intersect.

Opposites (ŏp′ ŭ zĭtz)   Two numbers on a number line which are the same distance from zero, such as $^-5$ and 5, $^-6\frac{2}{3}$ and $6\frac{2}{3}$, etc.

Origin (or′ ĭ jĭn)   Point of intersection of the coordinate axes in a rectangular-coordinate system; identified by the ordered pair (0, 0).

Osteomyelitis (ŏs tē ō mī ah lī′ tĭs)   Inflammation of the bone marrow.

Oxygen (ŏk′ sĭ jĕn)   Chemical element; a colorless, odorless gas that makes up about 20 percent of the atmosphere.

Parallel (păr′ ŭ lĕl) **(lines)**   Two (or more) lines in the same plane that have no points in common.

Parallelogram (păr′ ŭ lĕl′ ŭ gram)   Quadrilateral with opposite sides parallel.

Pentagon (pĕn′ tŭ gŏn)   Polygon with five sides.

Pentahedron (pĕn′ tŭ hē′ drŭn)   Polyhedron that has five faces.

Percent (pur sĕnt′)   Fraction with a denominator of 100, such as $\frac{7}{100} = 0.07 = 7\%$.

Percentage (pur sĕn′ tĭj)   Result of multiplying a percent times a number. That is, in $5\% \times 30 = 1.5$, the percentage is 1.5.

Perimeter (pĕ rĭm′ ŭ tur) **(of a polygon)**   Total length of all the sides of the polygon.

Periodic (pĭr ē ŭd′ ĭk)   Having repeated cycles.

Perpendicular (pur′ pĕn dĭk′ ŭ lur) **(lines)**   Two intersecting lines that form a right angle.

Plane (plān)   Flat surface (such as a table top) that extends infinitely in every direction.

Pneumococcal (nu mō′ kŏk kăl) **pneumonia** (nu mō′ nē ah)   Acute inflammation of the lung caused by pneumococcus.

Point   Location in space that has no thickness.

Polygon (pŏl′ ĭ gŏn)   Plane closed figure of three or more angles.

Polygonal (pŭ lĭg′ ŭ nŭl) **(region)**   Polygon and its interior.

Polyhedra (pŏl′ ĭ hē′ dră)   Plural of polyhedron.

Polyhedron (pŏl′ ĭ hē′ drŭn)   Geometric solid where surfaces are polygonal regions.

Positive (pŏz′ ĭ tĭv) **(number)**   Any number that is located to the right of zero on a horizontal number line.

Power (pow′ ur)   Expression used when referring to numbers with exponents, such as 3^5, "the fifth power of three."

Prime (prīm) **(number)**   Whole number greater than 1 divisible by exactly two whole-number factors, itself and 1.

Prism (prĭz'm)   Polyhedron that has two faces which have the same size and shape and which lie in parallel planes, and the remaining faces are parallelograms.

Product (prŏd'ŭkt)   Result of a multiplication, such as 15 is the product of 3×5.

Proper (prŏp'ur) **(fraction)**   Fraction that has a value less than 1.

Proportion (prŭ por'shun)   Statement of equality between two ratios.

Protractor (prō trăk'tur)   Instrument used to measure angles.

Pyramid (pĭr'ŭ mĭd)   Polygonal region (base), the surface made up of line segments connecting the polygon with a point outside the plane of the base (apex), and all interior points.

Pythagoras (Pŭ thag'or us)   Greek philosopher and mathematician.

Pythagorean (pŭ thag'ō rē ăn) **theorem** (thr'um)   Sum of the squares of the legs of a right triangle is equal to the square of the hypotenuse.

Quadrant (kwŏd'rănt)   Any of the four parts into which a plane is divided by rectangular coordinate axes lying in that plane.

Quadrilateral (kwŏd'rĭ lăt'ur ŭl)   Polygon with four sides.

Quantity (kwŏn'tĭ tē)   Indicates an expression that has been placed within parentheses or that is being considered in its entirety.

Quotient (kwō'shŭnt)   Result of a division, such as 5 is the quotient of $15 \div 3$.

Radical (răd'ĭ kŭl) **(sign)**   The symbol $\sqrt{}$ (used to indicate square root).

Radii (rā'dē ī) **(of a circle)**   Plural of radius.

Radium (rā'dē ŭm)   Rare, brilliant-white, luminescent, highly radioactive metallic element.

Radius (rā'dē ŭs) **(of a circle)**   Line segment connecting the center of a circle to any point on the circle.

Rankine (răng'kĭn)   Unit of measure of radiation.

Ratio (rā'shō)   Quotient of two quantities or numbers.

Rational (răsh'ŭn ŭl) **(number)**   Any number that can be written in the form $\frac{p}{q}$, where p and q are integers and $q \neq 0$.

Ray (rā)   Part of the line on one side of a point which includes the endpoint.

Rectangle (rĕk'tăng'g'l)   Parallelogram whose sides meet at right angles.

Rectangular (rĕk tăng'gū lur) **(coordinate system)**   Formed by crossing (intersecting) vertical and horizontal number lines.

Rectification (rĕk'tah fah kā'shun)   Process of changing alternating current to direct current.

Reduce (rŭ dōōs')   Process of dividing both numerator and denominator of a fraction by some common factor.

Regular (rĕg'ū lur)
    (polygon)   Polygon that has sides and angles of equal measure.
    (polyhedron)   Polyhedron that has faces which are regular polygons.

Remainder (rŭ mān'dur)   Amount left over when it is not possible to divide the dividend into an equal number of groups exactly.

Replacement set   Set of permissible values of a variable in an algebraic expression.

Respiration (rĕs pah rā′ shun)   Process of inhaling and exhaling.

Right
    (angle)   Any of the angles formed by two intersecting lines, where all four angles are equal (the measure of a right angle is 90°).
    (triangle)   Triangle with one angle of 90°.

Roentgen (rŭnt′ gahn)   Obsolete unit of measure of exposure to x-rays.

Roman (rō′ mahn) **(numerals)**   Numbers formed by specific arrangement of the symbols I (1), V (5), X (10), L (50), C (100), D (500), and M (1000).

Scalene (skā lēn′) **(triangle)**   Triangle that has no pair of sides equal.

Scientific (sī ahn tǐf′ ǐk) **(notation)**   Numbers written as a number greater than or equal to 1 but less than 10, times a power of 10.

Scruple (skroo′ pahl)   Unit of weight in the apothecaries' system (1 scruple = 20 grains).

Sector (sĕk′ tur) **(of a circle)**   Figure enclosed by a central angle and its intercepted arc.

Semicircle (sĕm′ ǐ sŭr kŭl)   Arc of a circle in which the end points of the arc are on a diameter of the circle.

Septic (sĕp′ tǐk) **arthritis** (ar thrī′ tǐs)   Imflammation of joint or joints.

Set (sĕt)   Well-defined (membership in the set is clear) collection of things.

(slant) height (hīt) **(of a right circular cone)**   Length of a line segment from the vertex to a point on the circle of the base.

Sphere (sfēr)   Set of points in space at a fixed distance (radius) from a given point (center).

Sphygmomanometer (sfǐg mō mah nǒm′ ah tur)   Instrument used to measure blood pressure.

Square (skwair)   Rectangle whose sides are of equal length.

Subset (sŭb′ sĕt)   Set in which each element is also an element of another set.

Subtract (sŭb trăkt′)

Subtraction (sŭb trăk′ shŭn)   Act of subtracting.

Sum (sŭm)   Result of an addition of two or more numbers.

Supplementary (sŭp′ lŭ mĕn′ tŭ rē) **(angles)**   Two or more angles whose measures added together result in a sum of 180°.

Systolic (sǐs′ tō lǐk) **(pressure)**   Pertaining to contraction of the heart.

Tachometer (tă kǒm′ ǐ tur)   Instrument used to measure the number of revolutions the shaft of a motor makes with respect to a unit of time.

Terms (tŭrmz)   Parts of an expression separated by an addition symbol.

Tetrahedron (tĕt′ rŭ hē′ drŭn)   Polyhedron that has four faces.

Thorax (thor′ ăks)   Part of the human body between the neck and the diaphragm.

Tibia (tǐb′ ē ah)   Shin bone.

Trapezoid (trăp′ ŭ zoid)   Quadrilateral in which only one pair of opposite sides are parallel.

Triangle (trī′ ăng′ g′l)   Polygon with three sides.

Variable (vair′ ǐ ŭ b′l)   Letter in an algebraic expression that can be replaced by any one of a set of many numbers.

Venereal (vah nǐr′ ē ahl) **(disease)**   Any of several contagious diseases, such as syphilis and gonorrhea.

Ventricle (ven′ trĭ k′l)   Small cavity of chamber, as of the brain or heart.

Vertex (vur′ tĕks) **(of an angle)**   Common endpoint of two rays that form an angle.

Vertical (vur′ tĭ kăl)
  axis (ăk′ sĭs) **(y axis)**   Number line that runs up and down in a rectangular coordinate system.
  (line)   Line perpendicular to the horizon.

Vertices (vur′ tĭ sēz)   Plural of vertex.
  (of a polygon)   Vertices of the sides of the polygon.
  (of a polyhedron)   Vertices of the faces of the polyhedron.

Vial (vī′ ahl)   Sealed glass vessel containing sufficient solution for multiple hypodermic injections.

Volt (vōlt)   Electromotive force which when steadily applied to a conductor whose resistance is one ohm will produce a current of one ampere.

Volume (vŏl′ yŭm)   Measure (in cubic units) of the space within a closed solid figure.

Watt (wŏt)   Unit of power equal to work done at a rate of one joule a second or to the rate of work represented by a current of one ampere under a pressure of one volt.

Whole (number)   Any number that is in the following list: 0, 1, 2, 3, . . . (the next whole number is formed by adding 1 to the previous whole number).

Drugs or chemicals:

Acetylsalicylic (ah sēt′l săl ah sĭl′ ĭl) **(acid)**

Acid (ăs′ ĭd)

Alkaline (ăl′ kah lĭn)

Arsenic (ar′ sah nĭk) **trioxide** (trī ŏk′ sīd)

Ascorbic (ah skor′ bik) **(acid)**

Aspirin (ăs′ pahr ĭn)

Atropine (ăt′ rah pēn) **sulfate** (sŭl′ fāt)

Bichloride   (bī klor′ īd)   **(of)**   **mercury** (mur′ kyah rē)

Boric (bor′ ĭk) **(acid)**

Caffeine (kă fēn′)

Calcium (kăl′ sē ahm)

Carbohydrate (kar bō hī′ drāt)

Carbon (kar′ bahn) **dioxide** (dī ŏk′ sīd)

Cocaine (kō kān′)

Codeine (kō′ dēn)

Cresol (krē′ sōl)

Digitalis (dĭj ah tăl′ ĭs)

Digitoxin (dĭj ah tŏk′ sĭn)

Ephedrine (ĕf′ ah drēn) **sulfate** (sŭl′ fāt)

Epinephrine (ĕp ah nĕf′ rĕn)

Formaldehyde (for măl′ dah hīd)

Furoxone (fur ŏk′ ōn)

Glucose (glo̅o̅′ kōs)

Glycerin (glĭs′ ahr ĭn)

Histaspan (hĭs′ tah spăn)

Lysol (lī′ sōl)

Magnesium (măg nē′ zē um) **sulfate** (sŭl′ fāt)

Morphine (mor′ fēn)

Penicillin (pĕn ĭ sĭl′ ĭn)

Phenol (fē′ nol)

Phosphorus (fos′ for us)

Placebo (plah sĕ′ bō)

Potassium (pō tăs′ ē um)
  citrate (sĭt′ rāt)
  permanganate (pur măn′ gah nāt)

Promazine (pro′ mah zēn)

Pseudorenin (sū dō′ rē nĭn)

Saline (sā′ lēn) **(solution)**

Sodium (sō′ dē ahm)
  benzoate (bĕn′ zō āt)
  bicarbonate (bī kar′ bah nāt)
  bromide (brō′ mīd)
  chloride (klor′ īd)

Silver (sĭl′ vur) **nitrate** (nī′ trāt)

Terramycin (tĕr ah mī′ sahn)

Tetracycline (tĕt rah sī′ klēn)

Thiamine (thī′ ah mēn)

INDEX